Parkinson's Disease

Current and Future Therapeutics and Clinical Trials

Parkinson's Disease

Current and Future Therapeutics and Clinical Trials

Edited by

Néstor Gálvez-Jiménez
Professor of Medicine (Neurology-Florida), Cleveland Clinic Lerner College of Medicine, Case Western Reserve University; Pauline M. Braathen Endowed Chair; Director, Neurological Center, Chairman, Department of Neurology, and Chief, Movement Disorders Unit, Cleveland Clinic Florida, Weston, FL, USA

Hubert H. Fernandez
Professor of Medicine (Neurology), Cleveland Clinic Lerner College of Medicine, Head of Movement Disorders, Centre for Neurological Restoration, Cleveland Clinic, Cleveland, OH, USA

Alberto J. Espay
Associate Professor of Neurology, Director and Endowed Chair James J and Joan A Gardner Center for Parkinson's Disease and Movement Disorders, University of Cincinnati Academic Health Center, Cincinnati, OH, USA

Susan H. Fox
Associate Professor of Neurology, University of Toronto; Associate Director of the Movement Disorders Clinic at Toronto Western Hospital, Staff Neurologist Division of Neurology, Department of Medicine, University Health Network, Toronto, Canada

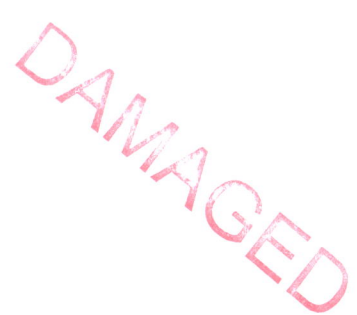

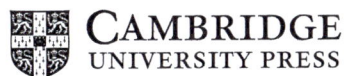

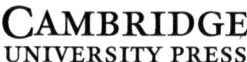

University Printing House, Cambridge CB2 8BS, United Kingdom

Cambridge University Press is part of the University of Cambridge.

It furthers the University's mission by disseminating knowledge in the pursuit of education, learning and research at the highest international levels of excellence.

www.cambridge.org
Information on this title: www.cambridge.org/9781107053861

© Cambridge University Press 2016

This publication is in copyright. Subject to statutory exception and to the provisions of relevant collective licensing agreements, no reproduction of any part may take place without the written permission of Cambridge University Press.

First published 2016

Printed in United Kingdom by Clays, St Ives plc

A catalogue record for this publication is available from the British Library

ISBN 978-1-107-05386-1 Hardback

Cambridge University Press has no responsibility for the persistence or accuracy of URLs for external or third-party internet websites referred to in this publication, and does not guarantee that any content on such websites is, or will remain, accurate or appropriate.

Every effort has been made in preparing this book to provide accurate and up-to-date information which is in accord with accepted standards and practice at the time of publication. Although case histories are drawn from actual cases, every effort has been made to disguise the identities of the individuals involved. Nevertheless, the authors, editors and publishers can make no warranties that the information contained herein is totally free from error, not least because clinical standards are constantly changing through research and regulation. The authors, editors and publishers therefore disclaim all liability for direct or consequential damages resulting from the use of material contained in this book. Readers are strongly advised to pay careful attention to information provided by the manufacturer of any drugs or equipment that they plan to use.

Contents

List of contributors vii
Acknowledgments xi

Section I: The Pharmacological Basis for Parkinson's Disease Treatment

1 **The pharmacological basis of Parkinson's disease therapy: an overview** 1
Néstor Gálvez-Jiménez, Hubert H. Fernandez, Alberto J. Espay and Susan H. Fox

2 **Anticholinergic agents in the management of Parkinson's disease** 5
Juan Carlos Giugni and Ramon L. Rodriguez-Cruz

3 **Amantadine and antiglutamatergic drugs in the management of Parkinson's disease** 13
Marco Onofrj, Valerio Frazzini, Laura Bonanni and Astrid Thomas

4 **Monoamine oxidase inhibitors in the management of Parkinson's disease** 23
Sven-Eric Pålhagen

5 **Oral dopamine agonists in the management of Parkinson's disease** 34
Javier Pagonabarraga, Juan Marín-Lahoz and Jaime Kulisevsky

6 **Subcutaneous, intranasal and transdermal dopamine agonists in the management of Parkinson's disease** 48
Antoniya Todorova and K. Ray Chaudhuri

7 **Oral and infusion levodopa therapy in the management of Parkinson's disease** 63
M. Angela Cenci-Nilsson and Per Odin

8 **Catechol-O-methyltransferase inhibitors in the management of Parkinson's disease** 76
Ilana Schlesinger and Amos D. Korczyn

9 **Experimental pharmacological agents in the management of Parkinson's disease** 83
Krishe Menezes, Lawrence W. Elmer and Robert A. Hauser

Section II: Management of Nonmotor Symptoms of Parkinson's Disease

10 **Management of autonomic dysfunction in Parkinson's disease** 93
Shen-Yang Lim and Ai Huey Tan

11 **Management of cognitive impairment in Parkinson's disease** 111
Dawn M. Schiehser, Eva Pirogovsky-Turk and Irene Litvan

12 **A neurobehavioralist approach to the management of cognitive impairment in Parkinson's disease** 122
Po-Heng Tsai

13 **Management of disease-related behavioral disturbances in Parkinson's disease** 127
Joseph H. Friedman

14 **Management of treatment-related behavioral disturbances in Parkinson's disease** 139
Mayur Pandya, Dimitrios A. Nacopoulos and Naveed Khokhar

15 **Management of sleep disorders in Parkinson's disease** 151
Daniela Calandrella and Alberto Albanese

16 **Management of pain and neuromuscular complications in Parkinson's disease** 162
John A. Morren

Section III: Surgical Management of Parkinson's Disease

17 **Thalamotomy, pallidotomy and subthalamotomy in the management of Parkinson's disease** 175
Malco Rossi, Daniel Cerquetti, Jorge Mandolesi and Marcelo Merello

18 **Deep-brain stimulation of the globus pallidus internus in the management of Parkinson's disease** 187
Lilia C. Lovera, Alberto J. Espay and Andrew P. Duker

19 **Deep-brain stimulation of the subthalamic nucleus in the management of Parkinson's disease** 195
David A. Schmerler, Alberto J. Espay and Andrew P. Duker

20 **Deep-brain stimulation of the thalamic ventral intermediate nucleus in the management of Parkinson's disease** 206
Diana Apetauerova, Jay L. Shils and Peter K. Dempsey

21 **Emerging targets and other stimulation-related procedures in the management of Parkinson's disease** 216
Tiago A. Mestre and Elena Moro

Section IV: Clinical Trials in Parkinson's Disease: Lessons, Controversies and Challenges

22 **Rating scales and clinical outcome measures in the evaluation of patients with Parkinson's disease** 231
Pablo Martinez-Martin and Carmen Rodríguez-Blázquez

23 **Functional imaging markers as outcome measures in clinical trials for Parkinson's disease** 242
Ryan R. Walsh

24 **Cerebrospinal fluid and blood biomarkers as outcome measures in clinical trials for Parkinson's disease** 249
Thomas F. Tropea and Claire Henchcliffe

25 **Lessons learned: neuroprotective trials in Parkinson's disease** 265
Isabelle Beaulieu-Boire and Anthony E. Lang

26 **Lessons learned: symptomatic trials in early Parkinson's disease** 280
Ramon Lugo-Sanchez and Néstor Gálvez-Jiménez

27 **Controversy: globus pallidus internus versus subthalamic nucleus deep-brain stimulation in the management of Parkinson's disease** 287
Sarah K. Bourne, Sean J. Nagel and Darlene A. Lobel

28 **Controversy: ablative surgery vs deep-brain stimulation in the management of Parkinson's disease** 297
Gian D. Pal and Leo Verhagen Metman

29 **Controversy: midstage vs advanced-stage deep-brain stimulation in the management of Parkinson's disease** 313
Mallory L. Hacker and David Charles

30 **Lessons and challenges of trials for cognitive and behavioral complications of Parkinson's disease** 325
Daniel Weintraub and Lama M. Chahine

31 **Lessons and challenges of trials for other nonmotor complications of Parkinson's disease** 337
Federico E. Micheli and Carlos Zúñiga-Ramírez

32 **Lessons and challenges of trials involving ancillary therapies for the management of Parkinson's disease** 349
Chris J. Hass, Elizabeth L. Stegemöller, Madeleine E. Hackney and Joe R. Nocera

Index 361
Color plate section between pp. 324 and 325

Contributors

Alberto Albanese MD
Department of Neurology, Istituto Neurologico Carlo Besta, Milan, Italy

Diana Apetauerova MD
Department of Neurology, Lahey Hospital and Medical Center, Burlington, MA, USA

Isabelle Beaulieu-Boire MD FRCPC
Department of Neurology, Toronto Western Hospital, Toronto, Ontario, Canada

Laura Bonanni MD PhD
Department of Neuroscience and Imaging, Università "G. D'Annunzio" Chieti-Pescara, Chieti, Italy

Sarah K. Bourne MD
Center for Neurological Restoration, Cleveland Clinic, Cleveland, OH, USA

Daniela Calandrella MD
Department of Neurology, Istituto Neurologico Carlo Besta, Milan, Italy

M. Angela Cenci-Nilsson MD PhD
Basal Ganglia Pathophysiology Unit, Department of Experimental Medical Science, Lund University, Lund, Sweden

Daniel Cerquetti Eng
Neuroscience Department, Raul Carrea Institute for Neurological Research, Buenos Aires, Argentina

Lama M. Chahine MD
Department of Neurology, University of Pennsylvania School of Medicine, Philadelphia, PA, USA

David Charles MD
Department of Neurology, Vanderbilt University, Nashville, TN, USA

K. Ray Chaudhuri FRCP DSc
National Parkinson Foundation Centre of Excellence, Department of Neurology, King's College Hospital, London, UK

Peter K. Dempsey MD
Department of Neurosurgery, Lahey Clinic and Medical Center, Burlington, MA, USA

Andrew P. Duker MD
Department of Neurology, University of Cincinnati Health Center, Cincinnati, OH, USA

Lawrence W. Elmer MD
Department of Neurology, University of Toledo, Toledo, OH, USA

Alberto J. Espay MD MSc
Department of Neurology, University of Cincinnati Academic Health Center, Cincinnati, OH, USA

Hubert H. Fernandez MD
Center for Neurological Restoration, Cleveland Clinic, Cleveland, OH, USA

Susan H. Fox MD PhD
Movement Disorders Clinic, Toronto Western Hospital, Toronto, Ontario, Canada

Valerio Frazzini MD PhD
Department of Neuroscience and Imaging, Università "G. D'Annunzio" Chieti-Pescara, Chieti, Italy

Joseph H. Friedman MD
Department of Neurology, Butler Hospital, Providence, RI, USA

Néstor Gálvez-Jiménez MD
Department of Neurology/Pauline M. Braathen Neurological Center, Cleveland Clinic Florida, Weston, FL, USA

List of contributors

Juan Carlos Giugni MD
Department of Neurology, University of Florida, Gainesville, FL, USA

Mallory L. Hacker PhD
Department of Neurology, Vanderbilt University, Nashville, TN, USA

Madeleine E. Hackney PhD
Atlanta VA Center for Visual & Neurocognitive Rehabilitation, Emory University School of Medicine, Atlanta, GA, USA

Chris J. Hass PhD
Department of Applied Physiology & Kinesiology, University of Florida, Gainesville, FL, USA

Robert A. Hauser MD MBA
Parkinson's Disease and Movement Disorders Center, NPF Center of Excellence, Department of Neurology, University of South Florida College of Medicine, Tampa, FL, USA

Claire Henchcliffe MD DPhil FANA
Department of Neurology & Neuroscience, Weill Medical College of Cornell University, New York, NY, USA

Naveed Khokhar MD
Department of Psychiatry, Cleveland Clinic, Cleveland, OH, USA

Amos D. Korczyn MD
Neurology Department, Tel Aviv Medical Center, Tel Aviv, Israel

Jaime Kulisevsky MD PhD
Department of Neurology, Sant Pau Hospital, Barcelona, Spain

Anthony E. Lang OC MD FRCPC
Division of Neurology, University of Toronto; Morton and Gloria Shulman Movement Disorders Clinic and the Edmond J. Safra Program in Parkinson's Disease, Toronto Western Hospital, Toronto, Ontario, Canada

Shen-Yang Lim MD FRACP
Division of Neurology, University of Malaya Medical Centre, Kuala Lumpur, Malaysia

Irene Litvan MD
Department of Neurosciences, University of California San Diego, La Jolla, CA, USA

Darlene A. Lobel MD
Center for Neurological Restoration, Cleveland Clinic, Cleveland, OH, USA

Lilia C. Lovera MD
Department of Neurology, University of Cincinnati Medical Center, Cincinnati, OH, USA

Ramon Lugo-Sanchez MD
Pauline M. Braathen Neurological Center, Cleveland Clinic Florida, Weston, FL, USA

Jorge Mandolesi MD
Department of Neurosurgery, Raul Carrea Institute for Neurological Research, Buenos Aires, Argentina

Pablo Martinez-Martin MD PhD
National Center of Epidemiology, Instituto de Salad Carlos III, Madrid, Spain

Juan Marín-Lahoz MD
Department of Neurology, Sant Pau Hospital, Barcelona, Spain

Krishe Menezes MD
Department of Neurology, University of Toledo, Toledo, OH, USA

Marcelo Merello MD PhD
Neuroscience Department, Raul Carrea Institute for Neurological Research, Buenos Aires, Argentina

Tiago A. Mestre MD
Division of Neurology, University of Ottawa Hospital, Ottawa, Ontario, Canada

Federico E. Micheli MD PhD
Neurology Service, José de San Martín Clinicas Hospital, Buenos Aires, Argentina

Elena Moro MD PhD
Department of Neurology, University Hospital Center of Grenoble, Grenoble, France

John A. Morren MD
Neuromuscular Center, Cleveland Clinic, Cleveland, OH, USA

Dimitrios A. Nacopoulos MD
Center for Neurological Restoration, Cleveland Clinic, Cleveland, OH, USA

Sean J. Nagel MD
Department of Neurosurgery, Cleveland Clinic, Cleveland, OH, USA

List of contributors

Joe R. Nocera PhD
Center for Visual & Neurocognitive Rehabilitation, Atlanta VA Medical Center, Emory University, Atlanta, GA, USA

Per Odin MD PhD
Department of Neurology, Skåne University Hospital, Lund, Sweden; Central Hospital, Bremerhaven, Germany

Marco Onofrj MD
Department of Neuroscience and Imaging, Università "G. D'Annunzio" Chieti-Pescara, Chieti, Italy

Javier Pagonabarraga MD PhD
Department of Neurology, Sant Pau Hospital, Barcelona, Spain

Gian D. Pal MD
Department of Neurology, Rush University Medical Center, Chicago, IL, USA

Sven-Eric Pålhagen MD PhD
Department of Clinical Neuroscience, Huddinge, Karolinska Institute, Stockholm, Sweden

Mayur Pandya DO
Center for Neurological Restoration, Cleveland Clinic, Cleveland, OH, USA

Eva Pirogovsky-Turk PhD
Department of Psychiatry, University of California San Diego, La Jolla, CA; Veteran's Affairs San Diego Health Care System, San Diego, CA, USA

Carmen Rodríguez-Blázquez PhD
National Center of Epidemiology, Instituto de Salud Carlos III, Madrid, Spain

Ramon L. Rodriguez-Cruz MD
Department of Neurology, University of Florida, Gainesville, FL, USA

Malco Rossi MD
Neuroscience Department, Raul Carrea Institute for Neurological Research, Buenos Aires, Argentina

Dawn M. Schiehser PhD
Department of Neurosciences, University of California San Diego, La Jolla, CA, USA

Ilana Schlesinger MD
Department of Neurology, Rambam Health Care Campus, Haifa, Israel

David A. Schmerler DO
Department of Neurology, University of Cincinnati Medical Center, Cincinnati, OH, USA

Jay L. Shils PhD
Department of Anesthesiology, Rush University Medical Center, Chicago, IL, USA

Elizabeth L. Stegemöller MT-BC PhD
Kinesiology Department, Iowa State University, Ames, IA, USA

Ai Huey Tan MD MRCP
Division of Neurology, University of Malaya Medical Centre, Kuala Lumpur, Malaysia

Astrid Thomas MD
Department of Neuroscience and Imaging, Università "G. D'Annunzio" Chieti-Pescara, Chieti, Italy

Antoniya Todorova PhD
National Parkinson Foundation Centre of Excellence, Department of Neurology, King's College Hospital, London, UK

Thomas F. Tropea DO MPH
Department of Neurology, NY Presbyterian Hospital, New York, NY, USA

Po-Heng Tsai MD
Lou Ruvo Center for Brain Health, Pauline M. Braathen Neurological Center, Cleveland Clinic Florida, Weston, FL, USA

Leo Verhagen Metman MD PhD
Department of Neurological Sciences, Rush University Medical Center, Chicago, IL, USA

Ryan R. Walsh MD PhD
Cleveland Clinic Lou Ruvo Center for Brain Health, Las Vegas, NV, USA

Daniel Weintraub MD
Department of Psychiatry, University of Pennsylvania School of Medicine, Philadelphia, PA, USA

Carlos Zúñiga-Ramírez MD
Department of Neurology, Hospital Civil de Guadalajara "Fray Antonio Alcalde," Guadalajara, Mexico

Acknowledgments

To Kassandra, Jessica and Nicholas. N.G.-J.

Section I: The Pharmacological Basis for Parkinson's Disease Treatment

Chapter 1: The pharmacological basis of Parkinson's disease therapy: an overview

Néstor Gálvez-Jiménez, Hubert H. Fernandez, Alberto J. Espay and Susan H. Fox

The "shaking palsy" was first recognized by James Parkinson in 1817 when he described a condition characterized by "involuntary tremulous motion, with lessened muscular power, in parts not in action and even when supported; with a propensity to bend the trunk forward, and to pass from a walking to a running pace [here he was referring to festination or more accurately referred to in that era as scelotyrbe festinans]: the sense and intellects being uninjured." In his writings, James Parkinson credits Galen as first noticing shaking of the limbs belonging to this disease and calling them "by an appropriate term: tremor." Parkinson further and correctly stated that "tremor can indeed only be considered as a symptom" and not a disease in itself. Since then, others have laid the foundations for the study and understanding of this condition. Freidrich Lewy described the body that now bears his name and the central focus of the science behind Parkinson's disease (PD). Froscher Tretiakoff localized the disease to the substantia nigra. Greenfield confirmed the scattered cellular changes in the locus coeruleus of the pontine tegmentum and substantia nigra. In his 1962 monograph on the *Basal ganglia*, Derek Denny-Brown described his clinical and pathological experience of PD patients, calling attention to the presence of the preponderance of thinning of the myelin sheaths as a consequence of nigral cell loss and pallor of the outer pallidum and ansa lenticularis. Arvid Carlsson, a Nobel Prize winner, recognized that the sole function of dopamine was not limited to the synthesis of norepinephrine, and, together with the work by Walter Birkmayer and Oleh Hornykiewicz, demonstrated that dopamine was decreased in the striatum in PD. George Cotzias successfully treated PD patients with levodopa (3,4-dihydroxyphenyl-L-alanine or L-DOPA), initiating the modern era of neurotherapeutics based on solid scientific data. Long gone are the days of blood letting and other treatment options that Parkinson himself recommended as the treatment of choice to "release the humors causing the condition." Recent advances in our understudying of the pathological distribution and progression in PD along with progress in genomics are constantly challenging our understanding and are providing hope for the future of the PD patient.

Since the first description and recognition of PD, many other movement disorders have been recognized. Oppenheimer first described dystonia muscular deformans in 1912, and tremor has been recognized since Galen times, and chorea was already recognized by the Romans. More recently, other abnormal involuntary movements were recognized at the turn of the 20th century. These seemingly disparate conditions were slowly recognized and were further defined and grouped conceptually into an emerging field called "movement disorders." Classically, movement disorders referred to conditions stemming from basal ganglia dysfunction. As advances in basal ganglia physiology and understanding of the underlying pathophysiology of such disorders accrued, it became clear that the term must also include conditions stemming from basal ganglia connections (reciprocal, fugal pathways, for example), along with other functionally related structures such as the thalamus, subthalamus, brainstem nuclei and pedunculopontine nuclei, and networks such as the reticular formation, cerebellum and its connections, the spinal cord and some disorders of peripheral nerve and muscle. Hence, in today's usage, the term movement disorders is quite broad, encompassing disorders of motor control, coordination, gait, abnormal involuntary movements and other seemingly "orphan" conditions such as cramps, spasms, restless legs syndrome and stiff person syndrome. Coupled with genomic

---

Parkinson's Disease: Current and Future Therapeutics and Clinical Trials, ed. Gálvez-Jiménez et al. Published by Cambridge University Press. © Cambridge University Press 2016.

advances, the field is going through a renaissance requiring the mastering of a broad area of neurological disorders and basic neurosciences, and further blurring the borders between neuromuscular diseases, epilepsy, dementias, praxis and other higher cortical conditions, and genetics.

Broadly, movement disorders may be categorized into akinetic–rigid syndromes, hyperkinetic movement disorders, gait disturbances, cerebellar diseases, psychogenic movement disorders and spasticity. It is important to recognize that the observed phenomenology may be due to a variety of secondary causes, and the proper observed phenomena must be placed in the overall context in which the process is occurring. A physician interested in movement disorders thus must first recognize the category or type of movement disorder, for example whether it is tremor, chorea or dystonia. The concept or "what is it?" is the first and often most important component of determining a cause, rather than the traditional neurological approach of "where is the lesion?" This latter point cannot be overstated, i.e. defining the broad category of movement disorders in a given patient must precede the classical approach of localization to help place into perspective the alterations observed. A careful history with particular attention to family history, consanguinity, pregnancy, labor and delivery, early developmental milestones, trauma, infections, medical and psychiatric comorbidities and psychological stressors, and exposure to illicit drugs or medications for the treatment of gastrointestinal and psychiatric disorders, especially neuroleptics, are particularly important when first evaluating a patient with abnormal involuntary movements. A detailed general medical and neurological examination with emphasis on oculomotor disturbances, the presence of saccadic intrusions, Kayser–Fleischer rings (betraying Wilson's disease), fundoscopic examination looking for retinopathies and optic nerve abnormalities (papillitis, papilledema or optic nerve atrophy suggesting a space-occupying lesion, normal-pressure hydrocephalus, demyelinating diseases, metabolic or mitochondrial cytopathies), organomegaly (metabolic or storage diseases) and skin discolorations and/or deposits (phakomatosis, xeroderma pigmentosum, vitaminosis, malabsorption) may prove rewarding. Once the abnormal movements have been classified, and the neurological accompaniments documented and placed in context, the cause may become apparent and proper ancillary testing may be undertaken.

It should be recognized that hyperkinetic and/or akinetic–rigid syndromes may coexist in different combinations, and some may be bizarre and difficult to classify properly. In these circumstances, a clear and detailed description of the observed abnormality is the best step to define what is observed and to share among colleagues. For example, the akinetic–rigid syndrome characteristic of the parkinsonian syndrome may be accompanied by tremor, early-morning foot dystonia, and medication-related abnormal involuntary dyskinesias in the same patient (see below). In addition to a careful neurological examination, a focused general physical examination must be carried out paying particular attention to the iris and sclera by fundoscopic examination looking for the presence of optic disk disease and retinopathies, the presence of hepatosplenomegaly, skin rashes or lesions, and tendon xanthomata, which may be indicators of a more systemic disorder such as lipid storage diseases, cholesterol disorders, mitochondria cytopathies, neurocutaneous syndromes, leukomyelodystrophies or other demyelinating diseases among others, all leading to parkinsonian syndrome. Many other disorders of movement have been described and are outside the scope of this work. The remainder of the discussion will center on the akinetic–rigid syndrome which is the topic of this monograph.

The akinetic–rigid syndromes are characterized by paucity of movement. Parkinson's disease and other parkinsonian syndromes are the classic examples of this syndrome, characterized by slowness of movement, stiffness or rigidity, gait disturbances and imbalance, and tremor. This can easily be recognized if the pneumonic TRAP is kept in mind – tremor, rigidity, akinesia (bradykinesia) and postural instability (gait disturbances) – which may be present in various combinations. The key symptom for defining a parkinsonian condition is the presence of bradykinesia. Many patients with PD will not exhibit a tremor. Overall, recognizing the presence of two of the four (especially two out of tremor, rigidity and bradykinesia) will help define on clinical grounds the presence of the parkinsonian syndrome in a given individual. Postural and gait disturbances usually develop late in the course of the illness. For example, early-onset postural instability and imbalance, falls and gait disturbances characterize progressive supranuclear palsy, the spinocerebellar ataxias and spastic paraplegias, whereas early-onset autonomic disturbances may herald the onset of multiple-system atrophy. Other features quite common in the parkinsonian patient include decreased facial expression (facial hypomimia), soft and at times slurred speech with or without start hesitation, occasional stuttering, apraxia of lid opening, blepharoclonus or blepharospasm, tremor of the tongue, jaw or lips, sialorrhea, and malar and forehead seborrheic dermatitis and may be present in various combinations. Decreased blinking and micrographia are common features in parkinsonism but are not unique to PD and may be present in other parkinsonian syndromes. An astonished facial expression due to frontalis muscle contraction may also be seen. A high, raspy, high-pitched voice can also be present. When these two latter features are present, other parkinsonian syndromes such as progressive supranuclear palsy, vascular parkinsonism, some instances of drug-induced parkinsonism, bilateral basal ganglia necrosis, mitochondrial cytopathies and the nigrostriatal form of multiple-system atrophy (currently known as multiple-system atrophy-P) should be considered. A rest tremor may be evident during the initial contact and may not be restricted to the upper extremity. Not infrequently, a foot tremor may also be evident. Although a rest tremor is usually asymmetric, it may have started on the one body side affected first and not infrequently is noticed only when occurring bilaterally, with the side at onset being the most affected over time. When tremor is suspected, it can be elicited with mental exercises, maintaining the hands resting on the thighs and asking the patient to close their eyes. It is important to allow the patient to feel comfortable and relaxed when testing for the presence of tremor, as any voluntary limb movement may eliminate the rest tremor. In many patients, the rest tremor becomes evident when holding the hands outstretched, especially when the hands have been brought into position and after a short period of finger and hand quiescence allowing for "resetting or reappearance of hand rest tremor." In spite of classical teachings, cogwheeling is not unique to PD but rather is a common phenomenon in other parkinsonian syndromes and conditions in which tremor is present, such as essential tremor. The key for the cogwheeling phenomena is the presence of tremor on increased tone. When the limb is tested for tone, cogwheeling may be noticed. Stooping may be evident when sitting but quite noticeable when standing. In severe cases, marked flexion at the waist resulting in camptocormia (bent spine) may be observed. Other abnormal postures such as a striatal hand and foot may be noticed (Figure 1.1) especially in the early-morning hours or when the levels of levodopa are at their lowest ("off" stage). In some cases, severe antecollis and bent spines may ensue, betraying marked extensor muscle atrophy/myopathy with fatty infiltration. Dystonic limb posturing may be associated with other abnormal involuntary movements during the peak or "on" time of levodopa effect (see below). Many patients will demonstrate gait abnormalities consisting of start hesitation or gait ignition failure, short stride, slow cadence, decreased arm swing, turning en bloc, occasional imbalance when turning and retropulsion when tested. Rigidity is often present bilaterally but may be asymmetric in the early stages of the disease. If rigidity is suspected and is not clearly evident during the examination, it may be "brought out" by using Froment's maneuver. This is especially helpful when looking for subtle neck rigidity and limb rigidity. Other maneuvers not frequently mentioned but helpful when assessing these patients include the pillow sign, the shaking of limbs and trunk rotation.

In the untreated patient, five stages may be identified. Stage 1 is characterized by mild unilateral symptoms. Tremor may be mild and intermittent in the presence of other subtle symptoms such as rigidity or slowness of movement. Gait is usually normal, but a decrease in arm swing may be noticeable on the most symptomatic side, with the upper limb carried slightly abducted at the shoulder and flexed at the elbow. Facial hypomimia may be present but may be confused with "normal for the person's age." There is usually subtle reduced manual dexterity and impaired rapid repetitive movements. For example, patients may complain of having difficulties with the computer keyboard or when using a computer mouse. Micrographia may be present, with poorly formed letters. As the disease advances to stage 2, there is usually bilateral involvement with onset of mild postural changes in some, but the key is worsening of the initial symptoms with progression to bilaterality. In this stage, the more classic phenotype is observed with clear reduced facial expression, stooping when standing, reduced arm swing on walking and en-bloc turning. There are definitive alterations in rapid alternating and repetitive movements. The patient's movements are clearly slow and deliberate. Some patients may begin to complain of fatigue and weakness at this time. Commonly heard is a sense of weakness in the most affected limb but lack of objective alteration when testing muscle power on examination. Fatigue may be quite disabling in many patients thus affected. Another observation is the

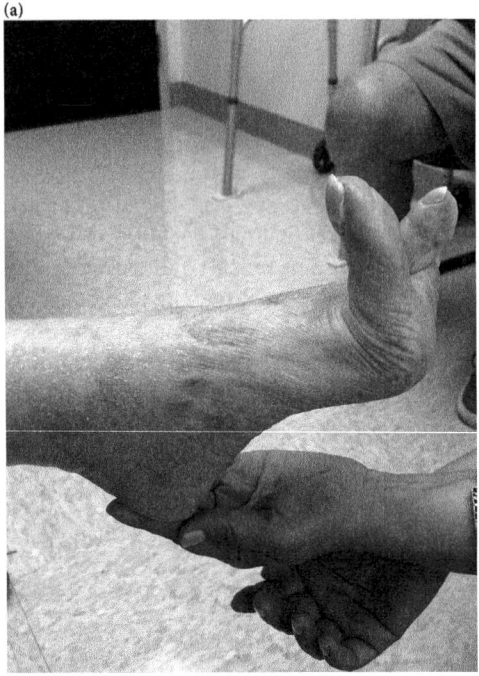
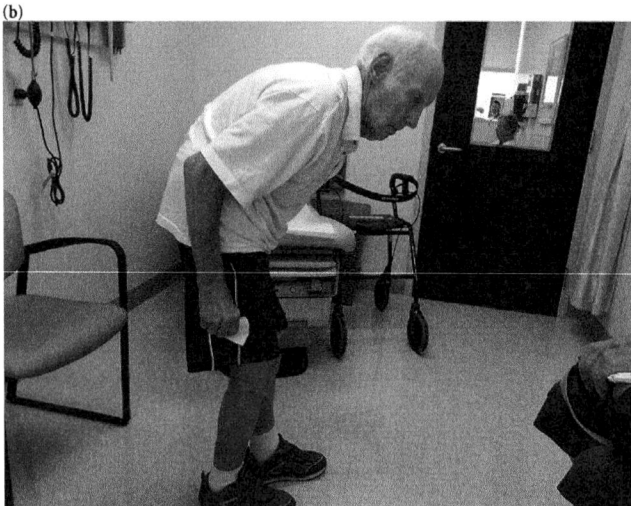

Figure 1.1 (a) A striatal foot, which may easily be confused with early-morning foot dystonia. In this particular case, there is a fixation of the joints exacerbated by a superimposed off-period worsening of great toe extension. (b) Camptocormia.

beginning of the development of the so-called striatal hand with dorsiflexion of the wrist, adducted fingers, flexed metacarpophalangeal and distal interphalangeal joints. Similarly, some patients may develop a striatal foot with clawing of the toes and varus foot posture. In stage 3, retropulsion and propulsion betray the onset of increasing impairment of postural reflexes and righting responses. Shuffling and festination of gait are noted. At this stage, the patient may require some assistance in the activities of daily living. With further progression, a more advanced stage, stage 4, is reached with severe disability, rigidity, bradykinesia and gait disturbances. Standing is unsteady, with severe retropulsion with falls if not caught by the examiner or a caregiver. Once the patient reaches an end stage with confinement to a wheelchair or bed, they are said to have reached stage 5. Drs Melvin Yahr and Margaret Hoehn carefully studied and documented the natural history of PD and developed an operational scale that bears their names arbitrarily dividing this disorder into five stages on which the above discussion was based. This scale provides a somewhat crude estimate of disease severity and progression.

Parkinson's disease is no longer considered only a motor disorder. It has become evident that the pathological changes are broad, and the progression seems to follow a pattern suggesting *trans*-synaptic transmission via propagation of proteins in a prion-like fashion, such that: (i) these pathological changes usually antedate by decades the motor symptoms; (ii) the process may have a portal of entry or origin at the gut or in the nasal passages; (iii) when the motor symptoms become evident the disease is fairly advanced; and (iv) any attempt to alter the natural history of the disease must be coupled with solid epidemiological data to identify those at risk before the disease becomes clinically manifest. These and other hot topics are the subject of this monograph and the editors hope the reader finds in these pages the necessary clinical and scientific foundations for an understanding of the disease, the underpinnings of the pathological processes and the foundations for solid therapeutics.

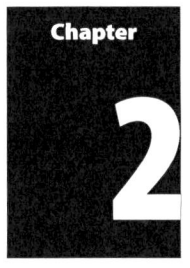

Chapter 2

Anticholinergic agents in the management of Parkinson's disease

Juan Carlos Giugni and Ramon L. Rodriguez-Cruz

Introduction

Anticholinergics had a leading role in the treatment of Parkinson's disease (PD) until the 1960s, when levodopa (L-DOPA) was introduced and proved to be a better treatment option to improve the cardinal symptoms of the disease. Since then, levodopa and dopaminergic agents have taken the leading role and have remained the most efficacious symptomatic treatment for PD. Despite the widespread use of dopaminergics drugs in PD, anticholinergics are still in use today and play a role in the treatment of PD. They are most commonly prescribed to alleviate symptoms in young patients with tremor-dominant PD and in those with PD-related dystonia. In this chapter, we describe the use, efficacy and side effects using anticholinergics for the management of PD.

Anticholinergics are substances that block the neurotransmitter acetylcholine, in both the central and peripheral nervous systems, and act on acetylcholine receptors in neurons through competitive inhibition. Anticholinergics are classified into two categories according to the receptors they act on: antimuscarinic and antinicotinic agents [1].

Antimuscarinic agents are named as such because they block muscarine, found in *Amanita muscaria*, a nonedible mushroom species. Muscarine is a toxic compound that competes with acetylcholine for the same receptors. The classic antimuscarinic agent atropine, a belladonna alkaloid, has been used for centuries to treat a variety of conditions, mainly gastrointestinal disorders. Centrally acting antimuscarinics such as trihexyphenidyl, benztropine, biperiden and procyclidine have been used in the management of PD, and were the first synthetic drugs for PD [2].

The use of anticholinergics dates back hundreds of years. In the Odyssey, Homer describes the lethal effects of *Datura stramonium*, commonly known now as jimsonweed. The antiparkinsonian effect of anticholinergics was initially described in 1867 by Ordenstein [3], one of Charcot's students, when he wrote his medical thesis on the treatment of parkinsonian tremor with belladonna alkaloids. At the time, Charcot's preferred treatment was hyoscyamine, derived from *Atropa belladonna*, for the treatment of PD [4]. As seen in a prescription located in the Philadelphia College of Physicians (Figure 2.1), the anticholinergic treatment used by Professor Charcot was usually combined with rye-based ergot products. These kinds of products are the predecessors some dopamine agonists that are currently in use [4]. In the 1940s, trihexyphenidyl (Artane®) was introduced as the first synthetic anticholinergic [2], replacing natural alkaloids.

The cholinergic system and Parkinson's disease

Some authors have postulated the theory of imbalance between acetylcholine and dopamine in the striatum as the origin of motor symptoms in PD [1, 5]. The dopaminergic and cholinergic systems are closely related and in constant balance. In PD, the degeneration of nigral neurons leads to decreased dopamine production, and this situation cause an imbalance between acetylcholine and dopamine. In PD, dopamine depletion blocks autoinhibition of acetylcholine release through muscarinic autoreceptors, leading to excessive acetylcholine release [5]. This hypothesis is supported by the fact that anticholinergics were the first treatment for PD [6].

The striatum is a nodal basal ganglia structure and is a major input station of the basal ganglia. Acetylcholine is an important neurotransmitter in the striatum based on its abundance [7]. The striatum is

---

Parkinson's Disease: Current and Future Therapeutics and Clinical Trials, ed. Gálvez-Jiménez *et al*. Published by Cambridge University Press. © Cambridge University Press 2016.

Section I: Pharmacological Basis for PD Treatment

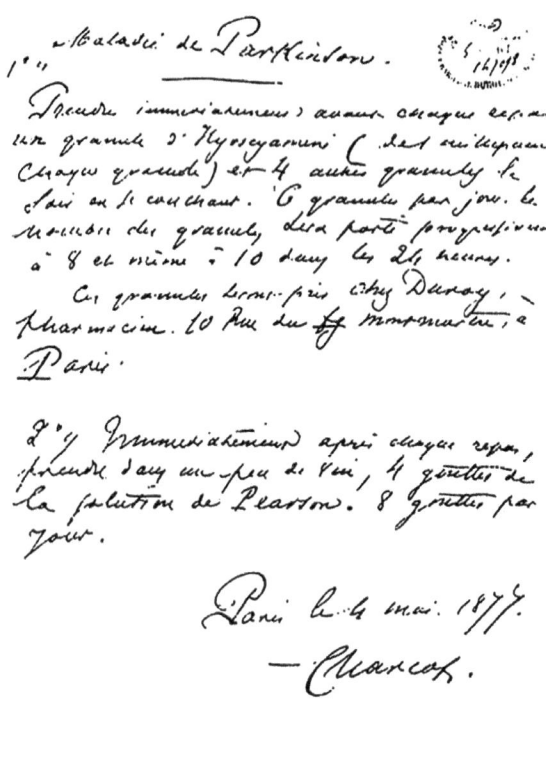

Figure 2.1 Prescription of anticholinergic treatment used by Professor Charcot, dated 1887 from the College of Physicians of Philadelphia Library.

subdivided into two regions, the matrix and the striosomes. Both compartments contain medium spiny neurons, which comprise nearly 95% of striatal neurons, and affect the direct and indirect pathways [8, 9]. The remaining striatal neurons are interneurons and only 1–3% are giant aspiny cholinergic interneurons. These interneurons have multifold arborizing axons [10, 11], and this explains the high expression of cholinergic markers in the striatum [7]. In the striatum, acetylcholine acts via muscarinic and nicotinic receptors, in postsynaptic and presynaptic targets, and contributes to the activity of the medium spiny neurons [12]. The primary effect of acetylcholine on medium spiny neurons is depolarization via muscarinic receptor M1. This facilitation occurs primarily on medium spiny neurons of the indirect pathway [13].

Multiple studies in PD have shown loss of cholinergic neurons in the pedunculopontine nucleus (PPN) in PD [14–16]. The PPN is located in the mesencephalic tegmentum and contains cholinergic, GABAergic and glutamatergic neurons [17]. Effects on the PPN in PD are narrowly related to gait disturbance, and the severity of cholinergic neuronal depletion in the PPN correlates with the severity of motor symptoms [14]. Another cholinergic system change in PD is an increase in the muscarinic binding sites in the globus pallidus internus, probably due to a compensatory upregulation in response to a decrease in cholinergic activity [18]. These changes result in elevated peaks of acetylcholine in the striatum, and may affect the indirect pathway [5]. Some authors believe that anticholinergics can correct this imbalance in PD, thereby reducing the degree of neurotransmission mediated by neostriatal acetylcholine [19].

Nicotinic receptors also play a role in PD. Nicotinic receptors are located at presynaptic terminals. Substantial evidence from studies of epidemiologic and animal PD models suggest a protective effect and an inverse relationship on the development of PD [20]. However, clinical trials have not shown similar results [21, 22].

Pharmacokinetics and pharmacodynamics

The anticholinergic drugs available for use in the treatment of PD provide a different mechanism of action, which is an alternative to relieve some of the bothersome motor symptoms, especially tremors.

The anticholinergic drugs used in the treatment of PD are competitive antagonists of muscarinic receptors. The most commonly used worldwide are trihexyphenidyl (Artane®), benztropine (Cogentin®), biperiden (Akineton®) and procyclidine (Kemadrin®).

The mechanism of action of anticholinergics is still not fully known but is suspected to be a result of blocking of the muscarinic receptors in the striatum, acting as strong inhibitors of the presynaptic carrier-mediated dopamine transport mechanism [23]. In addition to the muscarinic blockade, anticholinergics act as agonists at the noradrenergic synapse, and also have N-methyl-D-aspartate (NMDA) antagonist receptor activity [24].

In general, most anticholinergic drugs have good and rapid oral absorption through the gut. The average the time to maximal plasma concentration (T_{max}) is 2.5 h (1.5–3.5 h). The maximum plasma concentration (C_{max}) is dose dependent and is different for each drug,

Table 2.1 Properties of major anticholinergics used in Parkinson's disease

Drug	C_{max} (µg/l) for dose (mg)	T_{max} (h)	$t_{1/2}$ (h)	Preparations[a]	Initial daily dosage	Titration	Final daily dosage
Trihexyphenidyl	7 (10)	1.3	33	2–5 mg 0.4 mg/ml	1 mg	Increase 2 mg every 4–5 days	6–10 mg (2–3 mg tid)
Biperiden	4–6 (4)	1.5	18–24	2 mg 5 mg/ml	1 mg	Increase 1 mg every 4 days	6–9 mg (2–3 mg tid)
Benztropine	2.5 (1.5)		7	0.5, 1, 2 mg 1 mg/ml	0.5 mg	Increase 0.5 mg every 5–6 days	2–6 mg (1–2 mg tid)
Procyclidine	116 (10)	1	8–16	2.5–5 mg 2.5 mg/5 ml	2.5–3 mg		15–30 mg (5–10 mg tid)

Tid, three times daily.

[a]Available tablet and liquid forms are given.

with the exception of procyclidine as its plasma concentration is high even in small doses [25]. The half-life ($t_{1/2}$) is also different in each drug; for example, trihexyphenidyl has a C_{max} of 7 µg/l for a 10 mg dosage with a $t_{1/2}$ of 33 h, and biperiden has a C_{max} of 4–6 µg/l for 4 mg dosage with a $t_{1/2}$ of 18–24 h. The results for these and the other two commonly used drugs are illustrated in Table 2.1.

The bioavailability of anticholinergics ranges from 30 to 90%; for example, procyclidine and biperiden have an absolute bioavailability of 75% and 33%, respectively [25, 26]. The tissue distribution of anticholinergics has been observed in laboratory animals and has been reported to be large. For biperiden, a brain/plasma area-under-the-curve ratio of 7–12 ng/(h ml) has been reported [27]. These authors also showed that with an intravenous infusion of biperiden, maximal brain concentration was obtained within 3–10 min. The high concentrations of these drugs in the brain could be explained by their intensely lipophilic properties. Lipophilic biomolecules in the brain serve to promote the uptake of anticholinergics, and for trihexyphenidyl and biperiden, the uptake is also related to intralysosomal uptake of the drug [28]. The protein binding of anticholinergics has not been elucidated in humans, but in rats the binding of biperiden to plasma protein is approximately 90% [29].

For the most part, all anticholinergics are metabolized in the liver, and the pathways of excretion are urine and bile. There are some differences for each of these drugs. For trihexyphenidyl and procyclidine, the metabolism is due to hydroxylation of the alicyclic groups, and excretion is through urine and bile for trihexyphenidyl and through urine for procyclidine

Table 2.2 Commonly used drugs with secondary anticholinergic effects

Name of drug	Use
Diphenylhydramine	Antihistamine
Ipratropium bromide	Bronchospasm
Clozapine	Antipsychotic
Quetiapine	Antipsychotic
Olanzapine	Antipsychotic
Amitriptyline	Antidepressant
Nortriptyline	Antidepressant
Paroxetine	Antidepressant

[30]. Benztropine is metabolized by N-oxidation, N-dealkylation and ring hydroxylation [31].

The dosage and titration vary for each drug (Table 2.2), but in general, to avoid the adverse effects of these kinds of medication, initiation of treatment should be with low dosages and slow titration, especially in the older population.

Beyond the anticholinergic drugs, there are many others drugs used for different conditions in PD, especially psychiatric symptoms (such as depression, psychosis and hallucinations), as well as drugs used for general conditions like allergies that also have anticholinergic properties acting on cholinergic receptors [32].

Current use of anticholinergic drugs in the management of Parkinson's disease

While anticholinergic drugs were initially the most important drugs for treating PD, their use declined after the development of levodopa and most recently dopamine agonists. The occurrence of adverse effects also caused a decline in their use but to a much lesser extent. The current use of anticholinergics has been limited to the treatment of a PD resting tremor that is not responding satisfactorily to dopaminergics and PD-related dystonia [33]. One of the reasons beyond the advent of dopaminergic drugs and the presence of adverse events is the lack of clinical trials with anticholinergic drugs in recent years. The majority of studies in this class of drug were performed several decades ago, and most were conducted before the use of current clinical diagnostic criteria such as the UK Parkinson's Disease Society Brain Bank criteria [34] for idiopathic PD, and also before the use of the Unified Parkinson's Disease Rating Scale (UPDRS).

In the last Cochrane review of anticholinergics for symptomatic management of PD, the authors evaluated the efficacy and tolerability of anticholinergic drugs in the motor treatment of PD compared with placebo [35]. In the review, they included randomized controlled trials comparing anticholinergic drugs versus placebo or no treatment in new-onset or advanced PD, either as monotherapy or as adjunctive therapy. Initially, there were 14 potentially qualifying studies published from 1954 to 1986, and five were excluded for technical or methodological issues. The remaining nine studies, with a total of 221 patients participating, were included. The duration of the studies was between 5 and 20 weeks. Different drugs were investigated (benzhexol, orphenadrine, benztropine, bornaprine, benapryzine and methixine), and one study used two different anticholinergics drugs. All the studies reported improvement from baseline in at least one outcome measure with the exception of one study. Five studies reported both tremor and other parkinsonian motor manifestations as outcome measures, while the rest of the studies used disability and other parkinsonian signs but no tremor. All studies demonstrated anticholinergics to be better than placebo for improving motor symptoms as adjunct therapy or monotherapy. Neuropsychiatric and cognitive adverse events were described in six studies. Side effects, in particular cognitive and neuropsychiatric, were the most common reason for withdrawal. There is insufficient available data to compare efficacy or tolerability among anticholinergics.

There have been a few studies using anticholinergic drugs for PD in recent years, with most focusing on the management of sialorrhea and bladder dysfunction in PD. A randomized, double-blind, placebo-controlled study with ipratropium bromide in 17 patients with PD and troublesome drooling showed a mild improvement on a subjective measure of sialorrhea, without significant adverse events, although it did not affect objective measures of saliva production [36]. Most recently two randomized, double-blind, placebo-controlled crossover studies, one with glycopyrrolate for sialorrhea in 23 patients with PD, showed that 1 mg three times daily of glycopyrrolate, an anticholinergic drug with poor permeability across the blood–brain barrier, is safe and effective for sialorrhea in PD [37]. Another pilot study comprised 19 patients taking a single dose of oral, slow-dissolving thin films containing tropicamide. The results showed that 1 mg tropicamide resulted in a significant saliva reduction when compared with placebo, and without adverse events [38]. A 12-week dose-titration trial of controlled-release oxybutynin for neurogenic bladder concluded that controlled-release oxybutynin was safe and effective for this condition [39].

The first report of anticholinergics improving tremors was in 1949 [40], and this was followed by other studies confirming the benefits of anticholinergics [41, 42]. In our experience, we have seen improved tremor in similar PD patients with good tolerability, especially in young PD patients (under 60 years old). In those patients with medication-refractory tremors, we believe it is a good option to try anticholinergics before considering surgical interventions, although there is no evidence to argue in favor of a preferential effect of anticholinergics on tremor rather than other motor symptoms [35].

Another use of anticholinergic drugs in PD is to treat dystonia. Dystonia in PD, which occurs in different stages of the disease, is common in the early stage of young-onset PD and is most often seen as either a "wearing off" or a dyskinetic phenomenon, especially at peak dose, but also as biphasic dyskinesia in advanced PD [43]. End-of-dose dystonia is present most often as an early-morning and generally painful foot dystonia but can involve any part of the body. Dystonias as a dyskinetic phenomenon are most common as a facial dystonia. Anticholinergics are useful in the treatment of dystonia, especially DYT1 dystonia [44]. For PD dystonia, there have been no randomized trials with anticholinergics. There is a report of benefit from anticholinergics in wearing off of foot dystonia [45].

The benefits of anticholinergics to treat axial symptoms in PD were reported in a few trials [42, 46, 47]. A recent study showed that the anticholinergic agent trihexyphenidyl improved axial symptoms after deep-brain stimulation of the subthalamic nucleus [48]. Only a few reports have been published comparing dopaminergic therapy and anticholinergics directly with objective measures. In a small study, Koller [49] compared trihexiphenidyl and carbidopa/levodopa taken for 2 weeks and found improvement of tremors. Another study by Parkes et al. [50] demonstrated improvement of resting tremor, rigidity and bradykinesia with levodopa when compared with benzhexol. There was a more robust improvement of rigidity and tremors using levodopa after 6 months but only mildly after using benzhexol. Akinesia responded better to levodopa, with only a negligible improvement with benzhexol. In another single-dose study, Schrag et al. [51] compared biperiden intravenously and apomorphine on two consecutive days and found that both drugs were effective in reducing tremor in PD, although without evidence for selective anticholinergic responsiveness of parkinsonian tremor.

It is still unclear if there is a synergistic effect between levodopa and anticholinergics. One study found that combining anticholinergic drugs with levodopa could affect the profile of the levodopa concentration in plasma. Levodopa absorption was reduced because there was a delay in gastric emptying of levodopa, but the fluctuation in the plasma concentration was less after anticholinergics, which could be beneficial in fluctuating patients [52]. This synergistic effect has been reported by others authors [47, 50]. However, other reports found that the chronic use of anticholinergic agents may have a negative impact in levodopa absorption [53]. The same authors commented that patients stabilized on levodopa often present a severe deterioration after withdrawal of anticholinergics. In these patients, addition of benzhexol will produce improvement [54].

Adverse effects and contraindications of anticholinergic drugs

As we know, anticholinergics act by blocking the muscarinic receptor, in both the central and peripheral nervous systems; hence, they may be responsible for peripheral or nonneurological and central or neurological side effects (Table 2.3). Current evidence has shown that anticholinergics, when compared with other antiparkinsonian drugs, are associated with a higher risk of adverse effects, especially in the elderly, who seem to be more susceptible. Many factors may contribute to this, including increased permeability of the blood–brain barrier, pharmacodynamic changes related to aging, the fact that the aging brain is particularly sensitive to these medications, and the risk of polypharmacy and drug–drug interactions [55]. Although the use of anticholinergics in PD is low, there are many other drugs with anticholinergic properties (e.g. antidepressants, amantadine) [32] that PD patients receive that may cause anticholinergic side effects, mainly neurological side effects. These side effects may be uncomfortable for younger patients, but the effects in older patients could be devastating. The central adverse effects could be a serious problem too. Cognitive impairment and dementia are common problems observed in patients with PD [56]. Cholinergic deficits play an important role in the cortical neurochemical alterations in cognitive impairment [57]. Central anticholinergic side effects may be subtle but bothersome, such as sedation, the inability to concentrate and confusion, or more severe, such as agitation, hallucinations and cognitive decline. Ehrt et al. [58] reported a significant association of anticholinergic properties and the incidence of cognitive decline in a large cohort of PD patients followed for 8 years, with a rate of cognitive decline 6.5 times higher

Table 2.3 Common side effects and contraindications of anticholinergics

Central adverse effects	Peripheral adverse effects	Contraindications	Precautions
Sedation	Dry mouth	Bladder neck obstruction	Cardiovascular disease
Inability to concentrate	Sore throat	Myasthenia gravis	Gastrointestinal obstructions
Confusion	Anhidrosis	Uncontrolled arrhythmias	Glaucoma
Agitation	Tachycardia	Uncontrolled narrow-angle glaucoma	In the elderly
Cognitive decline	Urinary retention		Cognitive decline
Delirium	Constipation		Prostatic hyperplasia
Hallucinations	Increased intraocular pressure		
	Weakness		
	Blurred vision		

in the group using drugs with anticholinergic properties compared with those who were never exposed to them. The cognitive issues induced by anticholinergics are more related to executive function [59] and short-term memory [60].

Neurological signs of anticholinergic toxicity include ataxia, blurred vision, diplopia and in severe cases delirium, hallucinations, seizure coma and rarely death. This neurotoxicity is termed acute anticholinergic syndrome. This syndrome is usually reversible once all of the toxin has been excreted and usually no specific treatment is necessary, but in some severe cases use of physostigmine is necessary.

The peripheral adverse events of anticholinergics are due to parasympatholytic effects. These include dry mouth, which is very common but usually tolerated as many PD patients also have sialorrhea, and a sore throat due to decreased mucous production and cessation of perspiration (anhidrosis) leading to increased body temperature, which may be severe. One therapeutic option is to increase hydration and avoid hot weather and extreme exercise. Tachycardia is another possible side effect, and therefore it is good practice to have a cardiovascular evaluation and electrocardiogram before the onset of treatment. Urinary retention can happen, so elderly patients should be cautious, especially those with prostatic issues. Constipation is a common problem, and because it is almost always present in PD, it could be a problem for this population leading to discontinuity in the treatment with anticholinergics. Another potential severe side effect of anticholinergics is elevated intraocular pressure, which patients with narrow-angle glaucoma, or symptoms of, must avoid. In large doses or in susceptible patients, anticholinergics may cause weakness. Patients taking anticholinergics can also have blurring of vision due to accommodation problems and mydriasis.

Contraindications to the use of these drugs include patients with urinary retention due to bladder neck obstruction, patients with a diagnosis of myasthenia gravis, uncontrolled cardiac arrhythmias and narrow-angle glaucoma.

Future use of anticholinergic drugs

There are a few ongoing trials using anticholinergic agents in PD that are focused on the treatment of urinary issues and sialorrhea. However, there is increased interest in the cholinergic system, especially in the PPN for the axial symptoms in PD and the potential therapeutic use. Other interesting areas of research are the nicotinic receptors and their role in PD. Epidemiological and animal models in PD studies have shown substantial evidence that nicotine has a protective effect and an inverse relationship on the development of PD; despite this, clinical trial results have been negative. This is especially evident considering the modulation of dopamine release due to the α6 nicotinic acetylcholine receptor [61]. In another study with six PD patients who underwent ^{123}I-FP-CIT imaging prior to and at multiple intervals after nicotine therapy, imaging showed no significant decrease in binding potentials in the striatum over 1 year. This was slower than expected in parkinsonian patients and was inversely correlated with UPDRS-III, possibly representing a deceleration of neuronal loss [62].

Conclusions

There is evidence that anticholinergics can still play a role in improving motor function in PD, as monotherapy or as an adjunct to other antiparkinsonian drugs, but their use is limited by neuropsychiatric and cognitive adverse effects. In our experience, they are still an option to treat PD patients, mainly younger patients and those with severe tremor. The elderly population should be careful when using them, due to the presence and possibility of various adverse events. Future research may provide further insight about the better-tolerated drugs and optimal dosing.

References

1. Standaert DG, Roberson ED. Treatment of central nervous system degenerative disorders. In: Hardman JG, Molinoff PB, Ruddon RW and Gilman AG, eds. *Goodman and Gilman's The Pharmacological Basis of Therapeutics.* New York: McGraw-Hill, 1995; 503–19.
2. Schwab RS, Tillmann WR. Artane in the treatment of Parkinson's disease; a report of its effectiveness alone and in combination with benadryl and parpanit. *N Engl J Med*, 1949; **241**: 483–5.
3. Ordenstein L, *Sur la Paralysie Agitante et la Sclérose en Plaques Generalisée.*, 1867; Paris: Martinet (two leaves of color plates).
4. Goetz CG. The history of Parkinson's disease: early clinical descriptions and neurological therapies. *Cold Spring Harb Perspect Med* 2011; **1**: a008862.
5. Aosaki T. Miura M, Suzuki T, Nishimura K, Masuda M. Acetylcholine-dopamine balance hypothesis in the striatum: an update. *Geriatr Gerontol Int* 2010; **10** (Suppl. 1): S148–57.
6. Duvoisin, RC. Cholinergic-anticholinergic antagonism in parkinsonism. *Arch Neurol* 1967; **17**: 124–36.

7. Zhou FM, Liang Y, Dani JA. Endogenous nicotinic cholinergic activity regulates dopamine release in the striatum. *Nat Neurosci* 2001; **4**: 1224–9.

8. Graybiel AM. Neurochemically specified subsystems in the basal ganglia. *Ciba Found Symp* 1984; **107**: 114–49.

9. DeLong M, Wichmann T. Update on models of basal ganglia function and dysfunction. *Parkinsonism Relat Disord* 2009; **15** (Suppl. 3): S237–40.

10. Bolam JP. Synapses of identified neurons in the neostriatum. *Ciba Found Symp* 1984; **107**: 30–47.

11. Kawaguchi Y, Wilson CJ, Augood SJ, Emson PC. Striatal interneurones: chemical, physiological and morphological characterization. *Trends Neurosci* 1995; **18**: 527–35.

12. Pakhotin P, Bracci E. Cholinergic interneurons control the excitatory input to the striatum. *J Neurosci* 2007; **27**: 391–400.

13. Benarroch EE. Effects of acetylcholine in the striatum. Recent insights and therapeutic implications. *Neurology* 2012; **79**: 274–81.

14. Rinne JO, Ma SY, Lee MS, Collan Y, Röyttä M. Loss of cholinergic neurons in the pedunculopontine nucleus in Parkinson's disease is related to disability of the patients. *Parkinsonism Relat Disord* 2008; **14**: 553–7.

15. Jellinger K. The pedunculopontine nucleus in Parkinson's disease, progressive supranuclear palsy and Alzheimer's disease. *J Neurol Neurosurg Psychiatry* 1988; **51**: 540–3.

16. Benarroch EE. Pedunculopontine nucleus: functional organization and clinical implications. *Neurology* 2013; **80**: 1148–55.

17. Wang HL, Morales M. Pedunculopontine and laterodorsal tegmental nuclei contain distinct populations of cholinergic, glutamatergic and GABAergic neurons in the rat. *Eur J Neurosci* 2009; **29**: 340–58.

18. Griffiths PD, Sambrook MA, Perry R, Crossman AR. Changes in benzodiazepine and acetylcholine receptors in the globus pallidus in Parkinson's disease. *J Neurol Sci* 1990; **100**: 131–6.

19. Sweeney PJ. Parkinson's disease: managing symptoms and preserving function. *Geriatrics* 1995; **50**: 24–31.

20. Quik M, O'Leary K, Tanner CM. Nicotine and Parkinson's disease: implications for therapy. *Mov Disord* 2008; **23**: 1641–52.

21. Ebersbach G, Stöck M, Müller J, *et al.* Worsening of motor performance in patients with Parkinson's disease following transdermal nicotine administration. *Mov Disord* 1999; **14**: 1011–13.

22. Lemay S, Chouinard S, Blanchet P, *et al.* Lack of efficacy of a nicotine transdermal treatment on motor and cognitive deficits in Parkinson's disease. *Prog Neuropsychopharmacol Biol Psychiatry* 2004; **28**: 31–9.

23. Krueger BK. Kinetics and block of dopamine uptake in synaptosomes from rat caudate nucleus. *J Neurochem* 1990; **55**: 260–7.

24. McDonough JH Jr, Shih TM. A study of the N-methyl-D-aspartate antagonistic properties of anticholinergic drugs. *Pharmacol Biochem Behav* 1995; **51**: 249–53.

25. Whiteman PD, Fowle AS, Hamilton MJ, *et al.* Pharmacokinetics and pharmacodynamics of procyclidine in man. *Eur J Clin Pharmacol* 1985; **28**: 73–8.

26. Grimaldi, R, Perucca E, Ruberto G, *et al.* Pharmacokinetic and pharmacodynamic studies following the intravenous and oral administration of the antiparkinsonian drug biperiden to normal subjects. *Eur J Clin Pharmacol* 1986; **29**: 735–7.

27. Yokogawa, K, Nakashima E, Ishizaki J, *et al.* Brain regional pharmacokinetics of biperiden in rats. *Biopharm Drug Dispos* 1992; **13**: 131–40.

28. Ishizaki J, Yokogawa K, Nakashima E, Ohkuma S, Ichimura F. Influence of ammonium chloride on the tissue distribution of anticholinergic drugs in rats. *J Pharm Pharmacol* 1998; **50**: 761–6.

29. Nakashima E, Yokogawa K, Ichimura F, *et al.* Effects of fasting on biperiden pharmacokinetics in the rat. *J Pharm Sci* 1987; **76**: 10–13.

30. Paeme G, Van Bossuyt H, Vercruysse A. Phenobarbital induction of procyclidine metabolism: in vitro study. *Eur J Drug Metab Pharmacokinet* 1982; 7: 229–31.

31. He H, McKay G, Midha KK. Phase I and II metabolites of benztropine in rat urine and bile. *Xenobiotica* 1995; **25**: 857–72.

32. Chew ML, Mulsant BH, Pollock BG, *et al.* Anticholinergic activity of 107 medications commonly used by older adults. *J Am Geriatr Soc* 2008; **56**: 1333–41.

33. Lang AE. Treatment of Parkinson's disease with agents other than levodopa and dopamine agonists: controversies and new approaches. *Can J Neurol Sci* 1984; **11** (Suppl.): 210–20.

34. Hughes AJ, Daniel SE, Kilford L, Lees AJ. Accuracy of clinical diagnosis of idiopathic Parkinson's disease: a clinico-pathological study of 100 cases. *J Neurol Neurosurg Psychiatry* 1992; **55**: 181–4.

35. Katzenschlager R, Sampaio C, Costa J, Lees A. Anticholinergics for symptomatic management of Parkinson's disease. *Cochrane Database Syst Rev* 2003: CD003735.

36. Thomsen TR, Galpern WR, Asante A, Arenovich T, Fox SH. Ipratropium bromide spray as treatment for sialorrhea in Parkinson's disease. *Mov Disord* 2007; **22**: 2268–73.

37. Arbouw ME. Movig KL, Koopmann M, *et al.* Glycopyrrolate for sialorrhea in Parkinson disease: a randomized, double-blind, crossover trial. *Neurology* 2010; **74**: 1203–7.

38. Lloret SP, Nano G, Carrosella A, Gamzu E, Merello M. A double-blind, placebo-controlled, randomized, crossover pilot study of the safety and efficacy of multiple doses of intra-oral tropicamide films for the short-term relief of sialorrhea symptoms in Parkinson's disease patients. *J Neurol Sci* 2011; **310**: 248–50.
39. Bennett N, O'Leary M, Patel AS, et al. Can higher doses of oxybutynin improve efficacy in neurogenic bladder? *J Urol* 2004; **171**: 749–51.
40. Corbin KB. Trihexyphenidyl; evaluation of the new agent in the treatment of Parkinsonism. *J Am Med Assoc* 1949; **141**: 377–82.
41. Brumlik J, Canter G, Delatorre R, et al. A critical analysis of the effects of trihexyphenidyl (artane) on the components of the Parkinsonian syndrome. *J Nerv Ment Dis* 1964; **138**: 424–31.
42. Iivanainen M. KR 339 in the treatment of Parkinsonian tremor. *Acta Neurol Scand* 1974; **50**: 469–77.
43. Poewe WH, Lees AJ, Stern GM. Dystonia in Parkinson's disease: clinical and pharmacological features. *Ann Neurol* 1988; **23**: 73–8.
44. Jankovic J. Treatment of dystonia. *Lancet Neurol* 2006; **5**: 864–72.
45. Machado D, Jabbari B. Treatment of Parkinson's disease with anticholinergic medication. In: Pfeiffer RF., Wszolek ZK, Ebadi M, eds. *Parkinson's Disease*. Boca Raton: CRC Press, 2013; 811–18.
46. Cantello R, Riccio A, Gilli M, et al. Bornaprine vs placebo in Parkinson disease: double-blind controlled cross-over trial in 30 patients. *Ital J Neurol Sci* 1986; **7**: 139–43.
47. Tourtellotte WW, Potvin AR, Syndulko K, et al. Parkinson's disease: Cogentin with Sinemet, a better response. *Prog Neuropsychopharmacol Biol Psychiatry* 1982; **6**: 51–5.
48. Baba Y, Higuchi MA, Abe H, et al. Anti-cholinergics for axial symptoms in Parkinson's disease after subthalamic stimulation. *Clin Neurol Neurosurg* 2012; **114**: 1308–11.
49. Koller WC. Pharmacologic treatment of parkinsonian tremor. *Arch Neurol* 1986; **43**: 126–7.
50. Parkes JD, Baxter RC, Marsden CD, Rees JE. Comparative trial of benzhexol, amantadine, and levodopa in the treatment of Parkinson's disease. *J Neurol Neurosurg Psychiatry* 1974; **37**: 422–6.
51. Schrag A, Schelosky L, Scholz U, Poewe W. Reduction of Parkinsonian signs in patients with Parkinson's disease by dopaminergic versus anticholinergic single-dose challenges. *Mov Disord* 1999; **14**: 252–5.
52. Roberts, J, Waller DG, von Renwick AG, et al. The effects of co-administration of benzhexol on the peripheral pharmacokinetics of oral levodopa in young volunteers. *Br J Clin Pharmacol* 1996; **41**: 331–7.
53. Contin, M, Riva R, Martinelli P, et al. Combined levodopa-anticholinergic therapy in the treatment of Parkinson's disease. Effect on levodopa bioavailability. *Clin Neuropharmacol* 1991; **14**: 148–55.
54. Horrocks M, Vicary DJ, Rees JE, Parkes JD, Marsden CD. Anticholinergic withdrawal and benzhexol treatment in Parkinson's disease. *J Neurol Neurosurg Psychiatry* 1973; **36**: 936–41.
55. Tune LE, Anticholinergic effects of medication in elderly patients. *J Clin Psychiatry* 2001; **62** (Suppl. 21): 11–4.
56. Buter TC, van den Hout A, Matthews FE, et al. Dementia and survival in Parkinson disease: a 12-year population study. *Neurology* 2008; **70**: 1017–22.
57. Bohnen NI, Kaufer DI, Hendrickson R, et al. Cortical cholinergic denervation is associated with depressive symptoms in Parkinson's disease and parkinsonian dementia. *J Neurol Neurosurg Psychiatry* 2007; **78**: 641–3.
58. Ehrt U, Broich K, Larsen JP, Ballard C, Aarsland D. Use of drugs with anticholinergic effect and impact on cognition in Parkinson's disease: a cohort study. *J Neurol Neurosurg Psychiatry* 2010; **81**: 160–5.
59. Bedard MA, Pillon B, Dubois B, et al. Acute and long-term administration of anticholinergics in Parkinson's disease: specific effects on the subcortico-frontal syndrome. *Brain Cogn* 1999; **40**: 289–313.
60. Cooper JA, Sagar HJ, Doherty SM, et al. Different effects of dopaminergic and anticholinergic therapies on cognitive and motor function in Parkinson's disease. A follow-up study of untreated patients. *Brain* 1992; **115**: 1701–25.
61. Quik M, McIntosh JM. Striatal α6* nicotinic acetylcholine receptors: potential targets for Parkinson's disease therapy. *J Pharmacol Exp Ther* 2006; **316**: 481–9.
62. Itti E, Villafane G, Malek Z, et al. Dopamine transporter imaging under high-dose transdermal nicotine therapy in Parkinson's disease: an observational study. *Nucl Med Commun* 2009; **30**: 513–18.

Chapter 3

Amantadine and antiglutamatergic drugs in the management of Parkinson's disease

Marco Onofrj, Valerio Frazzini, Laura Bonanni and Astrid Thomas

Glutamatergic neurotransmission is the core excitatory activity in corticobasal circuits, directly intervening in thalamocortical, corticostriatal and subthalamo-pallidal transmission and [1], most likely, modulating dopamine release directly via presynaptic glutamate receptors or indirectly via nitric oxide production [2]. Alterations of glutamatergic balance are considered a core, hypothetical mechanism for the development of dyskinesias in Parkinson's disease (PD) [2–5] but also of addictive behaviors, including craving for abuse substances, and of repetitive stereotyped behaviors or impulse control disorders (ICDs) [2–5].

The most recent hypothesis on the origin of dyskinesias in PD or levodopa (L-DOPA)-induced dyskinesias (LIDs) suggests that these involuntary movements depend on the phosphorylation of glutamatergic postsynaptic receptors interacting with D2 dopamine receptors [2–6]. Furthermore, this hypothesis suggests that LIDs and behavioral alterations observed in dopamine dysregulation syndrome and ICD of PD [2–6], depend on a common mechanism involving alterations of glutamate homeostasis [7] with combined activation of sensitized dopamine and N-methyl-D-aspartate (NMDA) glutamatergic receptors (NMDARs). Pre- and postsynaptic mechanisms are implicated in the development of LIDs and ICDs, the first based on alteration of dopaminergic transmission because of chronic pulsatile instead of tonic dopamine release, and the second because of excessive expression and sensitization of D1 receptors in striatonigral neurons [2, 8]. The neural adaptation underlying an imbalance between synaptic and nonsynaptic glutamate activity results, hypothetically, in failure of prefrontal cortex control [9]. Therefore, a possible option for the treatment of LIDs but also of dopamine dysregulation syndrome, ICDs in PD, and ICDs or substance abuse in the non-PD population, is considered to be the use of antiglutamatergic drugs. MK-801 was the first antiglutamatergic drug to be modeled [10], and dextrometorphan [11], budipine [12], memantine (a drug that binds to glutamate receptors such as 2-amino-3-[5-methyl-3-oxo-1,2-oxazol-4-yl]propanoic acid receptors [AMPARs] and NMDARs) and acamprosate [13–17] were proposed shortly after. A case apart was amantadine, as this old drug was used serendipitously in PD [18, 19] and only lately was it discovered that its mechanism of action was not just based on enhancement of dopamine release or inhibition of reuptake but also on NMDAR blockade, modulating the activity of glutamatergic corticostriatal and subthalamo-pallidal pathways. Several Cochrane and meta-analyses studies have been performed demonstrating the reliability of antiglutamatergic drug effects [19–22].

In this chapter, we move from this background and discuss the consistency of findings related to different drugs.

Figure 3.1 shows a diagram illustrative of the corticostriatal circuits demonstrating the role of glutamatergic neurotransmission in motor, limbic and associative loops. The figure also shows the expression of different glutamate receptor subtypes in order to demonstrate the complexity expected in any attempt to modulate glutamate transmission. An early schematization of the dopaminergic/glutamatergic imbalance in PD and psychosis is also shown, as a tribute to the first pharmacologist who developed amantadine and memantine [23]. In this balancing diagram, it is evident that more than 20 years ago the conceptual framework had already predicted that antiglutamatergic activity might result in the improvement of motor symptoms but also in the occurrence of psychotic symptoms as observed with the psychotropic antiglutamatergic drug

Parkinson's Disease: Current and Future Therapeutics and Clinical Trials, ed. Gálvez-Jiménez *et al.* Published by Cambridge University Press. © Cambridge University Press 2016.

Section I: Pharmacological Basis for PD Treatment

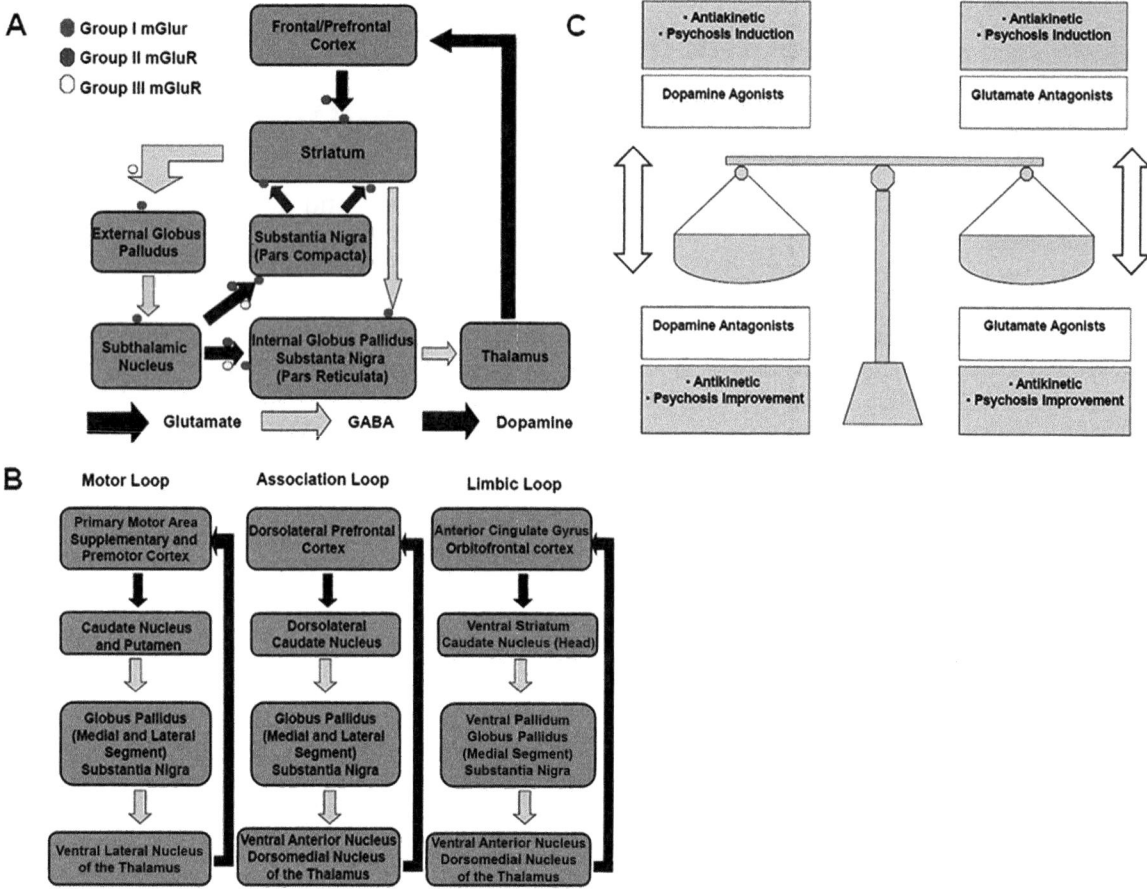

Figure 3.1 (A) Expression of different glutamate receptor subtypes, demonstrating the complexity expected in any attempt to modulate glutamatergic neurotransmission. (B) Illustration of the corticostriatal circuits, demonstrating the role of glutamatergic neurotransmission in motor, limbic and associative loops. (C) An early schematization of the dopaminergic/glutamatergic imbalance in Parkinson's disease and psychosis, as a tribute to the first pharmacologist who developed amantadine and memantine. (A black and white version of this figure will appear in some formats. For the color version, please refer to the plate section.)

phencyclidine (angel dust), which has no use beyond its recreational induction of psychosis and hallucinations. Figure 3.2 shows the receptor subtypes involved in glutamatergic transmission, and Table 3.1 summarizes the mechanisms of action of antiglutamatergic drugs.

Evidence-based results and meta-analyses

Evidence-based evaluations, promoted by scientific societies and by the Cochrane networks, by analyzing studies performed with blinded procedures versus placebo, concluded that amantadine is efficacious in reducing dyskinesias in PD [19, 20]. This evidence-based conclusion stems from the evaluation of several studies showing that amantadine reduces dyskinesias when administered orally at doses of 100–300 mg/day [24] or intravenously as single dose of 200 mg [25]. This evidence-based analysis included studies performed from 1998 to 2010 [19]. Effects were obtained in parallel-group or crossover designs. The duration of the studies was 2–6 weeks. Among the different studies in evidence-based and Cochrane reviews, only two protocols had prolonged follow-up of patients. These studies showed an apparent contradiction: one showed that after 6–8 months dyskinesias reoccurred, suggesting that tachyphylaxis superseded [24]. The other study reached a different conclusion: by withdrawing amantadine in patients, they observed an

Chapter 3: Amantadine and antiglutamatergic drugs in the management of PD

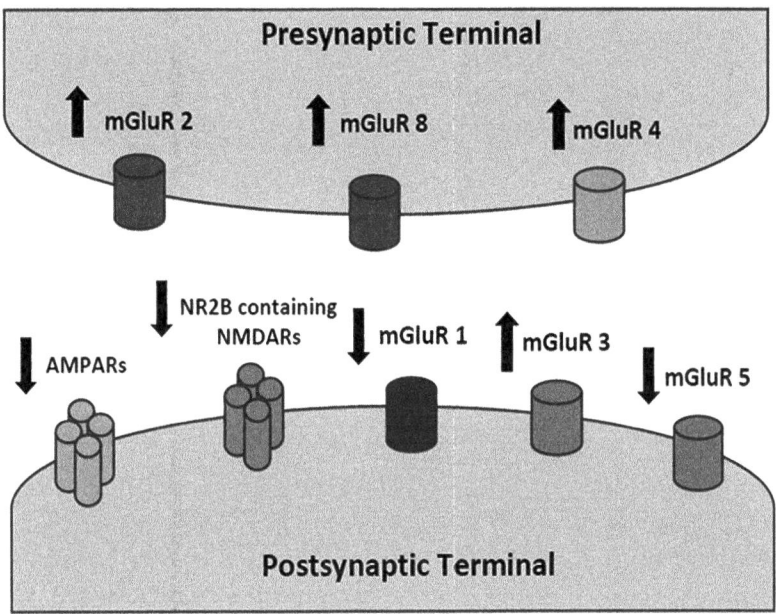

Figure 3.2 Schematic depiction of a glutamatergic synapse and localization of glutamate receptors. Arrows up or down indicate the possible receptor pharmacological modulation (activation vs inhibition). Glutamate receptors can be divided into two groups according to their molecular structure and pharmacodynamic mechanisms of activation. Ionotropic glutamate receptors (iGluRs) are ligand-gated ion channels activated by glutamate interaction with the receptor. Metabotropic glutamate receptors (mGluRs) indirectly modulate several neuronal targets (ion channels, transporters and intracellular enzymes) by the activation of intracellular signaling cascades. iGluRs have been classified, on the basis of their pharmacological profile, in AMPA, NMDA and kainate receptors. According to the more recent nomenclature, iGluR subunits can be classified as GluA1–4 (or GluR1–4) for AMPA receptors, GluK1–5 (or GluR5–7 and KA1 and KA2) for kainate receptors and GluN1–3 (or NR1–3) for NMDA receptors. mGluRs can be divided into three groups: group I (mGluR1 and 5) receptors are coupled to activation of phospholipase C; and group II (mGlu2 and –3) and group III (mGlu4, –6, –7 and –8) receptors are negatively coupled to adenylyl cyclase and inhibit cAMP formation.

Table 3.1 Summary of glutamatergic agents acting on ionotropic (A) and metabotropic (B) receptors and the pharmacodynamic mechanisms of each drug

(A)	AMPA receptors	GYKI-52466	Noncompetitive antagonist
		GYKI-53405	Noncompetitive antagonist
		NBQX	Competitive antagonist
		Perampanel	Noncompetitive antagonist
	AMPA/Kainate receptors	Tezampanel (LY293558)	Competitive antagonist
		Talampanel (LY300164)	Noncompetitive antagonist
	NMDA receptors	Amantadine	Noncompetitive antagonist
		MK-801	Noncompetitive antagonist
		Dextrophan	Noncompetitive antagonist
		MK-0657	Noncompetitive antagonist (NR2B subunit)
		APV	Competitive antagonist
		Ifenprodil	Noncompetitive antagonist (NR2B subunit)
		Traxoprodil	Noncompetitive antagonist (NR2B subunit)
		PAMQX	Competitive antagonist
		Remacemide	Noncompetitive antagonist

(continued)

Table 3.1 (cont.)

(B)	mGlu1 receptor	EMQMCM	Noncompetitive antagonist
	mGlu2 receptor	LY379268	Competitive agonist
	mGlu4 receptor	PHCCC	Positive allosteric modulator
		ADX88178	Positive allosteric modulator
		VU0155041	Positive allosteric modulator
	mGlu5 receptor	Dipraglurant (ADX48621)	Noncompetitive antagonist
		Mavoglurant (AFQ056)	Noncompetitive antagonist
		MPEP	Noncompetitive antagonist
		MRZ-8676	Noncompetitive antagonist
		MTEP	Noncompetitive antagonist
	mGlu7 receptor	AMN082	Positive allosteric modulator
	mGlu8 receptor	DCPG	Competitive agonist

increment of dyskinesias and conclude that this finding showed that amatadine has a persistent effect on dyskinesias [26]. However, the withdrawal effect and tachyphylaxis are due to different mechanisms and so should be considered separately for further discussion on other activities of the drug.

None of the other glutamatergic drugs received an evidence-based score for any effects. Evidence-based evaluation did not support the effect of amantadine on PD symptoms or progression.

A single meta-analysis [22] confirmed a statistically significant effect of amantadine in the reduction of dyskinesias, with a large effect size. This study also evaluated memantine, dextrometorphan and remacemide, and showed that these antiglutamatergic drugs are effective on dyskinesias, but the power and reliability reached by these other drugs were not statistically significant.

Minor studies

Dyskinesias

Beyond amantadine [27–32], reduction of dyskinesias has been described for dextromethorphan [11], remacemide [33] and memantine [13–17]. Dextromethorphan [11] administered alone at doses of 60–120 mg/day was tested in 18 patients and in 12 more patients in association with quetiapine sulfate: this combination is currently available only in the USA, but the US Food and Drug Administration (FDA) indication is only for emotional incontinence of pseudobulbar symptoms. Remacemide reduced dyskinesias at a dose of 150–600 mg/day in one study performed in 39 patients [33]. Memantine reduced dyskinesias in two patients as reported in two centers [13, 14], but an earlier study on 12 PD patients showed no effect [34].

Cognitive improvement

Amantadine has been used to improve cognition in patients affected by traumatic brain injury and minimally conscious state [35, 36]. A single case study described improvement following amantadine treatment in a patient in a vegetative state [37].

No evidence has been provided in PD, but in an observational study it was shown that amantadine reduced the incidence of dementia in a group of treated patients [38].

Memantine is used for the treatment of early- and late-stage of dementia. Three studies have described memantine effects in Lewy body dementia and PD with dementia [39–41].

Memantine improves the activities of daily living (ADL) and instrumental activities of daily living (IADL) but is limited by the same number needed to treat (NNT) ratio observed with cholinesterase inhibitors: one of seven treated patients [40] showed an appreciable improvement, i.e. the test score improvement was better than the single-item unit increment.

Akinetic crisis and neuroleptic malignant syndrome

Akinetic crisis, also termed malignant syndrome, parkinsonism–hyperpyrexia syndrome, neuroleptic-like malignant syndrome or acute akinesia, is a complication that appears in parkinsonism because of treatment manipulations or withdrawal, infectious disease, trauma or gastrointestinal tract disease [42, 43]. Akinetic crisis is the most severe complication of PD, occurring with an annual incidence of three cases per 1000 parkinsonian patients, and consist of worsening of acute motor symptoms characterized by an akinetic state with dysphagia, hyperthermia, an increase in serum creatine phosphokinase and myoglobin, dysautonomia, and transient unresponsiveness to the current antiparkinsonian treatment or to increase in dopaminergic doses [42]. Its symptoms are identical to the symptoms of neuroleptic malignant syndrome, and it was hypothesized that both represent idiosyncratic severe complications due to heterogeneous causes [44]. The guidelines of the German Neurologic Society suggest that amantadine sulfate should be used via intravenous injection at a dose of 200 mg to treat neuroleptic malignant syndrome and akinetic crisis. However, no evidence for this conclusion has been provided [45].

Psychosis induction

Anecdotal reports described the incidence of psychosis and hallucination in patients treated with amantadine and memantine [46–54]. A risk of psychosis induction was reported in cautionary guides for the side effects of this drugs, and reviews of safety show that the incidence is in the 1–5% range [19]. We found six reports of psychosis induced by amantadine [46–51] and three reports of psychosis induced by memantine [52–54], both administered at the current therapeutic dosages. A single case report described a complex psychosis with release of the maniac state and multiple ICDs in a patient treated with amantadine after several years of bipolar disorder (treated with antipsychotic drugs) and with late occurrence of PD [51].

Impulse control disorders and other compulsive disorders

Memantine is considered a possible option for the treatment of psychiatric disorders other than dementia: gambling [55], compulsive buying, binge-eating disorders [56], refractory obsessive-compulsive disorder [57] and pediatric obsessive-compulsive disorders [58] were improved in patients treated with memantine, but these studies are anecdotal, open label or have been presented in pilot studies or review.

Acamprosate is used for the treatment of alcohol craving at doses of 1200–2000 mg/day: for this compulsion, acamprosate is registered in Europe and other countries as its use has been supported by blinded studies [59].

There are no reports challenging the proposed effects of memantine or acamprosate on compulsive behaviors, while for amantadine, discussion of its possible effects on ICDs is more lively. A study designed as a double-blinded crossover with placebo and a washout period of the effect of 200 mg amantadine on gambling behavior in PD patients showed that amantadine reduced gambling (measured as Yale–Brown obsessive-compulsive scale scores and daily expenditure in gambling) in 17 patients [60]. A follow-up of this study suggested that the effect of amantadine was mediated by reduced risk-seeking behaviors [61]. An earlier anecdotal report showed that amantadine reduced gambling and punding behaviors in a lady affected by PD [62].

One further single case report showed that amantadine reduced gambling in one patient [63], and an open-label study suggested that amantadine may reduce punding [64].

As soon as the original study on gambling in PD was presented, two reports took a stand against the assumption that amantadine may reduce gambling or ICDs [65, 66]. The first one was a retrospective cross-sectional study that analyzed data from a study on dopamine agonist administration performed in order to understand the impact of these drugs on gambling and on ICDs in PD [65]. Data from this study were reanalyzed and the population treated with amantadine was compared with the untreated population; the study concluded that gambling was more common in patients who received amantadine and other drugs than in patients not receiving amantadine. However, this study provided no information and consistency of use (doses and timing, early or late add-ons, drug treatment duration) or other confounding factors of amantadine administration. The statistical results were significant only for part of the population – patients from the USA – and were not significant for patients from Canada, indicating a location bias. Moreover, in this study, dyskinesias that are reduced by amantadine, as shown by evidence-based reports [19], were more frequent in the in amantadine group than in the untreated group. This incongruity showed the confounding characteristics of any retrospective analysis that is unable to define the specific timing of treatment.

The second observational retrospective study [66] was presented as a comment on the crossover study on amantadine. In this study, gambling was also more common in the patients taking amantadine than in patients not exposed to the drug. Again in this study, the consistency and duration of treatment were not described. Dyskinesias were more frequent in the amantadine-treated group, yet even more relevant flaws could be shown in the statistical comparison, as no differences emerged from the treated and untreated groups if the comparison was adjusted for age, gender and disease duration and was restricted (as demanded by proper statistical methods) to patients with ICD.

Beyond the specific comments on these confutational reports [67], the essential element arising from this discussion is that a classical statistical epidemiological concept was not considered in either study, i.e. observational or cross-sectional studies cannot lead to cause-and-effect conclusions on drug efficacy because consistency of use, treatment duration and confounding by indication bias cannot be analyzed [68].

The confounding report of cross-sectional or observational studies can be exemplified by the experience with levodopa [69]. After the initial report by Cotzias, the use of levodopa was challenged by reports that showed no efficacy or only side effects [69]. The key to efficacy was patient selection and dose finding. Only after the appropriate PD staging systems were developed and the action mechanisms clarified did levodopa became the mainstay in PD treatment. Thus, our conclusion is that appropriate studies on the effects of amantadine and other antiglutamatergic drugs on ICDs should be designed and performed not just to provide a single indication for use, but mostly to highlight new research pathways [70]. Among the different antiglutamatergic drugs discussed in the present chapter, amantadine has several flaws that impinge on its chance of being involved again in prospective or blinded studies. Among these flaws is the fact that amantadine is an old drug [18, 20] with no patents forecasting revenues from the study, its production is not expensive and thus returns and costs are not important, and economical support for further studies is almost hopeless. A further flaw is that amantadine is an apparently well-known and widely used drug, even though its real mechanisms of action are poorly understood and guidelines suggest that it could worsen cognitive functions; it is nevertheless used for improving the outcome of brain trauma. It has a low dopaminergic activity but reduces dyskinesias. Cochrane and evidence-based reviews and treatment guidelines report insufficient evidence and low recommendations for the use of amantadine in early PD as properly blinded studies have not been performed [19]. The only class I level A studies were relative to amantadine use in late PD with dyskinesias [19]. Thus, amantadine use should not be undertaken lightly in early PD, yet it is still largely used, as shown by retrospective studies [66]. Exposition to amantadine is burdened by tachyphylaxis [24], but this effect is poorly studied, and its presence would imply that any study will require, as a prerequisite, absence of prior exposure to the drug.

Conclusion

In this chapter, we have emphasized controversial results and debates rather than focusing on the well-known effects of amantadine and antiglutamatergic drugs, which are described in detail by several previous reviews and analyses [19–21]. These reports are succinctly summarized, as widely known or available. All previous reviews concur in showing four main effects for antiglutamatergic drugs:

- Antiglutamatergic drugs may reduce dyskinesias, and the strongest statistical support of this effect has been produced for amantadine [19–22]. Other antiglutamatergic drugs may share the same effect, but none is supported by statistically sound studies.
- Antiglutamatergic drugs may improve cognition, but only the effect of memantine is statistically supported [39–41].
- Any antiglutamatergic drug may induce psychosis, and this effect may severely impinge our conclusion of studies inadequately supported by statistical analyses.
- Antiglutamatergic drugs may reduce ICDs and other compulsive disorders, but only acamprosate is registered and only for the treatment of alcohol cravings [59].

The first consideration provided by our review is focused instead on the controversial results, including no effects of memantine on dyskinesias, no effect of amantadine on ICDs and the controversial effects on cognition.

Our consideration is that, for any further study, adequate methodological approaches should be devised: patient selection should consider prior exposure to antiglutamatergic drugs, as complex tachyphylaxis and withdrawal effects have been described [24, 26]. Doses, duration of treatment and timing (i.e. antiglutamatergic administration before or after dopaminergic treatment) could clarify the proper approach to this class of drugs.

As a concluding hypothesis, we would like to focus on the peculiar cognition improvement/ICD reduction/psychosis induction pattern that can be identified, at least, for amantadine and memantine. We suggest that this pattern is dependent on an inverted U-shaped curve [71] of responses to this class of drugs: antiglutamatergic drugs, as shown by the apparently contradictory findings, may present with positive or negative effects.

Inverted U-shaped curves can be defined as a Yerkes–Dodson-type inverted U-shaped function [71], which represents a system that reaches its optimal function when the midrange level of a variable is reached, while both higher and lower levels are associated with impaired functions. Figure 3.3 shows examples of inverted U-shaped curves devised to explain the effects of dopaminergic drugs on behavior or on activity of the dorsal or ventral striatum. In the figure, we also propose an inverted U-shaped curve depicting the effect of antiglutamatergic drugs. In this case, mild levels of glutamatergic blockade may improve cognition by inhibiting the corticostriatothalamic loop (Figure 3.1) and by reducing recurrent behavior patterns. However, further blockade may excessively inhibit the cortical projections and release-stereotyped behaviors, interfering with cognition.

As described in the introduction, glutamatergic modulation is perhaps more complex than dopaminergic modulation: for the latter, several phenomena had to be identified and studied, such as priming [74] and the effects of continuous versus pulsatile administration

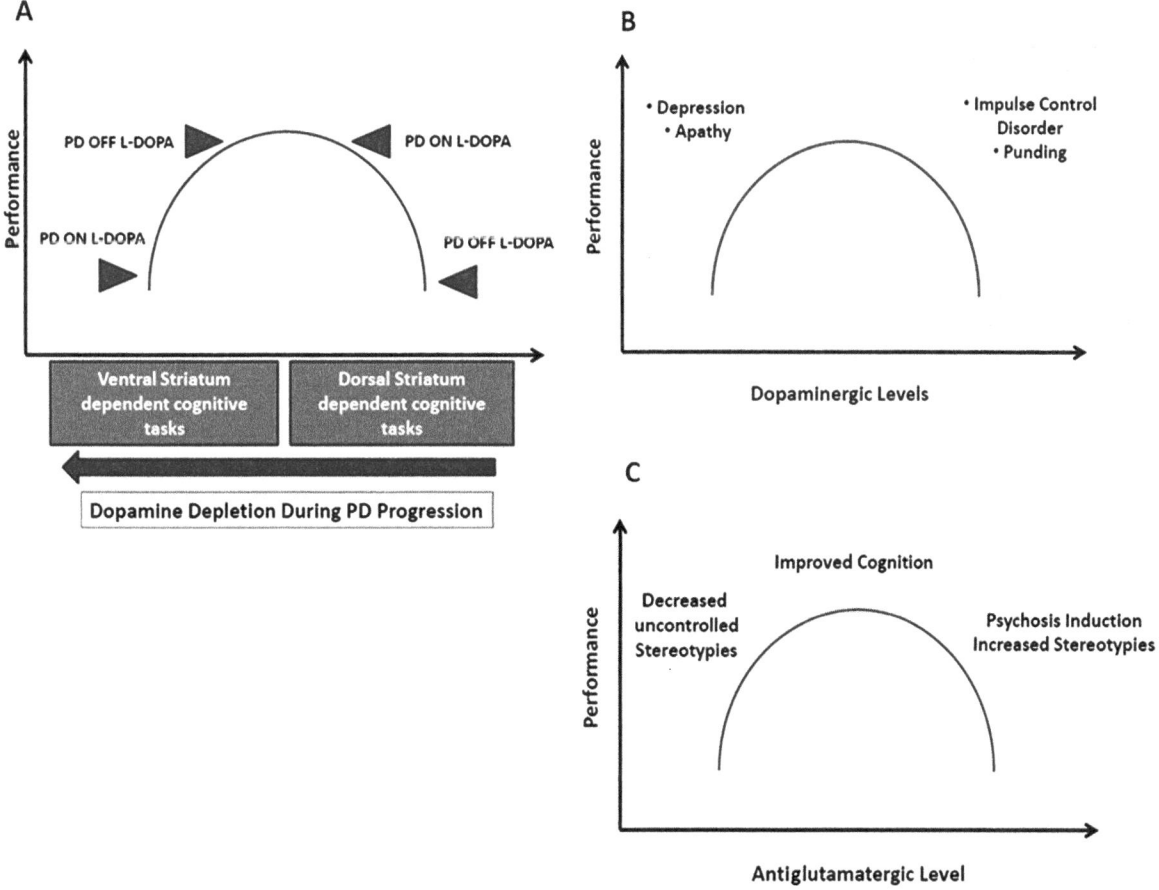

Figure 3.3 Examples of inverted U-shaped curves, focused on dopaminergic effects (A, B) and antiglutamatergic effects (C). (A and B are modified from Cools, 2006 [72], and Voon et al., 2011 [73], respectively.)

[75], in order to understand the mechanisms underlying erroneous predictions or results.

The clinical phenomenology of PD has also changed in recent years, from the plain motor phenotype to the complexities of mental disorders that were denied initially [76] and later became a core element in PD evaluation, to the point of classifying PD as a "neuropsychiatric disorder" [77]. In a temporal gradient, hallucinations and then depression and dementia, followed by ICDs and then functional overlays and somatoform disorders were identified [78]. In parallel, the idiopathic nature of PD was challenged by genetic evidence, to the point of proposing the concept of Parkinson's syndrome rather than PD [77].

We believe that understanding the effects of antiglutamatergic drugs in parkinsonism will require the same amount of conceptual and research efforts that were devoted to dopaminergic drugs.

The take-home message is that amantadine may be used for transient dyskinesia reduction, once other management options have been considered, as tachyphylaxis or complex effects of amantadine may play a role.

Memantine may be used for cognition improvement with the caveat that confusion or psychosis might worsen, rather than improve. However, the results of blinded studies on large patient populations suggest that the risk of these side effects is modest [39–41].

The presence of ICDs would suggest the use of antiglutamatergic drugs only as a speculative option. Add-ons of amantadine, memantine or acamprosate may reduce some compulsive behaviors, but our practical suggestion is that this approach should be used in a temporarily restricted frame, in order to slowly taper off dopamine agonist drugs and postpone/avoid the occurrence of the dopamine agonist withdrawal syndrome [80]. Clinical acumen will be needed to discern which patients are suitable for this mostly off-label trial, or for the use of antipsychotic drugs or for accelerated tapering of dopaminergic treatment. Confidence should come from properly designed studies on new drugs, and from characterization of responders and nonresponders.

References

1. Joel D. Open interconnected model of basal ganglia-thalamocortical circuitry and its relevance to the clinical syndrome of Huntington's disease. *Mov Disord* 2001; **16**: 407–23.
2. de la Fuente-Fernández R, Sossi V, Huang Z, *et al.* Levodopa-induced changes in synaptic dopamine levels increase with progression of Parkinson's disease: implications for dyskinesias. *Brain* 2004; **127**: 2747–54.
3. Lee JY, Lee EK, Park SS, *et al.* Association of DRD3 and GRIN2B with impulse control and related behaviors in disturbances in Parkinson disease. *Parkinsonism Relat Disord* 2009; **15**: 1803–10.
4. Calabresi P, Di Filippo M, Ghiglieri V, Tambasco N, Picconi B. Levodopa-induced dyskinesias in patients with Parkinson's disease: filling the bench-to-bedside gap. *Lancet Neurol* 2010; **9**: 1106–17.
5. Voon V, Fernagut PO, Wickens J, *et al.* Chronic dopaminergic stimulation in Parkinson's disease: from dyskinesias to impulse control disorders. *Lancet Neurol* 2009; **8**: 1140–9.
6. Linazasoro G. Dopamine dysregulation syndrome and levodopa-induced dyskinesias in Parkinson disease: common consequences of anomalous forms of neural plasticity. *Clin Neuropharmacol* 2009; **32**: 22–7.
7. Kalivas PW. The glutamate homeostasis hypothesis of addiction. *Nat Rev Neurosci* 2009; **10**: 561–72.
8. Cenci MA, Lundblad M. Post- versus presynaptic plasticity in l-DOPA-induced dyskinesia. *J Neurochem* 2006; **99**: 381–92.
9. van Eimeren T, Ballanger B, Pellecchia G, *et al.* Dopamine agonists diminish value sensitivity of the orbitofrontal cortex: a trigger for pathological gambling in Parkinson's disease? *Neuropsychopharmacology* 2009; **34**: 2758–66.
10. Allers KA, Bergstrom DA, Ghazi LJ, Kreiss DS, Walters JR. MK801 and amantadine exert different effects on subthalamic neuronal activity in a rodent model of Parkinson's disease. *Exp Neurol* 2005; **191**: 104–18.
11. Verhagen-Metman L, Blanchet PJ, van den Munckhof P, *et al.* A trial of dextromethorphan in parkinsonian patients with motor response complications. *Mov Disord* 1998; **13**: 414–17.
12. Spieker S, Loschmann PA, Klockgether T. The NMDA antagonist budipine can alleviate levodopa-induced motor fluctuations. *Mov Disord* 1999; **14**: 517–19.
13. Rabey JM, Nissipeanu P, Korczyn AD. Efficacy of memantine, an NMDA receptor antagonist, in the treatment of Parkinson's disease. *Neural Transm Park Dis Dement Sect* 1992; **4**: 277–82.
14. Varanese S, Howard J, Di Rocco A. NMDA antagonist memantine improves levodopa-induced dyskinesias and "on-off" phenomena in Parkinson's disease. *Mov Disord* 2010; **25**: 508–10.
15. Iderberg H, Rylander D, Bimpisidis Z, Cenci MA. Modulating mGluR5 and 5-HT1A/1B receptors to treat l-DOPA-induced dyskinesia: effects of combined treatment and possible mechanisms of action. *Exp Neurol* 2013; **250**: 116–24.
16. Vidal EI, Fukushima FB, Valle AP, Villas Boas PJ. Unexpected improvement in levodopa-induced dyskinesia and on-off phenomena after introduction of memantine for treatment of Parkinson's disease dementia. *J Am Geriatr Soc* 2013; **61**: 170–2.

17. Hanagasi HA, Kaptanoglu G, Sahin HA, Emre M. The use of NMDA antagonist memantine in drug-resistant dyskinesias resulting from l-dopa. *Mov Disord* 2000; **15**: 1016–17.
18. Rajput AH, Rajput A, Lang AE, et al. New use for an old drug: amantadine benefits levodopa-induced dyskinesia. *Mov Disord* 1998; **13**: 851.
19. Movement Disorders Society. Amantadine and other antiglutamate agents: management of Parkinson's disease. *Mov Disord* 2002; **17** (Suppl. 4): S13–22.
20. Crosby NJ, Deane KH, Clarke CE. Amantadine for dyskinesia in Parkinson's disease. *Cochrane Database Syst Rev* 2003: CD003467.
21. Higgins JPT, Green S (eds). *Cochrane Handbook for Systematic Reviews of Interventions*. Chichester: Wiley-Blackwell, 2008.
22. Elahi B, Phielipp N, Chen R. N-Methyl-d-Aspartate antagonists in levodopa induced dyskinesia: a meta-analysis. *Can J Neurol Sci* 2012; **39**: 465–72.
23. Riederer P, Kornhuber J, Gerlach M, et al. Glutamatergic-dopaminergic imbalance in Parkinson's disease and paranoid hallucinatory psychosis. In: Rinne UK, Nagatsu T, Horowski R (eds). *International Workshop Berlin: Parkinson's Disease*. The Netherlands: Medicom, 1991; 10–23.
24. Thomas A, Iacono D, Luciano AL, et al. Duration of amantadine benefit on dyskinesia of severe Parkinson's disease. *J Neurol Neurosurg Psychiatry* 2004; **75**: 141–3.
25. Metman LV, Del Dotto P, LePoole K, et al. Amantadine for levodopa-induced dyskinesias: a 1-year follow-up study. *Arch Neurol* 1999; **56**: 1383–6.
26. Wolf E, Seppi K, Katzenschlager R, et al. Long-term antidyskinetic efficacy of amantadine in Parkinson's disease. *Mov Disord* 2010; **25**: 1357–63.
27. Luginger E, Wenning GK, Bosch S, Poewe W. Beneficial effects of amantadine on l-dopa-induced dyskinesias in Parkinson's disease. *Mov Disord* 2000; **15**: 873–8.
28. Silva-Junior FP, Braga-Neto P, Sueli MF, de Bruin VM. Amantadine reduces the duration of levodopa-induced dyskinesia: a randomized, double-blind, placebo-controlled study. *Parkinsonism Relat Disord* 2005; **11**: 449–52.
29. Snow BJ, Macdonald L, McAuley D, Wallis W. The effect of amantadine on levodopa-induced dyskinesias in Parkinson's disease: a double-blind, placebo-controlled study. *ClinNeuropharmacol* 2000; **23**: 82–5.
30. Verhagen ML, Del Dotto P, van den Munckhof P, et al. Amantadine as treatment for dyskinesias and motor fluctuations in Parkinson's disease. *Neurology* 1998; **50**: 1323–6.
31. Rajput AH, Uitti RJ, Lang AE, et al. Amantadine ameliorates levodopa-induced dyskinesia. *Neurology* 1997; **48** (Suppl. 3): A328.
32. Sawada H, Oeda T, Kuno S, et al. Amantadine for dyskinesias in Parkinson's disease: a randomized controlled trial. *PLoS One* 2010; **5**: e15298.
33. Parkinson Study Group. Evaluation of dyskinesias in a pilot, randomized, placebo-controlled trial of remacemide in advanced Parkinson disease. *Arch Neurol* 2001; **58**: 1660–8.
34. Merello M, Nouzeilles MI, Cammarota A, Leiguarda R. Effect of memantine (NMDA antagonist) on Parkinson's disease: a double-blind crossover randomized study. *Clin Neuropharmacol* 1999; **22**: 273–6.
35. Mukherjee D, Patil CG, Palestrant D. Amantadine for severe traumatic brain injury. *N Engl J Med* 2012; **366**: 2427.
36. Zafonte RD, Watanabe T, Mann NR. Amantadine: a potential treatment for the minimally conscious state. *Brain Inj* 1998; **12**: 617–21.
37. Horiguchi J, Inami Y, Shoda T. Effects of long-term amantadine treatment on clinical symptoms and EEG of a patient in a vegetative state. *Clin Neuropharmacol* 1990; **13**: 84–8.
38. Inzelberg R, Bonuccelli U, Schechtman E, et al. Association between amantadine and the onset of dementia in Parkinson's disease. *Mov Disord* 2006; **21**: 1375–9.
39. Aarsland D, Ballard C, Walker Z, et al. Memantine in patients with Parkinson's disease dementia or dementia with Lewy bodies: a double-blind, placebo-controlled, multicentre trial. *Lancet Neurol* 2009; **8**: 613–18.
40. Ballard C, Kahn Z, Corbett A. Treatment of dementia with Lewy bodies and Parkinson's disease dementia. *Drugs Aging* 2011; **28**: 769–77.
41. Emre M, Tsolaki M, Bonuccelli U, et al. Memantine for patients with Parkinson's disease dementia or dementia with Lewy bodies: a randomised, double-blind, placebo-controlled trial. *Lancet Neurol* 2010; **9**: 969–77.
42. Onofrj M, Thomas A. Acute akinesia in Parkinson disease. *Neurology* 2005; **64**: 1162–9.
43. Thomas A, Onofrj M. Akinetic crisis, acute akinesia, neuroleptic malignant-like syndrome, Parkinsonism-hyperpyrexia syndrome, and malignant syndrome are the same entity and are often independent of treatment withdrawal. *Mov Disord* 2005; **20**: 1671; author reply 1671–2.
44. Margetić B, Aukst-Margetić B. Neuroleptic malignant syndrome and its controversies. *Pharmacoepidemiol Drug Saf* 2010; **19**: 429–35.
45. Eggert KM, Oertel WH, Reichmann H (eds). *Parkinson Syndrome – Diagnostik und Therapie. Leitlinien fuer Diagnostik und Therapie in der Neurologie*. Berlin: Deutsche Gesellschaft fuer Neurologie, 2012.
46. Smith EJ. Amantadine-induced psychosis in a young healthy patient. *Am J Psychiatry* 2008; **165**: 1613.
47. Harper RW, Knothe UC. Colored Lilliputian hallucinations with amantadine. *Med J Aust* 1973; **1**: 444–5.
48. Snoey ER, Bessen HA. Acute psychosis after amantadine overdose. *Ann Emerg Med* 1990; **19**: 668–70.

49. Stroe AE, Hall J, Amin F. Psychotic episode related to phenylpropanolamine and amantadine in a healthy female. *Gen Hosp Psychiatry* 1995; **17**: 457–8.

50. Flaherty JA, Bellur SN. Mental side effects of amantadine therapy: its spectrum and characteristics in a normal population. *J Clin Psychiatry* 1981; **42**: 344–5.

51. Walsh RA, Lang AE. Multiple impulse control disorders developing in Parkinson's disease after initiation of amantadine. *Mov Disord* 2012; **27**: 326.

52. Riederer P, Lange KW, Kornhuber J, Danielczyk W. Pharmacotoxic psychosis after memantine in Parkinson's disease. *Lancet* 1991; **338**: 1022–3.

53. Robles Bayón A, Gude Sampedro F. Inappropriate treatments for patients with cognitive decline. *Neurologia* 2012; **29**: 523–32.

54. Menendez-Gonzalez M, Calatayud MT, Blazquez-Menes B. Exacerbation of Lewy bodies dementia due to memantine. *J Alzheimers Dis* 2005; **8**: 289–91.

55. Grant JE, Chamberlain SR, Odlaug BL, Potenza MN, Kim SW. Memantine shows promise in reducing gambling severity and cognitive inflexibility in pathological gambling: a pilot study. *Psychopharmacology (Berl)* 2010; **212**: 603–12.

56. Gallini A, Sommet A, Salandini AM, *et al.* Weight-loss associated with anti-dementia drugs in a patient with Parkinson's disease. *Mov Disord* 2007; **22**: 1980–1.

57. Sani G, Serra G, Kotzalidis GD, *et al.* The role of memantine in the treatment of psychiatric disorders other than the dementias: a review of current preclinical and clinical evidence. *CNS Drugs* 2012; **26**: 663–90.

58. Stewart SE, Jenike EA, Hezel DM, *et al.* 2010; A single blinded case–control study of memantine insevere obsessive-compulsive disorder. *J Clin Psychopharmacol* 30: 34–9.

59. Pelc I, Verbanck P, Le Bon O, *et al.* Efficacy and safety of acamprosate in the treatment of detoxified alcohol-dependent patients. A 90-day placebo-controlled dose-finding study. *Br J Psychiatry* 1997; **171**: 73–7.

60. Thomas A, Bonanni L, Gambi F, Di Iorio A, Onofrj M. Pathological gambling in Parkinson disease is reduced by amantadine. *Ann Neurol* 2010; **68**: 400–4.

61. Cera N, Bifolchetti S, Martinotti G, *et al.* Amantadine and cognitive flexibility: decision making in Parkinson patients with severe pathological gambling and other impulse control disorders. *Neuropsychiatr Dis Treat* 2014; **10**: 1093–101.

62. Kashihara K, Imamura T. Amantadine may reverse punding in Parkinson's disease – observation in a patient. *Mov Disord* 2008; **23**: 129–30.

63. Pettorruso M, Martinotti G, Di Nicola M, *et al.* Amantadine in the treatment of pathological gambling: a case report. *Front Psychiatry* 2012; **3**: 102.

64. Fasano A, Ricciardi L, Pettorruso M, Bentivoglio AR. Management of punding in Parkinson's disease: an open-label prospective study. *J Neurol* 2011; **258**: 656–60.

65. Weintraub D, Sohr, M, Siderowf A, *et al.* Amantadine use associated with impulse control disorders in Parkinson disease. *Ann Neurol* 2010; **68**: 963–8.

66. Lee JY, Kim HJ, Jeon BS. Is pathological gambling in Parkinson's disease reduced by amantadine? *Ann Neurol* 2011; **69**: 213–14.

67. Onofrj M, Bonanni L, Di Iorio A, Thomas A. Is pathological gambling in Parkinson's disease reduced by amantadine? Reply *Ann Neurol* 2011; **69**: 214–15.

68. Wang O, Kilpatrick RD, Critchlow CW, *et al.* Relationship between epoetin alfa dose and mortality: findings from a marginal structural model. *Clin J Am Soc Nephrol* 2010; **5**: 182–8.

69. Fahn S. The history of dopamine and levodopa in the treatment of Parkinson's disease. *Mov Disord* 2008; **23**: S497–508.

70. Bastiaens J, Dorfman BJ, Christos PJ, Nirenberg MJ. Prospective cohort study of impulse control disorders in Parkinson's disease. *Mov Disord* 2013; **28**: 327–33.

71. Yerkes RM, Dodson JD. The relation of strength of stimulus to rapidity of habit-formation. *J Comp Neurol Psychol* 1908; **18**: 459–82.

72. Cools R. Dopaminergic modulation of cognitive function-implications for l-DOPA treatment in Parkinson's disease. *Neurosci Biobehav Rev* 2006; **30**: 1–23.

73. Voon V, Gao J, Brezing C, *et al.* Dopamine agonists and risk: impulse control disorders in Parkinson's disease. *Brain* 2011; **134**: 1438–46.

74. Jenner P. Molecular mechanisms of l-DOPA-induced dyskinesia. *Nat Rev Neurosci* 2008; **9**: 665–77.

75. Stocchi F, Vacca L, Ruggieri S, Olanow CW. Intermittent vs continuous levodopa administration in patients with advanced Parkinson disease: a clinical and pharmacokinetic study. *Arch Neurol* 2005; **62**: 905–10.

76. Chaudhuri KR, Schapira AH. Non-motor symptoms of Parkinson's disease: dopaminergic pathophysiology and treatment. *Lancet Neurol* 2009; **8**: 464–74.

77. Agid Y, Arnulf I, Bejjani P, *et al.* Parkinson's disease is a neuropsychiatric disorder. *Adv Neurol* 2003; **91**: 365–70.

78. Onofrj M, Bonanni L, Manzoli L, Thomas A. Cohort study on somatoform disorders in Parkinson disease and dementia with Lewy bodies. *Neurology* 2010; **74**: 1598–606.

79. Albin RL, Dauer WT. Parkinson syndrome. Heterogeneity of etiology; heterogeneity of pathogenesis? *Neurology* 2012; **79**: 202–3.

80. Rabinak CA, Nirenberg MJ. Dopamine agonist withdrawal syndrome in Parkinson disease. *Arch Neurol* 2010; **67**: 58–63.

Chapter 4

Monoamine oxidase inhibitors in the management of Parkinson's disease

Sven-Eric Pålhagen

Introduction

Monoamine oxidase B (MAO-B) inhibitors have again become relevant as a good option for the initial treatment of Parkinson's disease (PD) [1, 2], and there has been a recent reappraisal of the role for selegiline in PD treatment [3]. The main MAO-B inhibitors are still selegiline and rasagiline and therefore the emphasis in this chapter is on these drugs. A reported new formulation of selegiline, oral disintegrating tablets (ODT) is also discussed.

The purpose of this chapter is to emphasize treatment options for PD in light of evidence from randomized controlled clinical trials in order to develop practical recommendations for clinical therapeutics.

During the last 10 years, several guidelines have been produced by the Movement Disorders Society (MDS), the Cochrane Collaboration, the National Institute for Health and Clinical Excellence (NICE) and the American Academy of Neurology [4–10]. Monoamine oxidase B inhibitors are in all recommendations still an established option in the treatment of early PD as well as for symptomatic treatment of complications. Appendix I provides a summary of the European Federation of Neurological Societies (EFNS) classification scheme for therapeutic intervention and the evidence classification scheme for the rating of recommendations for a therapeutic intervention, as presented in 2004, which are the up-to-date recommendations from EFNS [11] – it is necessary to have this tabular form when interpreting the contents of the EFNS recommendations [12–14]. Likewise, Appendix II provides a description of the MDS definitions for their specific recommendations. The MDS recommendations in 2004 (based on [4, 5]) are still valid in the latest recommendations from 2011, shown in Appendix III [15], which presents comprehensive conclusions on the role of MAO-B inhibitors in evidence-based medicine methodology. Finally, the combined EFNS/MDS-European Section (ES) guidelines are summarized and presented as the 2013 Recommendations on Therapeutic Management of Parkinson's Disease in Appendix IV [16].

The pivotal studies for efficacy and possible neuroprotective potential of selegiline and rasagiline are presented in this chapter. The MAO-B inhibitors selegiline and rasagiline are both considered effective for symptomatic control of parkinsonism (level A), but for preventing motor complications, selegiline is ineffective (level A) and no there is no recommendation for rasagiline because of insufficient data.

Treatment with MAO-B inhibitors is simple and its side effects are well known and easily controllable. The relationship to treatment with serotonergic drugs requires attention but can be handled.

Background

The basis of symptomatic treatment for PD is dopamine replacement therapy and the golden standard therapy is levodopa (L-DOPA), the metabolic precursor of dopamine (in combination with carbidopa or benserazide, which are peripherally acting aromatic L-amino acid decarboxylase (AADC) or DOPA decarboxylase inhibitors, which are unable to cross the blood–brain barrier).

Dopamine is metabolized by intraneuronal monoamine oxidase A (MAO-A) and by MAO-A and MAO-B in glial and astrocyte cells. Monoamine oxidase A is found in the presynaptic neurons in the brain, while MAO-B is found predominantly localized to glia cells closest to dopaminergic synapses and controls both the release from storage and the free intraneuronal levels of

---

Parkinson's Disease: Current and Future Therapeutics and Clinical Trials, ed. Gálvez-Jiménez *et al*. Published by Cambridge University Press. © Cambridge University Press 2016.

dopamine. Monoamine oxidase B inhibition potentiates dopaminergic function in the brain and is a therapeutic option for patients with PD.

The identification of multiple forms of MAO and the discovery of selegiline as a selective, irreversible MAO-B inhibitor, which lacks the ability to potentiate the sympathomimetic effect of tyramine, i.e. without the "cheese effect," occurred in 1968 [17] and in the 1980s, this became a new treatment option for PD.

Selegiline

Selegiline (also known by the older name of L-deprenyl) is an irreversible inhibitor of MAO-B and has, for many years, been the reference agent of this class of drugs. Originally developed as a possible treatment for depression, the drug in fact exhibits no relevant activity in this condition when used at the low (<10 mg/day) doses effective in the treatment of PD. The inhibition of MAO-B that is the basis of selegiline's efficacy in PD appears to reside in the parent drug and its principal metabolite, desmethylselegiline. Selegiline has been credited, on the basis of preclinical observations, with a range of effects described under the umbrella term of "neuroprotective" [18–22], although the relevance of these actions to its clinical applications in PD remains uncertain, in part because it has proven difficult to differentiate accurately symptomatic and possible neuroprotective effects.

Efficacy

In 1985 [23], published by then well-established researchers in the field, including W. Birkmayer, J. Knoll, P. Riederer and M. Youdim, a long-term study (9 years) showed a significant increase in life expectancy resulting from the addition of selegiline to Madopar® (co-beneldopa). Even as an open-label, non-randomized trial, the results were remarkable. Earlier, in 1983 [24, 25] the discovery of 1-methyl-4-phenyl-1,2,3,6-tetrahydropyridine (MPTP) toxicity had been published, which produced selective loss of dopaminergic cells in the substantia nigra. When it was later shown that selegiline could inhibit the dopaminergic neurotoxicity of MPTP in monkeys [26], several clinical trials were prepared.

In 1993, Myllylä showed significant symptomatic benefit for selegiline as monotherapy in early PD compared with placebo [27]. The study also indicated that selegiline could significantly delay the need for supplementary levodopa treatment.

Neuroprotective potential

As early as 1987, the Parkinson Study Group initiated the Deprenyl and Tocopherol Antioxidant Treatment On Parkinson's disease (DATATOP) study. This study was the first clinical study that tried to detect a neuroprotective effect in PD. A total of 800 patients with early PD were randomized in a 2 × 2 factorial design to selegiline and/or the antioxidant vitamin E, tocopherol or placebo, and were evaluated clinically over 18+ months. There were no beneficial effects of tocopherol in comparison with placebo, but selegiline significantly delayed the onset of disability requiring levodopa by about 9 months, representing a 57% risk reduction of starting levodopa during the first year of treatment [28].

An extension study was carried out with 368 patients from the original DATATOP study who were on levodopa who agreed to continuing the selegiline treatment or changing to matching placebo under double-blinded conditions. During an average of 2 years follow-up, the patients treated with selegiline showed slower motor decline in terms of Unified Parkinson's Disease Rating Scale (UPDRS) scores, and total, activities of daily living, motor and on–off motor fluctuations or freezing of gait, but significantly more dyskinesias [29].

To further control for a possible symptomatic effect, a prospective, longitudinal, double-blinded controlled study of the effect of selegiline and levodopa on the progression of the signs and symptoms of PD over 14 months was performed [30]. A total of 101 untreated patients with mild PD were randomized to one of four treatment groups: group 1, selegiline and Sinemet® (carbidopa/levodopa); group 2, placebo-selegiline and Sinemet®; group 3, selegiline and bromocriptine; and group 4, placebo-selegiline plus bromocripitine. The primary endpoint was a change in motor score between an untreated baseline visit and an untreated final visit 2 months after withdrawal of the study drugs, i.e. selegiline or its placebo, and 7 days after withdrawal of Sinemet® or bromocriptine. The decline measured by UPDRS score with this study design was used as an index of disease progression. Placebo-treated patients deteriorated by 5.8 ± 1.4 points for the total UPDRS score and the deprenyl-treated patients by 0.4 ± 1.3 points ($P < 0.001$). The authors concluded that "these findings are not readily explained by the drug's symptomatic effects and are consistent with the hypothesis that selegiline has a neuroprotective effect." However, it is possible that the washout period was too short, so that a prolonged symptomatic effect may complicate the explanation of a neuroprotective effect.

In the MONOCOMB (Use of Selegiline as Monotherapy and in Combination with Levodopa in the Management of Parkinson's Disease) study [31–33], previously untreated patients with idiopathic PD ($n = 157$) were randomized to receive selegiline 10 mg/day or placebo until levodopa was required; experimental medication was then withdrawn for 8 weeks. Patients were then randomized to levodopa (50 mg/day, titrated in 50 mg/day increments to 150 mg/day) plus either selegiline or placebo. Treatment was continued until patients required additional antiparkinsonian therapy or up to 7 years after initial randomization. The impact of selegiline monotherapy on time to the start of levodopa therapy was first investigated, followed by a comparison of the progression of PD in patients treated with individualized levodopa plus selegiline or placebo. Selegiline significantly delayed the time when levodopa therapy became necessary during the monotherapy phase by more than 4 months, even though the mean total UPDRS scores at the time of initiation of levodopa were similar in both groups. In the combination therapy phase of the study, the use of selegiline as an adjunct to levodopa demonstrated a lower total consumption of levodopa. Patients treated with selegiline plus levodopa also exhibited a distinct ($P = 0.005$) slowing in the anticipated increase in the UPDRS scores over time, as, for example, shown by a mean UPDRS total score after 5 years that was 10 points lower than in patients on levodopa and placebo.

The MONOCOMB trial is among the largest and longest-duration placebo-controlled studies to report experience with selegiline monotherapy in the early phase of PD. The results of the MONOCOMB trial confirm that selegiline is effective in retarding the progression of early PD, that it has levodopa-sparing qualities in more advanced disease, and that it is reasonably well tolerated in long-term use.

Two meta-analyses in 2004 and 2005 [34, 6] addressed the effectiveness of MAO-B inhibitors in reducing the rate of progression and effective and safe symptomatic treatment.

Ives et al. [34] included 3525 people with PD in 17 randomized trials: 13 trials on selegiline, three on lazabemide (RO19-6327, a short-acting, reversible, highly selective inhibitor of MAO-B which, unlike selegiline, is not metabolized to active compounds) and one on rasagiline therapy. The result of the lazabemide studies were compatible with the results of the other therapies. All trials showed significantly improved scores in favor of selegiline versus controls, i.e. MAO-B inhibitors reduces disability, the need for levodopa and the incidence of motor fluctuations without significant side effects or increased mortality.

The Cochrane review on MAO-B inhibitors in 2005 [6] found similar results in 2514 PD patients from 12 trials, 11 on selegiline and one on lazabemide (several of these trials were also included in [34]). This Cochrane review also found significantly improved scores in favor of MAO-B inhibitors given from baseline to 1 year on treatment.

In the NICE guidelines of 2006 [7] for PD, recommendations based on the analyses by Ives et al. [34] and the Cochrane review [6] stated that "the benefits of MAOB inhibitors versus control in terms of rating scales were consistent with a known short-term symptomatic effect. There does not seem to be any clear increase or decrease in mortality with MAOB inhibitors" and that "further large trials with long-term follow-up are required to assess whether the MAOB inhibitors have neuroprotective properties in PD."

Rasagiline

In the 1990s, another MAO-B inhibitor, rasagiline, was developed for the treatment of both early PD as monotherapy and in more advanced disease as an adjunct to levodopa.

Rasagiline as an adjunct therapy to levodopa for motor fluctuations in PD

The efficacy of rasagiline was demonstrated in randomized, double-blinded clinical trials. Rasagiline as an adjunct therapy to levodopa has been tested in two separate multicenter, double-blind, parallel-group clinical trials, PRESTO and LARGO.

In the PRESTO (Parkinson Rasagiline: Efficacy and Safety in the Treatment of "Off") trial [35], 472 patients with at least 2.5 h of daily "off" time in spite of optimized treatment with other anti-PD medications (levodopa or concomitant medication such as dopamine agonists or entacapone) were randomized to receive rasagiline, either 1 or 0.5 mg/day, or placebo as an adjunct therapy over 26 weeks. A modest but significant reduction of "off" time was found from baseline by 1.85 h (29%) for the 1 mg/day dose and by 1.41 h (23%) for the 0.5 mg/day dose compared with a reduction of 0.49 h (15%) in the placebo group.

In the LARGO (Lasting effect in Adjunct therapy with Rasagiline Given Once daily) study [36], the investigators wanted to investigate the efficacy and safety of rasagiline compared with entacapone in levodopa-treated patients with PD and motor fluctuations. A total of 687 patients with at least 1 h of "off" time measured by a 24 h home diary were randomly assigned to either rasagiline 1 mg once daily or entacapone 200 mg with every levodopa dose or placebo for 18 weeks. The results showed a significant reduction of mean daily "off" time by 1.18 h for rasagiline and by 1.2 h for entacapone, and by 0.4 h for those patients on placebo, from baseline. This study also reported information that is useful for the physicians who treat the patients, i.e the mean daily "on" time without troublesome dyskinesias, and a modest but statistically significant increase of 0.85 h was found in patients on either rasagiline or entacapone compared with the placebo group.

Rasagiline in clinical trials for disease modification

The TEMPO (TVP-1012 in Early Monotherapy for PD Outpatients) study [37], was originally designed to evaluate the safety and efficacy of rasagiline given to patients not requiring dopaminergic therapy [29]. In this study, 404 patients with early PD were randomized to placebo or rasagiline 1 or 2 mg/day and followed 6 months. At the end of the study period, the rasagiline groups had a robustly improved UPDRS score in comparison with placebo, of 4.2 points ($P < 0.001$) for the rasagiline 1 mg/day group and 3.56 points ($P < 0.001$) for the rasagiline 2 mg/day group.

These promising data resulted in the 6-month study being extended for an additional 6 months for 380 patients [38]. The patients in the rasagiline groups remained on their original dose and the patients from the placebo group who wanted to participate were given rasagiline 2 mg/day. The primary endpoint was a change in total UPDRS score from baseline to week 52. The result for the whole 12-month period for the rasagiline groups on 1 or 2 mg/day and the delayed 2 mg/day were improvements of 3.0, 2.0 and 4.1 points, respectively, in their UPDRS scores. The 12-month rasagiline 2 mg/day group had a 2.29-point smaller increase in UPDRS total score compared with subjects treated with placebo for 6 month and then rasagiline 2 mg/day for 6 months. The conclusion was that subjects treated with rasagiline 2 or 1 mg/day for 12 months showed less functional decline than subjects whose treatment was delayed for 6 months. The TEMPO study was not initially designed as a disease modification trial but did provide the early data on which the planning for the ADAGIO study was based.

The ADAGIO (Attenuation of Disease Progression with Azilect GIven Once daily) study [39] was larger and longer but with a similar delayed-start design. In this double-blinded study, 1176 patients with early, untreated PD were randomized to four parallel arms: rasagiline at either 1 or 2 mg/day for a total of 72 weeks (i.e. the early-start groups), and placebo for 36 weeks followed by rasagiline 1 or 2 mg/day for another 36 weeks (i.e. delayed-start group). This study has been referred as "a land mark study in terms of size, design and outcome." It was the first to test prospectively the hypothesis that earlier rather than later use of a specific dopaminergic drug leads to an improvement in outcome that cannot be explained by a symptomatic effect alone [40] The primary analysis used to indicate significant disease modification required three hierarchical endpoints that the early-start group had to meet, based on the change in the total UPDRS score from baseline: (i) the superiority of early-start treatment versus placebo with respect to estimates of the rate of change from baseline in the total UPDRS score between weeks 12 and 36; (ii) superiority to delayed-start treatment in the change of the score from baseline to week 72; and (iii) the noninferiority of early-start treatment compared with delayed-start treatment in the rate of change of the score between weeks 48 and 72, i.e. that the rate of progression in the early-start group on 1 or 2 mg/day after week 12 must be significantly slower than the placebo group during the first 9 months showing effect and there had to be a significant difference at 18 months (end of the study) in UPDRS score for the early- and late-start patients indicating a long-lasting effect. However, the rate of progression for UPDRS scores during months 9–18 should also at least be parallel and should not converge.

The results showed that rasagiline 1 mg/day achieved all three hierarchical primary endpoints based on disease progression. However, the 2 mg/day dosage met the first but failed the second, and therefore did not meet all hierarchical primary endpoints as required. The authors pointed out that the early-start regimen with rasagiline 1 mg/day gave support to a possible disease-modifying effect, although 2 mg/day did not meet their endpoints.

Selegiline ODT (orally disintegrating tablets)

Studies presented in 2007 [41] with selegiline ODT in patients with PD and "wearing-off" symptoms in a double-blind, placebo-controlled, parallel-design trial showed no significant difference in improvement in percentage of daily "off" time with selegiline ODT (11.6%) versus placebo (9.8%). No data are currently available for selegiline ODT used as monotherapy in early PD.

Safety
Selegiline
Selegiline is a propargyl methamphetamine and undergoes extensive hepatic first-pass metabolism to L-methamphetamine and L-amphetamine. These amphetamine metabolites might be associated with cardiac or psychiatric adverse events. Interestingly, during the long-standing DATATOP study, no differences were noted between the groups with selegiline or placebo concerning serious adverse events, cardiovascular adverse events, discontinuation of therapy or mortality. However, the amphetamine metabolites of selegiline have potential cardiovascular effects and have been associated with aggravation of orthostatic hypotension in PD patients. Long-term postmarketing has revealed that psychiatric adverse effects such as nightmares and hallucinations have also been reported frequently in patients on selegiline [42]. In the UK, the PDRG (Parkinson's Disease Research Group) study showed, during a mean follow-up of 5.6 years, a 60% increase in mortality for patients on levodopa with selegiline compared with levodopa alone [43]. However, a population-based study of more than 12,000 patients with PD in the UK found no significant increase in the risk of mortality among patients on selegiline monotherapy or on combination levodopa/selegiline treatment [44].

Rasagiline
Rasagiline is not a propargyl amphetamine derivate and its principal metabolite, aminoindan, does not have an amphetamine-like chemical structure and therefore has no amphetamine-like adverse effects. The adverse events that more frequent with rasagiline than with placebo are more often gastrointestinal and dose related. In the TEMPO, LARGO and PRESTO studies, no significant differences were shown between rasagiline and placebo with respect to serious adverse events or discontinuations of active therapy.

In a postmarketing observational study [45] in patients with PD, overall 754 patients received rasagiline at a recommended dose of 1 mg/day under an observation period of 4 months. Both monotherapy and combination therapy improve parkinsonian symptoms such as reduced "off" time and improved quality of life, and tolerability was rated as "good" or "very good" in 97% in monotherapy patients and in 90% in combination therapy patients. The authors emphasized that "These results under every day clinical practice conditions provide additional support for the earlier findings of the pivotal rasagiline studies in clinical settings."

Comparison of selegiline and rasagiline in the symptomatic treatment of PD: indirect meta-analysis of randomized placebo-controlled clinical trials

No direct comparative randomized controlled study on comparison between selegiline and rasagiline in the symptomatic treatment of PD exists, but a indirect meta-analysis has been performed [46]. In a systematic literature review, a total of 83 publications on placebo-controlled studies (randomized controlled trials [RCTs]) were identified. For selegiline, there were 71 studies published between 1988 and 2009 with 38 different RCTs of which 15 were considered for analysis of efficacy and/or tolerability, and nine of the 15 met the inclusion criteria for the meta-analysis of efficacy and 12 of the 15 for analysis regarding safety and tolerability. All 12 studies for rasagiline met the criteria. Overall, rasagiline showed a "significant advantage in the primary endpoint UPDRS total scores." Risks for adverse events such as dizziness, hallucinations, diarrhea and syncope were lower with rasagiline than with selegiline ($P < 0.15$ for each).

Serotonin syndrome
Psychiatric symptoms are common in PD. It is believed that up to 60% of Parkinson's patients have depressive symptoms, which require periodic or continuous treatment with antidepressants such as tricyclic antidepressants, selective serotonin reuptake inhibitors (SSRIs) or serotonin norepinephrine reuptake inhibitors – all of these drugs have the possibility of developing serotonin syndrome. Symptoms of serotonin syndrome

include hyperthermia, rigidity, myoclonus, autonomic instability with possible rapid fluctuations of vital signs, and mental status changes such as confusion, irritability and extreme agitation progressing to delirium and coma. There is a theoretical risk in the use of antidepressants (in combination with MAO-B inhibitor), but, in practice, the incidence of serotonin syndrome is extremely rare [47]. In a recent review [48], pharmacological management of mood disorders in PD were reviewed. The authors reported the results of the RCT studies of SSRI treatment of depression in PD where only citalopram and paroxetine had a positive outcome, although with varying results. Regarding RCTs and tricyclic antidepressants used for depression in PD, nortryptiline and desipramine were shown to work. Regarding serotonin and norepinephrine reuptake inhibitors for the treatment of depression in PD, venlafaxine was effective.

One safety aspect that should be highlighted in the use of contraindicated antidepressants co-prescribed with MOA-B inhibitors is that velaflaxine and fluoxetine are contraindicated. Citalopram (up to 20 mg), escitalopram (up to 10 mg) or sertraline (up to 100 mg) can be used. Tricyclic antidepressants may be used with caution (amitriptyline up to 50 mg/day or trazodone up to 100 mg/day), and even paroxetine (up to 30 mg/day). It must be emphasized that venlafaxine/mirtazapine should not be used concomitantly with MAO-B inhibitors or within 2 weeks of discontinuation of MAO-B inhibitors. Similarly, approximately 2 weeks should be allowed to pass before a patient treated with venlafaxine/mirtazapine should be treated with MAO-B inhibitors.

Monoamine oxidase B inhibitors: future role

Levodopa represents the "gold standard" for treating the motor symptoms of PD, but when symptoms are mild, MAO-B inhibitors might be an appropriate alternative to avoid levodopa-related side effects. In PD patients with predominant postural instability and gait disability (PIGD-subtype of parkinsonism), it would be worthwhile in mild cases starting them on or adding MAO-B inhibitors [34, 49].

Monoamine oxidase B inhibitors like selegiline and rasagiline protect neuronal cells in animal models through intervention in the death signaling pathway in mitochondria [50]. It has been shown that selegiline and rasagiline increase the expression of antiapoptotic Bcl-2 protein family and neurotrophic factors, and both GDNF (glial cell line-derived neurotrophic factor) and BDNF (brain-derived neurotrophic factor) are induced by selegiline and rasagiline [50]. Rationally designed multitargeted drugs are being tested in studies as neuroprotective agents and neurorestorative drugs such as ladostigil and M30 derived from rasagiline [51].

Appendix I
EFNS Evidence Classification Scheme for a Therapeutic Intervention

Class I	An adequately powered prospective, randomized, controlled clinical trial with masked outcome assessment in a representative population or an adequately powered systematic review of prospective randomized controlled clinical trials with masked outcome assessment in representative populations
	The following are required: (a) randomization concealment (b) primary outcome(s) is/are clearly defined (c) exclusion/inclusion criteria are clearly defined (d) adequate accounting for dropouts and crossovers with numbers sufficiently low to have minimal potential for bias (e) relevant baseline characteristics are presented and substantially equivalent among treatment groups or there is appropriate statistical adjustment for differences
Class II	Prospective matched-group cohort study in a representative population with masked outcome assessment that meets (a)–(e) above or a randomized controlled trial in a representative population that lacks one of criteria (a)–(e)
Class III	All other controlled trials (including well-defined natural history controls or patients serving as own controls) in a representative population, where outcome assessment is independent of patient treatment
Class IV	Evidence from uncontrolled studies, case series, case reports or expert opinion

EFNS Evidence Classification Scheme for the Rating of Recommendations for a Therapeutic Intervention

Level A	(Established as effective, ineffective or harmful) requires at least one convincing class I study or at least two consistent, convincing class II studies
Level B	(Probably effective, ineffective or harmful) requires at least one convincing class II study or overwhelming class III evidence
Level C	(Possibly effective, ineffective or harmful) rating requires at least two convincing class III studies

From [11].

Appendix II
MDS definitions for specific recommendations

Efficacy conclusions	Definition	Required evidence
Efficacious	Evidence shows that the intervention has a positive effect on studied outcomes	Supported by data from at least one high-quality (score >75%) RCT without conflicting level I data
Likely efficacious	Evidence suggests, but is not sufficient to show, that the intervention has a positive effect on studied outcomes	Supported by data from any level I trial without conflicting level I data
Unlikely efficacious	Evidence suggests that the intervention does not have a positive effect on studied outcomes	Supported by data from any level I trial without conflicting level I data
Nonefficacious	Evidence shows that the intervention does not have a positive effect on studied outcomes	Supported by data from at least one high-quality (score >75%) RCT without conflicting level I data
Insufficient evidence	There is not enough evidence either for or against efficacy of the intervention in treatment of Parkinson's disease	All the circumstances not covered by the previous statements

Safety

Acceptable risk without specialized monitoring

Acceptable risk, with specialized monitoring

Unacceptable risk

Insufficient evidence to make conclusions on the safety of the intervention

Implications for clinical practice

Clinically useful	For a given situation, evidence available is sufficient to conclude that the intervention provides clinical benefit
Possibly useful	For a given situation, evidence available suggests, but is insufficient to conclude, that the intervention provides clinical benefit
Investigational	Available evidence is insufficient to support the use of the intervention in clinical practice, but further study is warranted
Not useful	For a given situation, available evidence is sufficient to say that the intervention provides no clinical benefit
Efficacy unlikely	Evidence suggests that the intervention does not have a positive effect on studied outcomes. Supported by data from any level I trial without conflicting level I data

Modified from [4] and [15].

Appendix III
Movement Disorders Society – Guidelines 2011

Selegiline	Efficacy	Insufficient evidence	Efficacious	Insufficient evidence	Insufficient evidence (F) Nonefficacious (D)	Insufficient evidence (F, D)
	Safety	Acceptable risk without specialized monitoring				
Practice implications	Investigational	Clinically useful	Investigational	Investigational (F) Not useful (D)	Investigational (F, D)	
Selegiline ODT	Efficacy	Insufficient evidence	Insufficient evidence	Insufficient evidence	Insufficient evidence (F, D)	Insufficient evidence (F, D)
	Safety	Acceptable risk without specialized monitoring				
Practice implications	Investigational	Investigational	Investigational	Investigational (F, D)	Investigational (F, D)	
Rasagiline	Efficacy	Insufficient evidence	Efficacious	Efficacious	Insufficient evidence (F, D)	Efficacious (F) Insufficient evidence (D)
	Safety	Acceptable risk without specialized monitoring				
Practice implications	Investigational	Clinically useful	Clinically useful	Investigational (F, D)	Clinically useful (F) Investigational (D)	

F, PD patients with fluctuations; D, PD patients with dyskinesias.
Modified from [15].

Appendix IV
EFNS/MDS-ES Guidelines 2012 Summary

MAO-B inhibitors		Prevention/delay of clinical progression	Symptomatic monotherapy	Symptomatic adjunct to levodopa	Prevention/delay of motor complications	Treatment of motor complications
Selegiline	Efficacy	Class I and II [26, 30, 31, 52, 53] Postpone need for dopaminergic treatment for several months	Effective level A Class I and II [53, 22] Meta-analysis [34] concluded a small symptomatic effect	No consistent beneficial effect Class I [53–58]	Ineffective level A Class I [59] Class II [29, 60]	No consistent effect on "off" time Class II [62, 63]
Rasagiline	Efficacy	TEMPO study; Class I [11, 12] patients with delayed start of 6 months showed greater worsening on UPDRS-III ADAGIO study, Class I [13] for early versus 9 months delayed start, the primary endpoint was reached for 1 mg – the result is considered compatible with the concept that rasagiline is possibly efficacious for disease modification	Effective level A Class I, [37–39] Showed a modest benefit	No recommendation/insufficient data	No recommendation/insufficient data	No recommendation/insufficient data
Selegiline and rasagiline	Safety	Dopaminergic adverse reactions may occur. The risk of tyramine-induced hypertension ("cheese effect") is low [61]. MAO-B inhibitors carry a small risk of serotonine syndrome, particularly when combined with other serotonergic agents				

Modified from [16].

References

1. Löhle M, Reichmann H. Clinical neuroprotection in Parkinson's disease – still waiting for the breakthrough. *J Neurol Sci* 2010; **289**: 104–14.
2. Löhle M, Reichmann H. Controversies in neurology: why monoamine oxidase B inhibitors could be a good choice for the initial treatment of Parkinson's disease. *BMC Neurol* 2011; **11**: 112.
3. Fabbrini G, Abbruzzese G, Marconi S, Zappia M. Selegiline: a reappraisal of its role in Parkinson disease. *Clinical Neuropharmacol* 2012; **35**: 134–40.
4. Goetz CG, Koller WC, Poewe W. Management of Parkinson's disease: an evidence-based review. *Mov Disord* 2002; **17** (Suppl. 4): S1–166.
5. Goetz CG, Poewe W, Rascol O, Sampaio C. Evidence-based medical review update: pharmacological and surgical treatments of Parkinson's disease: 2001 to 2004. *Mov Disord* 2005; **20**: 523–39.
6. Macleod A, Counsell C, Ives N, Stowe R. Monoamine oxidase B inhibitors for early Parkinson's disease. *Cochrane Database Syst Rev* 2005; **20**: CD004898.
7. National Collaborating Centre for Chronic Conditions. *Parkinson's Disease. National Clinical Guideline for Diagnosis and Management in Primary and Secondary Care. Guidelines for the NHS by NICE.* London: Royal College of Physicians, 2006.
8. Pahwa R, Factor SA, Lyons KE, et al. Practice parameter: treatment of Parkinson disease with motor fluctuations and dyskinesia (an evidence-based review): report of the Quality Standards Subcommittee of the American Academy of Neurology. *Neurology* 2006; **66**: 983–95.
9. Ryton BA, Liddle BJ. Implementing NICE clinical guidelines on Parkinson's disease *Clin Med* 2009; **9**: 436–40.
10. Caslake R, Macleod A, Ives N, Stowe R, Counsell C. Monoamine oxidase B inhibitors versus other dopaminergic agents in early Parkinson's disease. *Cochrane Database Syst Rev* 2009; (4): CD006661.
11. Brainin M, Barnes M, Baron JC, et al. Guidance for the preparation of neurological management guidelines by EFNS scientific task forces – revised recommendations 2004. *Eur J Neurol* 2004, **11**: 577–81.
12. Horstinka ME, Tolosa E, Bonuccelli U, et al. Review of the therapeutic management of Parkinson's disease. Report of a joint task force of the European Federation of Neurological Societies and the Movement Disorder Society–European Section. Part I: early (uncomplicated) Parkinson's disease. *Eur J Neurol* 2006; **13**: 1170–85.
13. Horstinka ME, Tolosa E, Bonuccelli U, et al. Review of the therapeutic management of Parkinson's disease. Report of a joint task force of the European Federation of Neurological Societies and the Movement Disorder Society–European Section. Part II: late(complicated) Parkinson's disease. *Eur J Neurol* 2006; **13**: 1186–202.
14. Leone MA, Brainin M, Boon P, et al. Guidance for the preparation of neurological management guidelines by EFNS scientific task forces – revised recommendations 2012. *Eur J Neurol* 2013; **20**: 410–19.
15. Fox S, Katzenschlager R, Lim SY, et al. The Movement Disorder Society Evidence-Based Medicine Review Update: treatments for the motor symptoms of Parkinson's disease. *Mov Dis* 2011; **26** (Suppl. 3): S2–41.
16. Ferreira JJ, Katzenschlager R, Bloem BR, et al. Summary of the recommendations of the EFNS/MDS-ES review on therapeutic management of Parkinson's disease. *Eur J Neurol* 2013; **20**: 5–15.
17. Knoll J, Vizi ES, Somogyi E. Phenylisopropyl-methylpropinylamine (E-250), a monoamine oxidase inhibitor antagonizing the effect of tyramine. *Drug Res* 1968; **18**: 109–12.
18. Szende B, Bokonyi G, Bocsi J, et al. Anti-apoptotic and apoptotic action of (–)-deprenyl and its metabolites. *J Neural Transm* 2001; **108**: 25–33.
19. Matsubara K, Senda T, Uezono T, et al. L-Deprenyl prevents the cell hypoxia induced by dopaminergic neurotoxins, MPP(+) and β-carbolinium: a microdialysis study in rats. *Neurosci Lett* 2001; **302**: 65–8.
20. Tatton W, Chalmers-Redman R, Tatton N. Neuroprotection by deprenyl and other propargy-lamines: glyceraldehyde-3-phosphate dehydrogenase rather than monoamine oxidase B. *J Neural Transm* 2003; **110**: 509–15.
21. Magyar K, Szende B. (–)-Deprenyl, a selective MAO-B inhibitor, with apoptotic and anti-apoptotic properties. *Neurotoxicology* 2004; **25**: 233–42.
22. Saravanan KS, Sindhu KM, Senthilkumar KS, Mohanakumar KP. L-Deprenyl protects against rotenone-induced, oxidative stress-mediated dopaminergic neurodegeneration in rats. *Neurochem Int* 2006; **49**: 28–40.
23. Birkmayer W, Knoll J, Riederer P, et al. Increased life expectancy resulting from addition of L-deprenyl to Madopar treatment in Parkinson's disease: a longterm study. *J Neural Transm* 1985; **64**: 113–27.
24. Blume E. Street drugs yield primate Parkinson's model. *JAMA* 1983; **250**: 13–14.
25. Langston JW, Ballard PA Jr. Parkinson's disease in a chemist working with 1-methyl-4-phenyl-1,2,5,6-tetrahydropyridine. *N Engl J Med* 1983; **309**: 310.
26. Tetrud JW, Langston JW. The effect of deprenyl (selegiline) on the natural history of Parkinson's disease. *Science* 1989; **245**: 519–22.
27. Myllylä VV, Sotaniemi KA, Aasly J, et al. An open multicenter study of the efficacy of MDL 72,974A,

a monoamine oxidase type B (MAO-B) inhibitor, in Parkinson's disease. *Adv Neurol* 1993; **60**: 676–80.

28. Parkinson Study Group. Effects of tocopherol and deprenyl on the progression and disability in early Parkinson's disease. *N Engl J Med* 1993; **328**: 176–83.

29. Shoulson I, Oakes D, Fahn S, et al. Impact of sustained deprenyl (selegiline) in levodopa-treated Parkinson's disease: a randomized placebo-controlled extension of the deprenyl and tocopherol antioxidative therapy of parkinsonism trial. *Ann Neurol* 2002; **51**: 604–12.

30. Olanow CW, Hauser RA, Gauger L, et al. The effect of deprenyl and levodopa on the progression of Parkinson's disease *Ann Neurol* 1995; **38**: 771–77.

31. Pålhagen S, Heinonen EH, Hägglund J, et al. Selegiline delays the onset of disability in de novo parkinsonian patients. Swedish Parkinson Study Group. *Neurology* 1998; **51**: 520–5.

32. Pålhagen S, Heinonen EH, Hägglund J, et al. Selegiline delays the onset of disability in de novo Parkinsonian patients. Swedish Parkinson Study Group. *Neurology* 1998; **51**: 520–5.

33. Pålhagen SE, Heinonen E. Use of selegiline as monotherapy and in combination with levodopa in the management of Parkinson's disease: perspectives from the MONOCOMB Study. *Prog Neurother Neuropsychopharmacol* 2008; **3**: 49–71.

34. Ives NJ, Stowe RL, Marro J, et al. Monoamine oxidase type B inhibitors in early Parkinson's disease: meta-analysis of 17 randomised trials involving 3525 patients. *BMJ* 2004; **329**: 593.

35. Parkinson Study Group. A randomized placebo controlled trial of rasagiline in levodopa-treated patients with Parkinson disease and motor fluctuations: the PRESTO study. *Arch Neurol* 2005; **62**: 241–8.

36. Rascol O, Brooks DJ, Melamed E, et al. Rasagiline as an adjunct to levodopa in patients with Parkinson's disease and motor fluctuations (LARGO, Lasting effect in Adjunct therapy with Rasagiline Given Once daily, study): a randomized, double-blind, parallel-group trial. *Lancet* 2005; **365**: 947–54.

37. Parkinson Study Group. A controlled trial of rasagiline in early Parkinson disease: the TEMPO Study. *Arch Neurol* 2002; **59**: 1937–43.

38. Parkinson Study Group. A controlled, randomized, delayed-start study of rasagiline in early Parkinson disease. *Arch Neurol* 2004; **61**: 561–6.

39. Olanow CW, Rascol O, Hauser R, et al. A double-blind, delayed-start trial of rasagiline in Parkinson's disease. *N Engl J Med* 2009; **361**: 1268–78.

40. Schapira A, Monoamine oxidase B inhibitors for the treatment of Parkinson's disease: a review of symptomatic and potential disease-modifying effects. *CNS Drugs* 2011; **25**: 1061–71.

41. Ondo WG, Sethi KD, Kricorian G. Selegilime orally disintegrating tablets in patient with Parkinson's disease and "wearing off" symptoms. *Clin Neuropharmacol* 2007; **30**: 295–300.

42. Montastruc JL, Chaumerliac C, Desboeuf K, et al. Adverse drug reactions to selegiline: a review of the French pharmaco vigilance database. *Clin Neuropharmacol* 2000; **23**: 271–5.

43. Lees AJ. Comparison of therapeutic effects and mortality data of levodopa and levodopa combined with selegiline in patients with early, mild Parkinson's disease. Parkinson's Disease Research Group of UK. *BMJ* 1995; **311**: 1602–7.

44. Thorogood M, Armstrong B, Nichols T, Hollowell J. Mortality in people taking selegiline; observational study. *BMJ* 1998; **327**: 252–4.

45. Reichmann H, Jost WH. Efficacy and tolerability of rasagiline in daily clinical use – a post-marketing observational study in patients with Parkinson's disease. *Eur J Neurol* 2010; **17**: 1164–71.

46. Jost W, Friede M, Schnitker J. Indirect meta-analysis of randomised placebo-controlled clinical trials on rasagiline and selegiline in the symptomatic treatment of Parkinson's disease. *Basal Ganglia* 2012; **2**: S17–26.

47. Richard IH, Kurland R, Tanner C, et al. Serotonin syndrome and the combined use of deprenyl and an antidepressant in Parkinson's disease. Parkinson Study Group. *Neurology* 1997; **48**: 1070–7.

48. Connolly BS, Fox SH. Drug treatments for the neuropsychiatric complications of Parkinson's disease. *Expert Rev Neurother* 2012; **12**: 1439–49.

49. Connolly BS, Lang AE. Pharmacological treatment of Parkinson disease. A review. *JAMA* 2014; **311**: 1670–83.

50. Naoi M, Maruyama W, Inaba-Hasegawa K. Revelation in the neuroprotective functions of rasagiline and selegiline: the induction of distinct genes by different mechanisms. *Expert Rev Neurother* 2013; **13**: 671–84.

51. Youdim MB. Multi target neuroprotective and neurorestorative anti-Parkinson and anti-Alzheimer drugs ladostigil and m30 derived from rasagiline. *Exp Neurobiol* 2013; **22**: 1–10.

52. Parkinson Study Group. Effect of deprenyl on the progression of disability in early Parkinson's disease. *N Engl J Med* 1989; **321**: 1364–71.

53. Myllylä VV, Sotaniemi KA, Vuorinen JA, Heinonen EH. Selegiline as initial treatment in de novo parkinsonian patients. *Neurology* 1992; **42**: 339–43.

54. Przuntek H, Kuhn W. The effect of R-(–)-deprenyl in de novo Parkinson patients on combination therapy with levodopa and decarboxylase inhibitor. *J Neural Transm Suppl* 1987; **25**: 97–104.

55. Sivertsen B, Dupont E, Mikkelsen B, *et al.* Selegiline and levodopa in early or moderately advanced Parkinson's disease: a double-blind controlled short- and long-term study. *Acta Neurol Scand Suppl* 1989; **126**: 147–52.

56. Nappi G, Martignoni E, Horowski R, *et al.* Lisuride plus selegiline in the treatment of early Parkinson's disease. *Acta Neurol Scand* 1991; **83**: 407–10.

57. Lees AJ. Comparison of therapeutic effects and mortality data of levodopa and levodopa combined with selegiline in patients with early, mild Parkinson's disease. Parkinson's Disease Research Group of the United Kingdom. *BMJ* 1995; **311**: 1602–7.

58. Larsen JP, Boas J. The effects of early selegiline therapy on long-term levodopa treatment and parkinsonian disability: an interim analysis of a Norwegian–Danish 5-year study. Norwegian–Danish Study Group. *Mov Disord* 1997; **12**: 175–82.

59. Larsen JP, Boas J, Erdal JE. Does selegiline modify the progression of early Parkinson's disease? Results from a five-year study. The Norwegian–Danish Study Group. *Eur J Neurol* 1999; **6**: 539–47.

60. Parkinson's Disease Research Group in the United Kingdom. Comparisons of therapeutic effects of levodopa, levodopa and selegiline, and bromocriptine in patients with early, mild Parkinson's disease: three year interim report. *BMJ* 1993; **307**: 469–72.

61. Heinonen EH, Myllylä V. Safety of selegiline (deprenyl) in the treatment of Parkinson's disease. *Drug Saf* 1998; **19**: 11–22.

62. Lieberman AN, Gopinathan G, Neophytides A, Foo SH. Deprenyl versus placebo in Parkinson disease: a double-blind study. *NY State J Med* 1987; **87**: 646–9.

63. Golbe LI, Lieberman AN, Muenter MD, *et al.* Deprenyl in the treatment of symptom fluctuations in advanced Parkinson's disease. *Clin Neuropharmacol* 1988; **11**: 45–55.

Chapter 5
Oral dopamine agonists in the management of Parkinson's disease

Javier Pagonabarraga, Juan Marín-Lahoz and Jaime Kulisevsky

Introduction and history

In 1960 and 1967, Hornykiewicz and Cotzias opened a new era in the management of neurodegenerative diseases by the demonstration of decreased levels of dopamine in the striatum and the indisputable effects of oral levodopa (L-DOPA) on parkinsonian motor symptoms [1, 2]. Nevertheless, within a few years of the introduction of levodopa, clinicians recognized several problems associated with its continued use. If the chronic use of levodopa was not associated with the development of motor complications – either motor fluctuations or dyskinesias – levodopa would still stand as the drug to use in patients with Parkinson's disease (PD). Other dopaminergic agents most likely would not have been developed, and the progressive impairment of dopamine-dependent PD motor deficits would be well controlled by increasing doses of levodopa. However, as has been well established, PD patients in monotherapy with levodopa develop motor complications after 5–10 years of treatment onset. In community-based studies of patients treated with levodopa, disabling motor complications develop in up to 80% of PD patients after 10 years of disease onset [3].

In fact, levodopa is still the most effective symptomatic treatment of PD. In the early stages of the disease, the response to levodopa is sustained during both the daytime and nighttime, despite its relatively short half-life. Even though more than 50% of neurons in the substantia nigra pars compacta are already lost when parkinsonian motor symptoms emerge, the remaining neurons preserve enough presynaptic nerve terminals so as to store and release for 24 h the available endogenous and exogenous dopamine. As the disease progresses, the beneficial effect of each dose of levodopa progressively shortens, and postsynaptic striatal receptors need to change their conformation and sensitivity to dopamine to maintain the effects of dopamine on dopamine for as long as possible receptors [4, 5]. The combination of pre- and postsynaptic changes progressively leads to more unpredictable motor fluctuations and the development of dyskinesias [4, 6, 7].

To overcome the limitations in the use of levodopa, new drugs with longer pharmacokinetic properties have been explored. Monoamine oxidase B (MAO-B) inhibitors and dopamine agonists (DAs) had longer half-lives and improved motor function in animal models [8, 9]. In addition, since DAs act directly on dopamine receptors, their efficacy was not supposed to be modified by the degenerating dopaminergic cells. Both the MAO-B inhibitor selegiline, and the DA bromocriptine entered into the clinical field, but the higher efficacy of bromocriptine on motor symptoms placed DAs as the drug family to complement levodopa in the management of PD [10, 11].

Compared with levodopa, treatment of parkinsonism with bromocriptine – either alone or in combination – resulted in fewer fluctuations and peak-dose dyskinesias after 3–5 years of treatment [11, 12]. Monotherapy with bromocriptine appeared to be a less effective stimulant than levodopa, but in combination achieved similar therapeutic responses with fewer motor complications [13, 14].

It is worth noting that psychiatric complications have appeared as a limiting factor in DA use since the first clinical trials. Hallucinations, anxiety, psychomotor agitation and vivid dreams were related to the administration of high doses and bromocriptine and lisuride [12, 15]. These complications were related to dose effects and were controlled by adjusting effective therapeutic ranges, but they stress the specific effects that DAs have on limbic structures, and the deleterious complications this may entail.

After bromocriptine, newer ergot-derived DAs emerged. Pergolide was an extremely potent and effective DA, and cabergoline, due to its long half-life, stood as a very good drug to deliver continuous dopaminergic stimulation. However, restrictive valvular heart disease and serositis appeared as adverse events common to all ergot-derived DAs, so that changing to a nonergot DA was advised [16, 17]. The nonergot-derived pramipexole and ropinirole have since been the most commonly used oral DAs, having proven to be beneficial to patients at all stages of the disease. Piribedil is also used in some countries, and rotigotine, a DA delivered through a silicone-based transdermal patch that is administered once daily, provides a stable drug release throughout the 24 h patch application [18].

During the last decade, the growing description of impulse control disorders (ICDs) in PD associated with the use of DAs [19, 20] – at both low and high doses – may alert physicians to remain cautious in their use, trying to select which patients may benefit.

In this chapter, we will review the evidence of the effectiveness and safety of pramipexole, ropinirole, piribedil and rotigotine in the management of PD.

Rationale for the use of dopamine agonists in Parkinson's disease

The National Institute for Health and Clinical Excellence (NICE) guidelines stated in 2011 that "there is no single drug choice for the initial pharmacotherapy of early PD" [21]. In the evidence-based reviews of the American Academy of Neurology, DAs have enough evidence to consider their use in both the symptomatic treatment of patients with early PD [22] and for the prevention and management of motor complications [23]. In addition, due to the higher risk of motor complications and the greater expectation of life of younger patients, there is a strong argument for using DAs as first-line therapy in patients younger than 60 years.

In the elderly patient, the use of DAs is not contraindicated but a balance between efficacy and adverse events must be taken into account. As indicated before, the description of ICDs in younger patients must be now carefully considered, and the relevant information given to patients when DAs are indicated. Nevertheless, the fact that DAs are currently one of the most relevant drug families in the management of PD is because they have given clear evidence in favor of delaying and even decreasing the prevalence of motor complications, as reported when levodopa was used in monotherapy [3].

The longer half-lives of available DAs seems almost certainly the reason why motor fluctuations and dyskinesias are less prevalent. Beyond age and genetic factors, the more continuous dopaminergic stimulation a drug may achieve seems a major variable for preventing motor fluctuations [24]. Levodopa-related motor complications in PD are associated with nonphysiological, discontinuous or pulsatile stimulation of striatal dopamine receptors, and can be prevented or reversed by long-acting dopaminergic drugs, such as DAs, that provide more continuous stimulation of striatal dopamine receptors.

That the long life of available DAs is crucial for the prevention of motor complications was reinforced by studies using experimental DAs with short half-lives. The use in animal models of intermittent injections of the short-acting DAs, such as apomorphine or U-91356A, rapidly induced dyskinesias, whereas continuous infusion of the same drug did not. Thus, the same drug may or may not induce motor complications depending only on its pharmacokinetic properties [25, 26].

Laboratory findings could be transferred to clinical studies. In patients with early PD, prospective double-blinded, controlled trials have shown that patients randomized to initiate therapy with long-acting DAs had a lower risk of developing motor complications in comparison with patients initiating treatment with levodopa. Initial pramipexole treatment resulted in significantly less development of wearing off, dyskinesias, or "on–off" motor fluctuations (28%) compared with levodopa (51%) after a follow-up of 2 years [27]. Using ropinirole, Rascol et al. [28] found that the cumulative incidence of dyskinesias after 5 years of treatment onset was significantly lower in the ropinirole group (20%) compared with levodopa (45%), and Whone et al. [29] obtained similar results after a follow-up of only 2 years, with significantly fewer patients in the ropinirole group (3.4%) developing dyskinesias compared with the levodopa group (26.75%).

Compelling data have recently come from prospective studies of patients who initiated treatment with bromocriptine 14 years ago. Whereas the majority of the patients were on combined treatment with bromocriptine and levodopa after 3–5 years of follow-up, the protective effects of bromocriptine for preventing the development of motor complications as a result of having initiated treatment with a DA were maintained for up to 10 years [30]. Even more interestingly, the prevalence of both disabling motor fluctuations and dyskinesias after 14 years of follow-up was much lower than that registered in previous historical community-based studies [3]. In the study by Schrag et al. [3] – in which nearly all patients had initiated treatment with levodopa – motor fluctuations and dyskinesias were present in 63 and 53% of PD patients with more than 10 years of disease evolution. In comparison, only 35% developed either motor fluctuations or dyskinesias in the 14-year study [30]. One possible reason for this important and clinically relevant difference is that in clinical series of patients following treatment with both levodopa and DAs, the total daily requirements of levodopa after 10–15 years of disease are significantly lower, which would protect patients from the uncontrolled oscillations in striatal and synaptic dopamine concentrations provoked by the pulsatile stimulation of the short-acting exogenous levodopa.

Pharmacology

Pharmacodynamics: dopamine receptors

Pharmacodynamics is the study of the effects of drugs in the body at any level. Understanding the effects of DAs requires a basic knowledge of dopamine receptors (Table 5.1). There are two classes of dopamine receptors: D1 (constituted by D1 and D5 subtypes) and D2 (constituted by D2, D3 and D4 subtypes). D1 class receptors are coupled to a Gs protein, which activates adenylyl cyclase mediating an excitatory response in the postsynaptic neuron. D2 class receptors are coupled to a Gi protein, which inhibits adenylyl cyclase leading to inhibition in the postsynaptic neuron. The D1 and D2 subtypes are located in the striatum forming the nigrostriatal pathway. D1 mainly excites the direct pathway, while D2 inhibits the indirect pathway. This implies that activating any of these receptors can relieve bradykinesia caused by dopaminergic depletion [31]. D2 also has a major role in the tuberoinfundibular pathway inhibiting prolactin release and in the area postrema leading to nausea and vomiting. This effect can be blocked without affecting other central D2 effects, with antidopaminergics unable to cross the blood–brain barrier as the area postrema is located outside of it [32].

In the peripheral nervous system, the D1 main effects are vasodilatation and natriuresis leading to hypotension, while D2 decreases noradrenaline release, indirectly lowering blood pressure. This peripheral side effect could also be related to peripheral edema, and a clinical trial was designed to avoid this with domperidone, but the study was terminated due the lack of recruitment [33].

D3, D4 and D5 act mainly in the mesolimbic and mesocortical pathways. D3 is the best studied and has been implied in addiction, psychosis and depression. D4 is mostly known for its implication in attention-deficit hyperactivity disorder and novelty-seeking traits [34]. D5 is distributed mainly in the prefrontal cortex. Its effects are less well known because no selective agonists are known; therefore, studies of dopamine effects on the prefrontal cortex usually do not differentiate between the D1 and D5 subtypes.

Aside from these five subtypes, heteromeric D1/D2 receptors are known in rodents. Interestingly, their main effect differs from both subtypes, as they are coupled to Gq proteins, which increase intracellular Ca^{2+} concentration [35]. D2 receptors are expressed in two forms: high affinity and low affinity. An increase in high-affinity D2 receptors has been shown in animal models of several disorders with dopamine hypersensitivity. Nevertheless, there have been no clinical studies yet [36]. Probably there are more forms of dopamine receptors (either heteromeric or produced by alternative splicing) and these discoveries may have potential implications for new DAs or even for choosing better among the current ones.

Each DA has a different affinity for each dopamine receptor, but it should be noted that ligands for D1 also

Table 5.1 Affinities of dopamine agonists to various receptors

	D1	D2	D3	D4	D5	α2	Other
Piribedil	0	++	+++	–	?	–	0
Pramipexole	0	+++	+++	++	0	+/–	0
Ropinirole	0	+++	+++	0	0	+/–	+/–5HT2
Rotigotine	+	++	+++	++	++	–	5HT1a*

+, Agonist; –, antagonist; +/–, very low affinity; 0, no affinity; ?, unknown; *, partial agonist.

have a high affinity for D5 and, in general, ligands for D2 also join D3 and D4. Nowadays, all DAs indicated for PD have D2 agonist activity varying in the degree to which they activate D1 and D3. No D1 selective agonist is in use for PD because of low bioavailability and a strong hypotensive effect, although they have proven antiparkinsonian effects in nonhuman primate models [37].

Pharmacokinetics

Pharmacokinetics is the study of the processes undergone by a drug from its administration to its complete elimination from the body. Pramipexole, ropinirole and piribedil are rapidly absorbed after oral administration reaching peak plasma concentration in 1–2 h (Table 5.2). Food delays cause peak plasma concentrations but do not affect the extent of absorption. Rotigotine is administered transdermally.

Rotigotine and ropinirole have a half-life of 5–7 h. Piribedil has a half-life of 1.7 to 6.7 h and that of pramipexole is about 8–12 h. Cabergoline and pergolide have much longer half-lives, which allow a single daily dose, but all nonergoline DAs need to be taken several times per day. Modified-release formulations are available for all of the nonergoline agonist, also allowing a single dose, except in the case of piribedil, which still needs to be taken three to five times per day.

It should be noted that, in advanced fluctuating PD, motor control is sometimes improved by splitting the dose of an extended-release agonist taken four times daily into two separated extended-release doses. This has been studied for ropinirole [38] but may apply to other extended-release agonists (author's observation).

Ropinirole, piribedil and rotigotine are metabolized in the liver, while pramipexole is excreted intact.

Rotigotine plasma protein binding is high, potentially leading to protein displacement interactions. Ropinirole binding is intermediate, while pramipexole and piribedil binding are lower. Dopamine agonists are usually titrated for several weeks, although their half-life is much shorter. Therefore, the time needed to reach a steady state depends mainly on the length of the titration period.

Dopamine agonists most commonly used in daily practice

Details of the levodopa-equivalent doses and therapeutic ranges for the DAs most commonly used in daily practice are given in Table 5.3.

Pramipexole

Mechanism of action

The nonergot DA pramipexole was approved for the treatment of PD in 1997 in the US and in 1998 in most European countries. Pramipexole acts as a potent agonist at D2 (K_i = 3.9 nM), D3 (K_i = 0.5 nM) and D4 (K_i = 5.1 nM) dopamine receptors, but has negligible affinity (>10,000 nM) for D1 and D5 receptors. Unlike the ergot DA, pramipexole has little or no interaction with adrenergic or serotonergic receptors [39]. The preferential affinity of pramipexole for the D3 receptor subtype has been (i) claimed to contribute to the efficacy of the drug for the treatment of affective disorders in PD; (ii) the base for exploring the efficacy of pramipexole in the treatment of primary major depression; and (iii) also advocated as one of the main sites responsible for the development of ICDs in patients with PD [20] or restless legs syndrome [40].

Pramipexole shows linear pharmacokinetics. It is rapidly and completely absorbed, with peak concentrations appearing in the bloodstream within 2 h of oral administration. It can be administered without regard to meals, and excretion is primarily renal. Of particular interest, pramipexole is not appreciably metabolized by the cytochrome P450 system, which minimizes drug–drug interactions in elderly populations [43].

Table 5.2 Pharmacokinetics of dopamine agonists

Drug	Bioavailability	Protein binding	Half-life	Metabolism	Excretion
Piribedil	Low	Low	1.7–6.9 h	Hepatic	Renal 68%, fecal 25%
Pramipexole	>90%	15%	8–12 h	None	Urine 90%, fecal 2%
Ropinirole	50%	40%	5–6 h	Hepatic (CYP1A2)	Renal
Rotigotine	37% transdermal	92%	5–7 h	Hepatic (several CYP)	Urine 71%, fecal 23%

Table 5.3 Levodopa-equivalent doses and therapeutic range

Drug	Dose for 100 mg levodopa	Conversion factor	Therapeutic range
Levodopa	100	×1	150–1200 mg
Bromocriptine	10	×10	20–60 mg
Pergolide	1	×100	3–8 mg
Piribedil	60–100	×1–1.67	150–250 mg
Pramipexole	0.7	×140	0.7–4.5 mg
Ropinirole	6	×17	8–24 mg
Rotigotine	3.3–4.5	×22–30	6–16 mg

Drug (mg) × conversion factor = levodopa-equivalent dose. Levodopa dosing is always considered in conjunction with a DOPA decarboxylase (carbidopa or benserazide) [41, 42].

Efficacy on motor symptoms

Clinical trials of pramipexole have included over 1200 patients, with 700 patients receiving pramipexole for up to 4 years, with doses ranging from 0.375 to 4.5 mg/day. As sustained by evidence, pramipexole can be used to improve motor impairments and disability in early PD patients, to reduce dyskinesias and total daily levodopa dose in advanced patients, and to reduce "off" time in patients with wearing off. These conclusions are based on short- and medium-term trials (up to 24 weeks) [44].

In early and fluctuating PD patients, treatment onset with pramipexole treatment has been shown to improve both the Unified Parkinson's Disease Rating Scale (UPDRS) II (daily disability) and UPDRS-III (motor severity) sum scores by 30%, and to decrease "off" times by approximately 2.5 h/day. Differences between groups are achieved, since daily doses of 0.75 mg/day of pramipexole, but increasing doses up to 4 mg/day are accompanied by further amelioration of symptoms [45]. In advanced patients, pramipexole not only improved fluctuations but has also proven to reduce the severity of motor dysfunction (UPDRS-III) during "off" periods [46].

The CALM-PD (Comparison of the Agonist Pramipexole versus Levodopa on Motor complications of Parkinson's Disease) trial explored the potential benefits of pramipexole for preventing the development of motor complications after a follow-up of 4 years. Patients could start treatment with either pramipexole 0.5 mg three times daily or levodopa 100 mg three times daily, and during the follow-up, levodopa supplementation was permitted, as required. Time to the first occurrence of dopaminergic complications (wearing off, dyskinesias, "on–off" or freezing) was determined. After 2 years, the prevalence of motor complications was significantly lower in patients with initial pramipexole treatment compared with the levodopa group (28 vs 51%; hazards ratio = 0.45; $P < 0.001$), and these benefits were maintained at 4 years (52 vs 74%; hazards ratio = 0.48; $P < 0.001$). The results at 6 years were also published, with PD patients who started treatment with pramipexole still showing both less wearing off (44.4 vs 58.8%; $P = 0.01$) and fewer dyskinesias (20.4 vs 36.8%; $P = 0.004$) [47]. Interestingly, the UPDRS total and motor scores, and scores on disability (Schwab and England scores) and Parkinson's Disease Quality of Life (PDQUALIF) scales did not differ significantly.

In patients with advanced PD and motor fluctuations, pramipexole has a proven efficacy for (i) improving 30–40% UPDRS total and motor scores when compared with placebo; (ii) decreasing levodopa daily doses in up to 30% of patients; and (iii) reducing daily "off" times in 30% of patients [45, 46]. In particular, when compared with entacapone, pramipexole was found to be significantly more efficacious for both improving UPDRS scores and for diminishing daily "off" times [48].

In terms of neuroprotection, study designs based on dopamine transporter imaging with single-photon-emission computed tomography (DAT-SPECT) reuptake changes have not been conclusive (CALM-PD trial) [49]. Following the methodology of a randomized, double-blind, placebo-controlled, delayed-start trial – as had been used previously to disclose the potential neuroprotective benefits of rasagiline – the PROUD (Pramipexole On Underlying Disease) study did not find pramipexole to delay the progression of motor symptoms in early PD patients treated for 6–9 months [50, 51]. As a result, it remains an open question as to whether pramipexole may confer additional neuroprotective effects.

Efficacy on nonmotor symptoms

The affinity of pramipexole on D3 dopamine receptors was used first in psychiatry to explore whether this drug might have antidepressant properties in monotherapy or as an add-on treatment in patients with primary major depression [52].

In PD patients, observational and open-label studies in which pramipexole has been used as an add-on therapy to levodopa have consistently shown significant improvements in depressive scales [53, 54]. In addition, in a double-blind, placebo-controlled study, pramipexole was shown to improve depressive symptoms through a direct antidepressant effect, independent from motor symptoms alleviation [55]. In a comparative study of pramipexole versus sertraline, both drugs achieved significant improvements in depressive symptoms, but in the pramipexole group, the proportion of patients with remission from depression was significantly higher [56]. Pramipexole has also achieved improvements in studies using specific scales for anhedonia [57]. In contrast, due to the lack of use of specific scales, the effects of pramipexole on apathy are still inconclusive. However, as assessed by the motivational items in the UPDRS-I and the Non-Motor Symptoms Scale (NMSS), pramipexole clearly improved apathy [53]. It must be noted that none of the studies that analyzed the antidepressant effect of pramipexole used scales to measure depression and apathy separately [55], making it difficult to determine whether pramipexole improved sadness and negativity, or whether changes in depression scales were more related to the alleviation of loss of interest and blunted affect [58, 59].

Regarding cognition, no studies have assessed the issue properly, but no changes were observed in the long follow-up of the CALM-PD trial.

Ropinirole

Mechanism of action

Ropinirole is a D2 and D3 agonist with no effect on D1, D4 and D5 subtypes. It has no affinity for other receptor families. Ropinirole immediate release is absorbed quickly, reaching peak plasma concentrations in 1–2 h. It has a half-life of 5.5 h, requiring three immediate-release doses per day. Modified-release presentations are commercialized, allowing one only dose per day. Nevertheless, a study has shown improvement in wearing-off control by splitting the dose into two extended-release pills, at least according to patients' impression [38]. Bioavailability is 50% in both cases, and transition from immediate release to extended release is performed easily overnight (just add up the daily dose of immediate release and substitute with the extended-release formulation with the closest dose).

Hepatic CYP1A2 is the major P450 enzyme metabolizing ropinirole. Therefore, the drug interacts with CYP1A2 inhibitors (including but not limited to fluoroquinolones, fluvoxamine, verapamil, caffeine and grapefruit) and inducers (including but not limited to omeprazole, tobacco, broccoli and modafinil) [60]. It is usually titrated up to 8 mg/day (or 9 mg in three divided doses) over 8 weeks. The maximum dosage is 24 mg/day.

Efficacy on motor symptoms

Ropinirole appeared superior to placebo in a double-blinded trial on early PD. Patients in the active group had better motor scores and fewer required levodopa during the 6-month treatment. It has also been proven to delay motor complications in a 5-year follow-up [28] and to prevent changes in postsynaptic availability of D2 receptors on positron emission tomography (PET) studies [29].

Ropinirole was also studied in PD with motor fluctuations for the reduction of levodopa dose and duration of "off" periods. Both were lowered in active and control groups, but the reductions were greater in patients treated with ropinirole [61].

Efficacy on nonmotor symptoms

In an open-label study, ropinirole was shown to relieve depression and anxiety in PD patients suffering motor complications, but no improvement was observed in patients without motor complications [62].

Ropinirole side effects are similar to other nonergoline DAs. Meta-analysis of clinical trials [63] has shown fewer cognitive adverse effects than other agonists, while another meta-analysis showed a higher risk for nausea, dizziness and somnolence than pramipexole although fewer hallucinations and less confusion (although the results were not significant) [64]. An indirect comparison in early PD against pramipexole showed more gastrointestinal and fewer cognitive adverse effects [63]. Nevertheless, the frequency of ICDs is similar to other DAs [20].

Rotigotine

Mechanism of action

A rotigotine transdermal patch was approved by the regulatory authorities for use in all stages of PD in 2007, at doses of 2–8 mg/day in early PD or 4–16 mg/day in advanced patients. After some problems with crystal formation in the patches, they were reformulated and reintroduced in 2012.

Rotigotine is analogous to 7-OH-DPAT and UH-232, all three of which are aminotetralin derivatives. These compounds are similar in structure to dopamine, likely underlying their pharmacology. Rotigotine has agonistic activity on all dopamine-receptor subtypes (D1–D5), but demonstrates its highest affinity for the D3 receptor ($K_i = 0.71$ nM), and acts as a potent agonist at D4 ($K_i = 3.9$ nM), D5 ($K_i = 5.4$ nM) and D2 ($K_i = 13.5$ nM); affinity for D1 receptors is lower ($K_i = 83$ nM). Rotigotine also possesses antagonistic activities at the α2-adrenergic receptor, and is a partial agonist at the serotonin 5-HT1A receptor [65].

In 70 patients with early PD who were treated with rotigotine at up to 18 mg/day, mean plasma concentrations decreased slightly after application of a new patch but concentrations remained similar independent of the application site, and stable drug blood levels were stable over a 24-h period. Rotigotine's pharmacokinetics are dose proportional and are not affected by renal impairment, and because of the transdermal administration route, food and/or gastrointestinal conditions do not influence the pharmacokinetics of the drug. The majority of the rotigotine dose is excreted in the urine (71%), with approximately 23% excreted in the feces [66].

Efficacy on motor symptoms

Published clinical studies with rotigotine include three large-scale phase III studies in early PD, two large-scale phase III studies in advanced PD, and five smaller phase 2 trials in early and advanced PD [66].

In the first open-label uncontrolled dose-escalation study of rotigotine monotherapy in early PD, patients received rotigotine to a maximum dose of 18 mg/day, which resulted in significant improvement of motor function (-4.62 ± 5 points on UPDRS-III; $P < 0.0001$) and functional disability (-2.76 ± 3 points on UPDRS-II; $P = 0.0001$) [67].

Three double-blind, placebo-controlled studies were then carried out. In early PD, significant improvements were observed from doses of 2 mg/day, reaching a response plateau at 8 mg in 24 h. One of these studies compared the efficacy of rotigotine with ropinirole over a 37-week period, showing a similar rate of responders for rotigotine ≤8 mg/day (52%) and ropinirole ≤24 mg/day (68%), and noninferiority to ropinirole, with UPDRS-II + -III mean decrease of −7.2 versus −11.0 points. It must be noted that the mean dose of ropinirole used in this trial was unusually high compared with other published clinical trials, and when post-hoc analysis compared rotigotine 8 mg with ropinirole 12 mg, the improvement in UPDRS-III was more similar (−7.2 versus −7.6) [68].

In large double-blinded controlled studies in advanced PD patients, rotigotine 8–12 mg/day significantly improved the UPDRS-II score by 2.7–3.5 points and UPDRS-III by 5.3–5.9 points, as well as the quality of life as assessed by the 39-Item Parkinson's Disease Questionnaire (PDQ-39) [69, 70]. In PD patients with motor complications, the CLEOPATRA-PD (Clinical Efficacy of Pramipexole and Transdermal Rotigotine in Advanced PD) study showed noninferiority of rotigotine (13 mg/day) against pramipexole (3.1 mg/day), with similar improvements in motor and disability scales, and significant reductions in daily "off" time, achieving responder rates (≥30% reduction in "off" time) of 60% for rotigotine and 67% for the pramipexole group [70].

In the double-blind, placebo-controlled RECOVER (Randomized Evaluation of the 24-Hour Coverage: Efficacy of Rotigotine) study, early-morning motor function was assessed by the UPDRS-III before a new dose of rotigotine was administered. At the end of the maintenance period, rotigotine significantly improved the UPDRS-III score by 7 points, with parallel improvements in quality-of-life scales [71].

Efficacy of nonmotor symptoms

The RECOVER study also assessed important nonmotor aspects of PD. The PD Sleep Scale (PDSS-2), NMSS and the Beck Depression Inventory (BDI) were administered to explore potential significant benefits compared with placebo. The NMSS represents a set of 30 questions about the severity and frequency of nonmotor symptoms in several domains. A greater and significant improvement was seen in NMSS total scores in the rotigotine group ($P = 0.015$). These results were evaluated in more detail in a post-hoc analysis, which concluded that total score NMSS changes were explained mainly by the significant amelioration of specific items assessing the degree of sleep, fatigue, sadness, anhedonia, and loss of interest in surroundings or in doing things [72]. The significant improvement in global sleep quality measured by the PDSS-2 was observed to cover different sleep disturbances, with significant and more specific changes in restless legs-like symptoms, motor nocturnal disability (uncomfortable and immobile postures, muscle cramps, pain in arms and legs, breathing problems) and early-morning parkinsonism (waking tremor and painful posturing). Mood changes were reinforced by the parallel improvement observed in BDI total scores ($P = 0.01$) [71, 73]. Rotigotine's effects on cognitive impairment have not been assessed yet in this or other studies.

Piribedil

Mechanism of action

Piribedil is the oldest nonergoline dopamine agonist still in use. It was introduced in the 1970s and, in addition to PD, it was approved in some countries for moderate cognitive impairment not constituting dementia, peripheral vasculopathies and retinal. Currently, it is still in use for PD, both in monotherapy and as adjunctive therapy. It activates D2 and D3 receptors and also inhibits α2 receptors.

Piribedil is absorbed rapidly after oral administration. It has the shortest half-life among the oral DAs requiring several doses per day, even for the extended-release formulation. In monotherapy, its titration is performed by increasing a 50 mg extended-release pill weekly. The common therapeutic range is 150–250 mg/day. When supplementing levodopa, 20 mg of piribedil is given per 100 mg of levodopa and the common range is 80–140 mg/day. Piribedil is metabolized in the liver, although the exact pathway is unknown. It is excreted in both bile and urine [74, 75].

Efficacy of motor symptoms

Clinical trials have proven motor improvement against placebo and the ability to delay levodopa use. Piribedil has been proven to be useful in combination with levodopa, as it diminishes wearing off and levodopa-induced dyskinesias. It is also available as an injectable formulation (not bioequivalent to the oral formulation).

Piribedil was compared with bromocriptine in a double-blinded study for motor scores and cognitive performance. There were no significant differences.

However, there are no direct comparisons against nonergoline DAs. An indirect comparison considered it better because of its usefulness in every state of PD and because its titration is faster than other DAs (3–7 weeks) [76]. Nevertheless, it should be noted that, even using a retard formulation, three to five doses need to be taken per day.

Efficacy of nonmotor symptoms

Piribedil has shown antidepressant activity in both PD and non-PD patients [77–79] and improvement of apathy after deep-brain stimulation in PD patients [79]. Alpha2 antagonism has been related in the case of other drugs with the appearance of rapid eye movement (REM) sleep behavior disorder [80]. Piribedil decreases REM sleep and increases its latency [81].

Aside from its effects on REM sleep, piribedil side effects are comparable to nonergoline DAs. It may cause hallucinations, psychosis, excessive daytime sleepiness, sleep attacks, hypotension, vomiting and impulse control disorders. Its action on α receptors could lower hypotensive effect, but clinical data is lacking. It could also diminish sleepiness, and consequently this side effect is less reported with piribedil than with other DAs [76].

Adverse events

Systemic and neuropsychiatric clinically relevant adverse events have been consistently reported during the past 20 years. For every adverse event, it has been an effort to determine whether it was related to a particular DA, or whether it was a class effect of DAs.

As has been mentioned above, serositis (pleuritis, pericarditis) and restrictive valvular heart disease are adverse events related to the use of ergot-derived DAs (bromocriptine, pergolide, cabergoline and lisuride) [16, 17, 82].

Apart from this systemic complication, common adverse events for all DAs include sleep disturbances, gastrointestinal symptoms (nausea, constipation), orthostatic hypotension, peripheral (pedal) edema, an increase in body weight, psychosis (hallucinations and delusions) and ICDs [64].

Increased excessive daytime somnolence and the development of attacks of sudden onset of sleep were initially attributed to PD patients on treatment with pramipexole [83]. These authors described the appearance of sudden, irresistible attacks of sleep while patients were driving, causing accidents. In this first description, eight patients were taking pramipexole and one ropinirole, five experienced no warning before falling asleep, and the attacks ceased when the drugs were stopped. The presence of sleep attacks was seen to be intimately associated with increased daytime somnolence, as assessed by the Epworth Sleepiness Scale (ESS). When it has been evaluated prospectively in open-label extension studies, 55% of patients receiving pramipexole reported somnolence as an adverse event, 20% reported falling asleep while driving, and 5% had had minor motor vehicle accidents [84]. In subsequent studies, however, it has been shown that the risk of daytime somnolence and sleep attacks is not specific for pramipexole users but is present at the same prevalence and severity in patients taking other DAs [85–87]. Happe et al. [88] replicated these findings, and found that sedation in PD may be a class effect of DAs, with no difference between ergot and nonergot DAs. In conclusion, the available evidence shows that somnolence, while being part of PD itself, can be induced by all dopaminergic drugs – DAs as well as levodopa itself.

Pedal and peripheral edemas were also initially related to pramipexole [89]. Further research, however, has found that lower-limb edemas are common to all DAs (with similar frequency and severity), and are actually more related to some comorbidities, such as a history of smoking, a history of coronary artery disease and a history of diabetes mellitus. No relationship between the dose of pramipexole or ropinirole and the incidence or severity of pedal edema has been seen, whereas a more rapid development of edema is related to a history of coronary artery disease. In all cases, peripheral edema is rapidly abated with discontinuation of therapy, and in all cases it rapidly returns if the DA is challenged again [89, 90].

Orthostatic hypotension is common to all DAs. Although levodopa is also associated with a higher frequency of hypotension, both the frequency and severity of decrease in blood pressure, and symptoms of postural hypotension (dizziness, light-headedness, nausea, headache or "coat hanger" pain) are higher in patients taking DAs [91, 92]. No adequate comparative study has been performed, but the description for each DA is very similar [92, 93].

Since the introduction of DAs, psychosis has been observed as an adverse event common to all of them. Given its reversibility, and the high impact that psychosis may have on quality of life, awareness of this cause-and-effect relationship is crucial for patient management. Although some meta-analyses have found a higher frequency of psychosis for pramipexole users [64, 94], when studies are compared in terms of age, disease duration and concomitant dopaminergic treatments, all DAs seem to predispose to psychosis at the same level [95, 96]. In particular, retrospective clinicopathological studies have shown that other factors – as has been shown for the occurrence of peripheral edema – are major contributors to the development of hallucinations in PD [97, 98]. The development of hallucinations and delusions is also considered part of PD itself, independently associated with age and the degree of cognitive dysfunction, depression and axial rigidity. When controlled for all these factors, the dopaminergic drugs that have been found to impose a higher risk of psychosis are selegiline and DAs [97].

Since the first description in 2000, the number of described ICDs has been growing exponentially, confirming their relationship to DAs, and clearly establishing this adverse event as maybe the most severe and disabling complication that DAs may cause. After their description in PD, ICDs have been also described in relevant frequencies in non-PD populations (restless legs syndrome, prolactinoma, fibromyalgia [40, 99–101]), indicating that this side effect is not only a class effect of DAs but that a personal predisposition also plays a role. Among the risk factors that have been found to predispose to ICDs are: younger age, better cognitive functioning, current smoking, family or personal history of gambling, personal history or current depression, and being single [19, 20]. The use of DAs, however, is the principal responsible for ICDs in PD.

It is worth of noting that two follow-up studies performed in different countries (USA and Spain) found very similar data on the evolution of ICDs after the withdrawal of the offending drug [102, 103]. After a follow-up of 1 and 2.5 years, both studies found that, in those patients in whom the DA could be totally withdrawn, the ICDs remitted completely. There was 17–20% of patients, however, who did not tolerate the absence of the DA. In this group of patients (where DA doses were lowered and levodopa was optimized), 14 and 17% of patients still manifested addictive behaviors [102, 103]. In addition, in a clinical series of six Canadian patients who had developed pathological gambling, although they initially stopped playing when the DA was withdrawn, after a follow-up of 2 years, four out of the six patients had resumed playing, even though these patients were only on levodopa or on minimal doses of the DA [104]. In a double-blind, within-subject study using functional MRI in healthy subjects, pramipexole increased the activity of the nucleus accumbens (NAcc), and enhanced the interaction between the NAcc and the anterior insula, weakening the interaction between the NAcc and the prefrontal cortex [105]. These findings indicate that, although ICDs are reversible in many patients, plastic changes induced by DAs in the neural network of reward anticipation may remain in some subjects [105].

In addition, changes in reward networks are also supposed to be responsible for apathetic or symptoms similar to addictive drug withdrawal observed after stopping treatment with DAs. In a structured longitudinal study of PD patients withdrawing from DAs, 15.5% developed anxiety, panic attacks, dysphoria, depression, agitation, irritability, suicidal ideation and drug cravings [106, 107]. This collection of symptoms is called DA withdrawal syndorme (DAWS). The main risk factor for the appearance of DAWS is the development of ICDs during DA treatment, and it has recently been observed that, while in some patients DAWS is transient, others have a protracted withdrawal syndrome lasting months to years. In this scenario, patients are unable to discontinue DA therapy, and ICDs reappear. As a result, patients who are unable to discontinue DA therapy may experience chronic ICDs [108, 109].

Thus, the potential development of ICDs when DAs are initiated stands today as a major adverse event to be considered in any single patient.

Conclusions

The ability of DAs to decrease and delay the appearance of motor complications – either motor fluctuations or dyskinesias – in comparison with patients treated with levodopa in monotherapy has established their generalized use for the management of motor symptoms in PD. They still are in every algorithm for the pharmacological treatment of PD, even though psychiatric complications related to their use are currently known not only to have a potential great impact on quality of life but also to be irreversible in some instances. It is possible that the delineation of risk factors for the development of ICDs may change current considerations for choosing a DA as a proper agent to treat motor symptoms in PD.

References

1. Hornykiewicz OD. Physiologic, biochemical, and pathological backgrounds of levodopa and possibilities for the future. *Neurology* 1970; **20** (Suppl.): 1–5.
2. Cotzias GC, Van Woert MH, Schiffer LM. Aromatic amino acids and modification of parkinsonism. *N Engl J Med* 1967; **276**: 374–9.
3. Schrag A, Quinn N. Dyskinesias and motor fluctuations in Parkinson's disease. A community-based study. *Brain* 2000; **123**: 2297–305.
4. Fabbrini G, Brotchie JM, Grandas F, Nomoto M, Goetz CG. Levodopa-induced dyskinesias. *Mov Disord* 2007; **22**: 1379–89; quiz 1523.
5. Linazasoro G. Pathophysiology of motor complications in Parkinson disease: postsynaptic mechanisms are crucial. *Arch Neurol* 2007; **64**: 137–40.
6. Nandhagopal R, Kuramoto L, Schulzer M, et al. Longitudinal evolution of compensatory changes in striatal dopamine processing in Parkinson's disease. *Brain* 2011; **134**: 3290–8.
7. de la Fuente-fernández R, Schulzer M, Mak E, Calne DB, Stoessl AJ. Presynaptic mechanisms of motor fluctuations in Parkinson's disease: a probabilistic model. *Brain* 2004; **127**: 888–99.
8. Hall TR, Figueroa HR, Yurgens PB. Effects of inhibitors on monoamine oxidase activity in mouse brain. *Pharmacol Res Commun* 1982; **14**: 443–53.
9. Dolphin AC, Jenner P, Sawaya MC, Marsden CD, Testa B. The effect of bromocriptine on locomotor activity and cerebral catecholamines in rodents. *J Pharm Pharmacol* 1977; **29**: 727–34.
10. Birkmayer W. Long term treatment with L-deprenyl. *J Neural Transm* 1978; **43**: 239–44.
11. Lees AJ, Stern GM. Sustained bromocriptine therapy in previously untreated patients with Parkinson's disease. *J Neurol Neurosurg Psychiatry* 1981; **44**: 1020–3.
12. Parkes JD, Debono AG, Marsden CD. Bromocriptine in Parkinsonism: long-term treatment, dose response, and comparison with levodopa. *J Neurol Neurosurg Psychiatry* 1976; **39**: 1101–8.
13. Montastruc JL, Rascol O, Senard JM, Rascol A. A randomised controlled study comparing bromocriptine to which levodopa was later added, with levodopa alone in previously untreated patients with Parkinson's disease: a five year follow up. *J Neurol Neurosurg Psychiatry* 1994; **57**: 1034–8.
14. Rinne UK. Early combination of bromocriptine and levodopa in the treatment of Parkinson's disease: a 5-year follow-up. *Neurology* 1987; **37**: 826–8.
15. Schachter M, Sheehy MP, Parkes JD, Marsden CD. Lisuride in the treatment of Parkinsonism. *Acta Neurol Scand* 1980; **62**: 382–5.
16. Massel D, Suskin N. Pergolide and cabergoline increased risk for valvular heart disease in Parkinson disease. *ACP J Club* 2007; **146**: 75–6.
17. Van Camp G, Flamez A, Cosyns B, et al. Treatment of Parkinson's disease with pergolide and relation to restrictive valvular heart disease. *Lancet* 2004; **363**: 1179–83.
18. Zhou CQ, Li SS, Chen ZM, Li FQ, Lei P, Peng GG. Rotigotine transdermal patch in Parkinson's disease: a

19. Voon V, Sohr M, Lang AE, et al. Impulse control disorders in Parkinson disease: a multicenter case – control study. *Ann Neurol* 2011; **69**: 986–96.
20. Weintraub D, Koester J, Potenza MN, et al. Impulse control disorders in Parkinson disease: a cross-sectional study of 3090 patients. *Arch Neurol* 2010; **67**: 589–95.
21. NICE. Parkinson's disease: Diagnosis and Management in Primary and Secondary Care. NICE guidelines [CG35]. National Institute for Health and Care Excellence, 2011. Available at: https://www.nice.org.uk/guidance/cg35.
22. Miyasaki JM, Martin W, Suchowersky O, Weiner WJ, Lang AE. Practice parameter: initiation of treatment for Parkinson's disease: an evidence-based review: report of the Quality Standards Subcommittee of the American Academy of Neurology. *Neurology* 2002; **58**: 11–7.
23. Pahwa R, Factor SA, Lyons KE, et al. Practice Parameter: treatment of Parkinson disease with motor fluctuations and dyskinesia (an evidence-based review): report of the Quality Standards Subcommittee of the American Academy of Neurology. *Neurology* 2006; **66**: 983–95.
24. Olanow CW, Obeso JA, Stocchi F. Continuous dopamine-receptor treatment of Parkinson's disease: scientific rationale and clinical implications. *Lancet Neurol* 2006; **5**: 677–87.
25. Blanchet PJ, Calon F, Martel JC, et al. Continuous administration decreases and pulsatile administration increases behavioral sensitivity to a novel dopamine D2 agonist (U-91356A) in MPTP-exposed monkeys. *J Pharmacol Exp Ther* 1995; **272**: 854–9.
26. Bibbiani F, Costantini LC, Patel R, Chase TN. Continuous dopaminergic stimulation reduces risk of motor complications in parkinsonian primates. *Exp Neurol* 2005; **192**: 73–8.
27. Parkinson Study Group. Pramipexole vs levodopa as initial treatment for Parkinson disease: A randomized controlled trial. *JAMA* 2000; **284**: 1931–8.
28. Rascol O, Brooks DJ, Korczyn AD, et al. A five-year study of the incidence of dyskinesia in patients with early Parkinson's disease who were treated with ropinirole or levodopa. 056 Study Group. *N Engl J Med* 2000; **342**: 1484–91.
29. Whone AL, Watts RL, Stoessl AJ, et al. Slower progression of Parkinson's disease with ropinirole versus levodopa: the REAL-PET study. *Ann Neurol* 2003; **54**: 93–101.
30. Katzenschlager R, Head J, Schrag A, et al. Fourteen-year final report of the randomized PDRG-UK trial comparing three initial treatments in PD. *Neurology* 2008; **71**: 474–80.
31. Tan EK, Jankovic J. Choosing dopamine agonists in Parkinson's disease. *Clin Neuropharmacol* 2001; **24**: 247–53.
32. Tonini M, Cipollina L, Poluzzi E, et al. Review article: clinical implications of enteric and central D2 receptor blockade by antidopaminergic gastrointestinal prokinetics. *Aliment Pharmacol Ther* 2004; **19**: 379–90.
33. Fox S. Domperidone as a treatment for dopamine agonist-induced peripheral edema in patients with Parkinson's disease. *ClinicalTrials.gov* 2012; NCT00305331.
34. Gizer IR, Ficks C, Waldman ID. Candidate gene studies of ADHD: a meta-analytic review. *Hum Genet* 2009; **126**: 51–90.
35. Rashid AJ, So CH, Kong MM, et al. D1-D2 dopamine receptor heterooligomers with unique pharmacology are coupled to rapid activation of Gq/11 in the striatum. *Proc Natl Acad Sci U S A* 2007; **104**: 654–9.
36. van Wieringen JP, Booij J, Shalgunov V, Elsinga P, Michel MC. Agonist high- and low-affinity states of dopamine D2 receptors: methods of detection and clinical implications. *Naunyn Schmiedebergs Arch Pharmacol* 2013; **386**: 135–54.
37. Zhang J, Xiong B, Zhen X, Zhang A. Dopamine D1 receptor ligands: where are we now and where are we going. *Med Res Rev* 2009; **29**: 272–94.
38. Yun JY, Kim HJ, Lee JY, et al. Comparison of once-daily versus twice-daily combination of ropinirole prolonged release in Parkinson's disease. *BMC Neurol* 2013; **13**: 113.
39. Kvernmo T, Härtter S, Burger E. A review of the receptor-binding and pharmacokinetic properties of dopamine agonists. *Clin Ther* 2006; **28**: 1065–78.
40. Tippmann-Peikert M, Park JG, Boeve BF, Shepard JW, Silber MH. Pathologic gambling in patients with restless legs syndrome treated with dopaminergic agonists. *Neurology* 2007; **68**: 301–3.
41. Thobois S. Proposed dose equivalence for rapid switch between dopamine receptor agonists in Parkinson's disease: a review of the literature. *Clin Ther* 2006; **28**: 1–12.
42. Tomlinson CL, Stowe R, Patel S, et al. Systematic review of levodopa dose equivalency reporting in Parkinson's disease. *Mov Disord* 2010; **25**: 2649–53.
43. Wright CE, Sisson TL, Ichhpurani AK, Peters GR. Steady-state pharmacokinetic properties of pramipexole in healthy volunteers. *J Clin Pharmacol*. 1997; **37**: 520–5.
44. Clarke CE, Speller JM, Clarke JA. Pramipexole for levodopa-induced complications in Parkinson's disease. *Cochrane Database Syst Rev* 2000; **3**: CD002261.
45. Moller JC, Oertel WH, Koster J, Pezzoli G, Provinciali L. Long-term efficacy and safety of pramipexole in

advanced Parkinson's disease: results from a European multicenter trial. *Mov Disord* 2005; **20**: 602–10.

46. Lieberman A, Ranhosky A, Korts D. Clinical evaluation of pramipexole in advanced Parkinson's disease: results of a double-blind, placebo-controlled, parallel-group study. *Neurology* 1997; **49**: 162–8.

47. Parkinson Study Group CALM Cohort Investigators. Long-term effect of initiating pramipexole vs levodopa in early Parkinson disease. *Arch Neurol* 2009; **66**: 563–70.

48. Inzelberg R, Carasso RL, Schechtman E, Nisipeanu P. A comparison of dopamine agonists and catechol-O-methyltransferase inhibitors in Parkinson's disease. *Clin Neuropharmacol* 2000; **23**: 262–6.

49. Herrero MT, Pagonabarraga J, Linazasoro G. Neuroprotective role of dopamine agonists: evidence from animal models and clinical studies. *Neurologist* 2011; **17** (Suppl. 1): S54–66.

50. Olanow CW, Rascol O, Hauser R, et al. A double-blind, delayed-start trial of rasagiline in Parkinson's disease. *N Engl J Med* 2009; **361**: 1268–78.

51. Schapira AH, McDermott MP, Barone P, et al. Pramipexole in patients with early Parkinson's disease (PROUD): a randomised delayed-start trial. *Lancet Neurol* 2013; **12**: 747–55.

52. Ostow M. Pramipexole for depression. *Am J Psychiatry* 2002; **159**: 320–1.

53. Leentjens AF, Koester J, Fruh B, et al. The effect of pramipexole on mood and motivational symptoms in Parkinson's disease: a meta-analysis of placebo-controlled studies. *Clin Ther* 2009; **31**: 89–98.

54. Rektorova I, Rektor I, Bares M, et al. Pramipexole and pergolide in the treatment of depression in Parkinson's disease: a national multicentre prospective randomized study. *Eur J Neurol* 2003; **10**: 399–406.

55. Barone P, Poewe W, Albrecht S, et al. Pramipexole for the treatment of depressive symptoms in patients with Parkinson's disease: a randomised, double-blind, placebo-controlled trial. *Lancet Neurol* 2010; **9**: 573–80.

56. Barone P, Scarzella L, Marconi R, et al. Pramipexole versus sertraline in the treatment of depression in Parkinson's disease: a national multicenter parallel-group randomized study. *J Neurol* 2006; **253**: 601–7.

57. Lemke MR, Brecht HM, Koester J, Kraus PH, Reichmann H. Anhedonia, depression, and motor functioning in Parkinson's disease during treatment with pramipexole. *J Neuropsychiatry Clin Neurosci* 2005; **17**: 214–20.

58. Kirsch-Darrow L, Marsiske M, Okun MS, Bauer R, Bowers D. Apathy and depression: separate factors in Parkinson's disease. *J Int Neuropsychol Soc* 2011; **17**: 1058–66.

59. Mayberg HS. Limbic-cortical dysregulation: a proposed model of depression. *J Neuropsychiatry Clin Neurosci* 1997; **9**: 471–81.

60. Kaye CM, Nicholls B. Clinical pharmacokinetics of ropinirole. *Clin Pharmacokinet* 2000; **39**: 243–54.

61. Lieberman A, Olanow CW, Sethi K, et al. A multicenter trial of ropinirole as adjunct treatment for Parkinson's disease. Ropinirole Study Group. *Neurology* 1998; **51**: 1057–62.

62. Rektorova I, Balaz M, Svatova J, et al. Effects of ropinirole on nonmotor symptoms of Parkinson disease: a prospective multicenter study. *Clin Neuropharmacol* 2008; **31**: 261–6.

63. Zagmutt FJ, Tarrants ML. Indirect comparisons of adverse events and dropout rates in early Parkinson's disease trials of pramipexole, ropinirole, and rasagiline. *Int J Neurosci* 2012; **122**: 345–53.

64. Kulisevsky J, Pagonabarraga J. Tolerability and safety of ropinirole versus other dopamine agonists and levodopa in the treatment of Parkinson's disease: meta-analysis of randomized controlled trials. *Drug Saf* 2010; **33**: 147–61.

65. Scheller D, Ullmer C, Berkels R, Gwarek M, Lubbert H. The in vitro receptor profile of rotigotine: a new agent for the treatment of Parkinson's disease. *Naunyn Schmiedebergs Arch Pharmacol* 2009; **379**: 73–86.

66. Reynolds NA, Wellington K, Easthope SE. Rotigotine: in Parkinson's disease. *CNS Drugs* 2005; **19**: 973–81.

67. Guldenpfennig WM, Poole KH, Sommerville KW, Boroojerdi B. Safety, tolerability, and efficacy of continuous transdermal dopaminergic stimulation with rotigotine patch in early-stage idiopathic Parkinson disease. *Clin Neuropharmacol* 2005; **28**: 106–10.

68. Giladi N, Boroojerdi B, Korczyn AD, et al. Rotigotine transdermal patch in early Parkinson's disease: a randomized, double-blind, controlled study versus placebo and ropinirole. *Mov Disord* 2007; **22**: 2398–404.

69. LeWitt PA, Lyons KE, Pahwa R. Advanced Parkinson disease treated with rotigotine transdermal system: PREFER Study. *Neurology* 2007; **68**: 1262–7.

70. Poewe WH, Rascol O, Quinn N, et al. Efficacy of pramipexole and transdermal rotigotine in advanced Parkinson's disease: a double-blind, double-dummy, randomised controlled trial. *Lancet Neurol* 2007; **6**: 513–20.

71. Trenkwalder C, Kies B, Rudzinska M, et al. Rotigotine effects on early morning motor function and sleep in Parkinson's disease: a double-blind, randomized, placebo-controlled study (RECOVER). *Mov Disord* 2011; **26**: 90–9.

72. Ray Chaudhuri K, Martinez-Martin P, Antonini A, et al. Rotigotine and specific non-motor symptoms of Parkinson's disease: post hoc analysis of

RECOVER. *Parkinsonism Relat Disord* 2013; **19**: 660–5.
73. Ghys L, Surmann E, Whitesides J, Boroojerdi B. Effect of rotigotine on sleep and quality of life in Parkinson's disease patients: post hoc analysis of RECOVER patients who were symptomatic at baseline. *Expert Opin Pharmacother* 2011; **12**: 1985–98.
74. Sarati S, Guiso G, Garattini S, Caccia S. Kinetics of piribedil and effects on dopamine metabolism: hepatic biotransformation is not a determinant of its dopaminergic action in rats. *Psychopharmacology (Berl)* 1991; **105**: 541–5.
75. Emile J, Chanelet J, Truelle JL, Bastard J. Action of piribedil in Parkinson's disease: I.V. test and oral treatment. *Adv Neurol* 1975; **9**: 409–13.
76. Lebrun-Frenay C, Borg M. Choosing the right dopamine agonist for patients with Parkinson's disease. *Curr Med Res Opin*. 2002; **18**: 209–14.
77. Ziegler M, Rondot P. [Action of piribedil in Parkinson disease. Multicenter study]. *Presse Med* 1999; **28**: 1414–18 (in French).
78. Post RM, Gerner RH, Carman JS, et al. Effects of a dopamine agonist piribedil in depressed patients: relationship of pretreatment homovanillic acid to antidepressant response. *Arch Gen Psychiatry* 1978; **35**: 609–15.
79. Thobois S, Lhommée E, Klinger H, et al. Parkinsonian apathy responds to dopaminergic stimulation of D2/D3 receptors with piribedil. *Brain* 2013; **136**: 1568–77.
80. Nash JR, Wilson SJ, Potokar JP, Nutt DJ. Mirtazapine induces REM sleep behavior disorder (RBD) in parkinsonism. *Neurology* 2003; **61**: 1161; author reply 1161.
81. Passouant P, Besset A, Billiard M, Negre C. [Effect of piribedil on nocturnal sleep (author's transl)]. *Rev Electroencephalogr Neurophysiol Clin* 1978; **8**: 326–34.
82. Peralta C, Wolf E, Alber H, et al. Valvular heart disease in Parkinson's disease vs. controls: An echocardiographic study. *Mov Disord* 2006; **21**: 1109–13.
83. Frucht S, Rogers JD, Greene PE, Gordon MF, Fahn S. Falling asleep at the wheel: motor vehicle mishaps in persons taking pramipexole and ropinirole. *Neurology* 1999; **52**: 1908–10.
84. Hauser RA, Gauger L, Anderson WM, Zesiewicz TA. Pramipexole-induced somnolence and episodes of daytime sleep. *Mov Disord* 2000; **15**: 658–63.
85. Etminan M, Samii A, Takkouche B, Rochon PA. Increased risk of somnolence with the new dopamine agonists in patients with Parkinson's disease: a meta-analysis of randomised controlled trials. *Drug Saf* 2001; **24**: 863–8.
86. Paus S, Brecht HM, Koster J, et al. Sleep attacks, daytime sleepiness, and dopamine agonists in Parkinson's disease. *Mov Disord* 2003; **18**: 659–67.
87. Avorn J, Schneeweiss S, Sudarsky LR, et al. Sudden uncontrollable somnolence and medication use in Parkinson disease. *Arch Neurol* 2005; **62**: 1242–8.
88. Happe S, Berger K. The association of dopamine agonists with daytime sleepiness, sleep problems and quality of life in patients with Parkinson's disease – a prospective study. *J Neurol* 2001; **248**: 1062–7.
89. Kleiner-Fisman G, Fisman DN. Risk factors for the development of pedal edema in patients using pramipexole. *Arch Neurol* 2007; **64**: 820–4.
90. Tan EK. Peripheral edema and dopamine agonists in Parkinson disease. *Arch Neurol* 2007; **64**: 1546–7; author reply 1547.
91. Senard JM, Rai S, Lapeyre-Mestre M, et al. Prevalence of orthostatic hypotension in Parkinson's disease. *J Neurol Neurosurg Psychiatry* 1997; **63**: 584–9.
92. Perez-Lloret S, Rey MV, Fabre N, et al. Factors related to orthostatic hypotension in Parkinson's disease. *Parkinsonism Relat Disord* 2012; **18**: 501–5.
93. Kujawa K, Leurgans S, Raman R, Blasucci L, Goetz CG. Acute orthostatic hypotension when starting dopamine agonists in Parkinson's disease. *Arch Neurol* 2000; **57**: 1461–3.
94. Etminan M, Gill S, Samii A. Comparison of the risk of adverse events with pramipexole and ropinirole in patients with Parkinson's disease: a meta-analysis. *Drug Saf* 2003; **26**: 439–44.
95. Onofrj M, Thomas A, D'Andreamatteo G, et al. Incidence of RBD and hallucination in patients affected by Parkinson's disease: 8-year follow-up. *Neurol Sci.* 2002; **23** (Suppl. 2): S91–4.
96. Kamakura K, Mochizuki H, Kaida K, et al. Therapeutic factors causing hallucination in Parkinson's disease patients, especially those given selegiline. *Parkinsonism Relat Disord* 2004; **10**: 235–42.
97. Williams DR, Lees AJ. Visual hallucinations in the diagnosis of idiopathic Parkinson's disease: a retrospective autopsy study. *Lancet Neurol* 2005; **4**: 605–10.
98. Harding AJ, Stimson E, Henderson JM, Halliday GM. Clinical correlates of selective pathology in the amygdala of patients with Parkinson's disease. *Brain* 2002; **125**: 2431–45.
99. Holman AJ. Impulse control disorder behaviors associated with pramipexole used to treat fibromyalgia. *J Gambl Stud* 2009; **25**: 425–31.
100. Almanzar S, Zapata-Vega MI, Raya JA. Dopamine agonist-induced impulse control disorders in a patient with prolactinoma. *Psychosomatics* 2013; **54**: 387–91.
101. Schreglmann SR, Gantenbein AR, Eisele G, Baumann CR. Transdermal rotigotine causes impulse control disorders in patients with restless legs syndrome. *Parkinsonism Relat Disord* 2012; **18**: 207–9.

102. Avila A, Cardona X, Martin-Baranera M, Bello J, Sastre F. Impulsive and compulsive behaviors in Parkinson's disease: a one-year follow-up study. *J Neurol Sci* 2011; **310**: 197–201.

103. Mamikonyan E, Siderowf AD, Duda JE, *et al.* Long-term follow-up of impulse control disorders in Parkinson's disease. *Mov Disord* 2008; **23**: 75–80.

104. Dang D, Cunnington D, Swieca J. The emergence of devastating impulse control disorders during dopamine agonist therapy of the restless legs syndrome. *Clin Neuropharmacol* 2011; **34**: 66–70.

105. Ye Z, Hammer A, Camara E, Munte TF. Pramipexole modulates the neural network of reward anticipation. *Hum Brain Mapp* 2011; **32**: 800–11.

106. Pondal M, Marras C, Miyasaki J, *et al.* Clinical features of dopamine agonist withdrawal syndrome in a movement disorders clinic. *J Neurol Neurosurg Psychiatry* 2013; **84**: 130–5.

107. Rabinak CA, Nirenberg MJ. Dopamine agonist withdrawal syndrome in Parkinson disease. *Arch Neurol* 2010; **67**: 58–63.

108. Nirenberg MJ. Dopamine agonist withdrawal syndrome: implications for patient care. *Drugs Aging* 2013; **30**: 587–92.

109. Edwards MJ. Dopamine agonist withdrawal syndrome (DAWS): perils of flicking the dopamine 'switch'. *J Neurol Neurosurg Psychiatry* 2013; **84**: 120.

Chapter 6

Subcutaneous, intranasal and transdermal dopamine agonists in the management of Parkinson's disease

Antoniya Todorova and K. Ray Chaudhuri

Introduction

Dopamine agonists (DAs) are widely used in clinical practice and are an established part of therapeutic strategies to treat Parkinson's disease (PD), as initiating agents, as adjunctive agents and in advanced disease as infusional therapies.

Dopamine agonists are generally indicated as monotherapy in early PD and as adjunctive therapy to levodopa (L-DOPA) at all stages of PD. Despite the "gold-standard" status of levodopa for controlling motor symptoms, dopamine agonists have potential advantages, including the pharmacokinetic advantage of their longer half-lives and an effect on reducing dyskinesias and promoting a "levodopa-sparing" strategy [1]. The latter effect may be mediated through selectivity in their binding to dopamine receptors, permitting a reduction in dyskinesias, by use of agonists selective for D2-like receptors [2–4].

In this chapter, we will focus on nonoral delivery of DAs – DAs used by the subcutaneous (SC), transdermal and intranasal route. An additional benefit of these routes entails the implementation of the strategy of continuous drug delivery (CDD), regarded as an effective and possibly physiological way of delivering dopaminergic treatment in PD, associated with motor benefits, reduction of motor complications and, more recently, nonmotor benefits as well, largely mediated by reducing nonmotor fluctuations [5–7].

Continuous drug delivery

A large body of evidence (preclinical and clinical) suggests that pulsatile drug delivery and receptor stimulation are involved in the emergence of motor complications in PD [8]. In addition, it is now established that the majority of motor fluctuations are also associated with nonmotor fluctuations and nonmotor symptoms [7]. The concept of continuous dopaminergic stimulation, as can be delivered by CDD strategies, appears to prevent or attenuate motor complications, ameliorate or reverse them once established in advanced disease, and also help in reversing nonmotor fluctuations. Thus, CDD appears to have a beneficial role in PD both in early (by delaying or preventing the onset of motor complications) and advanced stages [9].

Several methods of delivering nonoral treatments in PD exist and these are summarized in Table 6.1.

Transdermal dopamine agonists

Transdermal delivery of DAs is a promising therapeutic concept, which aims to deliver the drug in a continuous manner and to decrease the severity of the motor fluctuations in PD. The transdermal route avoids fluctuating gastrointestinal absorption due to delayed gastric emptying and avoids hepatic first-pass effects, a common and often underappreciated problem in early and advanced PD [10]. Also, if side effects occur, the patch easily can be removed. In addition, it has recently been suggested that compliance with medication is an issue in the care of PD, and to many patients, transdermal patches (once daily) may be a more acceptable method of delivering medication [11]. A further advantage is that the patch formulation may be more suitable than oral therapy in a small population of patients with dysphagia or severe dribbling of saliva, or in those undergoing surgery.

Table 6.1 Nonoral strategies (excluding levodopa intrajejunal infusion)

Route	Agent	Clinical positioning in Parkinson's disease
Transdermal	Rotigotine	In routine clinical use as monotherapy as well as adjunctive therapy
	Apo-MTD (apomorphine included in a microemulsion and administered by transdermal route)	One study describes clinical motor efficacy and long action
	Lisuride	Preliminary clinical data on motor complications available
	Piribedil	One clinical study with no significant beneficial effect on motor symptoms reported
Intranasal	Apomorphine	Not in use due to side effects such as nasal congestion, crusting and vestibulitis
Subcutaneous	Apomorphine	In clinical use usually as injections for predictable motor "off" and infusion as advanced therapy
	Lisuride	Not in widespread clinical use
		Discontinued in the UK and USA
	Rotigotine polyoxazoline conjugate SER-214	In development, and clinical studies in rat models reported

Transdermal delivery

Skin penetration of the active drug can be achieved in various manner and by different routes of skin penetration as shown in Table 6.2.

Rotigotine transdermal system

Rotigotine is structurally similar to dopamine but with increased lipid solubility (Figure 6.1). It can be applied in several formulations, intravenous, subcutaneous and transdermal and the rotigotine transdermal system (RTS) is now widely used as a licensed treatment for PD. Rotigotine is the first and only transdermal patch currently available in routine clinical practice that contains a nonergot, selective D2-receptor active DA.

Pharmacokinetics

Rotigotine has a broad spectrum of action across the D1–D5 receptors (Table 6.3) [12]. This, particularly its D1 activity, is in theory an advantage.

In addition to D3 activity, rotigotine also has considerable affinity for the D1 receptor, unlike other DAs, and this may be important because D1 activity is proposed to synergistically enhance the effect mediated via D2-like receptors [13]. Furthermore, studies suggest that D1 agonism may underlie an antidyskinetic effect as well as a beneficial effect on bladder function, often affected in PD [14].

Rotigotine also binds to serotonin receptors 5-HT1A and 5-HT7, and is an antagonist at α2B receptors. It has been suggested that the action of rotigotine on 5-HT1A and α2B receptors may contribute to other beneficial effects, such as an antidepressant effect (5-HT1A agonistic action) and also antidyskinetic action (α2B antagonistic action) [15, 16]. Furthermore, its lack of affinity for 5-HT2B receptors provides safety in terms of cardiac valvulofibrosis, a problem with ergot-derived DAs.

Rotigotine's absorption and other pharmacokinetic properties, and also comparison with the other

Table 6.2 Various routes of skin penetration described in clinical practice

Patch-like devices and ointment-like products intended for the delivery of active pharmaceutical ingredients (APIs)

Traditional drug-in-adhesive and reservoir type of product

Chemically enriched developments:
Use of novel permeation enhancers
Use of better and multifunctional adhesives stabilizers for APIs and formulations

Physical methods (different mechanical forces and means to break the natural barrier of the human skin):
Microneedles
Electric current
Heat
Ultrasound
Radiofrequency

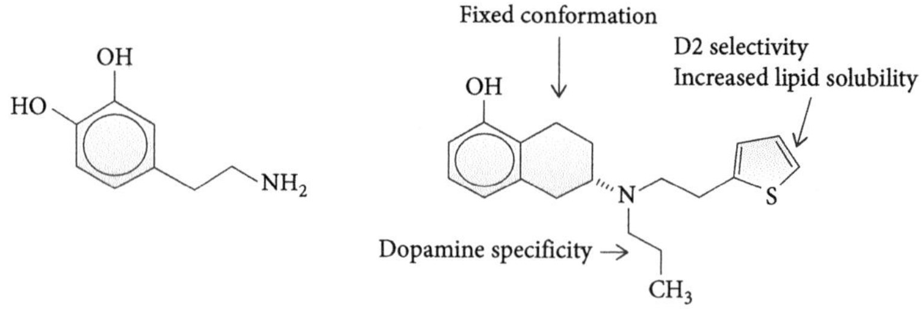

Figure 6.1 Structure of dopamine and rotigotine. (A black and white version of this figure will appear in some formats. For the color version, please refer to the plate section.)

commonly used DAs ropinirole and pramipexole, are shown in Table 6.4 [17].

In terms of composition, rotigotine is dispersed in a silicone adhesive and then spread evenly across a silicone backing. This permits uniform release of the drug delivery at a constant rate (Figure 6.2). In 2008 concern was raised about crystals developing within the patch which could be avoided by cold storage of the patch [11]. More recently, the need for cold storage of the patch has been reevaluated and the product is now applicable without cold storage.

Effect on motor function and nonmotor symptoms

Several large, multicenter, randomized, controlled trials, providing a level I evidence base, have demonstrated the safety and efficacy of 24-h RTS for the treatment of motor symptoms associated with both early and advanced PD.

In two placebo-controlled studies [18, 19] transdermal rotigotine, adjunctive to levodopa, showed efficacy

Table 6.3 Receptor-binding profile of rotigotine

Affinity for dopamine receptors		Affinity for nondopamine receptors	
D1	++	5HT1A	++
D2	++	α2B	++
D3	++++		
D4	+++		
D5	+++		

From [12].

Table 6.4 Pharmacokinetic profile of rotigotine and comparison with ropinirole and pramipexole

	Rotigotine transdermal patch	Ropinirole (oral)	Pramipexole (oral)
Absorption			
Absorption rate	Linear/24 h	Rapid	Rapid
T_{max}	Hours	1–2 h	2 h
Food interaction	None	T_{max}: +2.5 h	T_{max}: +1 h
First-pass effect	None	Yes	Minimal
Distribution			
Protein binding	89.5%	40%	15%
Metabolism			
Metabolic pathways	Extensive	Extensive	None
CYP450 system	Multiple	CYP1A2	None
Active metabolites	None	None	None
Elimination			
Renal excretion	71%	<10%	90% (tubular secretion)
$T_{½}$	5–7 h	6–8 h	8–10 h

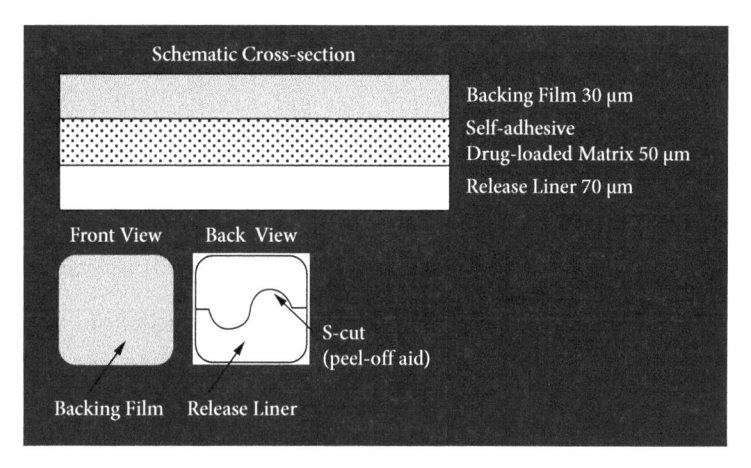

Figure 6.2 Structure of a rotigotine patch.

for motor complications in advanced PD, as evidenced by significant reductions in "off" time (average 2.5 h) and increases in "on" time without troublesome dyskinesias. In one of the studies [19], a third treatment arm permitted head-to-head comparisons between the rotigotine patch and pramipexole immediate release given three times per day. Even with the rotigotine patch being administered once in the morning, improvements in "off" time, "on" time without troublesome dyskinesias and other outcomes showed no significant differences between these two treatments.

Nonmotor effects
Nonmotor symptoms of PD are a key unmet need, and increasingly clinical trials are required to show nonmotor outcome benefits in addition to motor benefits [6]. A recent large-scale, double-blind, randomized study (RECOVER, Randomized Evaluation of the 24-Hour Coverage: Efficacy of Rotigotine) was the first to investigate early-morning motor function and sleep as co-primary outcome measures in PD [20]. In this study, 24-h transdermal rotigotine treatment was associated with significant benefits versus placebo in terms of early-morning motor impairment and nocturnal sleep disturbances. At 12 weeks, early-morning motor dysfunction as measured by Unified Parkinson's Disease Rating Scale (UPDRS) III scores and sleep disturbance as measured by the PD Sleep Scale (PDSS-2) total scores showed significantly greater improvements in the active-treatment group. Difficulty in falling asleep, and feeling tired and sleepy in the morning were among the ten items showing significant improvement. The RECOVER study was also the first large-scale trial to extensively investigate nonmotor symptoms of PD using the Non-Motor Symptoms Scale (NMSS). Significantly greater improvements with rotigotine were seen in NMSS total score, with significant changes on the sleep/fatigue and mood/apathy domains. In addition, the authors reported greater improvements with rotigotine than placebo on depression scores of Beck Depression Inventory (BDI) II, as well as quality of life.

Following the RECOVER study, a post-hoc analysis investigated the effects of rotigotine on individual nonmotor symptoms [21]. This post-hoc analysis suggested that RTS may have a positive effect on fatigue and mood disturbances (symptoms of depression, anhedonia) and apathy in patients with PD.

In another post-hoc analysis of RECOVER, using an 11-point Likert pain scale, authors evaluated the effect of rotigotine on pain [22]. They concluded that pain was improved in patients with PD treated with rotigotine, and this may be partly attributable to benefits in motor function and sleep disturbances.

Further studies addressing the effect of rotigotine patch therapy versus placebo on depression and anxiety are currently under way.

Long-term effect of RTS
The long-term effect of rotigotine in PD was studied in a 1-year study designed as an open-labeled extension of the RECOVER trial. At the end of the maintenance phase, rotigotine was well tolerated; the most common adverse events were application site reactions (24%), somnolence and hallucinations (13% each), nausea (12%), and dizziness and dyskinesias (11% each),

most of which were mild or moderate in intensity and resolved at the end of the trial. The beneficial effects of RTS on motor function and sleep disturbances were sustained for up to 1 year [23].

Side effects
Rotigotine is generally well tolerated, and a survey of DA trials suggested that adverse events are similar to those of other DAs, such as nausea, dizziness and somnolence [24]. In clinical trials, the rotigotine transdermal patch was associated with an incidence of application site reaction of 39–44% [25], although only a small subset had a severe reaction. The risk of skin reactions is reduced by daily rotation of the application site, and there is evidence of a lower rate of skin reactions when the rotations are strictly undertaken [25].

Role in impulse control disorders
Impulse control disorders (ICDs) such as compulsive gambling, shopping or hypersexuality are being increasingly recognized in PD patients as adverse effects of DA therapy and pose a major therapeutic challenge [26]. A recent postmarketing observational multicenter European study (the DAICE-ET survey) conducted in Europe has suggested that the risk of developing ICDs may be significantly lower for the rotigotine patch (4.9%) than for shorter-acting agonists, where the rates are considerably higher [27]. The pathophysiological basis of this observation is unclear and may be related to a possible "ICD-sparing" action of the CDD strategy compared with the pulsatile delivery associated with short-acting agents given orally.

Other transdermal DAs
Several other DAs have been developed into a transdermal form, with only apomorphine showing promising results and with a possibility to be used in the future. Two DAs, a lisuride patch and transdermal piribedil, have been discontinued since they failed to show superior efficacy.

Apomorphine transdermal patch
As mentioned above, a transdermal form of apomorphine included in a microemulsion and administered by the transdermal route (Apo-MTD) has also been developed. However, there is only one study showing its effects on PD. Priano *et al.* [28] studied 21 PD patients who were treated with levodopa plus oral DAs, with levodopa alone or with levodopa plus Apo-MTD. The authors reported steady therapeutic plasma levels, improved UPDRS motor scores and a reduced total duration of "off" periods in the group treated with the Apo-MTD patch. They also concluded that the epicutaneous–transdermal route is able to provide sustained release of the drug and, importantly, therapeutic plasma levels for a period of time that is longer than other DA preparations and is comparable to continuous infusion of apomorphine [28]. However, there have been no further recent developments in this area.

Lisuride transdermal patch
Lisuride patches have been under development for PD in the past. However, they have not been studied extensively because of the drug's side effects, particularly neuropsychiatric issues. A small open-label study of eight patients showed efficacy and tolerability in the treatment of motor complications in PD [29]. Assessment of "motor changing rate" was performed and it was shown that lisuride patch application significantly ($P = 0.023$) improved the motor changing rate compared with baseline. The authors noted side effects of transient skin irritations in four patients [29]. Another randomized, placebo-controlled study of 20 PD patients reported (in an abstract form) a significant reduction in motor fluctuations, improved quality of life, decreased daytime somnolence and increased duration of nighttime sleep [30]. Skin irritation was reported as a side effect in this study as well. Currently, therefore, a robust evidence base to support the use of lisuride patches in clinical practice is lacking.

Piribedil transdermal patch
Piribedil is a dopaminergic agonist active on all central dopaminergic pathways, essentially by stimulating postsynaptic D2 receptors [31]. Clinical studies with piribedil administered orally or intravenously have shown its efficacy in PD. However, through the oral route, the drug undergoes a major hepatic first-pass effect and bioavailability is consequently low, at less than 10%. To minimize the hepatic first-pass effect and achieve stable effective plasma concentrations, a 50 mg transdermal patch formulation was developed. However, a single-center, randomized, double-blinded study of 27 PD patients during 3 weeks of treatment administered to three different groups – placebo, one piribedil patch and two piribedil patches – showed no clinical efficacy on the motor symptoms or UPDRS scores [32]. The main adverse events noted in this study were nausea (11%), vomiting (7.4%) and malaise (7.4%); however, these effects were observed mainly in the placebo group (four of seven patients) and the

authors reported good local acceptability of the transdermal system. Although the transdermal patch has several advantages (local tolerance, good patch adhesion), it is not currently being actively developed.

Intranasal dopamine agonists

The intranasal administration of solutions has been recognized as a promising route of delivery of therapeutic compounds. It is convenient, with rapid absorption, bioavailability and quality of response for drugs penetrating mucous membranes such as apomorphine.

Apomorphine

Several small open-label studies using intranasal apomorphine were published in the 1990s (Table 6.5) [33–40]. In all of these, intranasal apomorphine improved the motor function of the patients, reducing daily "off" time by 19–50% and improving the motor scores. In two studies, the effect was reported to be comparable to oral levodopa [37] or subcutaneous apomorphine injections [35].

However, in most of the studies, patients experienced significant adverse events. These were not only the common apomorphine side effects such as nausea, vomiting and orthostatic hypotension, but also nasal congestion, crusting and vestibulitis, some of which were severe (in ten cases altogether) and eventually led to discontinuation of the treatment.

Subcutaneously administered dopamine agonists

Apomorphine infusion and injection

Apomorphine (10,11-dihydroxyapomorphine) is the most potent short-acting DA at D1 and D2 dopamine receptors, and it was proposed as an antiparkinsonian drug more than a century ago. Since apomorphine cannot be absorbed when administered orally, it needs to be given by the subcutaneous route, either intermittently as an injection or as a continuous infusion.

Apomorphine was first used by veterinary physicians in animals to treat behavioral vices before its emetic properties were exploited as a treatment for poisoning. At high doses, apomorphine caused involuntary movement and stereotyped behavior similar to punding, but at lower doses it had a robust beneficial motor effect and this was evidence that different doses of apomorphine could produce different outcomes in the context of PD [41].

Schwab and colleagues in the USA were the first to demonstrate the antiparkinsonian properties of apomorphine in 1951 [42] and showed that apomorphine relieved rigidity and tremor for periods of up to 30–40

Table 6.5 Summary of studies using intranasal apomorphine

Reference	n	Dose	Clinical findings	Adverse events
Kapoor et al. (1990) [33]	8	6 mg (0.6 ml)	50% decrease in off scores	None
Kleedorfer et al. (1991) [34]	5	4.3 mg	Decrease of "off" time	Transient nasal congestion Vestibulitis (n = 2) Orthostatic hypotension (n = 4)
van Laar et al. (1992) [35]	7	1–10 mg	Improved motor response Similar to s.c. injections	Nasal congestion and crusting (n = 3) Vestibulitis (n = 1)
Sam et al. (1995) [36]	7	5.3 mg	Achieved "on" response	Not described
Dewey et al. (1996) [37]	11	2–5 mg	Similar to oral levodopa Relieves "off" state	Nausea and vomiting (n = 3), Orthostatic hypotension (n = 1)
Esteban Muñoz et al. (1997) [38]	9		SC vs intranasal route Reduced daily "off" hours Improved "off" dystonia improved dyskinesias	Nasal crusting Vestibulitis Poor tolerability in intranasal group
Dewey et al. (1998) [39]	9	4.1 mg	Improvement in motor scores	Nausea (n = 2) Orthostatic hypotension (n = 2) Nasal irritation (n = 5)
Wickremaratchi et al. (2003) [40]	6	5 mg	Induced "on" response	None

min. Subsequently, Cotzias *et al.* [43] suggested that apomorphine improved tremor refractory to dopamine and may have an antidyskinetic effect.

The development of ambulatory mini pumps for the management of brittle diabetes mellitus and use of the peripheral dopamine antagonist domperidone were utilized to define the role of apomorphine single injections as a "rescue" therapy for patients with predictable "off" periods. In the UK, work from the group of Lees and colleagues and others showed that continuous waking day subcutaneous apomorphine delivered by a Graseby™ dynamics pump resulted in a dramatic reduction in the frequency and duration of "off" periods (a reduction of 10 h "off"/day to 3–4 h "off" per day) [44, 45]. These data suggest that apomorphine, to this day, is the only clinically available DA that is equipotent to levodopa.

Currently, apomorphine continuous infusion is generally used when continuous dopaminergic stimulation is required in PD patients with increasing or prolonged "off" periods, motor fluctuations and/or moderate to severe levodopa-induced dyskinesias. Apomorphine can now be delivered via a small, portable pump (APO-go® pump) worn by the patient using a low-impact Neria™ line for subcutaneous delivery (Figure 6.3).

A portable pump permits continuous infusion of the drug into the subcutaneous fatty tissue of the abdomen, thighs or arms [46], and in Europe and parts of Asia and Australia, this specific delivery method using Neria™ lines is available. After long-term usage, however, inflammatory skin nodules may form, which may interfere with drug absorption [47], and active and continuing skin care is an essential part of apomorphine therapy (Table 6.6).

Pharmacokinetics of subcutaneous apomorphine

The pharmacokinetics of apomorphine are shown in Table 6.7.

Effect on motor complications: dyskinesias and "off" periods

In a range of clinical trials, apomorphine has been shown to have equivalent efficacy to oral levodopa [41]. The injection formulation comprises apomorphine hydrochloride 10 mg/ml for subcutaneous injection in a multidose, disposable pen. This formulation is intended for use by PD patients who are experiencing refractory periods, which occur when oral medications start to fail (see Table 6.6). It is recommended

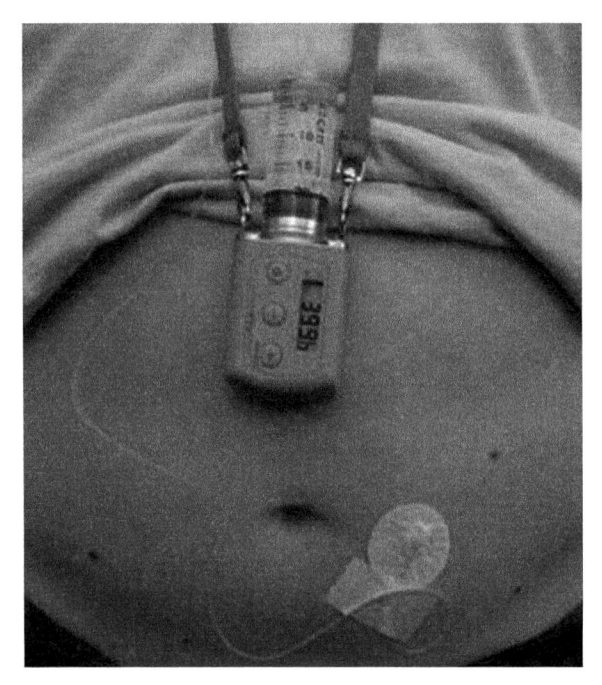

Figure 6.3 Patient with an apomorphine pump.

Table 6.6 Indications for using an apomorphine pen or pump

Pen	Pump
• Anticipated rescue when required • When absorption of oral levodopa is impaired • To treat delayed "on" period • To treat early-morning motor problems (akinesia and dystonia)	• Patient considers that rescue doses required too frequently • Dyskinesias limit further therapy optimization • Nonmotor symptoms associated with "off" periods • To simplify complex PD dosing regimens to improve convenience and compliance with therapy • As an alternative to surgical therapy or levodopa/carbodopa intestinal gel if these are contraindicated or because of patient preference • Absorption of oral levodopa is impaired

Table 6.7 Pharmacokinetic profile of apomorphine

Rapidly absorbed and correlates with rapid onset of clinical effect
Peak levels achieved after 3–5 min
Absorption of apomorphine varies among patients (5–10-fold difference)
Half-life in distribution phase of ~5 min
Biological half-life in elimination phase of ~33 min
Brief clinical effect is accounted for by the rapid clearance of apomorphine

as a rescue treatment for those patients experiencing only a few "off" episodes per day, as an adjunct to oral medications. Apomorphine injection has a rapid onset (4–12 min) and a duration of action of about 1 h. In an open-label study, PD patients were switched from subcutaneous to intravenous apomorphine (delivered by indwelling venous catheter) in patients with refractory motor fluctuations and severe dyskinesias [48]. There was a dramatic reduction in dyskinesias with virtual complete elimination of the "off" period (mean reduction from 5.4 to 0.5 h; $P < 0.05$); however, severe and serious side effects including cardiovascular ones resulted in discontinuation of the study. In this study, plasma apomorphine levels did not correlate well with dosage level or with motor function and response. However, in a small study of two PD patients, plasma apomorphine levels again showed weak correlation with motor function, although cerebrospinal fluid apomorphine levels showed a strong correlation with motor function [49]. Clinical studies addressing the effects of apomorphine in PD are shown in Table 6.8.

Several long-term, open-label, uncontrolled studies evaluated the efficacy of continuous subcutaneous apomorphine infusions in monotherapy or as an add-on to levodopa therapy in advanced PD (Table 6.8) [44, 45, 52, 54, 57–62, 66]. These studies showed that subcutaneous apomorphine infusions are successful in aborting "off" periods (often not amenable to oral treatment), reducing dyskinesias and improving PD motor scores [41, 57, 62, 66, 68].

Most of the studies [44, 52, 54, 58, 59] reported mainly large reductions (50–72%) in daily "off" time in patients treated with continuous apomorphine infusion (as in Table 6.8). In addition, a marked and sustained reduction (43–64%) in dyskinesias has been reported in those patients who achieve a substantial reduction in their oral dopaminergic therapy [57, 60–62, 66, 68]. However, this observation has not been supported in two open-label, nonrandomized studies and a 5-year prospective study that compared apomorphine with deep-brain stimulation of the subthalamic nucleus [67, 70, 72]. While a similar efficiency in reducing "off" time (51–76%) was observed in both groups, dyskinesia duration and severity was reduced only in the deep-brain stimulation group.

Nonmotor effects of apomorphine

While there is a reasonable body of evidence that confirms the efficacy of apomorphine on motor function in PD, as well as a possible antidyskinetic effects [45], there have also been reports of the possible beneficial effect of apomorphine on nonmotor symptoms in PD stretching back to Cotzias suggesting an antipsychotic effect. Given that nonmotor symptoms are now recognized to be almost universal across all stages of PD [6] and are also the key determinant of quality of life of people with PD [69], a closer examination of the nonmotor effects of apomorphine is justified. In a recent review, Todorova and Chaudhuri [73] produced a summary of the possible beneficial nonmotor effects of apomorphine in PD.

A controlled comparative study (not blinded and nonrandomized) addressing apomorphine and nonmotor symptoms was performed by Martinez-Martin et al. [69] using the NMSS as one primary outcome variable in addition to standard motor outcomes. The authors compared 17 patients receiving subcutaneous apomorphine infusion with a patient group on conservative therapy with motor, nonmotor and quality-of-life measures being assessed at initiation of therapy and at a 6-month follow-up as part of the routine clinical practice in a real-life study. Apomorphine infusion was found to improve NMSS total score significantly ($P = 0.0003$), quality of life as measured by the 8-Item Parkinson's Disease Questionnaire (PDQ-8) and motor state as measured by UPDRS-III and -IV scores. When the NMSS domains were subanalyzed, moderate to large improvements in effect size of apomorphine were observed in sleep (mainly related to nocturnal restless legs-type symptoms and insomnia), attention, mood, apathy, fatigue, urinary (urgency, nocturia) and gastrointestinal (dribbling, constipation) domains of the NMSS [69]. Importantly, quality-of-life scores deteriorated significantly in the group maintained on optimal oral therapy versus the apomorphine group where a significant benefit in quality of life was observed.

Some have argued that the piperidine moiety contained in the structure of apomorphine may have some antipsychotic properties. In specific studies addressing this issue, Chaudhuri et al. [74] and Ellis et al. [75] published a total of 15 case reports on PD patients with previous drug-related neuropsychiatric problems, confirming the possible role of the use of apomorphine in PD patients with neuropsychiatric problems. Contrary to common perception, apomorphine therapy can be tolerated in patients experiencing visual hallucinations and delusions, as well as in patients with paranoid ideations [69]. Apomorphine infusion was well tolerated in PD patients experiencing hallucinations [75, 76]. Some authors have even suggested that apomorphine may

Table 6.8 Summary of studies (mostly open label) using apomorphine infusion in Parkinson's disease

Reference	n	Follow-up period (months)	Daily time in "off" period (%)	Dyskinesia intensity (%)
Stibe et al. (1988) [44]	11	8	−62	
Chaudhuri et al. (1988) [45]	7	11	−85	−45
Frankel et al. (1990) [50]	25	22	−55	
Pollak et al. (1990) [51]	9	10	−67	−20
Hughes et al. (1993) [52]	22	36	−59	
Stochhi et al. (1993) [53]	10	12	−58	−40
Poewe et al. (1993) [54]	18	20	−58	
Kreczy-Kleedorfer et al. (1993) [55]	14	26	−77	
Gancher et al. (1995) [56]	7	3	−58	
Colzi et al. (1998) [57]	19	35	−72	−65
Pietz et al. (1998) [58]	25	44	−50	−14
Wenning et al. (1999) [59]	16	57	−55	
Stocchi et al. (2001) [60]	30	60		
Kanovsky et al. (2002) [61]	12	24	−80	
Manson et al. (2002) [62]	64	34	−49	−57
Di Rosa et al. (2003) [63]	12	12	−40	−37
Morgante et al. (2004) [64]	12	24	−60	−48
Tyne et al. (2004) [65]	80	25		
Katzenschlager et al. (2005) [66]	12	6	−38	−31
De Gaspari et al. (2006) [67]	13	12	−51	No change
Garcia-Ruiz et al. (2008) [68]	82	20	−80	−32
Martinez-Martin et al. (2011) [69]	17	6	−65	
Antonini et al. (2011) [70]	12	60	−49	No change
Drapier et al. (2012) [71]	23	12	−36	
Summary (total number of patients; mean reduction of time in "off" period and dyskinesia scores)	552		−59.3	−32.4

improve visual processing in PD patients with visual hallucinations, in particular increasing contrast sensitivity and decreasing reaction time [76]. These observations have never been studied in a controlled fashion and thus remain controversial.

Gastroparesis is emerging as a key problem in PD, both early and advanced [77], and there is evidence that nonoral therapies such as apomorphine infusion or a rotigotine patch in this scenario are particularly effective. Preliminary data (shown in an abstract form) from the AM IMPAKT (Apokyn for Motor Improvement of Morning Akinesia Trial) study (a phase 4, multicenter, open-label study to investigate the rapid and reliable improvement of motor symptoms with APOKYN® in PD patients with morning akinesia resulting from delayed or unreliable onset of levodopa action) showed that apomorphine provided rapid and reliable turning on for patients with morning akinesia, and had a significant impact on PD patients who experience delayed "on" to levodopa in the early morning.

In relation to other gastrointestinal symptoms, two studies have reported on defecatory dysfunction, and in both studies, apomorphine showed a positive effect on anorectal dysfunction in PD [78, 79]. Tison et al. [80] studied the effects of apomorphine on liquid swallowing using videofluoroscopy and found that apomorphine improved swallowing abnormalities in a subgroup of PD patients with swallowing disorders.

There are only a few case reports on apomorphine in restless legs syndrome (RLS). In a patient with idiopathic RLS and another with PD and RLS, an overnight infusion with apomorphine improved nocturnal discomfort and leg movements [81], and resulted in a rapid and significant (55%) improvement in subjective RLS symptoms and an almost immediate cessation of periodic limb movements [82].

Apomorphine and ICDs

No proper studies have been undertaken showing the relationship between apomorphine and ICD. A small study by Magennis *et al.* [83] showed improvement of ICDs in five patients after they were commenced on apomorphine infusion. In a recent observational study by Todorova *et al.* [84] of 41 patients receiving apomorphine infusion, seven had preexisting ICDs that resolved or attenuated after the initiation of therapy. Six new ICDs developed, including excessive eating, compulsive shopping and internet use, hypersexuality and punding. The authors concluded that apomorphine infusion appears to have a relatively low risk for the development of ICDs, with discontinuation of therapy required in only 2.4%. These data on low rates of ICDs on apomorphine are also indirectly supported by a large-scale multicenter national study conducted by Garcia-Ruiz *et al.* [68] of 82 patients on chronic apomorphine infusion therapy. At a mean follow-up period of 19.9 ± 16.3 months, only one had developed severe hypersexuality, while the overall rate was 8%. These preliminary studies, currently largely restricted to abstract-based and open-label information, suggest a substantially lower rate of development of ICDs with the use of the CDD strategy. However, this observation needs to be examined in a controlled manner with large-scale international studies.

Side effects

Skin nodules are a common problem with apomorphine infusion, with a longer duration being associated with a greater occurrence of nodules. However, several studies, long term as well as cumulative clinical experience of centers in Europe, with long-term experience in apomorphine therapy, report that skin nodules are seldom a reason for discontinuation of therapy as long as good skin hygiene is followed and the rates are lowered further with the use of the new atraumatic needles of the Neria™ line and dilution of the apomorphine concentration delivered. Nevertheless, in some cases, an infection at the injection site and nodules may occur, and this may lead to discontinuation of treatment.

Nausea is another unavoidable problem with apomorphine infusion and injection; however, there is tachyphylaxis with prolonged use. In Europe and many other countries, oral domperidone is successfully used, as originally suggested by Corsini *et al.* [85], as pretreatment prophylaxis against nausea and vomiting and also during the first 2–3 weeks of treatment. Recent concern about domperidone safety has led to the suggestion that doses lower than 40 mg/day should be used and caution needs to be exercised in those over 60 years of age, with close monitoring of cases on high-dose oral domperidone. In countries, where domperidone is not routinely available, alternative antiemetics may need to be used.

Effects of long-term apomorphine therapy

There are four studies reporting the long-term efficacy of apomorphine infusions and injections in PD patients. In 1993, Hughes *et al.* [52] published a 5-year follow-up study of the efficacy and safety of daytime infusion or intermittent injections in 71 PD patients with response fluctuations. They reported a 50% decrease in "off" time for apomorphine and no tolerance issues. In 2002, Manson *et al.* [62] reported another study of apomorphine monotherapy in the treatment of refractory motor fluctuations in 64 PD patients followed up for a mean period of 3 years. The results confirmed that apomorphine monotherapy can reset the peak-dose dyskinesia threshold in levodopa-treated patients and further reduce "off"-period disability. In 2004, Tyne *et al.* [65] published a 10-year retrospective audit of long-term apomorphine use in 107 PD patients treated with subcutaneous apomorphine injections or infusions. The authors reported only two cases of hypotension, three of confusion and five of hallucination, which confirmed that apomorphine was well tolerated and has a low incidence of side effects.

In 2008, Garcia Ruiz *et al.* [68] studied the evolution of 82 PD patients with severe motor fluctuations treated for a mean period of 3 years with continuous subcutaneous apomorphine infusion. The authors found a significant reduction in "off" hours, total and motor UPDRS scores, and dyskinesia severity. No serious side effects were observed. Hypersexuality as an adverse effect was reported in only seven patients (8%).

Other subcutaneous DAs

Lisuride

Lisuride, a potent soluble DA, was the first drug to be used for chronic subcutaneous treatment in PD [86]. Lisuride is a water-soluble, ergoline derivative with mixed D1/D2 agonist properties. It has been used in PD for more than 20 years. Having a short half-life, good solubility and low oral bioavailability, the drug is suitable for continuous subcutaneous infusion, which provides stable serum concentrations [87].

A prospective comparison of oral levodopa versus lisuride infusion showed that patients receiving lisuride infusions experienced a significant reduction in both motor fluctuations and dyskinesias (41% reduction in severity) compared with patients receiving standard dopaminergic therapies [88]. In several other studies [89–91] where patients were treated with subcutaneous lisuride infusion in addition to oral levodopa, "off" periods and parkinsonian disability in "off" and "on" were reduced significantly.

Few studies have addressed the long-term efficacy and adverse event profile of lisuride infusion. Long-term experience with 24 h continuous infusion in advanced PD confirmed its favorable impact on motor function [92]. Despite its beneficial effect on motor fluctuations, a significant number of patients treated with lisuride reported neuropsychiatric side effects, particularly hallucinations, thus reducing its therapeutic usefulness [91, 92]. However, a small study of five patients showed that these psychiatric adverse effects can be reduced by lowering of the dose of lisuride without a significant increase in motor fluctuations [93].

Lisuride was considered relatively safe; unlike other ergot derivatives, it was thought to carry no risk of cardiac valvulopathy [94] and had even been under investigation as a patch for treatment of PD. However, its use has been discontinued in many countries, including the UK and USA.

Role of combined subcutaneous and transdermal therapies in Parkinson's disease

Often a 24 h infusion regime may be ideal, as this has been shown to reduce troublesome dyskinesias, and overnight infusion is also beneficial for nocturnal problems causing sleep disruption in PD. The concept of combining daytime apomorphine infusion with nocturnal rotigotine patch use is therefore attractive, although with a potential risk of side effects such as ICDs, and has only been explored in two studies. A small case study of six patients by Canesi et al. [95] showed that this combination was well tolerated and was an effective treatment in patients with advanced PD, reducing nocturnal disability and ameliorating sleep disorders without inducing undesirable dopaminergic effects. Recently, Todorova et al. [96] investigated the use of apomorphine infusion and a rotigotine patch as an alternative CCD approach in the treatment of PD during a follow-up period extending to 2 years. The authors reported significant improvement of motor and nonmotor states and quality of life at 2 years compared with baseline. In particular, significant improvements were noted and sustained at 2 years in relation to the sleep/fatigue and mood/apathy domains of NMSS.

Combining apomorphine infusion with a rotigotine patch appears to be a useful of way of extending the beneficial effects of infusion with good tolerability and improved aspects of sleep and mood sustained at 2 years in advanced PD with an overall beneficial effect on quality of life in these patients.

Conclusions

Nonoral therapies in PD are going to be increasingly important in the future given recent data support the growing evidence of gastrointestinal dysfunction, in particular issues related to gastric emptying problems even in early PD, rendering oral therapies to be of unpredictable effect. An added issue is silent aspiration in many patients with continuing oral therapies and gastric medication overload in many patients requiring oral treatment for a number of comorbid conditions. Transdermal therapy with a rotigotine patch and subcutaneous apomorphine infusion currently represent two robust therapeutic options in this regard, and the data suggest that, in addition to motor benefits, there is also growing evidence that these therapies affect nonmotor symptoms of PD as a key determinant of quality of life. Further studies and developments in these areas are likely to enhance a holistic quality of care in PD.

Acknowledgements

KRC receive salary support from the National Institute for Health Research (NIHR) Mental Health Biomedical Research Centre and Dementia Unit at South London and Maudsley NHS Foundation Trust and King's College London, UK. The views expressed are those of the authors and not necessarily those of the NHS, the NIHR or the Department of Health.

References

1. Kvernmo T, Härtter S, Burger E. A review of the receptor-binding and pharmacokinetic properties of dopamine agonists. *Clin Ther* 2006; **28**: 1065–78.
2. Jenner P. Preventing and controlling dyskinesia in Parkinson's disease – a view of current knowledge and future opportunities. *Mov Disord* 2008; **23** (Suppl. 3): S585–8.
3. Chase TN, Baronti F, Fabbrini G, et al. Rationale for continuous dopaminomimetic therapy of Parkinson's disease. *Neurology* 1989; **39** (Suppl. 2): 7–10.
4. Mouradian MM, Heuser IJ, Baronti F, Chase TN. Modification of central dopaminergic mechanisms by continuous levodopa therapy for advanced Parkinson's disease. *Ann Neurol* 1990; **27**: 18–23.
5. Brotchie J, Jenner P. New approaches to therapy. In: Brotchie J, Bezard E, Jenner P, eds. *Pathophysiology, Pharmacology, and Biochemistry of Dyskinesia*. San Diego: Elsevier Academic Press, 2011; 123–50.
6. Chaudhuri KR, Schapira AH. Non-motor symptoms of Parkinson's disease: dopaminergic pathophysiology and treatment. *Lancet Neurol* 2009; **8**: 464–74.
7. Storch A, Schneider CB, Wolz M, et al. Nonmotor fluctuations in Parkinson disease: severity and correlation with motor complications. *Neurology* 2013; **80**: 800–9.
8. Ray Chaudhuri K, Rizos A, Sethi K. Motor and nonmotor complications in Parkinson's disease: an argument for continuous drug delivery? *J Neural Transm* 2013; **120**: 1305–20.
9. Mouradian MM. Scientific rationale for continuous dopaminergic stimulation in Parkinson's disease. *Eur Neurol Rev* 2006; 62–6.
10. Marinnan S, Emmanuel A, Burn D. Delayed gastric emptying in Parkinson's disease. *Mov Disord* 2014; **29**: 23–32.
11. Naidu Y, Ray Chaudhuri K. Transdermal rotigotine: a new non-ergot dopamine agonist for the treatment of Parkinson's disease. *Expert Opin Drug Deliv* 2007; **4**: 111–18.
12. Jenner P. A novel dopamine agonist for the transdermal treatment of Parkinson's disease. *Neurology* 2005; **65** (Suppl. 1): S3–5.
13. Paul ML, Graybiel AM, David JC, Robertson HA. D1-like and D2-like dopamine receptors synergistically activate rotation and c-fos expression in the dopamine-depleted striatum in a rat model of Parkinson's disease. *J Neurosci* 1992; **12**: 3729–42.
14. Albanese A, Jenner P, Marsden CD, Stephenson JD. Bladder hyperreflexia induced in marmosets by 1-methyl-4-phenyl-1,2,3,6-tetrahydropyridine. *Neurosci Lett.* 1988; **87**: 46–50.
15. Tomiyama M, Kimura T, Maeda T, et al. A serotonin 5-HT1A receptor agonist prevents behavioral sensitization to L-DOPA in a rodent model of PD. *Neurosci Res* 2005; **52**: 185–94.
16. Srinivasan J, Schmidt WJ. Treatment with $\alpha2$ – adrenoceptor antagonists, 2 methoxy idazaoxan, protects 6- hydroxydopamine induced Parkinsonian symptoms in rats: neurochemical and behavioral evidence. *Behav Brain Res* 2004; **154**: 353–63.
17. Cawello W, Braun M, Boekens H. Absorption, disposition, metabolic fate, and elimination of the dopamine agonist rotigotine in man: administration by intravenous infusion or transdermal delivery drug metabolism and disposition. *Drug Metab Dispos* 2009; **37**: 2055–60.
18. LeWitt PA, Lyons KE, Pahwa R, SP 650 Study Group. Advanced Parkinson disease treated with rotigotine transdermal system: PREFER study. *Neurology* 2007; **68**: 1262–7.
19. Poewe WH, Rascol O, Quinn N, et al. Efficacy of pramipexole and transdermal rotigotine in advanced Parkinson's disease: a double-blind, double-dummy, randomised controlled trial. *Lancet Neurol* 2007; **6**: 513–20.
20. Trenkwalder C, Kies B, Rudzinska M, et al. Rotigotine effects on early morning motor function and sleep in Parkinson's disease: a double-blind, randomized, placebo-controlled study (RECOVER). *Mov Disord* 2011; **26**: 90–9.
21. Ray Chaudhuri K, Martinez-Martin P, Antonini A, et al. Rotigotine and specific non-motor symptoms of Parkinson's disease: post hoc analysis of RECOVER. *Parkinsonism Relat Disord* 2013; **19**: 660–5.
22. Kassubek J, Ray Chaudhuri K, Zesiewicz T, et al. Rotigotine transdermal system and evaluation of pain in patients with Parkinson's disease: a post hoc analysis of the RECOVER study. *BMC Neurology* 2014; **14**: 42.
23. Trenkwalder C, Kies B, Dioszeghy P, et al. Rotigotine transdermal system for the management of motor function and sleep disturbances in Parkinson's disease: results from a 1-year, open-label extension of the RECOVER study. *Basal Ganglia* 2012; **2**: 79–85.
24. Chen JJ, Swope DM, Dashtipour K, Lyons KE. Transdermal rotigotine: a clinically innovative dopamine-receptor agonist for the management of Parkinson's disease. *Pharmacotherapy* 2009; **29**: 1452–67.
25. Metta V, Muzerengi S, Ray Chadhuri K. Rotigotine: first dopamine agonist transdermal patch. *Prescriber* 2007; **18**: 19–30.
26. Weintraub D, Nirenberg MJ. Impulse control and related disorders in Parkinson's disease. *Neurodegener Dis* 2013; **11**: 63–71.
27. Rizos A, Martinez-Martin P, Martin A, et al. European multicentre survey of tolerability rates and impulse

28. Priano L, Albani G, Brioschi A, et al. Transdermal Apomorphine permeation from microemulsions: a new treatment in Parkinson's disease. *Mov Disord* 2004; **19**: 937–42.
29. Woitalla D, Müller T, Benz S, Horowski R, Przuntek H. Transdermal lisuride delivery in the treatment of Parkinson's disease. *J Neural Transm Suppl* 2004; **68**: 89–95.
30. Dimitrova T, Bara-Jiminez W, Thomas M, et al. Continuous dopaminergic stimulation with lisuride TTS (patch) in moderately advanced parkinsonian patients. *Neurology* 2006; **66** (Suppl. 2): A185.
31. Corrodi H, Farnebo LO, Fuxe K, Hamberger B, Ungerstedt U. ET 495 (piribedil) and brain catecholamine mechanisms: evidence for stimulation of dopamine receptors. *Eur J Pharmacol* 1972; **20**: 195–204.
32. Montastruc JL, Ziegler M, Rascol O, Malbezin M. A randomized, double-blind study of a skin patch of a dopaminergic agonist, piribedil, in Parkinson's disease. *Mov Disord* 1999; **14**: 336–41.
33. Kapoor R, Turjanski N, Frankel J, et al. Intranasal apomorphine: a new treatment in Parkinson's disease. *J Neurol Neurosurg Psychiatry* 1990; **53**: 1015.
34. Kleedorfer B, Turjanski N, Ryan R, et al. Intranasal apomorphine in Parkinson's disease. *Neurology* 1991; **41**: 761–2.
35. van Laar T, Jansen EN, Essink AW, Neef C. Intranasal apomorphine in parkinsonian on–off fluctuations. *Arch Neurol* 1992; **49**: 482–4.
36. Sam E, Jeanjean AP, Maloteaux JM, Verbeke N. Apomorphine pharmacokinetics in parkinsonism after intranasal and subcutaneous application. *Eur J Drug Metab Pharmacokinet.* 1995; **20**: 27–33.
37. Dewey RB Jr, Maraganore DM, Ahlskog JE, Matsumoto JY. Intranasal apomorphine rescue therapy for parkinsonian "off" periods. *Clin Neuropharmacol* 1996; **19**: 193–201.
38. Esteban Muñoz J, Martí MJ, Marín C, Tolosa E. Long-term treatment with intermittent intranasal or subcutaneous apormorphine in patients with levodopa-related motor fluctuations. *Clin Neuropharmacol* 1997; **20**: 245–52.
39. Dewey RB Jr, Maraganore DM, Ahlskog JE, Matsumoto JY. A double-blind, placebo-controlled study of intranasal apomorphine spray as a rescue agent for off-states in Parkinson's disease. *Mov Disord* 1998; **13**: 782–7.
40. Wickremaratchi M, Hadjikoutis S, Weiser R, et al. Efficacy and tolerability of intranasal apomorphine powder (INAP) 5mg as rescue therapy in subjects with Parkinson's disease (PD) complicated by motor fluctuations. *J Neurol Neurosurg Psychiatry* 2003; **74**: 1448–60.
41. Deleu D, Hanssens Y, Northway MG. Subcutaneous apomorphine: an evidence-based review of its use in Parkinson's disease. *Drugs Aging* 2004; **21**: 687–709.
42. Schwab RS, Amador LV, Lettvin JY. Apomorphine in Parkinson's disease. *Trans Am Neurol Assoc* 1951; **56**: 251–3.
43. Cotzias GC, Papavasiliou PS, Tolosa ES, Mendez JS, Bell-Midura M. Treatment of Parkinson's disease with apomorphines. Possible role of growth hormone. *The N Engl J Med* 1976; **294**: 567–72.
44. Stibe CM, Lees AJ, Kempster PA, Stern GM. Subcutaneous apomorphine in parkinsonian on–off oscillations. *Lancet* 1988; **331**: 403–6.
45. Chaudhuri KR, Critchley P, Abbott RJ, Pye IF, Millac PAH. Subcutaneous apomorphine for on–off oscillations in Parkinson's disease. *Lancet* 1988; **332**: 1260.
46. LeWitt PA. Subcutaneously administered apomorphine: pharmacokinetics and metabolism. *Neurology* 2004; **62** (Suppl. 4): S8–11.
47. Nicolle E, Pollak P, Serre-Debeauvais F, et al. Pharmacokinetics of apomorphine in parkinsonian patients. *Fundam Clin Pharmacol* 1993; **7**: 245–52.
48. Manson AJ, Hanagasi H, Turner K, et al. Intravenous apomorphine therapy in Parkinson's disease: clinical and pharmacokinetic observations. *Brain* 2001; **124**: 331–40.
49. Hofstee DJ, Neef C, van Laar T, Jansen EN. Pharmacokinetics of apomorphine in Parkinson's disease: plasma and cerebrospinal fluid levels in relation to motor responses. *Clin Neuropharmacol* 1994; **17**: 45–52.
50. Frankel JP, Lees AJ, Kempster PA, Stern GM. Subcutaneous apomorphine in the treatment of Parkinson's disease. *J Neurol Neurosurg Psychiatry* 1990; **53**: 96–101.
51. Pollak P, Champay AS, Gaio JM, et al. [Subcutaneous administration of apomorphine in motor fluctuations in Parkinson's disease]. *Rev Neurol (Paris)* 1990; **146** : 116–22 (in French).
52. Hughes AJ, Bishop S, Kleedorfer B, et al. Subcutaneous apomorphine in Parkinson's disease: response to chronic administration for up to five years. *Mov Disord* 1993; **8**: 165–70.
53. Stocchi F, Bramante L, Monge A, et al. Apomorphine and lisuride infusion. A comparative long-term study. *Adv Neurol* 1993; **60**: 653–5.
54. Poewe W, Kleedorfer B, Wagner M, Bosch S, Schelosky L. Continuous subcutaneous apomorphine infusions for fluctuating Parkinson's disease. Long-term follow-up in 18 patients. *Adv Neurol* 1993; **60**: 656–9.
55. Kreczy-Kleedorfer B, Wagner M, Bösch S, Poewe W. [Long-term results of continuous subcutaneous apomorphine pump therapy in patients with advanced Parkinson disease]. *Nervenarzt* 1993; **64**: 221–5 (in German).

56. Gancher ST, Nutt JG, Woodward WR. Apomorphine infusional therapy in Parkinson's disease: clinical utility and lack of tolerance. *Mov Disord* 1995; **10**: 37–43.
57. Colzi A, Turner K, Lees AJ. Continuous subcutaneous waking day apomorphine in the long term treatment of levodopa induced interdose dyskinesias in Parkinson's disease. *J Neurol Neurosurg Psychiatry* 1998; **64**: 573–6.
58. Pietz K, Hagell P, Odin P. Subcutaneous apomorphine in late stage Parkinson's disease: a long-term follow-up. *J Neurol Neurosurg Psychiatry* 1998; **65**: 709–16.
59. Wenning GK, Bösch S, Luginger E, Wagner M, Poewe W. Effects of long-term, continuous subcutaneous apomorphine infusions on motor complications in advanced Parkinson's disease. *Adv Neurol* 1999; **80**: 545–8.
60. Stocchi F, Vacca L, De Pandis MF, et al. Subcutaneous continuous apomorphine infusion in fluctuating patients with Parkinson's disease: long-term results. *Neurol Sci.* 2001; **22**: 93–4.
61. Kanovsky P, Kubova D, Bares M, et al. Levodopa-induced dyskinesias and continuous subcutaneous infusions of apomorphine: results of a two-year, prospective follow-up. *Mov Disord* 2002; **17**: 188–91.
62. Manson AJ, Turner K, Lees AJ. Apomorphine monotherapy in the treatment of refractory motor complications of Parkinson's disease: long-term follow-up study of 64 patients. *Mov Disord* 2002; **17**: 1235–41.
63. Di Rosa AE, Epifanio A, Antonini A, et al. Continuous apomorphine infusion and neuropsychiatric disorders: a controlled study in patients with advanced Parkinson's disease. *Neurol Sci* 2003; **24**: 174–5.
64. Morgante L, Basile G, Epifanio A, et al. Continuous apomorphine infusion (CAI) and neuropsychiatric disorders in patients with advanced Parkinson's disease: a follow-up of two years. *Arch Gerontol Geriatr Suppl* 2004; **9**: 291–6.
65. Tyne HL, Parsons J, Sinnott A, et al. A 10 year retrospective audit of long-term apomorphine use in Parkinson's disease. *J Neurol* 2004; **251**: 1370–4.
66. Katzenschlager R, Hughes A, Evans A, et al. Continuous subcutaneous apomorphine therapy improves dyskinesias in Parkinson's disease: a prospective study using single-dose challenges. *Mov Disord* 2005; **20**: 151–7.
67. De Gaspari D, Siri C, Landi A, et al. Clinical and neuropsychological follow up at 12 months in patients with complicated Parkinson's disease treated with subcutaneous apomorphine infusion or deep brain stimulation of the subthalamic nucleus. *J Neurol Neurosurg Psychiatry* 2006; **77**: 450–3.
68. Garcia Ruiz PJ, Sesar Ignacio A, Ares Pensado B, et al. Efficacy of long-term continuous subcutaneous apomorphine infusion in advanced Parkinson's disease with motor fluctuations: a multicenter study. *Mov Disord* 2008; **23**: 1130–6.
69. Martinez-Martin P, Reddy P, Antonini A, et al. Chronic subcutaneous infusion therapy with apomorphine in advanced Parkinson's disease compared to conventional therapy: a real-life study of non-motor effect. *J Parkinson's Dis* 2011; **1**: 197–203.
70. Antonini A, Isaias IU, Rodolfi G, et al., A 5-year prospective assessment of advanced Parkinson disease patients treated with subcutaneous apomorphine infusion or deep brain stimulation, *J Neurol* 2011; **258**: 579–85.
71. Drapier S, Gillioz AS, Leray E, et al. Apomorphine infusion in advanced Parkinson's patients with subthalamic stimulation contraindications. *Parkinsonism Relat Disord* 2012; **18**: 40–4.
72. Alegret M, Valldeoriola F, Marti M, et al. Comparative cognitive effects of bilateral subthalamic stimulation and subcutaneous continuous infusion of apomorphine in Parkinson's disease. *Mov Disord* 2004; **19**: 1463–9.
73. Todorova A. Ray Chaudhuri K. Subcutaneous apomorphine and non motor symptoms in Parkinson's disease. *Parkinsonism Relat Disord* 2013; **19**: 1073–8.
74. Ray Chaudhuri K, Abbott RJ, Millac PAH. Subcutaneous apomorphine for parkinsonian patients with psychiatric side effects on oral treatment. *J Neurol Neurosurg Psychiatry* 1991; **54**: 372–3.
75. Ellis C, Lemmens G, Parkes JD, et al. Use of apomorphine in parkinsonian patients with neurospsychiatric complications of oral treatment. *Parkinsonism Relat Disord* 1997; **3**: 103–7.
76. van Laar T, Postuma AG, Drent M. Continuous subcutaneous infusion of apomorphine can be used safely in patients with Parkinson's disease and pre-existing visual hallucinations. *Parkinsonism Relat Disord* 2010; **16**: 71–2.
77. Issacson S, Ray Chaudhuri K. Morning akinesia and the potential role of gastroparesis – managing delayed onset of first daily dose of oral levodopa in patients with Parkinson's disease. *European Neurological Review* 2013; **8**: 82–4.
78. Mathers SE, Kempster PA, Law PJ, et al. Anal sphincter dysfunction in Parkinson's disease. *Arch Neurol* 1989; **46**: 1061–4.
79. Edwards LL, Quigley EM, Harned RK, Hofman R, Pfeiffer RF. Defecatory function n Parkinson's disease: response to apomorphine. *Ann Neurol* 1993; **33**: 490–3.
80. Tison F, Wiart L, Guatterie M, et al. Effects of central dopaminergic stimulation by apomorphine on swallowing disorders in Parkinson's disease. *Mov Disord* 1996; **11**: 729–32.
81. Reuter I, Ellis CM, Ray Chaudhuri K. Nocturnal subcutaneous apomorphine infusion in Parkinson's disease and restless legs syndrome. *Acta Neurol Scand* 1999; **100**: 163–7.

82. Tribl GG, Sycha T, Kotzailias N, Zeitlhoger J, Auff E. Apomorphine in idiopathic restless legs syndrome: an exploratory study. *J Neurol Neurosurg Psychiatry* 2005; **76**: 181–5.
83. Magennis B, Cashell A, O'Brien D, Lynch T. An audit of apomorphine in the management of complex idiopathic Parkinson's disease in Ireland. *Mov Disord* 2012; **27** (Suppl. 1): S44.
84. Todorova A, Martin A, Okai D, et al. Assessment of impulse control disorders in Parkinson's patients with infusion therapies: a single centre experience. *Mov Disord* 2013; **28** (Suppl. 1): S133.
85. Corsini GU, Del Zompo M, Gessa GL, Mangoni A. Therapeutic efficacy of apomorphine combined with an extracerebral inhibitor of dopamine receptors in Parkinson's disease. *Lancet* 1979; **313**: 954–6.
86. Stocchi F, Ruggieri S, Antonini A, et al. Subcutaneous lisuride infusion in Parkinson's disease: clinical results using different modes of administration. *J Neural Transm* 1988; **27**: 27–33.
87. Krause W, Nieuweboer B, Ruggieri S, Stocchi F, Suchy I. Pharmacokinetics of lisuride after subcutaneous infusion. *J Neural Transm Suppl* 1988; **27**: 71–4.
88. Stocchi F, Ruggieri S, Vacca L, Olanow CW. Prospective randomized trial of lisuride infusion versus oral levodopa in patients with Parkinson's disease. *Brain* 2002; **125**: 2058–66.
89. Heinz A, Suchy I, Klewin I, et al. Long-term observation of chronic subcutaneous administration of lisuride in the treatment of motor fluctuations in Parkinson's disease. *J Neural Transm Park Dis Dement Sect* 1992; **4**: 291–301.
90. Obeso JA, Luquin MR, Vaamonde J, Martinez Lage JM. Subcutaneous administration of lisuride in the treatment of complex motor fluctuations in Parkinson's disease. *J Neural Transm Suppl* 1988; **27**: 17–25.
91. Critchley PH, Grandas Perez F, Quinn NP, Parkes JD, Marsden CD. Continuous subcutaneous lisuride infusions in Parkinson's disease. *J Neural Transm Suppl*. 1988; **27**: 55–60.
92. Vaamonde J, Luquin MR, Obeso JA. Subcutaneous lisuride infusion in Parkinson's disease. Response to chronic administration in 34 patients. *Brain* 1991; **114**: 601–17.
93. Hayashi R, Tako K, Makishita H, Koyama J, Yanagisawa N. Efficacy of a low-dose subcutaneous lisuride infusion in Parkinson's disease. *Intern Med* 1998; **37**: 444–8.
94. Hofmann C, Penner U, Dorow R, et al. Lisuride, a dopamine receptor agonist with 5-HT2B receptor antagonist properties: absence of cardiac valvulopathy adverse drug reaction reports supports the concept of a crucial role for 5-HT2B receptor agonism in cardiac valvular fibrosis. *Clin Neuropharmacol* 2006; **29**: 80–6.
95. Canesi M, Mariani C, Isaias IU, Pezzoli G. Night-time use of Rotigotine in advanced Parkinson's disease. *Funct Neurol* 2010; **25**: 201–3.
96. Todorova A, Martinez-Martin P, Martin A, et al. Daytime apomorphine infusion combined with transdermal Rotigotine patch therapy is tolerated at 2 years: a 24-h treatment option in Parkinson's disease. *Basal Ganglia* 2013; **3**: 127–30.

Chapter 7

Oral and infusion levodopa therapy in the management of Parkinson's disease

M. Angela Cenci-Nilsson and Per Odin

Introduction

The clinical diagnosis of Parkinson's disease (PD) is based on the identification of bradykinesia and at least one additional feature among rigidity, resting tremor and postural instability. These clinical features have been estimated to appear when at least 50% of the nigral dopamine neurons and 70% of putaminal dopamine tissue contents are lost [1]. Dopaminergic imaging suggests that at least 30% of the dopamine storage capacity (measured by ^{18}F-DOPA uptake) and 50% of putamen dopamine transporters have been lost by the onset of contralateral limb bradykinesia and rigidity [2]. In addition to the above motor symptoms, a number of nonmotor symptoms are associated with PD. These include gastrointestinal, cardiovascular, urological and psychiatric symptoms, as well as problems with vision, pain and sleep [3].

There is general agreement that the typical motor features of PD depend on putaminal dopamine depletion. Indeed, these features respond well to dopaminergic treatments, the most effective being levodopa (L-DOPA), a dopamine precursor that can cross the blood–brain barrier. Treatment with levodopa contributes significantly to improvements in the quality of life of people with PD and increases their expected life length (reviewed in [4]). Moreover, treatment with peroral levodopa is relatively well tolerated and inexpensive [5]. Many of nonmotor symptoms may also respond to levodopa treatment [3]. Because of the above reasons, levodopa is currently considered the "gold standard" for the symptomatic treatment of PD [4, 5]. However, the response to levodopa changes with disease progression, becoming complicated by motor fluctuations and dyskinesias in a majority of patients within a few years. As will be discussed below, these motor complications can become disabling, calling for a reduction in oral levodopa dosage and/or for its replacement with advanced invasive treatments. Moreover, levodopa is poorly effective against clinical features that mainly depend on the degeneration of nondopaminergic systems. These include some nonmotor symptoms as well as motor features that occur in advanced disease stages, such as freezing of gait and falls [6]. In this chapter, we will review the history of levodopa pharmacotherapy in PD, the complications of this therapy, the options currently available to optimize oral treatment with levodopa, and recent advances in developing methods for a more continuous levodopa delivery.

History of levodopa therapy in Parkinson's disease

The discovery of dopamine as a central neurotransmitter at the end of the 1950s represents a pivotal moment in the modern pharmacotherapy of PD [7]. Soon after this basic discovery, Hornykiewicz reported dopamine deficiency in the brains of PD patients [8]. In 1961, Hornykiewicz and Birkmayer performed a trial with intravenous levodopa in a group of 20 patients and reported that levodopa dramatically improved akinetic motor deficits [9]. At the same time, and independently, a research group in Montreal evaluated the effects of oral levodopa administration in PD patients, reporting a beneficial effect of the treatment on the parkinsonian symptom of rigidity [10]. The breakthrough for levodopa as a therapeutic agent in PD came in 1967, when George Cotzias in New York introduced a high-dose levodopa regimen with gradual dose increments [11], whose principles are still applied today. Levodopa received US Food and Drug Administration approval in 1970. The addition of inhibitors of peripheral DOPA decarboxylases to the amino acid preparations [12] represented an important milestone toward the development of a better therapy. Indeed, inhibitors of peripheral DOPA decarboxylases (such as carbidopa and benserazide) reduce the peripheral side effects of levodopa (e.g. nausea and vomiting), increase the proportion of the active amino acid that is available to the brain and allow a significant overall reduction in drug dosage (reviewed in [4]). The advent of levodopa revolutionized the treatment of PD by greatly improving the symptoms and increasing the life expectancy of the patients (reviewed in [4, 5]). It soon became apparent, however, that this treatment was not devoid of complications. Already at the beginning of the 1970s, abnormal involuntary movements (dyskinesia) were reported as a common dose-limiting side effect of levodopa. Involuntary movements could occur very early after the initiation of levodopa treatment, but their incidence and severity were reported to increase with time [12].

Levodopa: biochemistry, pharmacokinetics and pharmacodynamics

3,4-Dihydroxyphenyl-L-alanine (abbreviated to L-DOPA but commonly referred to as levodopa) is the immediate precursor of dopamine, to which it is converted in one enzymatic reaction catalysed by aromatic L-amino acid decarboxylase (also referred to as DOPA decarboxylase). In contrast to dopamine, levodopa can cross the blood–brain barrier, utilizing the endothelial transporter for aromatic amino acids (reviewed in [13]). Once in the brain, levodopa becomes decarboxylated to dopamine also in the very advanced stages of PD, as documented by positron emission tomography studies of in vivo dopamine release in human subjects (reviewed in [13]). In contrast, in advanced PD the ability of levodopa to be decarboxylated to dopamine is reduced [13].

Following oral administration, levodopa is rapidly absorbed from the small intestine, but its absorption depends both on the rate of gastric emptying and on the pH and amino acid concentration of the gastric contents (reviewed in [4, 5]). Indeed, levodopa is mainly absorbed via the plasma membrane transporter for aromatic amino acids in the intestinal mucous epithelium. An amino acid-rich meal would therefore delay the absorption of levodopa due to competition between the drug and dietary amino acids for transepithelial transport mechanisms. Plasma levodopa concentrations usually peak between 1 and 2 h after an oral dose, and the plasma half-life is usually between 1.5 and 3 h (reviewed in [4]).

In early disease stages, treatment with levodopa produces a sustained motor benefit, lasting over hours or days, which is referred to as the "long-duration response" [14]. As the disease becomes more advanced, the long-duration response diminishes, the effect of each levodopa dose become shorter and the patient's motor status becomes highly dependent on the actual plasma levels of the drug. The patient can now feel that the benefit "wears off" and symptoms reappear a few hours after taking the medication [14]. At these stages, a close correlation can be established between the pharmacokinetic profile of levodopa and the fluctuating symptomatology (Table 7.1) [15].

The first-line strategy to manage motor fluctuations is to divide the daily levodopa dose into several smaller doses. The dose fractionation results in a more continuous supply of levodopa and more stable plasma concentrations [17]. This strategy is, however, only partially effective because of poorer treatment compliance and

Table 7.1 Impact of disease progression on levodopa pharmacokinetics and pharmacodynamics. The table summarizes observations performed in Parkinson's disease patients on chronic levodopa therapy after standard test doses.

Levodopa plasma kinetics	
$t_{1/2}$a	Unchanged
$t_{1/2}$	Unchanged
C_{max}	Unchanged
T_{max}	Unchanged
Levodopa dynamics	
Latency to response	Shorter
Duration of response	Shorter
Magnitude of response	Unchanged or stronger
Levodopa concentration–effect relationship	
$t_{1/2}$eq	Shorter
E_{max}	Unchanged or increased
EC_{50}	Stronger
N	Larger

$t_{1/2}$a, absorption half-life; $t_{1/2}$, elimination half-life; C_{max}, peak plasma drug concentration; T_{max}, time to peak plasma drug concentration; $t_{1/2}$eq, equilibration half-life between plasma drug concentration and effect; EC_{50}, concentration producing 50% of maximum effect; E_{max}, maximum effect; N, Hill coefficient.

Modified from [16].

gastrointestinal factors. Indeed, the reduced gastrointestinal motility associated with PD can cause delays in the absorption of levodopa, and small levels of intestinal bacterial overgrowth can contribute to levodopa malabsorption as a consequence of an inflammation in the intestinal mucosa [18]. These phenomena are likely to contribute, at least in part, to the motor fluctuations (see below), and particularly to the "delayed on" and the "unpredictable on–off" phenomena.

Motor complications of dopamine replacement therapy

As PD gets more severe, it may become difficult to find a dose range at which levodopa relieves parkinsonian motor symptoms without inducing dyskinesias and abrupt fluctuations in the patient's clinical state. These motor complications have a clear negative impact on the health-related quality of life [19].

The most common pattern of levodopa-induced dyskinesia consists of choreiform movements that are most severe at the time when the drug is producing the maximal relief of parkinsonian motor symptoms, hence the term "peak-of-dose" or "on" dyskinesia. Dyskinesias can also occur at the beginning and end of a dose cycle (diphasic dyskinesias). A third type of dyskinesia is known as "off"-period dystonia; this commonly affects the foot and can be rather painful (reviewed in [4, 20]). Motor fluctuations are often rapid transitions between periods of good motor function ("on" phase) and periods of severe parkinsonian immobility ("off" phase). The earliest and most common type of motor fluctuation consists of a decreased duration of the effect of single levodopa doses, termed "wearing-off phenomenon" or "end-of-dose deterioration." With time, fluctuations between "on" and "off" phases can become unpredictable, and the effect of single doses may come with a delay ("delayed on") [14].

Meta-analyses of published studies indicate that these motor complications affect approximately 40% of PD patients after 4–6 years of levodopa therapy and up to 90% of the patients by 10 years of treatment (reviewed in [4]). A study comparing different assessment methods has shown that response fluctuations can be detected relatively early (< 5 years' disease duration) in a majority of levodopa-treated patients using questionnaires, particularly when both motor and nonmotor symptoms are considered [21].

The levodopa dose, the duration of levodopa treatment and the age of the patient seem to be key risk factors for developing motor fluctuations and dyskinesias. In the ELLDOPA (Early versus Later Levodopa in Parkinson Disease) trial, de novo patients were treated with 150, 300 or 600 mg of levodopa daily or placebo [22]. Already within the first 40 weeks of the trial, 29.7 and 16.5% of the patients in the group receiving 600 mg of levodopa daily developed wearing-off fluctuations and dyskinesias, respectively. In contrast, the incidence of fluctuations and dyskinesias were considerably lower in the groups receiving 300 and 150 mg of levodopa daily. In the latter group, the incidence of dyskinesias was similar to that in the placebo arm [22, 23].

The STRIDE-PD (Stalevo Reduction in Dyskinesia Evaluation in Parkinson's Disease) study is among the largest and longest double-blinded studies where dyskinesias and wearing off have been monitored over time [24]. The results from this study have been analyzed concerning the risk factors for motor complications, and it was confirmed that levodopa dosage represents the single most important risk. The factors most predictive of development of dyskinesias were, in order of impact: young age, high levodopa dose and low body weight. The most important predictive factors for wearing-off fluctuations were: young age, high levodopa dose and living in North America. The correlation between levodopa dose and dyskinesia incidence was almost linear. That the levodopa dose is an important factor for dyskinesia development had already been indicated by retrospective analyses. In addition to confirming these previous assumptions, the ELLDOPA and STRIDE-PD studies have also demonstrated the importance of levodopa dose for the risk of wearing off- fluctuations.

Nonmotor complications of dopamine replacement therapy

Dopamine replacement therapy in PD is also associated with neuropsychiatric complications, including confusion, hallucinations and sleep problems. Psychiatric complications appear in less than 5% of de novo patients on levodopa monotherapy [25]. This type of complication seems to be less common with levodopa than with other antiparkinsonian agents. Monotherapy with levodopa is, therefore, generally preferred to treat parkinsonian motor symptoms in patients presenting with dementia or hallucinations.

Patients on dopaminergic therapies may also experience impulse control disorders [26]. Large studies indicate that the prevalence of this group of complications is up to 17% when dopamine agonists are used, and only 6–7% when dopamine replacement therapy does not include dopamine agonists [26]. Levodopa has, however, been associated with the development of dopamine dysregulation syndrome [27], a condition whereby patients develop a craving for levodopa and self-medicate with much higher doses than needed for adequate control of their motor features. This condition appears to develop in patients with a particular vulnerability, and its prevalence has been estimated not to exceed 3–4% [27]. Punding is a characteristic behavioral feature often connected with impulse control disorders or dopamine dysregulation syndrome. The definition applies to patients engaging in repetitive and seemingly purposeless activities (usually examining, sorting or dismantling objects) for many hours. Its prevalence has been estimated to be about 1.5% [28].

At present, specific treatments for the above behavioral problems are lacking, and management strategies consist of modifying the regimen of dopamine replacement therapy (in particular, reducing or stopping the administration of dopamine agonists).

Finally, it has recently become recognized that motor complications are often accompanied by fluctuations in the severity of many nonmotor symptoms. When ten nonmotor symptoms (dysphagia, anxiety, depression, fatigue, excessive sweating, inner restlessness, pain, concentration/attention, dizziness and bladder urgency) were quantified in PD patients with motor fluctuations, it was demonstrated that all of these features, except for dysphagia, excessive sweating and bladder urgency, fluctuated in conjunction with the motor symptomatology, being generally more severe in motor "off" compared with "on" periods [29]. The temporal pattern of nonmotor fluctuations was, however, complex, and some nonmotor symptoms could be as severe (or even more severe) in the "on" state.

Oral levodopa treatment with standard immediate-release preparations

Standard levodopa pharmacotherapy consists of tablets for oral administration, which are usually taken from three to eight times per day depending on the individual response and disease stage (Figure 7.1). All levodopa preparations that are used today also contain an inhibitor of DOPA decarboxylases that does not cross the blood–brain barrier, such as carbidopa or benserazide. Treatment is commonly initiated with a daily dosage of 300–400 mg divided into three to four dose administrations. Most PD patients respond well to a levodopa dosage between 300 and 600 mg/day. Some patients may, however, require a much higher dose for a good effect. Unresponsiveness to levodopa can indicate that the patient does not have idiopathic PD but rather atypical parkinsonism (for example, multiple-system atrophy, progressive supranuclear palsy or corticobasal degeneration). To establish that the patient is unresponsive, it is recommended that levodopa dosage is titrated to at least 1000 mg/day, continuing this treatment for at least 8 weeks. The dosage ought to be increased slowly in order to avoid dopaminergic side effects. In the absence of antiparkinsonian effects, great attention should be paid to the occurrence of central side effects, such as somnolence, dyskinesias, mood changes or even worsening of motor symptoms, which can give an indication that the levodopa has been adequately absorbed and distributed.

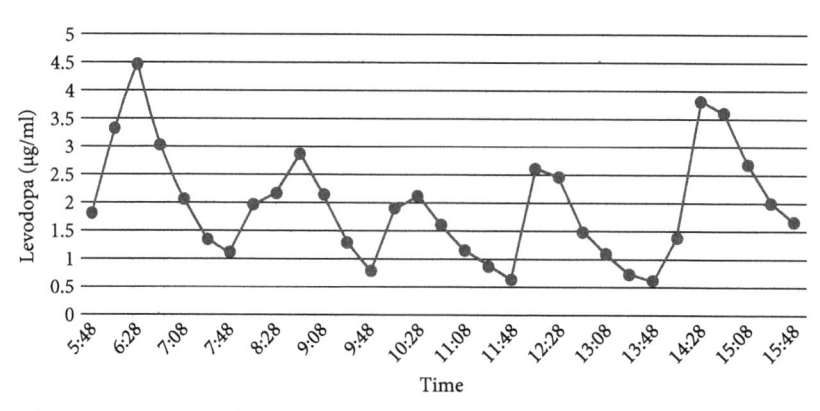

Figure 7.1 Levodopa plasma concentrations with standard oral therapy, for a patient taking five daily doses of levodopa/carbidopa perorally (100 + 100 + 75 + 75 + 100 mg every second hour).
Graph published with permission from Dag Nyholm.

A fast way of establishing whether levodopa has had an effect in the individual patient is to perform a so-called levodopa test. The patient is kept without PD medication for some hours (normally overnight) and then administered a standard peroral dose of levodopa. The effect of this dose on the motor symptomatology is monitored by clinical observation/examination, often including quantitative measurements of movement speed. A positive levodopa test is a good predictor of the effect of long-term dopaminergic treatment and aids in the diagnosis of idiopathic PD [30]. To define the levodopa test as positive, the recommended cut-off value consists of an improvement of the Unified Parkinson's Disease Rating Scale (UPDRS) III motor score by 14.5% to predict a good effect of long-term dopaminergic treatment or by 18% (to diagnose idiopathic PD) [30]. A negative test must be interpreted with caution, since many patients with a negative test may still respond to long-term dopaminergic therapy. A negative levodopa test should therefore never exclude a trial with dopaminergic treatment.

Sustained-release levodopa preparations

Controlled-release levodopa formulations were developed during the 1980s and became available in 1991. Controlled-release formulations consist of levodopa combined with either carbidopa or benserazide in a matrix designed to delay the release of the active substance. Compared with standard immediate-release tablets, controlled-release formulations have a longer T_{max} (time to maximum plasma concentration) and longer $t_{1/2}$ (biological half-life) [31, 32]. Plasma concentration profiles are less fluctuating and bioavailability is more unpredictable but generally lower than with immediate-release formulations, necessitating a 20–30% higher levodopa dose [33, 34]. Controlled-release formulations have a longer symptomatic effect, but this is counterpoised by a slower onset (Table 7.2).

The controlled-release formulations are seldom used in fluctuating patients because of their unpredictable absorption. Indeed, the irregularity of gastric emptying associated with PD becomes even more of a problem with controlled-release formulations compared with standard levodopa tablets, since the former have a lower administration frequency. Controlled-release formulations can be combined with immediate-release formulations to give a faster onset of effect, and this is especially common with the first dose of the day.

Table 7.2 Pharmacokinetics and pharmacodynamics of levodopa in controlled-release levodopa formulations versus standard-release formulations

Levodopa pharmacokinetics	
T_{max}	Longer (2–3-fold)
C_{max}	Lower (2–3-fold)
$t_{1/2}$	Unchanged
C4-h post-dose	Higher (2-fold)
Levodopa pharmacodynamics	
Latency to response	Longer
Duration of response	Unchanged or shorter
Magnitude of response	Unchanged or less
Dyskinesias	Unchanged or more

T_{max}, time to peak plasma concentration following dose administration; C_{max}, maximum plasma drug concentration after a single-dose administration; $t_{1/2}$, plasma elimination half-life; C4-h post-dose, concentration 4 h after dose administration.

Modified from [16].

In some dyskinetic PD patients, the controlled-release formulations have been reported to generate prominent dyskinesias toward the end of the day [33].

Results concerning the efficacy of controlled-release-based treatments versus standard therapy have varied among studies. Two trials have described an improved effect of controlled-release formulations on daily "off" time and/or activities of daily living [35, 36], another trial reported no difference regarding "on" time without dyskinesias [37], and a long-term study in de novo-treated patients could not demonstrate any advantage of the controlled-release formulations with respect to the incidence of motor fluctuations and dyskinesias [38]. In the clinical practice, controlled-release formulations are seldom used for daytime therapy but are often given as a late evening dose to cover the night hours.

Levodopa and catechol-*O*-methyltransferase inhibitors

Peripheral inhibition of the metabolism of levodopa via catechol-*O*-methyltransferase (COMT) prolongs the drug's elimination half-life and raises its central bioavailability (Table 7.3). This inhibition can be achieved using the COMT inhibitors entacapone or tolcapone, both in use since the late 1990s (reviewed in [5]). Tolcapone seems to be slightly more effective than entacapone but has a limited use due to the risk

Table 7.3 Main effects of catechol-O-methyltransferase inhibitors intake on levodopa pharmacokinetics and pharmacodynamics

Levodopa pharmacokinetics	
T_{max}	Unchanged or longer
C_{min}	Higher
C_{max}	Unchanged or higher
$t_{1/2}$	Longer (25–50%)
AUC	Larger (40%)
Levodopa pharmacodynamics	
Latency to response	Unchanged or longer
Duration of response	Unchanged or longer
Magnitude of response	Unchanged
Dyskinesias	Unchanged or stronger

T_{max}, time to peak plasma concentration following dose administration; C_{min}/C_{max}, minimum/maximum plasma drug concentration after a single-dose administration; $t_{1/2}$, plasma elimination half-life; AUC, area under the plasma concentration–time curve.

Modified from [16].

of potentially fatal hepatotoxicity. Tolcapone is mostly recommended for patients who have not had a satisfactory effect with entacapone. The use of tolcapone also necessitates regular laboratory liver function tests.

With repeated dosing in clinical routine use, COMT inhibition increases the relative bioavailability and plasma elimination half-life of levodopa. Both C_{min} and C_{max} are increased, and the degree of fluctuations is relatively unchanged [39, 40]. A slow increase in C_{max} during the day has also been reported upon repeated dosing [40]. The clinical benefit of adding a COMT inhibitor therefore mainly consists in decreasing "off" time and increasing "on" time accordingly [41–43]. If the COMT inhibitor is added to an unchanged levodopa dosage in patients with dyskinesias, the latter might increase in severity. Therefore, levodopa should be reduced by 20–30% when adding a COMT inhibitor [41–43].

Since 2003, a combination of levodopa/carbidopa/entacapone in one tablet has been available. The STRIDE-PD study was performed to investigate whether the use of levodopa/carbidopa/entacapone tablets in early-stage untreated patients could reduce the risk of developing dyskinesias [24]. Unexpectedly, initiating treatment with the combined formulation failed to delay or reduce dyskinetic complications of levodopa therapy. In fact, the use of levodopa/carbidopa/entacapone was associated both with a shorter time to onset and with an increased frequency of dyskinesias. These results might depend on the fact that the administration frequency (four doses per day) failed to provide a continuous dopaminergic stimulation and that, moreover, the group treated with the combined formulation received larger levodopa dose equivalents [24].

A new COMT inhibitor in clinical development is opicapone, which provides a very sustained effect making a once-daily administration possible. In a potential clinical application of this treatment, it would be advisable to carefully adjust the levodopa dosage in order to compensate for the relatively enhanced levodopa levels that opicapone will afford [44].

Levodopa and monoamine oxidase type B inhibitors

As an alternative to the approach described above, inhibitors of monoamine oxidase type B (MAO-B, the enzyme that degrades dopamine) can be used to prolong the central effects of levodopa. Two compounds producing a selective and irreversible inactivation of MAO-B are selegiline and rasagiline, both of which are currently used in the treatment of PD (reviewed in [4]). Although there are no direct comparative studies, indirect comparisons would seem to indicate that rasagiline is slightly more effective and better tolerated than selegiline. In a large, double-blinded trial performed in levodopa-treated patients with motor fluctuations, once-daily administration of rasagiline was found to reduce mean daily "off" time and improve PD motor symptoms, an effect similar to that of entacapone [45]. In addition to prolonging the effect of levodopa, MAO-B inhibitors have mild efficacy against PD motor symptoms when used as a monotherapy (reviewed in [4, 5]). In various in vivo and in vitro models of dopamine neuron injury, MAO-B inhibitors exhibited antiapoptotic and antioxidant properties that associated with neuroprotective effects (partly reviewed in [4]). A clinical trial in untreated PD patients has attempted to assess the potential disease-modifying properties of rasagiline using a delayed-start study design. While early treatment with rasagiline at a dose of 1 mg/day provided benefits suggestive of a possible disease-modifying effect, early treatment with 2 mg/day of rasagiline did not [46]. Because the two very similar drug doses were associated with different outcomes, the results of this study cannot support the hypothesis that rasagiline has disease-modifying properties in PD.

Levodopa and dopamine agonists

Based on their chemical structure, dopamine agonists are divided into two main categories, namely, ergot derivative (e.g. bromocriptine, lisuride, pergolide, cabergoline) and nonergot-type (e.g. ropinirole, pramipexole, rotigotine) compounds. With the exception of apomorphine, all dopamine agonists have a much longer elimination half-life than levodopa and preferential activity at D2/D3 receptors (reviewed in [4]). Accumulating evidence has indicated that some ergot derivatives increase the risk of fibrosis, i.e. an excess formation of connective tissue in organs and body structures (see, for example, the recent statement entitled "Restrictions on use of medicines containing ergot derivatives" issued by the European Medicines Agency at http://www.ema.europa.eu/). Because of this risk, nonergot dopamine agonists are commonly preferred today.

Dopamine agonists are effective as a monotherapy in early disease stages [47, 47]. They are also effective in early combination with levodopa, allowing for a reduction in levodopa dosage. For some of these substances, it has been shown that their late combination with levodopa can improve motor fluctuations [49, 50]. Studies comparing early monotherapy with dopamine agonists versus levodopa have consistently shown than de novo treatment with dopamine agonists gives significantly fewer dyskinesias during a period of 3–5 years [51, 52]. Whether this benefit would persist for a period of longer than 5 years is currently unknown. It is also unknown whether initiating treatment with dopamine agonists will protect from dyskinesia development when levodopa is added later on in the course of PD. Indeed, the addition of levodopa must be taken into consideration at later disease stages, given that dopamine agonist monotherapy may not suffice to manage a more severe parkinsonian syndrome. A number of basic experimental studies have provided indications that dopamine agonists may exert neuroprotective or neurorestorative effects (partly reviewed in [4]), but no clinical study are currently available to support the potential disease-modifying properties of this class of compounds. Dopamine agonists have specific side effects that might limit their clinical usability, including daytime tiredness, impulse control disorders, psychotic symptoms, and heart and lung fibrosis (for ergot-type compounds) (reviewed in [4]).

Levodopa and amantadine

Amantadine was originally developed as a prophylactic treatment against Asian influenza, although it is no longer recommended for this indication. Serendipitous observations in the 1960s indicated that amantadine could reduce parkinsonian symptoms. An early double-blind, placebo-controlled trial of amantadine monotherapy in PD patients concluded that amantadine provided a significant although very mild benefit over placebo, and that this substance could be effective in the long-term treatment of some patients [53]. Today, the most common indication of amantadine in PD is the treatment of levodopa-induced dyskinesias. Indeed, amantadine was the only pharmacological agent to be recognized as efficacious for this indication in a recent evidence-based medicine review [54]. The antidyskinetic and antiparkinsonian properties of amantadine are generally attributed to its antagonistic action at N-methyl-D-aspartate (NMDA) glutamate receptors (reviewed in [4]), although this compound can potentially interact with a number of additional molecular targets.

Novel levodopa formulations in the pipeline

New oral levodopa formulations and prodrugs are currently in different phases of clinical development. A new extended-release formulation of levodopa/carbidopa is IPX066. This product consists of beads, containing levodopa/carbidopa, that dissolve at various rates to allow intestinal absorption to occur over a longer period of time than with standard levodopa/carbidopa tablets. This formulation was compared with standard levodopa/carbidopa in 27 patients in a randomized crossover study over 8 + 8 days [55]. While plasma levodopa concentrations increased at a similarly rapid rate following a single dose of IPX066 versus standard levodopa, the former resulted in significantly more sustained plasma levels [55]. In a recent study, the drug was compared with immediate-release levodopa in 393 patients with fluctuations, and IPX066 was shown to significantly reduce "off" time [56].

Other treatments under clinical development include a sustained-release levodopa prodrug (XP21279), a carbidopa subcutaneous patch (ND0611), a mixed MAO-B and glutamate inhibitor (safinamide) and inhalable levodopa (reviewed in [57]).

Like IPX066, XP21279 aims to overcome the pharmacokinetic limitations of levodopa and to provide more continuous exposure. However, in contrast to IPX066, XP21279 employs a prodrug that is absorbed by high-capacity nutrient transporters expressed throughout the gastrointestinal tract, which will be enzymatically converted to levodopa inside the body. The engagement of a more widespread transport mechanism is meant to give a larger interface and more time for drug absorption. A phase 2 trial of XP21279 in PD patients with motor fluctuations demonstrated that XP21279 provides less variability in levodopa concentration than the standard oral tablets, and that XP21279-treated subjects had a 30% reduction in mean daily "off" time [58].

ND0611 is a continuously delivered carbidopa solution administered subcutaneously by a pump patch with a number of microneedles [57]. Preclinical studies have suggested that co-administration of ND0611 with standard oral levodopa results in more sustained plasma levels of levodopa. In a phase 1 study in healthy volunteers, ND0611 was administered with levodopa/carbidopa immediate-release preparations, and was found to improve the levodopa half-life, area under the curve, trough levels and time with concentrations above 1000 ng/ml (reviewed in [57]). Further developments of this method consist of combining levodopa and carbidopa in the pump patch. A phase 1, double-blind, placebo-controlled trial in healthy people has shown that this combination is well tolerated and that adequate plasma concentrations are reached (reviewed in [57]).

Fast-acting levodopa formulations can be an aid to the management of motor fluctuations (particularly the "delayed on" phenomenon). An orally administered formulation of levodopa/carbidopa that disintegrates rapidly on the tongue and does not require swallowing is available in some countries (Parcopa®, see http://www.drugs.com/pro/parcopa.html). In addition, effervescent tablets containing the water-soluble levodopa methyl ester melevodopa hydrochloride have been developed recently. It has so far not been possible to demonstrate a significant advantage of these formulations in reducing "off" time above standard levodopa/carbidopa tablets, although trends favoring the fast-acting formulations have been reported by some clinical trials (e.g. [59]). Fast-acting formulations may therefore be useful in certain patients or for particular purposes (e.g. to shorten the interval from drug administration to clinical improvement).

A microtablet formulation containing 5 mg of levodopa and 1.25 mg of carbidopa is being launched in Sweden. This preparation aims to afford a more individualized levodopa dosage, as 5 mg dosing steps can be used. The tablets are delivered by an electronic dose dispenser, making frequent dosing feasible, and also enabling symptom registration by integrating a diary in the portable dispenser. The system has been compared with levodopa/carbidopa/entacapone in a recent phase 1 study. A total of 300 mg of levodopa was given to healthy volunteers either as microtablets every 2 h and 24 min (75 + 45 + 45 + 45 + 45 + 45 mg) or as levodopa/carbidopa/entacapone (100/25/200 mg) every 6 h. The microtablet treatment resulted in significantly more stable levodopa plasma concentrations [60].

Levodopa infusion therapy

The first studies describing intravenous delivery of levodopa were published in 1975 [61] and were soon followed by several other reports showing an improvement of motor fluctuations [62]. In most cases the patients were, however, only treated for a few days. It proved practically difficult to give levodopa intravenously over longer times. The first experiences with intraduodenal levodopa infusion were published in 1986 [63], reporting an effect comparable to intravenous levodopa delivery. This was later confirmed in several other studies (reviewed in [64]). Duodenal delivery methods for broad clinical application have been developed mainly in two different centers, the University of New Brunswick (NB, Canada) and the University of Uppsala (Sweden). A collaboration between the Department of Neurology and the Department of Galenic Pharmacy at the University of Uppsala led to the development of levodopa/carbidopa intestinal gel (LCIG) (reviewed in [65]). This is a combination of levodopa (20 mg/ml) and carbidopa (5 mg/ml) in the form of a pseudoplastic cellulose-based gel and is delivered with a portable infusion pump. For short-term therapy, a nasoduodenal catheter is used. For long-term treatment, a catheter is inserted into the duodenum by surgical intervention (percutaneous endoscopic gastrostomy or jejunostomy, the latter being performed in only a few cases) (Figure 7.2). Open and randomized controlled studies have shown that LCIG achieves stabilization of both plasma levodopa concentrations and clinical status, producing a strong reduction in motor fluctuations and an overall increase in time spent in the "on" phase (reviewed in [65]). A blinded, randomized, crossover study comparing LCIG monotherapy with

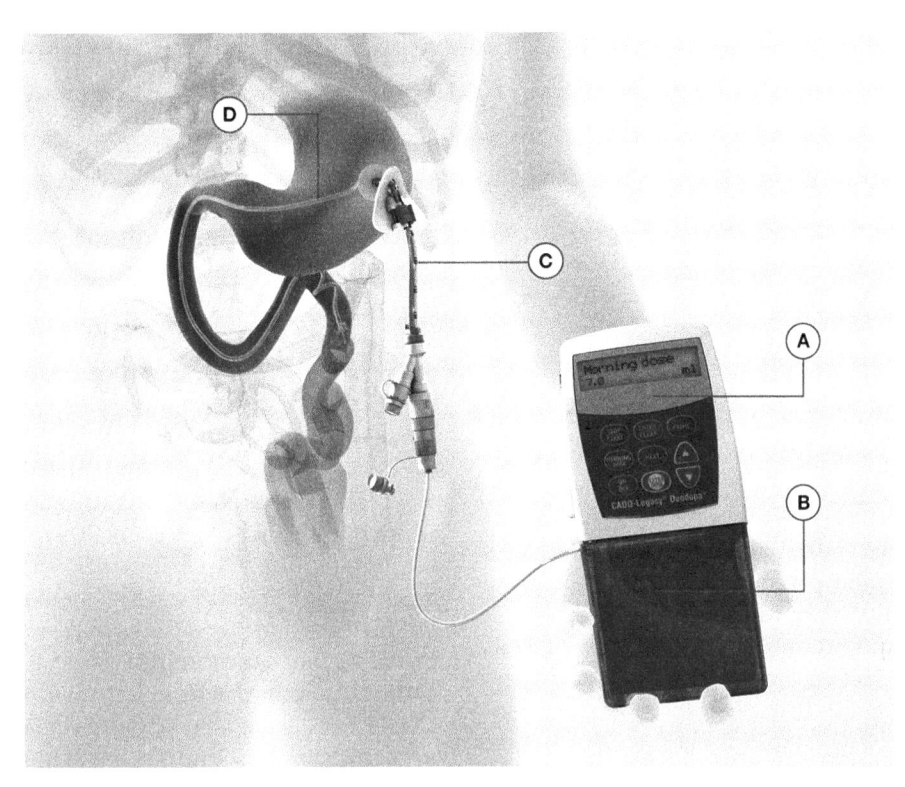

Figure 7.2 The levodopa/carbidopa gel (LCIG) infusion system. (A) Pump. (B) LCIG cassette. (C) Percutaneous endoscopic gastrostomy. (D) Intestinal tube. (A black and white version of this figure will appear in some formats. For the color version, please refer to the plate section.) (Permission for publication from AbbVie Inc.)

individually optimized peroral therapy has demonstrated an increase in daily "on" time from 81 to 100% and an improvement in health-related quality of life upon treatment with LCIG (reviewed in [65]). In a second randomized, double-blind, double-dummy study, 71 patients were randomized to active pump or active levodopa/carbidopa standard therapy [66]. The use of LCIG reduced "off" time and increased "on" time without dyskinesias significantly more than tablet treatment. Health-related quality of life improved significantly more in the LCIG group. A large, open-label study of 192 patients receiving LCIG treatment over 1 year demonstrate improvements in "off" time, "on" time without dyskinesias and health-related quality of life similar to those reported in the randomized controlled study [67]. Preliminary data indicate that moving from peroral levodopa to infusion therapy can also improve nonmotor symptomatology [68].

Treatment with LCIG is initially given only during the daytime. In patients experiencing nighttime problems with parkinsonism symptoms and suboptimal sleep, a 24 h treatment can bring significant improvement without inducing further side effects or tolerance [69]. Adverse events of LCIG therapy are related to the infusion method. These include peritonitis, dislocation or occlusion of the duodenal catheter, and leakage in the infusion system. Acute or chronic neuropathies and reversible encephalopathies have been reported in some patients receiving LCIG treatment, and a link has been suggested between these conditions and adverse metabolic effects of the treatment, such as deficiency of vitamin B6 or B12 and/or elevated plasma homocysteine levels (reviewed in [5]). However, the pathogenic mechanisms underlying the observed neuropathies/encephalopathies remain to be clarified. The main drawback associated with levodopa infusion therapy does not lie in these infrequent potential complications but rather in its high costs, which would become prohibitive for the healthcare systems in most countries if this treatment were to be prescribed routinely to PD patients with motor fluctuations.

Summary of current treatment strategies in early Parkinson's disease

There are several expert reviews and consensus documents giving detailed advice on the clinical management PD, for example evidence-based reviews commissioned by the Movement Disorders Society [54, 70] and the European Federation of Neurological Societies (EFNS) [71], and the guidelines issued by the UK National Institute for Health and Care Excellence (NICE). In this and the following section, we shall summarize and expand concepts and conclusions that have already been expressed in different sections of this chapter.

A common strategy is to start the treatment with substances other than levodopa in order to delay the development of motor fluctuations and dyskinesias. Often, this is the preferred option in young-onset PD patients. As long as levodopa is not given, the risk for fluctuations and dyskinesias is very low. However, it is not clear whether starting without levodopa reduces the long-term risk for motor fluctuations and dyskinesias. This strategy includes using MAO-B inhibitors (also as monotherapy in the beginning, when the patients have very slight symptomatology), dopamine agonists and amantadine, separately or in combinations. Levodopa is added when a stronger symptomatic effect is needed. It should, however, be considered that dopamine agonists entail other types of side effects, including daytime tiredness and impulse control disorders. An alternative is to introduce levodopa early but in small doses (preferably below 400 mg daily to avoid motor complications). In older patients, therapy is most often started with levodopa. If dopamine replacement therapy does not include levodopa, at least 50% of the patients will need addition of levodopa within a couple of years. If a fast and strong control of PD motor symptoms is needed, levodopa can also be considered for early treatment in young patients, but the dosage should be kept low and the addition of other types of medications should be considered. Since there is no evidence for an advantage of early treatment with either sustained-release levodopa or combined levodopa and COMT inhibition, the standard immediate-release levodopa/carbidopa tablets can be used from the start. Studies are currently being performed to establish whether and how different types of dopamine replacement therapy may affect nonmotor symptoms. In the future, the results of these studies might affect the individual choice of PD treatment, especially in early disease phases.

Summary of current treatment strategies in advanced-stage Parkinson's disease

In PD patients exhibiting motor fluctuations and dyskinesias, the most effective approach to therapy seems to consist of a more continuous and individually titrated dopaminergic stimulation. A common first step in this direction is to divide the levodopa dose into a larger number of small doses (dose fragmentation). The doses must, however, be large enough to achieve a significant effect on PD motor symptoms. It must also be considered that a large number of drug administrations may lead to worse patient compliance.

A common problem is early-morning akinesia, which refers to the occurrence of PD symptoms early in the morning before the first medication dose produces an effect. This problem can be counteracted by using fast-acting dopaminergic drugs in the morning and/or by adding long-acting dopaminergic drugs in the late evening (sustained-release levodopa, levodopa plus COMT inhibitor or long-acting dopamine agonists).

As explained in other sections of this chapter, dose failures and a delayed "on" period often result from an interaction between medication and food intake, because of the competition between levodopa and aromatic amino acids for transepithelial (and transendothelial) transport mechanisms. The patient will therefore be advised to take their medication separately from larger meals. In some cases, a dietary protein restriction might become necessary. In addition to these measures, it is often valuable to present the patient with the possibility of using a fast-acting dopaminergic drug upon demand. This can be either soluble levodopa orally (effect onset after 20–40 min) or subcutaneous injections of the dopamine agonist apomorphine with injection pens (effect onset after 5–15 min).

Dyskinesias normally improve by levodopa dosage fragmentation or by dose reductions that are afforded by combined treatment with dopamine agonists, MAO-B inhibitors or COMT inhibitors. If dyskinesias remain a problem, the addition of drugs with antidyskinetic properties, i.e. amantadine or clozapine, can be considered (reviewed in [4]).

In patients with significant motor fluctuations and/or dyskinesias in spite of optimized peroral/transdermal therapy, the so-called advanced PD therapies can be considered. These include subcutaneous infusion of apomorphine with portable pumps, intraduodenal infusion of LCIG with portable pumps and deep-brain stimulation. The latter is also indicated when the patient has a tremor that does not respond in a satisfactory way to pharmacological therapy.

Nonpharmacological approaches to continuous dopaminergic stimulation, such as dopamine cell transplants or gene therapy for enzyme replacement, are currently at the stage of late preclinical/early clinical development (reviewed in [4]). However, whether these novel approaches will be devoid of motor complications remains to be seen. For example, clinical trials of intrastriatal dopamine cell grafting in PD have shown that transplants can induce a new form of dyskinesia that is unrelated to the timing of levodopa administration, which has been termed graft-induced dyskinesia (reviewed in [4]).

References

1. Fearnley JM, Lees AJ. Ageing and Parkinson's disease: substantia nigra regional selectivity. *Brain* 1991; **114**: 2283–301.
2. Brooks DJ, Frey KA, Marek KL, et al. Assessment of neuroimaging techniques as biomarkers of the progression of Parkinson's disease. *Exp Neurol* 2003; **184** (Suppl. 1): S68–79.
3. Chaudhuri KR, Odin P, Antonini A, Martinez-Martin P. Parkinson's disease: the non-motor issues. *Parkinsonism Relat Disord* 2011; **17**: 717–23.
4. Cenci MA, Ohlin KE, Odin P. Current options and future possibilities for the treatment of dyskinesia and motor fluctuations in Parkinson's disease. *CNS Neurol Disord Drug Targets* 2011; **10**: 670–84.
5. Salat D, Tolosa E. Levodopa in the treatment of Parkinson's disease: current status and new developments. *J Parkinsons Dis* 2013; **3**: 255–69.
6. Heremans E, Nieuwboer A, Vercruysse S. Freezing of gait in Parkinson's disease: where are we now? *Curr Neurol Neurosci Rep* 2013; **13**: 350.
7. Carlsson A, Lindqvist M, Magnusson T. 3,4-Dihydroxyphenylalanine and 5-hydroxytryptophan as reserpine antagonists. *Nature* 1957; **180**: 1200.
8. Hornykiewicz O. Die Topische Lokalisation und das Verhalten von Noradrenalin und Dopamin in der Substantia Nigra des normalen und Parkinsonkranken Menschen. *Wien Klin Wochenschr* 1963; **75**: 309–12.
9. Birkmayer W, Hornykiewicz O. Der L-Dioxyphenylalanin (=DOPA – Effekt bei der Parkinson-akinase. *Wien Klin Wschr* 1961; **73**: 787–8.
10. Barbeau A, Sourkes TL, Murphy GF. Les catécholamines dans la maladie de Parkinson. In: de Ajuriaguerra J, ed. *Monoamines et Systéme Nerveaux Central*. Geneva: Georg & Cie SA; 1962; 247–62.
11. Cotzias G, Van Woert M, Schiffer L. Aromatic amino acids and modification of parkinsonism. *N Engl J Med* 1967; **276**: 374–9.
12. Calne DB, Reid JL, Vakil SD et al. Idiopathic Parkinsonism treated with an extracerebral decarboxylase inhibitor in combination with levodopa. *BMJ* 1971; **3**: 729–32.
13. Cenci MA, Lundblad M. Post- versus presynaptic plasticity in L-DOPA-induced dyskinesia. *J Neurochem* 2006; **99**: 381–92.
14. Nutt JG, Holford NH. The response to levodopa in Parkinson's disease: imposing pharmacological law and order. *Ann Neurol* 1996; **39**: 561–73.
15. Nyholm D, Lennernas H, Gomes-Trolin C, Aquilonius SM. Levodopa pharmacokinetics and motor performance during activities of daily living in patients with Parkinson's disease on individual drug combinations. *Clin Neuropharmacol* 2002; **25**: 89–96.
16. Contin M, Martinelli P. Pharmacokinetics of levodopa. *J Neurol* 2010; **257** (Suppl. 2): S253–61.
17. Nyholm D, Stepien V. Levodopa fractionation in Parkinson's disease. *J Parkinsons Dis* 2014; **4**: 89–96.
18. Fasano A, Bove F, Gabrielli M, et al. The role of small intestinal bacterial overgrowth in Parkinson's disease. *Mov Disord* 2013; **28**: 1241–9.
19. Chapuis S, Ouchchane L, Metz O, Gerbaud L, Durif F. Impact of the motor complications of Parkinson's disease on the quality of life. *Mov Disord* 2005; **20**: 224–30.
20. Fabbrini G, Brotchie JM, Grandas F, Nomoto M, Goetz CG. Levodopa-induced dyskinesias. *Mov Disord* 2007; **22**: 1379–89; quiz 523.
21. Stacy M, Bowron A, Guttman M, et al. Identification of motor and nonmotor wearing-off in Parkinson's disease: comparison of a patient questionnaire versus a clinician assessment. *Mov Disord* 2005; **20**: 726–33.
22. Fahn S. Parkinson disease, the effect of levodopa, and the ELLDOPA trial. Earlier vs later L-DOPA. *Arch Neurol* 1999; **56**: 529–35.
23. Fahn S. A new look at levodopa based on the ELLDOPA study. *J Neural Transm Suppl* 2006: 419–26.
24. Stocchi F, Rascol O, Kieburtz K, et al. Initiating levodopa/carbidopa therapy with and without entacapone in early Parkinson disease: the STRIDE-PD study. *Ann Neurol* 2010; **68**: 18–27.
25. Castro-Garcia A. [Psychiatric complications of L-dopa: physiopathology and treatment]. *Rev Neurol.* 1997; **25** (Suppl. 2): S157–62.
26. Weintraub D, Koester J, Potenza MN, et al. Impulse control disorders in Parkinson disease: a cross-sectional study of 3090 patients. *Arch Neurol* 2010; **67**: 589–95.
27. O'Sullivan SS, Evans AH, Lees AJ. Dopamine dysregulation syndrome: an overview of its epidemiology,

mechanisms and management. *CNS Drugs* 2009; **23**: 157–70.
28. Spencer AH, Rickards H, Fasano A, Cavanna AE. The prevalence and clinical characteristics of punding in Parkinson's disease. *Mov Disord* 2011; **26**: 578–86.
29. Storch A, Schneider CB, Wolz M, et al. Nonmotor fluctuations in Parkinson disease: severity and correlation with motor complications. *Neurology* 2013; **80**: 800–9.
30. Rossi P, Colosimo C, Moro E, Tonali P, Albanese A. Acute challenge with apomorphine and levodopa in Parkinsonism. *Eur Neurol.* 2000; **43**: 95–101.
31. Cedarbaum JM, Kutt H, McDowell FH. A pharmacokinetic and pharmacodynamic comparison of Sinemet CR (50/200) and standard Sinemet (25/100). *Neurology* 1989; **39** (Suppl. 2): 38–44; discussion 59.
32. MacMahon DG, Sachdev D, Boddie HG, et al. A comparison of the effects of controlled-release levodopa (Madopar CR) with conventional levodopa in late Parkinson's disease. *J Neurol Neurosurg Psychiatry* 1990; **53**: 220–3.
33. Gauthier S, Amyot D. Sustained release antiparkinson agents: controlled release levodopa. *Can J Neurol Sci* 1992; **19** (Suppl.): 153–5.
34. Sage JI, Mark MH. Pharmacokinetics of continuous-release carbidopa/levodopa. *Clin Neuropharmacol* 1994; **17** (Suppl. 2): S1–6.
35. Block G, Liss C, Reines S, Irr J, Nibbelink D. Comparison of immediate-release and controlled release carbidopa/levodopa in Parkinson's disease. A multicenter 5-year study. The CR First Study Group. *Eur Neurol* 1997; **37**: 23–7.
36. Wolters EC, Tesselaar HJ. International (NL-UK) double-blind study of Sinemet CR and standard Sinemet (25/100) in 170 patients with fluctuating Parkinson's disease. *J Neurol* 1996; **243**: 235–40.
37. Jankovic J, Schwartz K, Vander Linden C. Comparison of Sinemet CR4 and standard Sinemet: double blind and long-term open trial in parkinsonian patients with fluctuations. *Mov Disord* 1989; **4**: 303–9.
38. Koller WC, Hutton JT, Tolosa E, Capilldeo R. Immediate-release and controlled-release carbidopa/levodopa in PD: a 5-year randomized multicenter study. Carbidopa/Levodopa Study Group. *Neurology* 1999; **53**: 1012–9.
39. Baas H, Zehrden F, Selzer R, et al. Pharmacokinetic-pharmacodynamic relationship of levodopa with and without tolcapone in patients with Parkinson's disease. *Clin Pharmacokinet* 2001; **40**: 383–93.
40. Kuoppamaki M, Korpela K, Marttila R, et al. Comparison of pharmacokinetic profile of levodopa throughout the day between levodopa/carbidopa/entacapone and levodopa/carbidopa when administered four or five times daily. *Eur J Clin Pharmacol* 2009; **65**: 443–55.

41. Adler CH, Singer C, O'Brien C, et al. Randomized, placebo-controlled study of tolcapone in patients with fluctuating Parkinson disease treated with levodopa-carbidopa. Tolcapone Fluctuator Study Group III. *Arch Neurol* 1998; **55**: 1089–95.
42. Deane KH, Spieker S, Clarke CE. Catechol-O-methyltransferase inhibitors for levodopa-induced complications in Parkinson's disease. *Cochrane Database Syst Rev* 2004; CD004554.
43. Kurth MC, Adler CH, Hilaire MS, et al. Tolcapone improves motor function and reduces levodopa requirement in patients with Parkinson's disease experiencing motor fluctuations: a multicenter, double-blind, randomized, placebo-controlled trial. Tolcapone Fluctuator Study Group I. *Neurology* 1997; **48**: 81–7.
44. Rocha JF, Santos A, Falcao A, et al. Effect of moderate liver impairment on the pharmacokinetics of opicapone. *Eur J Clin Pharmacol* 2014; **70**: 279–86.
45. Rascol O, Brooks DJ, Melamed E, et al. Rasagiline as an adjunct to levodopa in patients with Parkinson's disease and motor fluctuations (LARGO, Lasting effect in Adjunct therapy with Rasagiline Given Once daily, study): a randomised, double-blind, parallel-group trial. *Lancet* 2005; **365**: 947–54.
46. Olanow CW, Rascol O, Hauser R, et al. A double-blind, delayed-start trial of rasagiline in Parkinson's disease. *N Engl J Med* 2009; **361**: 1268–78.
47. Adler CH, Sethi KD, Hauser RA, et al. Ropinirole for the treatment of early Parkinson's disease. The Ropinirole Study Group. *Neurology* 1997; **49**: 393–9.
48. Shannon KM, Bennett JP Jr, Friedman JH. Efficacy of pramipexole, a novel dopamine agonist, as monotherapy in mild to moderate Parkinson's disease. The Pramipexole Study Group. *Neurology* 1997; **49**: 724–8.
49. Fahn S, Oakes D, Shoulson I, et al. Levodopa and the progression of Parkinson's disease. *N Engl J Med* 2004; **351**: 2498–508.
50. Rinne UK, Bracco F, Chouza C, et al. Cabergoline in the treatment of early Parkinson's disease: results of the first year of treatment in a double-blind comparison of cabergoline and levodopa. The PKDS009 Collaborative Study Group. *Neurology* 1997; **48**: 363–8.
51. Oertel WH, Wolters E, Sampaio C, et al. Pergolide versus levodopa monotherapy in early Parkinson's disease patients: The PELMOPET study. *Mov Disord* 2006; **21**: 343–53.
52. Rascol O, Brooks DJ, Korczyn AD, et al. A five-year study of the incidence of dyskinesia in patients with early Parkinson's disease who were treated with ropinirole or levodopa. 056 Study Group. *N Engl J Med* 2000; **342**: 1484–91.
53. Butzer JF, Silver DE, Sahs AL. Amantadine in Parkinson's disease. A double-blind,

placebo-controlled, crossover study with long-term follow-up. *Neurology* 1975; **25**: 603–6.

54. Fox SH, Katzenschlager R, Lim SY, *et al.* The Movement Disorder Society Evidence-Based Medicine Review Update: Treatments for the motor symptoms of Parkinson's disease. *Mov Disord* 2011; **26** (Suppl. 3): S2–41.

55. Hauser RA, Ellenbogen AL, Metman LV, *et al.* Crossover comparison of IPX066 and a standard levodopa formulation in advanced Parkinson's disease. *Mov Disord* 2011; **26**: 2246–52.

56. Hauser RA, Hsu A, Kell S, *et al.* Extended-release carbidopa-levodopa (IPX066) compared with immediate-release carbidopa-levodopa in patients with Parkinson's disease and motor fluctuations: a phase 3 randomised, double-blind trial. *Lancet Neurol* 2013; **12**: 346–56.

57. Hauser RA. Future treatments for Parkinson's disease: surfing the PD pipeline. *Int J Neurosci.* 2011; **121** (Suppl. 2): 53–62.

58. LeWitt PA, Huff FJ, Hauser RA, *et al.* Double-blind study of the actively transported levodopa prodrug XP21279 in Parkinson's disease. *Mov Disord* 2014; **29**: 75–82.

59. Stocchi F, Zappia M, Dall'Armi V, *et al.* Melevodopa/carbidopa effervescent formulation in the treatment of motor fluctuations in advanced Parkinson's disease. *Mov Disord* 2010; **25**: 1881–7.

60. Nyholm D, Ehrnebo M, Lewander T, *et al.* Frequent administration of levodopa/carbidopa microtablets vs levodopa/carbidopa/entacapone in healthy volunteers. *Acta Neurol Scand* 2013; **127**: 124–32.

61. Shoulson I, Glaubiger GA, Chase TN. On–off response. Clinical and biochemical correlations during oral and intravenous levodopa administration in parkinsonian patients. *Neurology* 1975; **25**: 1144–8.

62. Quinn N, Marsden CD, Parkes JD. Complicated response fluctuations in Parkinson's disease: response to intravenous infusion of levodopa. *Lancet* 1982; **320**: 412–5.

63. Kurlan R, Rubin AJ, Miller C, *et al.* Duodenal delivery of levodopa for on–off fluctuations in parkinsonism: preliminary observations. *Ann Neurol* 1986; **20**: 262–5.

64. Nyholm D. Enteral levodopa/carbidopa gel infusion for the treatment of motor fluctuations and dyskinesias in advanced Parkinson's disease. *Expert Rev Neurother* 2006; **6**: 1403–11.

65. Fernandez HH, Odin P. Levodopa-carbidopa intestinal gel for treatment of advanced Parkinson's disease. *Curr Med Res Opin.* 2011; **27**: 907–19.

66. Olanow CW, Kieburtz K, Odin P, *et al.* Continuous intrajejunal infusion of levodopa-carbidopa intestinal gel for patients with advanced Parkinson's disease: a randomised, controlled, double-blind, double-dummy study. *Lancet Neurol* 2014; **13**: 141–9.

67. Fernandez HH, Vanagunas A, Odin P, *et al.* Levodopa-carbidopa intestinal gel in advanced Parkinson's disease open-label study: interim results. *Parkinsonism Relat Disord* 2013; **19**: 339–45.

68. Honig H, Antonini A, Martinez-Martin P, *et al.* Intrajejunal levodopa infusion in Parkinson's disease: a pilot multicenter study of effects on nonmotor symptoms and quality of life. *Mov Disord* 2009; **24**: 1468–74.

69. Busk K, Nyholm D. Long-term 24-h levodopa/carbidopa gel infusion in Parkinson's disease. *Parkinsonism Relat Disord* 2012; **18**: 1000–1.

70. Seppi K, Weintraub D, Coelho M, *et al.* The Movement Disorder Society Evidence-Based Medicine Review Update: treatments for the non-motor symptoms of Parkinson's disease. *Mov Disord* 2011; **26** (Suppl. 3): S42–80.

71. Ferreira JJ, Katzenschlager R, Bloem BR, *et al.* Summary of the recommendations of the EFNS/MDS-ES review on therapeutic management of Parkinson's disease. *Eur J Neurol* 2013; **20**: 5–15.

Chapter 8
Catechol-*O*-methyltransferase inhibitors in the management of Parkinson's disease

Ilana Schlesinger and Amos D. Korczyn

The introduction of 3,4-dihydroxyphenylalanine (DOPA) to the treatment of Parkinson's disease (PD) has been a major scientific and clinical breakthrough in the treatment of this devastating disease. This can be seen from two aspects. The primary one is, of course, the enormous benefit to patients, but in addition there is the realization that understanding the biochemical deficits can provide a clue as to how replacement therapy can be successfully employed even in neurodegenerative diseases, providing significant symptomatic benefit if not cure. This has had a great impact on attempts to treat other neurodegenerative disorders, particularly Alzheimer's disease. Unfortunately, in spite of miraculous effects on patients with early and advanced PD and the motor benefits afforded to them, it became clear that DOPA does not slow the neurodegenerative process and its effects are purely symptomatic. Consequently, the dose of drug that is needed to control the motor manifestations has to be increased gradually as the disease progresses. It quickly became clear also that of the two DOPA isomers, only the levorotatory stereoisomer, L-DOPA (levodopa), was able to afford therapeutic benefits, and chemical means to separate the isomers were developed. In practice, only levodopa is now used in the treatment of PD, resulting in an improved safety profile. Soon after came the recognition that some of the adverse effects associated with the drug were the result of peripheral, rather than central, conversion of levodopa to dopamine, which, unlike levodopa, has significant autonomic activity [1]. Unlike levodopa, dopamine does not cross the blood–brain barrier, and thus this metabolite does not contribute to the clinical benefits afforded by levodopa, and in fact causes significant adverse effects, particularly autonomic.

The enzyme involved in the transformation of levodopa to dopamine, L-amino acid decarboxylase (L-AAD, also called DOPA decarboxylase), is widespread in the body, with high concentrations present in the liver. Two agents were developed that could inhibit this enzyme, and both are still in use – carbidopa and benserazide. At present, practically all patients who require treatment with levodopa receive it in a fixed-dose combination with one of these inhibitors. Of course, as it is essential that levodopa be converted to dopamine in the brain, the L-AAD inhibitors should not cross the blood–brain barrier.

The inhibition of peripheral L-AAD had another result, at first unappreciated, namely a prolongation of the biological half-life of levodopa (and therefore also of dopamine in the brain). The importance of this effect is manifested in advanced PD. Early on in PD, there is a dramatic beneficial effect of levodopa, known as the "honeymoon period." As the disease progresses and additional dopaminergic neurons are lost, there is a need to compensate for this by increasing the daily dose of levodopa. This is first manifested by shortening of the duration of action of individual levodopa doses, called the "end-of-dose" effect or "wearing off." Later on, other manifestations appear including "peak-of-dose" dyskinesias and erratic responses to levodopa (so-called unexpected "on–off", or yo-yoing). While the exact mechanism responsible for this erratic response is still elusive, it is at least partly dependent on pharmacokinetic factors such as plasma levels of levodopa. In particular, the phenomenon of wearing off, where the initial prolonged response to individual doses of levodopa is no longer maintained [2], limits patients' independence. Wearing off probably results from a combination of peripheral and central mechanisms. Peripheral mechanisms include delayed gastric emptying and impaired absorption due to dietary protein, and central mechanisms are mainly due to impaired

Parkinson's Disease: Current and Future Therapeutics and Clinical Trials, ed. Gálvez-Jiménez *et al.* Published by Cambridge University Press. © Cambridge University Press 2016.

capacity of the nigrostriatal dopaminergic neurons and their terminals to uptake, store and release dopamine. This problem becomes more severe as gastric emptying becomes more sluggish and more dopaminergic terminals degenerate [2]. Blockade of peripheral L-AAD, which prolongs the biological half-life of the drug, can only incompletely compensate for this

An alternative metabolic pathway for levodopa, in the brain and in the periphery, is through the activity of another enzyme, catechol-O-methyltransferase (COMT). Like L-AAD, this enzyme is widespread in the body, with high concentrations occurring particularly in the liver. Notably, when levodopa tablets are used, the chemical reaches the liver at high concentration through the portal system and is there exposed to enzymatic degradation. This so-called "first-pass effect" is of crucial importance in reducing the concentration of levodopa that reaches the brain. Inhibition of COMT results in slightly higher, and particularly more prolonged, plasma levels of levodopa, manifested as elevation of the area under the curve of the time–concentration curve to a given dose of levodopa. Inhibition of these two enzymes, L-AAD and COMT, does not have a direct antiparkinsonian effect, and they are used only as co-medications, or co-drugs. In particular, the prolongation of serum levels of levodopa offers a valuable benefit to patients with the wearing-off phenomenon [3].

In the brain, COMT is an extracellular enzyme that metabolizes the conversion of levodopa to 3-O-methyldopa and of dopamine to 3-methoxytyramine. It is associated with dopaminergic synapses but actually occurs outside the synapse. Its main physiological action is probably to limit diffusion of the biologically active neurotransmitter, dopamine (as well as norepinephrine), outside the desired site of action. Thus, COMT helps to maintain neurochemical stability in the central nervous system. The metabolism of levodopa by COMT results in its conversion to 3-O-methyldopa, which is inactive as a neurotransmitter but has a long biological half-life and can be converted back to levodopa (and consequently to dopamine). Thus, it may function as a depot prolonging the action of levodopa. Moreover, 3-O-methyldopa may compete with levodopa in uptake through the blood–brain barrier, and thus limit the availability of levodopa for conversion of dopamine centrally.

Normally, no or only very small amounts of levodopa exist in the central nervous system, but this situation is altered dramatically when levodopa is given as a drug and gets into the brain, causing huge amounts to accumulate in the extracellular space. Under these conditions levodopa may be degraded by COMT (and other enzymes), thus limiting the amount available for neuronal uptake and transformation into the active metabolite, dopamine.

The normal release of dopamine from nigrostriatal terminals in the striatum is primarily tonic. Conversely, levodopa administration results in fluctuations in serum and brain levels and pulsatile stimulation of brain dopamine receptors. The smoothing of fluctuations in serum levels of levodopa, provided by inhibition of L-AAD and of COMT, may theoretically reduce the motor fluctuations characteristic of advanced PD by providing more continuous dopaminergic stimulation. More importantly, the unnatural fluctuations of dopamine levels in the brain when levodopa is given to PD patients may contribute to receptoral or post-receptoral changes in the striatum or elsewhere in the brain, which may induce fluctuations that are pharmacodynamic, not pharmacokinetic, in nature. If this still unproven assumption is correct, then treatment with levodopa together with its two metabolic inhibitors might delay the appearance of these manifestations of advanced PD. Based on this speculation, treatment with both inhibitors as soon as levodopa is first prescribed was hypothesized to delay the appearance of motor fluctuations.

Four inhibitors of COMT have been developed, entacapone, tolcapone, opicapone and nebicapone. At present, only tolcapone and entacapone are available on the market. Tolcapone, entacapone and opicapone have a short half-life of 1.4–3.6 h. The standard dose of entacapone is 200 mg, and of tolcapone is 100 mg, and no titration is needed. The dose of opicapone is as yet undetermined and will be either 25 or 50 mg. Nebicapone has not yet been put on the market. Of the four COMT inhibitors, tolcapone and nebicapone inhibit brain COMT [4], whereas entacapone and opicapone do not cross the blood–brain barrier and thus are unable to inhibit COMT in the brain. It is unclear what exactly the consequences of this difference are, but they are unlikely to be large. Because dopamine itself is also a COMT substrate, COMT inhibition is expected to prolong even further the duration of action of a given levodopa dose. As stated above, COMT metabolizes dopamine into 3-O-dopamine. As the latter does not contribute directly to the antiparkinsonian effect of levodopa, and may even block dopamine receptors,

COMT inhibitors acting both in the periphery and centrally are theoretically advantageous.

To date, entacapone has been the most extensively studied COMT inhibitor. It is a peripherally acting, selective, reversible inhibitor of COMT. It prolongs the action of levodopa and indeed increases "on" time in patients with motor fluctuations. The main pharmacokinetic effect of COMT inhibitors is to prolong the biological half-life (i.e. the duration of action) of levodopa. Therefore, the area under the curve of the serum concentration of levodopa almost doubles. However, it may cause slight elevation of C_{max} (peak levodopa concentration). This may result in dopaminergic hyperstimulation, manifested as dyskinesias. The latter can usually be treated by reducing the individual levodopa dose [5]. Nausea, a side effect of levodopa, which is partly a central and partly a peripheral action, may also be increased. If this occurs, it can be managed by either dose reduction or the addition of domperidone. Because of the mechanism of action, entacapone (as well as the other COMT inhibitors) is ineffective unless given concomitantly with levodopa.

In repeated dosed, entacapone reduces the peak-to-trough variations of levodopa in the plasma, and thus presumably provides a more evenly sustained dopaminergic stimulation to the brain. The COMT(HH) genotype in PD patients enhances the effect of entacapone on the pharmacodynamics and pharmacokinetics of levodopa. The response to entacapone after repeated administrations and in heterozygous patients remains to be determined [6], as upregulation of the enzyme has been observed in red blood cells after 3 months of administration, suggesting that long-term administration may limit its efficacy [7]. The main indication for the use of COMT inhibitors is in the more advanced stages of the disease, when wearing off appears [8–13]. Based on the considerations mentioned above, the primary indication for COMT inhibitors is advanced PD, when patients have developed "end-of-dose" effects, "peak-of-dose" dyskinesias necessitating reduction of individual doses of the drug or severe response fluctuations. One point is patient selection. Patients recruited to the pivotal studies were mostly those with advanced disease with motor fluctuations. There are many ways to try and reduce the fluctuations, and it is not clear to what extent an attempt had been made to exploit alternatively methods before the patients were included in the studies.

Unfortunately, most of the pivotal studies cannot really be considered as double blind as entacapone causes urinary discoloration. Thus, to minimize the consequences of unblinding, later studies added an independent evaluator, a clinician, who was involved in the patients' care and who simply measured the relevant endpoints, such as the United Parkinson Disease Rating Scale (UPDRS) or time spent "off."

Several of the pivotal studies suffered from additional serious shortcomings. For example, the FILOMEN study [14] included patients at different disease stages and on different dosing regimens, ranging from two to ten times daily levodopa and entacapone administration. Obviously improvement cannot be expected for patients who need levodopa only twice daily, or if they take the medication every 1–2 h while awake. The fact that most patients received continuous-release preparations and many were also taking dopamine agonists further masks the potential benefits of entacapone.

The long-term benefits of entacapone are still not completely clear. Even though the clinical effects of COMT inhibitors are clear, data on long-term use are meager. In the NOMESAFE study, only 60% of patients continued to be treated for the full 3 years (including 30 months of open-label treatment) [15–16]. For example, in the NOMESAFE (Nordic Multicenter Study on Entacapone) study [16], while patients initially improved on entacapone, this benefit gradually diminished after 3 years, so that the duration of benefit from the first morning dose of levodopa, 2.1 h at baseline, extended initially to 2.8 h but then declined again to 2.5 h at the last evaluation. This could be the result of a reduced effect of the drug or a reflection of the progression of the disease, as would be expected after 3 years.

These studies, showing a clinically beneficial effect of entacapone, prompted studies that examined the benefits to PD patients with and without fluctuations. For instance, the UK–Irish Entacapone Study Group found entacapone to be beneficial in both fluctuating and nonfluctuating patients with PD in a randomized, placebo-controlled, double-blind, 6-month study [11].

Most patients suffering from PD are elderly and have comorbid conditions. Consequently, they consume a number of medications. The need to add COMT inhibitors is therefore an impediment, and may confuse the patients and decrease compliance. The practical solution to this problem was to design a tablet that contains the three elements: levodopa, carbidopa and entacapone. This combination, under the trade name Stalevo®, is now available in many countries. The short half-life of entacapone (about 2 h) is consistent with this procedure. One problem, however, is that inhibition of the enzyme is not immediate, and the short latency period may allow some levodopa still to be metabolized.

The encouraging results with entacapone, the concept that continuous dopaminergic stimulation may delay the appearance of motor fluctuations if started early in the disease course and the ease of use of Stalevo® were the driving force behind the STRIDE-PD (Stalevo Reduction in Dyskinesia Evaluation in Parkinson's Disease) study [17]. The study was an international, multicenter, randomized, double-blind, parallel-group, active-controlled study. Surprisingly, the study found that patients taking Stalevo® had a shorter time to onset of dyskinesia (hazards ratio, 1.29; $P=0.04$) and increased frequency at week 134 (42 vs 32%; $P=0.02$). This study has discouraged the initiation of Stalevo® as a first-line therapy in PD.

Thus, it appears that entacapone is efficacious in PD patients with motor fluctuations but nonefficacious as a symptomatic adjunct to levodopa in nonfluctuating patients and nonefficacious in the prevention and delay of motor complications [18]. Importantly, STRIDE-PD raised safety issues regarding the long-term use of Stalevo®. Before this study, it was appreciated that diarrhea is a relatively specific adverse effect of entacapone. Its underlying mechanism is unclear. Appearing in up to 14% of treated patients, diarrhea is the most significant adverse event associated with entacapone and may lead to discontinuation of therapy in as many as half of cases. The diarrhea usually appears within the first few weeks of therapy, but not immediately, and typically disappears soon after withdrawal [8]. As PD patients frequently suffer from constipation, the diarrhea, if mild, is not necessarily a problem. Future pharmacogenetic studies might identify patients susceptible to this effect.

In the STRIDE-PD study, 11 males developed prostate cancer, of whom nine had received Stalevo®. The odds ratio for the occurrence of prostate cancer in males taking Stalevo® was 4.19 (95% Confidence Interval: 0.90–19.63). Healthcare professionals were advised to be aware of this possible risk and follow current guidelines for prostate cancer screening. Furthermore, the US Food and Drug Administration stated that meta-analysis of several studies "appeared to show an increase in the risk of heart attack, stroke, and cardiovascular death for people taking" Stalevo® but also stated "findings were not clear." No recommendations regarding this possible side effect were issued [19]. Other less common side effects of entacapone include sleep attacks.

As stated above, an important pathway for the metabolism of levodopa is methylation by COMT. In this reaction, COMT uses S-adenosylmethionine as a methyl-group donor. Demethylation of S-adenosylmethionine forms S-adenosyl-homocysteine, which is hydrolyzed to homocysteine. Thus, the methylation of levodopa may interfere with homocysteine metabolism, leading to hyperhomocysteinemia. Although inhibition of COMT should theoretically prevent or reduce levodopa-induced hyperhomocysteinemia, results from several prospective studies are conflicting, possibly owing to differences in vitamin status of the study participants. In patients with low or low–normal folate levels, levodopa administration is associated with a greater increase in homocysteine and concomitant entacapone administration is associated with a greater reduction in homocysteine [20].

Interestingly, entacapone is a metal chelator and may therefore deplete the body of several metals, particularly iron. However, to date there are no reports of clinical problems due to this effect.

Tolcapone inhibits COMT in the brain as well as in the periphery. Meta-analysis of studies using COMT inhibitors has suggested that it may be more efficacious than entacapone [21]. This has been shown in studies such as the Entacapone to Tolcapone Switch Study where patients receiving entacapone switched to tolcapone or continued to receive entacapone [22]. However, its efficacy was overshadowed by its side effects. Patients receiving this medication had elevation of serum levels of liver enzymes and in some also overt evidence of hepatotoxicity. Elevation of liver enzymes occurred in 1–3% of patients receiving tolcapone; this may disappear even on continued treatment, and in most patients after drug withdrawal. However, a few cases of fatal acute fulminant hepatic failure have occurred. This resulted in almost total elimination of tolcapone from the market for a few years. It was reintroduced with a black box warning regarding hepatotoxicity [23]. It was deemed necessary that patients provide informed consent prior to being treated with this medication. The medication should not be initiated if the patient exhibits clinical evidence of liver disease or serum liver enzymes greater than the upper limit of normal. Liver function tests are recommended at baseline and periodically (i.e. every 2–4 weeks) for the first 6 months of therapy. After the first 6 months, periodic monitoring is recommended. Patients who fail to show substantial clinical benefit within 3 weeks of initiation of treatment should be withdrawn from tolcapone because of the risk of hepatotoxicity with no apparent improvement. After the medication was reintroduced, the company distributing the medication (Valeant Pharmaceuticals International) claimed that severe hepatocellular damage occurred in only 0.04% of patients, mostly with no clinical signs or symptoms. The mechanism underlying tolcapone-induced hepatotoxicity is not known.

Tolcapone can also cause diarrhea, constipation, headache, abdominal pain and urine discoloration.

Nebicapone, a peripheral and central COMT inhibitor showed promising results in preliminary studies. In 250 PD patients with motor fluctuations treated with levodopa/carbidopa or levodopa/benserazide (four to eight daily doses) given different doses of the medication or placebo, "off" time decreased significantly compared with placebo with 150 mg of nebicapone [24]. However, clinically relevant elevation in liver enzymes was observed in four of 46 patients with the nebicapone 150 mg dose. No further studies with this medication have been reported.

Opicapone, a peripheral COMT inhibitor, has shown no hepatotoxicity. It was evaluated in a phase 3 trial where it was compared with placebo and entacapone in PD patients suffering from end-of-dose motor fluctuations. A clinical benefit of opicapone has been reported in the company's website but has yet to be published in medical journals.

Based on the considerations mentioned above, the primary indication for COMT inhibitors is advanced PD, when patients have developed "end-of-dose" effects, "peak-of-dose" dyskinesias necessitating reduction of individual doses of the drug or severe response fluctuations. However, the option of using COMT inhibitors must be seen against other possibilities of dealing with these situations.

Several options are available for the treatment of PD patients in the more advanced stages. When wearing off appears, more frequent dosing of levodopa, long-acting levodopa preparations, and the addition of selegiline or rasagiline as well as longer-acting dopamine agonists [25] have all shown efficacy. However, most of these methods have drawbacks. The addition of yet another agent increases the possibility of confusion as well as of interaction with any of the many other drugs the patient may take (for neurological or other indications), and therefore the addition of a drug that will prolong the action of levodopa itself is expected to benefit these patients. This is particularly so as levodopa remains the most potent of all antiparkinsonian drugs.

As mentioned above, several of the theoretical or actual benefits of more stable levodopa delivery can also be achieved through other means, such as duodenal infusion of levodopa. However, this is technically difficult and may cause severe complications and so has not achieved popularity. A more appealing option is to use direct-acting drugs such as cabergoline [26]. However, dopamine agonists are not selective to the brain, and their peripheral actions may cause significant side effects such as nausea and autonomic changes, particularly orthostatic hypotension [27], and those that are ergot derivatives may cause complications such as cardiac valve fibrosis. They are also considerably less potent than levodopa. The most effective agonist, apomorphine, is also not user friendly because of its poor gastrointestinal absorption and the need for repeated daily injections or a pump connected by a subcutaneous needle. The transdermal absorption of drugs such as rotigotine [28] is appealing, with similar efficacy to other dopamine agonists but with application site reactions [29]. Dopamine agonists may increase sleep time, and the reduced "off" time does not necessarily lead to functional improvement.

Several drug studies have so far been conducted in an attempt to answer some of the questions posed above [8–14, 30, 31]. While confirming the relative safety of both agents, they have not fully addressed relevant issues.

There is only limited information concerning comparisons between entacapone and dopamine agonists as no head-to-head study has been performed. In an open-label, multicenter study, tolcapone was compared with bromocriptine and was found to be somewhat more effective in advanced cases, although the differences were not very large and in many cases failed to reach statistical significance [16]. Recent results suggest that rasagiline is active in this situation. Although comparisons with COMT inhibitors still need to be made, available data from the LARGO study [32] suggest that the two drugs have similar efficacy. Since the two agents act through completely different mechanisms, it may be logical and interesting to study the effect of combining these therapies. Recent meta-analysis has in fact suggested that dopamine agonist therapy may be more effective than COMT inhibitor and monoamine oxidase type B (MAO-B) inhibitor therapy, which have comparable efficacy [21].

The relative advantages, if any, of entacapone versus long-acting dopamine agonists such as cabergoline or the transdermal preparations [22] will have to be studied. In addition, the notion that the longer half-life of levodopa afforded by the addition of COMT inhibitors prevents motor deterioration and the development of dyskinesias (particularly unexplained motor fluctuations) needs to be confirmed by future prospective studies with more attention to the dose of levodopa.

While entacapone currently dominates the market (being practically the only player), several pharmaceutical companies are attempting to develop other COMT inhibitors. One modification could be irreversible "suicide"-type inhibitors, which will require only once daily administration.

Levodopa combined with L-AAD inhibitors and COMT inhibitors should not be used, or only with extreme caution, in patients who receive nonspecific monoamine oxidase inhibitors (MAOIs) such as phenelzine, tranylcypromine or nialamid, because dietary tyramine will not be metabolized and could cause a severe sympathetic storm with extreme hypertension (the "cheese reaction"). Because of the long duration of activity of MAOIs, they should be stopped at least 2 weeks before L-AAD inhibitors are given. This precaution still applies to patients taking COMT inhibitors. On the other hand, selective MAO-B inhibitors are not contraindicated in this situation. Although still not studied formally, the combination of inhibitors of the three enzymes involved in dopamine metabolism may be advantageous and may result in an even longer effect of a given dose of levodopa.

If the dose of 150 mg levodopa is to be increased, for example to 200 mg, a combination of different Stalevo® tablets can be used, but this may not be the correct approach. Stalevo® is marketed with fixed-dose entacapone (200 mg), varying doses of levodopa ranging from 50 to 200 mg and varying doses of carbidopa ranging from 12.5 to 50 mg. The dose of 200 mg entacapone that is contained in any Stalevo® tablet causes maximal enzyme inhibition. In such cases, the addition of levodopa/carbidopa or levodopa/benserazide without additional entacaopone is more logical. Moreover, the safety of individual doses of entacapone exceeding 200 mg has not been assured.

Other drugs may also be metabolized by COMT inhibitors. These include all catechlamines (dopamine, norepinephrine, epinephrine, isoprenaline, dobutamine), as well as α-methyldopa, apomorphine, isoetherine and bitolterol. The effect of these agents may well be enhanced when co-administered with COMT inhibitors, and they should be used carefully, starting with lower doses than commonly recommended.

The addition of COMT inhibitors reduces the peripheral side effects of levodopa (nausea, vomiting and orthostatic hypotension) but, because COMT inhibitors allow more levodopa to be delivered to the brain, will not improve central side effects, which might even be worsened. In particular, the occurrence of dyskinesias may demand reduction of individual levodopa doses.

In conclusion, COMT inhibitors, and particularly entacapone, seem to be effective and safe additions to the armamentarium available for the treatment of advanced PD, resulting in a more continuous dopaminergic stimulation, which avoids exposing striatal (and other) dopamine receptors to alternating high and low concentrations of dopamine, thus reducing the effects and minimizing the risk of late motor complications. In particular, they diminish end-of-dose deterioration in the effect of individual doses, thus prolonging "on" time while decreasing "off" periods. Importantly, the reduced "off" time is due to increased "on" time.

References

1. Korczyn AD, Keren O. The effect of dopamine on the papillary diameter in mice. *Life Sci* 1980; **26**: 757–63.
2. Korczyn AD. Pathophysiology of drug-induced dyskinesias. *Neuropharmacology* 1973; **11**: 601–7.
3. Routtinen HM, Rinne UK. Entacapone prolongs levodopa response in one-month double-blind study in Parkinsonian patients with levodopa-related fluctuations. *J Neurol Neurosurg Psychiatry* 1996; **60**: 36–40.
4. Ceravalo R, Piccini P, Bailey DL, et al. ^{18}F-dopa PET evidence that tolcapone acts as a central COMT inhibitor in Parkinson's disease. *Synapse* 2002; **43**: 201–7.
5. Jorga KM. COMT inhibitors: pharmacokinetics and pharmacodynamic comparisons. *Clin Neuropharmacol* 1998; **21** (Suppl.): S9–16.
6. Corvol JC, Bonnet C, Charbonnier-Beaupel F, et al. The COMT Val158Met polymorphism affects the response to entacapone in Parkinson's disease: a randomized crossover clinical trial. *Ann Neurol* 2011; **69**: 111–8.
7. Maltête D, Cottard AM, Mihout B, Costentin J. Erythrocytes catechol-O-methyl transferase activity is up-regulated after a 3-month treatment by entacapone in parkinsonian patients. *Clin Neuropharmacol* 2011; **34**: 21–3.
8. Agid Y, Destée A, Durif F, et al. Tolcapone, bromocriptine, and Parkinson's disease. French Tolcapone Study Group. *Lancet* 1997; **350**: 712–13.

9. Baas H, Beiske AG, Ghika J. COMT inhibitors with tolcapone reduces 'wearing-off' phenomenon and levodopa requirements in fluctuating Parkinsonian patients. *J Neurol Neurosurg Psychiatry* 1997; **63**: 421–8.

10. Adler CH, Singer C, O'Brien C., et al. Randomized placebo-controlled study of tolcapone in patients with fluctuating Parkinson's disease treated with levodopa carbidopa. *Arch Neurol* 1998; **55**: 1089–95.

11. Brooks DJ, Sagar H, UK–Irish Entacapone Study Group. Entacapone is beneficial in both fluctuating and non-fluctuating patients in Parkinson's disease: a randomized, placebo controlled, double-blind, six months study. *J Neurol Neurosurg Psychiatry* 2003; **74**: 1071–9.

12. Fenelon G, Gimenez-Roldan S, Monstrut JL, et al. Efficacy and tolerability of entacapone in patients with Parkinson's disease treated with levodopa plus a dopamine agonist and experiencing wearing-off motor fluctuations. A randomized, double-blind, multicentre study. *J Neural Transm* 2008; **110**: 239–51.

13. Parkinson Study Group. Entacapone improves motor fluctuations in levodopa-treated Parkinson's disease patients. *Ann Neurol* 1997; **42**: 747–55.

14. Myllylä VV, Kultalahti ER, Haapaniemi H, Leinonen M, FILOMEN Study Group. Twelve-month safety of entacapone in patients with Parkinson's disease. *Eur J Neurol* 2001; **8**: 53–60.

15. Larsen JP, Worm-Petersen J, Sideo A, et al. The tolerability and efficacy of entacapone over 3 years in patients with Parkinson's disease. *Eur J Neurol* 2008; **10**: 137–46.

16. Rinne UK, Larsen JP, Siden A, et al. Entacapone enhances the response to levodopa in Parkinsonian patients with motor fluctuations. *Neurology* 1998; **51**: 1309–14.

17. Stocchi F, Rascol O, Kieburtz K, et al. Initiating levodopa/carbidopa therapy with and without entacapone in early PD: the STRIDE-PD study. *Ann Neurol* 2010; **68**: 18–27.

18. Fox SH, Katzenschlager R, Lim SY, et al. The Movement Disorder Society Evidence-Based Medicine Review Update: treatments for the motor symptoms of Parkinson's disease. *Mov Disord* 2011; **26** (Suppl. 3): S2–41.

19. US FDA. FDA Drug Safety Communication: ongoing safety review of Stalevo (entacapone/carbidopa/levodopa) and possible development of prostate cancer. Available at: http://www.fda.gov/Drugs/DrugSafety/PostmarketDrugSafetyInformationforPatientsandProviders/ucm206363.htm.

20. Zesiewicz TA, Wecker L, Sullivan KL, Merlin LR, Hauser RA. The controversy concerning plasma homocysteine in Parkinson disease patients treated with levodopa alone or with entacapone: effects of vitamin status. *Clin Neuropharmacol* 2006; **29**: 106–11.

21. Stowe R, Ives N, Clarke CE, et al. Meta-analysis of the comparative efficacy and safety of adjuvant treatment to levodopa in later Parkinson's disease. *Mov Disord* 2011; **26**: 587–98.

22. Entacapone to Tolcapone Switch Study Investigators. Entacapone to tolcapone switch: multicenter double-blind, randomized, active-controlled trial in advanced Parkinson's disease. *Mov Disord* 2007; **22**: 14–19.

23. Valeant Pharmaceuticals. TASMAR® (tolcapone). Available at: http://www.accessdata.fda.gov/drugsatfda_docs/label/2013/020697s004lbl.pdf.

24. Ferreira JJ, Rascol O, Poewe W, et al. A double-blind, randomized, placebo and active-controlled study of nebicapone for the treatment of motor fluctuations in Parkinson's disease. *CNS Neurosci Ther* 2010; **16**: 337–47.

25. Korczyn AD, Nisipeanu P, Newer therapies for Parkinson's disease. *Neurol Neurochir Pol* 1996; **30** (Suppl. 2): 105–11.

26. Inzelberg R, Nisipeanu P, Rabey JM, et al. Double-blind comparison of caberigolineand bromocriptine in Parkinson's disease patients with motor fluctuations. *Neurology* 1996; **47**: 785–8.

27. Rascol O, Brooks DJ, Korczyn AD, et al. A five year study of the incidence of dyskinesia in patients with early Parkinson's disease who were treated with ropinirole or levidopa. *N Engl J Med* 2000; **342**: 1484–91.

28. Parkinson Study Group. A controlled trial of rotigotine monotherapy in early Parkinson's disease. *Arch Neurol* 2003; **60**: 1721–8.

29. Korczyn AD. Transdermal therapy in Parkinson's disease. *Lancet Neurol* 2007; **6**: 475–6.

30. Kurth MC, Adler CH, Saint Hilaire MH. Tolcapone improves motor function and reduces levodopa requirement in patients with Parkinson's disease experiencing motor fluctuations: a multicenter, double-blind, randomized, placebo-controlled trial. *Neurology* 1997; **48**: 81–7.

31. Rajput AH, Martin W, Saint Hilaire MH, Dorflinger E, Pedder S. Tolcapone improves motor function in Parkinsonian patients with the 'wearing-off' phenomenon: a double-blind, placebo-controlled, multicenter trial. *Neurology* 1997; **49**: 1066–71.

32. Rabey M, Sagi I, Huberman M, et al. Rasagiline mesylate, a new MAO-B inhibitor for the treatment of Parkinson's disease. *Clin Neuropharmacol* 2000; **23**: 324–30.

Chapter 9

Experimental pharmacological agents in the management of Parkinson's disease

Krishe Menezes, Lawrence W. Elmer and Robert A. Hauser

Introduction

On the contrary, there appears to be sufficient reason for hoping that some remedial process may ere long be discovered, by which, at least, the progress of the disease may be stopped.

James Parkinson, Royal College of Surgeons, *An Essay on the Shaking Palsy*, 1817.

Levodopa (3,4-dihydroxyphenyl-L-alanine or L-DOPA) has been the mainstay of treatment of Parkinson's disease (PD) for almost 5 decades, now in combination with a peripherally acting DOPA decarboxylase inhibitor such as benserazide or carbidopa. Levodopa typically produces a robust clinical response with reduction of classic motor symptoms of PD but over time is associated with motor fluctuations and drug-induced dyskinesias, both of which may be quite debilitating. Several drug classes, such as catechol-*O*-methyl transferase (COMT) inhibitors, monoamine oxidase type B (MAO-B) inhibitors and dopamine agonists (DAs) are used as adjuncts to prolong the effects of levodopa. When MAO-B inhibitors or DAs are used as initial monotherapy for PD, studies have demonstrated a delay in the development of both dyskinesias and motor fluctuations, but these drugs alone are insufficient to provide adequate clinical benefit without the addition of levodopa over a period of more than a few years. While strategies exist for managing long-term complications of levodopa therapy, only amantadine has demonstrated definitive clinical efficacy in suppressing dyskinesias without worsening PD symptoms. The future of PD management using agents that bypass the dopaminergic system holds the hope of helping to optimize clinical benefits while avoiding the development of motor complications [1].

The ideal therapy would treat motor and nonmotor symptoms of PD without serious side effects and would also slow or stop the disease progression. While deep-brain stimulation (DBS) provides a powerful tool in the treatment of motor symptoms in PD, it is nevertheless not a cure, nor does it remove the need for pharmacological therapy in the vast majority of cases. In addition, DBS introduces other limitations, including surgical risk. The indications, use and outcome of DBS are covered in Chapters 18–20 (this volume). Finally, it should be noted that the actual benefits of DBS are frequently compared with the clinical benefits of levodopa therapy. In other words, the use of "electrical levodopa" can help supplant the need for increasing and/or repetitive doses of levodopa containing drugs, allowing an absolute reduction in the total daily dose of levodopa while concomitantly decreasing motor symptoms and complications. It seems fitting, therefore, to begin our discussion with strategies under development to improve the effectiveness of levodopa.

Novel approaches to levodopa delivery

As discussed in earlier chapters, levodopa remains the mainstay of effective PD treatment. However, as the disease progresses, multiple variables impair its ability to maintain control of PD symptoms. Therefore, other methods of levodopa delivery have emerged.

Levodopa/carbidopa intestinal gel

Levodopa/carbidopa intestinal gel (LCIG or Duodopa®) is a new formulation that utilizes a novel delivery system [1–3]. It utilizes a pump to deliver a gel formulation of levodopa/carbidopa via a gastrostomy tube into the duodenum to provide a steady, continuous release of levodopa, thereby reducing motor fluctuations and levodopa-induced dyskinesias (LIDs) [2, 4, 5]. The rationale, design, studies and effectiveness of LCIG are described extensively in Chapter 7 (this volume), so only a brief review of its status in the drug development pipeline will be described here.

Several large multinational clinical trials of LCIG have recently been completed. The use of LCIG is currently approved and in use in over 30 countries outside the USA. Compared with orally administered levodopa, LCIG shows reduced plasma levodopa fluctuations (14 vs 34%) [6]. The stabilization of plasma (and presumably brain levels) appears to correlate with reductions in "off" time and dyskinesias, and provides benefit for quality of life [7].

A 12-week, prospective, multicenter, placebo-controlled, parallel-group, double-blind, double-dummy, double-titration study comparing carbidopa/levodopa immediate release (IR) versus LCIG was recently completed in Germany, New Zealand and the USA [8]. Participants were patients with advanced PD experiencing a minimum of 3 h of "off" time per day based on home diaries. In addition, patients were judged to be unsatisfactorily controlled despite optimized medical therapy.

From baseline to 12 weeks, mean "off" time decreased by 4.04 h for 35 patients allocated to the LCIG group compared with a decrease of 2.14 h for 31 patients allocated to carbidopa/levodopa IR (difference of −1.91 h; $P = 0.0015$). In addition, a significant treatment benefit was seen in secondary efficacy measures including increased "on" time without troublesome dyskinesias (4.11 h/day for LCIG vs 2.24 h/day for carbidopa/levodopa IR, $P = 0.0059$) and "on" time without dyskinesias (3.37 h/day for LCIG vs 1.09 h/day for carbidopa/levodopa IR, $P = 0.0142$).

Quality-of-life measures using the 39-item Parkinson's Disease Questionnaire (PDQ-39) were also significantly improved in favor of the LCIG group (−10.9 for LCIG vs −3.9 for carbidopa/levodopa IR, $P = 0.0155$). Adverse events in this 12-week prospective study frequently involved device complications (92% in the LCIG group vs 85% in the carbidopa/levodopa IR group). Other adverse events included abdominal pain (51% LCIG vs 32% carbidopa/levodopa IR), nausea (30% LCIG vs 21% carbidopa/levodopa IR) and procedural pain (30% LCIG vs 35% carbidopa/levodopa IR).

Side effects of LCIG are frequently related to the surgical procedure and hardware. In a multicenter, retrospective study of LCIG therapy with an average duration of 18 months, the following gastrointestinal/mechanical adverse events were observed: peritonitis, 4.3%; inner tube disconnection and leakage, 20%; inner tube pulled out, 18%; inner tube occlusion, 17%; and inner tube displacement and migration, 21% [1]. Interim results of an open-label study have also shown pain to be an issue. Abdominal pain was seen in 30.7%, and procedural pain was seen in 17.7% [9, 10]. For further details of this investigational approach to delivering levodopa, please refer to Chapter 7 (this volume).

IPX066

IPX066 is a novel, extended-release oral preparation of carbidopa/levodopa. It has been studied extensively for the treatment of PD in both early patients ("levodopa naïve") as well as more advanced patients on commercially available formulations of levodopa, but with inadequate clinical response due to motor fluctuations. In an open-label study, both carbidopa/levodopa IR and IPX066 provided similar times to "on," but IPX066 maintained significantly better motor score improvements from 3 to 6 h after administration [11].

A phase 3, randomized, double-blind, double-dummy, parallel-group study comparing IPX066 with carbidopa/levodopa IR was performed in North America and Europe [12]. Parkinson's disease patients were required to have at least 2.5 h/day of "off" time in order to qualify for the study. Other inclusion criteria required subjects to be on a stable regimen of carbidopa/levodopa IR for at least 4 weeks prior to screening with a total daily dose of levodopa of at least 400 mg along with a dosing frequency of at least four times per day. Patients were allowed to be receiving other agents including dopamine agonists, MAO-B inhibitors, amantadine and anticholinergic medications as long as they were maintained at stable doses of these medications during the study.

The study design required the patients undergo a 3-week open-label carbidopa/levodopa IR dose adjustment. During that time, investigators were allowed to adjust both the dose and the frequency, with the goal of achieving optimum motor function. This dose-adjustment period was followed by a 6-week open-label IPX066 dose conversion and optimization. Following this, patients were randomly allocated to 13 weeks of double-blind, double-dummy treatment with either IPX066 or carbidopa/levodopa IR using the dosage regimens achieved during the open-label optimization periods.

At the end of 22 weeks, the treatment group receiving IPX066 (mean of 3.6 doses per day) experienced

1.17 h less "off" time per day compared with the individuals who received carbidopa/levodopa IR (mean of 5.0 doses per day) ($P < 0.0001$). In addition, "on" time without troublesome dyskinesia was also significantly more increased in the IPX066 group (by 0.93 h). Other secondary efficacy measures, including global improvement scores and motor scores, were also significantly more improved with IPX066.

The most common adverse events reported during the study included insomnia, nausea, falls and dizziness, but these were of low frequency, between 1 and 3% for both groups. This study suggests that IPX066 may be considered as a replacement for conventional carbidopa/levodopa in patients with motor fluctuations.

IPX066 was also evaluated in early PD versus placebo in a multicenter, multinational, randomized, double-blind, parallel-group, fixed dose, 30-week study. Eligible subjects were randomized 1:1:1:1 to placebo or one of three different dosages of IPX066. The three doses in the active-treatment arm were 145, 245 or 390 mg. Each of these doses was taken three times daily, approximately 6 h apart [13]. Participants were required to be levodopa naïve. Some medications, including anticholinergics, amantadine and MAO-B inhibitors, were permitted, but the doses had to be stable for 4 weeks prior to study entry. The doses of these medications also had to remain unchanged throughout the study. A total of 361 patients were enrolled, and 300 patients completed the study.

The primary efficacy measure was a mean improvement in the Unified Parkinson's Disease Rating Scale (UPDRS) II plus III at 30 weeks compared with baseline. Results demonstrated significant improvement in all three IPX066 treatment arms compared with placebo. The total improvement in the placebo arm was 0.6 points compared with 11.7, 12.9 and 14.9 points for the three IPX066 dosages, respectively. A secondary efficacy measure, the PDQ-39, was also improved for all IPX066 dosages compared with placebo. The most commonly reported adverse events in this study included nausea, headache, dizziness and insomnia. Overall, the 245 mg three times daily dosage appeared to provide the best balance between efficacy and adverse events.

This study demonstrated the effectiveness and tolerability of IPX066 in patients with early PD [13]. There is interest as to whether IPX066 might be able to reduce the development of dyskinesias compared with carbidopa/levodopa IR by delivering levodopa in a smoother, more continuous fashion, but this remains to be evaluated in a prospective clinical trial.

XP21279

One of the challenges in the use of levodopa (L-DOPA) as a therapeutic agent in the management of PD is its limited geographical absorption. Levodopa is actively absorbed through amino acid transporters in the duodenum and jejunum, a relatively short segment of the small intestine. XP21279 is a levodopa prodrug that utilizes a nutrient moiety attached to levodopa and, when combined with carbidopa, has been shown to be absorbed throughout the entire gastrointestinal tract. This allows a greater proportion of the levodopa dose to be absorbed over a longer period of time.

A phase 2, randomized, double-blind, double-dummy, crossover study examining the efficacy, safety and pharmacokinetic profile of XP21279/carbidopa versus carbidopa/levodopa IR was performed in patients with PD who were experiencing motor fluctuations. A total of 35 patients were randomized, and 28 patients completed the study. There was an open-label dose, random-ordered optimization phase for carbidopa/levodopa IR and XP21279/carbidopa followed by a double-blind, double-dummy treatment phase in which subjects were on each active treatment for 2 weeks [14].

The primary efficacy measure was change from baseline in total daily "off" time at the end of each double-blinded treatment. The total reduction in "off" time was 2.7 h with carbidopa/levodopa IR and 3.0 h for XP21279/carbidopa (nonsignificant). However, XP21279/carbidopa was administered three times daily whereas carbidopa/levodopa IR was administered four or five times daily.

A secondary analysis that excluded outliers found that XP21279/carbidopa reduced "off" time by 0.9 h more than carbidopa/levodopa IR ($P = 0.016$). In addition, there was a statistically significant improvement in the change in total "on" time without troublesome dyskinesias in favor of XP21279/carbidopa. Adverse events were mild and were similar between the two treatment arms. Participants at two sites also underwent pharmacokinetic analysis, the results of which demonstrated a significant reduction in the variability of levodopa concentrations with XP21279/carbidopa compared with carbidopa/levodopa IR [14]. These results suggest that XP21279/carbidopa may be a potential option for the management of advanced PD with motor fluctuations, but phase 3 studies are required.

Other levodopa formulations

Several additional novel methods of delivering levodopa are in development, including an accordion pill, a gastric-retentive pill and an intrapulmonary formulation for inhalation of levodopa. Phase 2 studies of all these agents have been published in abstract form.

Accordion Pill™ (AP) carbidopa/levodopa incorporates a unique gastroretentive formulation to provide stable levodopa plasma levels analogous to those seen with LCIG. A phase II, multicenter, open-label, two-way randomized crossover, multiple-dose study with active control groups was completed in PD patients with motor fluctuations [15]. Twice daily administration of AP carbidopa-levodopa provided therapeutic plasma levels of levodopa. A total of 18 patients completed the study according to the protocol. In these patients, a statistically significant reduction in total daily "off" time was recorded using home diaries, from an average of 5.1 h/day to 2.8 h/day with AP carbidopa/levodopa ($P < 0.0001$). Adverse events were reported as "mild."

A gastroretentive formulation, DM-1992, administered twice daily, was studied in comparison with carbidopa/levodopa IR given three to eight times daily (median of times per day) in an open-label, randomized, crossover design study involving 34 patients with PD [16, 17]. At baseline, patients recorded an average of 5.5 h of "off" time per day. During the treatment phase, DM-1992 demonstrated a statistically significant reduction in "off" time of 0.9 h/day compared with an increase of 0.1 h/day of "off" time in the carbidopa/levodopa IR group ($P = 0.047$).

Pharmacokinetic studies on the final day using DM-1992 administered once daily compared with carbidopa/levodopa IR given multiple times per day demonstrated similar levodopa C_{max} and area-under-the-curve values. In addition, the ratio of C_{max}/C_{min} was significantly lower in the DM-1992 once daily group, consistent with a more stable levodopa plasma concentration. Adverse events were reported in 35% of the patients in the DM-1992 group compared with 14.7% in the carbidopa/levodopa IR group, although no consistent pattern of adverse events was demonstrated and most adverse events were reported as mild.

Finally, a novel method of administering levodopa has been developed as a "bridging" therapy. CVT-301 is an inhaled formulation of levodopa administered as a fine-particle dose (FPD). A double-blind, placebo-controlled, crossover study of CVT-301 was performed in 24 patients experiencing more than 2 h/day of "off" time [18]. Patients were maintained on their usual doses of carbidopa/levodopa and the study drug versus placebo was administered approximately 4–5 h after their first morning dose of carbidopa/levodopa. While two doses of CVT-301 (25 and 50 mg of FPD) were studied in comparison with placebo, only the 50 mg FPD resulted in statistically significant improvements in motor performance compared with placebo. However, these changes were seen within 5 min post-dose, suggestive of rapid increases in plasma and brain levodopa levels. There were no serious adverse events and no discontinuations. In addition, there were no changes in spirometry measures compared with baseline in either of the two CVT-301 dosages.

Adenosine A_{2a} antagonists

Adenosine A_{2a} receptors are highly concentrated in the basal ganglia, and co-localize with D2 receptors on the striatal outflow tracts of the "indirect" pathway. A_{2a} receptors couple through stimulatory G proteins to increase adenyl cyclase, whereas D_2 receptors couple through inhibitory G proteins to reduce adenyl cyclase. Thus, A_{2a} and D_2 stimulation have balancing effects on striatopallidal outflow. In models of PD, antagonism of A_{2a} receptors suppresses the overactivity of striatopallidal firing induced by the dopamine deficiency, thereby resulting in a reduction in parkinsonian symptoms [19]. In animal models of PD, A_{2a} antagonists have been demonstrated to provide antiparkinsonian benefit without causing dyskinesias and to enhance the antiparkinsonian effect of levodopa without worsening preexisting dyskinesias [20]. Neuroprotection has also been demonstrated in monkey and mouse models of PD [21, 22].

Istradefylline

Istradefylline (KW-6002) is the most extensively studied A_{2a} antagonist and is currently approved in Japan as an adjunct to levodopa. The complete history of this compound's development was documented in a review published in 2013 [23]. Istradefylline consistently and significantly reduced "off" time in a series of exploratory and phase 2 studies in patients experiencing motor fluctuations on levodopa [24–26]. These were then followed by two large phase 3 studies that yielded mixed results [27, 28].

The KW-6002-US-013 study was a phase 3, 12-week, multicenter, placebo-controlled, double-blind, randomized study of istradefylline 20 mg/day compared with placebo as an adjunct to levodopa in PD patients with motor fluctuations. Patients were required to be experiencing at least 3 h of daily "off" time per day as documented in home diaries [27]. A total of 231 participants were randomized 1:1 to the addition of istradefylline or placebo. Total daily "off" time was reduced by 0.7 h more in the istradefylline group compared with the placebo group (P = 0.03). Common reported adverse events included dyskinesias (istradefylline vs placebo: 22.6 vs 12.2%), light-headedness (7.8 vs 3.5%), decreased weight (6.1 vs 2.6%) and constipation (5.2 vs 0.9%). Overall, istradefylline provided a small but significant reduction in "off" time and was generally well tolerated.

The KW-6002-US-018 study was a phase 3, 12-week, North American, multicenter, placebo-controlled, double-blind, paralle-group, randomized study examining the efficacy of istradefylline 10, 20 and 40 mg/day compared with placebo in patients with PD treated with levodopa and experiencing motor complications. A total of 610 patients were randomized 1:1:1:1 to the addition of placebo or one of the three different dosages of istradefylline [28]. Patients were required to be taking at least three doses/day of levodopa but were allowed to be receiving other adjunctive therapies including dopamine agonists, MAO-B inhibitors, COMT inhibitors and amantadine. The results demonstrated no statistically significant change from baseline to the end of the study in the primary efficacy measure of percentage of awake time per day spent in the "off" state. However, some of the secondary efficacy measures were significantly improved in favor of istradefylline, including UPDRS motor scores in the highest dose group, and the 36-Item Short Form Health Survey (SF-36) mental component score in the two highest dose groups. The most common reported adverse events (istradefylline 40 mg vs placebo) included dyskinesia (26.3 vs 19.2%), headache (7.2 vs 4.2%) and light-headedness (7.2 vs 3.3%).

One possible explanation for the failure of istradefylline to demonstrate a significant difference in reduction in "off" time compared with placebo included a higher-than-average placebo effect. One factor that may have contributed to a large placebo effect was the relatively high number of active-treatment arms [3] and the relatively low likelihood of a patient being randomized to placebo (25%) [28].

Despite this result, a subsequent Japanese phase 3 study found a reduction in "off" time compared with placebo of 0.65 h with istradefylline 20 mg/day (P = 0.013) and 0.92 h with 40 mg/day (P < 0.001), and istradefylline was approved for the management of motor fluctuations in Japan in March 2013 [23].

Preladenant

Preladenant was the second adenosine A_{2a} receptor antagonist to enter clinical development for the treatment of motor fluctuations in PD. An international phase 2, randomized dose-finding trial was performed to evaluate the efficacy and safety of preladenant in patients with PD receiving levodopa and other antiparkinsonian medications but experiencing motor fluctuations. Subjects were required to have a minimum of at least 2 h of "off" time per day based on home diaries. Eligible patients were randomized 1:1:1:1:1 to preladenant 1, 2, 5 or 10 mg or matching placebo dosed twice daily. The primary efficacy measure was the change in mean daily "off" time from baseline to week 12 as determined by home diaries [29]. A total of 44 sites in 15 countries recruited 253 patients, of which 246 received at least one dose of the study drug.

Mean daily "off" time from baseline to week 12 was significantly reduced versus placebo in patients on 5 mg preladenant twice daily and 10 mg preladenant twice daily. The preladenant 5 mg twice daily group experienced a 1.0 h greater reduction in "off" time compared with placebo (P = 0.049), and the preladenant 10 mg BID group experienced a 1.2 h reduction in "off" time (P = 0.019). Common adverse events in the preladenant 10 mg twice daily group versus placebo included somnolence (13 vs 6%) and dizziness (11 vs 2%).

Unfortunately, a large phase 3 study of preladenant as an adjunct to levodopa was negative produced negative results [30] and further development was recently discontinued.

Tozadenant

A third adenosine A_{2a} receptor antagonist, tozadenant, has been evaluated in a small phase 2, randomized, placebo-controlled, double-blind, crossover study involving a total of 26 patients. Two different dosages of either 20 or 60 mg twice daily were given in a crossover fashion with placebo, and patients were evaluated before and after intravenous levodopa infusion. With the highest dose of tozadenant (60 mg twice daily), there was a significant improvement in motor function as determined by tapping speed [31].

A larger phase 2/3 study of patients with PD and motor fluctuations has been completed using tozadenant. Study participants on stable dosages of levodopa were required to be experiencing at least 2.5 h of "off" time per day based on home diaries. A total of 420 patients were randomized to receive 60, 120, 180 or 240 mg of tozadenant twice daily or matched placebo in an international, 12-week, double-blinded study. Of the 420 patients randomized, 337 completed the study. The primary efficacy measure was change from baseline to week 12 in total daily "off" time as determined by home diaries [32].

Compared with placebo, there were statistically significant reductions in total daily "off" time in the 120 mg twice daily (−1.1 h, $P = 0.0039$) and the 180 mg twice daily (−1.2 h, $P = 0.0039$) tozadenant groups. The most common adverse events reported in the combined tozadenant groups were dyskinesias, nausea, dizziness, constipation, worsening of Parkinson's symptoms, insomnia and falls. This study suggested that tozadenant at a daily dosage of 120 or 180 mg twice daily may be effective in the treatment of advanced PD with motor fluctuations. Phase 3 trials are awaited.

Thus, experience to date indicates that A_{2a} antagonists have demonstrated efficacy as adjuncts to levodopa in PD patients with motor fluctuations to reduce "off" time in phase 2 studies. However, preladenant failed in phase 3, and istradefylline yielded mixed results. This probably reflects the difficulty of scaling up from smaller phase 2 studies, typically performed at expert centers, to phase 3 trials, which require many more sites and investigators.

Although A_{2a} antagonists demonstrated antiparkinsonian efficacy as monotherapy in animal models [33], clinical trials of A_{2a} antagonists as monotherapy in patients with early PD have so far been negative. These include one istradefylline trial [28] and one preladenant trial [30].

Miscellaneous symptomatic agents: safinamide

Safinamide is an α-aminoamide with novel multifunctional properties including MAO-B inhibition, dopamine reuptake inhibition, inhibition of glutamate release and antagonism of activity-dependent sodium channel activity. Two large, multicenter studies have demonstrated clinical efficacy of this compound in patients with both early and advanced PD.

Study 015 was a 24-week, randomized, double-blind, placebo-controlled, parallel-group study conducted at centers in Italy, Spain, the UK, India, Argentina, Chile and Columbia. Patients had to be within 5 years of their original diagnosis and receiving a stable dose of a single dopamine agonist. Subjects were randomized to the addition of safinamide 100 or 200 mg/day or matching placebo in a 1:1:1 ratio [34].

A total of 270 patients were randomized, and 232 patients completed the study. Twice the number of patients ($n = 19$) discontinued the study drug in the safinamide 200 mg/day group compared with either the safinamide 100 mg/day group ($n = 9$) or the placebo group ($n = 9$).

The primary efficacy measure was the mean change in UPDRS-III (motor subscale) scores at week 24 compared with baseline, assessed in a hierarchical fashion. Safinamide 200 mg/day was compared with placebo and, if that result was positive, the second comparison was safinamide 100 mg/day versus placebo.

In the comparison of safinamide 200 mg/day versus placebo, there was no significant difference between the drug and placebo at week 24 versus baseline with respect to changes in the UPDRS-III total score. A comparison of safinamide 100 mg versus placebo showed some improvement from baseline to week 24 in the UPDRS-III motor score with a reduction of 2.4 points after correcting for placebo (raw $P = 0.0419$) [35].

Study 016 was a phase 3, multicenter, randomized, double-blind, placebo-controlled, parallel-group study that evaluated safinamide as an adjunct to levodopa in patients with motor fluctuations [29]. The design included a 4-week levodopa stabilization period and a 24-week treatment period, followed by a 1-week taper. Participants had to have had a diagnosis of PD for at least 3 years and more than 1.5 h of "off" time per day, as determined by home diaries. Patients were randomized to safinamide 50 or 100 mg/day or matching placebo in a 1:1:1 ratio. The primary efficacy measure was change in mean daily "on" time without troublesome dyskinesias as measured by home diaries.

A total of 669 patients were randomized and 594 completed the study. The 75 discontinuations were fairly equally divided between the three treatment arms. At week 24, safinamide 50 mg/day increased "on" time without troublesome dyskinesias by 0.51 h compared with placebo ($P = 0.0223$) and 100 mg/day increased "on" time without troublesome dyskinesias by 0.55 h ($P = 0.0130$). Safinamide was generally well tolerated, although dyskinesias were reported as an adverse event in 12.6% of placebo subjects, 21.1% of safinamide 50 mg/day subjects and 18.3% of safinamide 100 mg/day subjects. This study suggests that safinamide may be helpful in the management of motor fluctuations. It was hoped that safinamide might also be useful to decrease dyskinesias but this has not yet been seen clinically.

Antidyskinetic agents

A common side effect in the treatment of PD is levodopa-induced dyskinesias (LIDs). If we had a highly effective medication to prevent the development of dyskinesias or to symptomatically reduce their expression, we would be free to utilize levodopa more aggressively to improve parkinsonian signs and reduce motor fluctuations. Amantadine IR is currently available and has been demonstrated to be clinically effective in the treatment of LID but has a relatively narrow therapeutic window, is only partially effective and produces common side effects such as hallucinations, confusion and edema [36].

A long-acting formulation of amantadine, ADS-5102, was studied in a large, randomized, double-blind, placebo-controlled, parallel-group study of PD patients with troublesome LID. Three separate doses of ADS-5102 of 260, 340 and 420 mg were administered daily in comparison with placebo. The primary efficacy measure was the Unified Dyskinesia Rating Scale (UDysRS) [37].

Both 340 and 420 mg of ADS-5102 demonstrated significantly reduced LID scores compared with placebo as measured by UDysRS at 8 weeks of treatment compared with baseline ($P = 0.004$ and $P = 0.0004$, respectively).

The most common adverse events reported at the two highest doses (340/420 mg) included constipation (23.8/15 vs 9.1% for placebo), dizziness (28.6/15 vs 4.5% for placebo), dry mouth (19/10 vs 0% for placebo) and visual hallucinations (14.3/10 vs 0% for placebo).

The results of this study suggest that ADS-5102 is effective in treating LID at dosages of 340 and 420 mg, but withdrawals were higher in the 420 mg dose group.

Fipamezole

One mechanism of action thought to be responsible for LID includes overstimulation of α2 adrenergic receptors. Fipamezole is a potent and effective α2 adrenergic receptor antagonist that decreased LID in ten patients with PD in a proof-of-concept study at doses of 60 and 90 mg/day [38]. In another study involving 21 patients with moderate to advanced PD, subjects were administered various doses of fipamezole as a buccal spray. Dosages of 60 and 90 mg were found to reduce dyskinesias by 23 and 31%, respectively, and prolong the levodopa effect by 41 min at the 90 mg dose [39]. No benefit was observed when the drug was evaluated as monotherapy.

Fipamezole was then evaluated in a 4-week, phase 2, multicenter, randomized, placebo-controlled, double-blind, dose-escalating study in patients with PD who were experiencing LID. A total of 33 centers including 26 in the USA and seven in India were involved. Patients were required to have LID for a minimum of 25% of their waking hours as recorded in home diaries. Dyskinesias had to be at least moderately disabling. Subjects were randomized to the addition of fipamezole 30, 60 or 90 mg/day or matching placebo in a 1:1:1:1 ratio [38].

A total of 180 subjects were randomized, and 173 patients completed the study. In the primary analysis, there was no difference in reduction of dyskinesias between fipamezole and placebo-treated subjects. However, the US and Indian cohorts did not behave similarly. Unlike the total group, the US cohort demonstrated a dose–response relationship regarding changes in dyskinesias. Furthermore, in the US population, fipamezole 90 mg significantly reduced dyskinesias compared with placebo (1.9 LID points, $P = 0.047$). Adverse events resulted in very few discontinuations. Common adverse events (fipamezole vs placebo) included nausea (22.5 vs 6.0%) dysgeusia (17.1 vs 4.0%) and oral hypoesthesia (9.3 vs 0%.). Although this study provided a signal of potential efficacy for the treatment of LID, it is unclear whether fipamezole will undergo further clinical development.

AFQ056

Antagonism of the metabotropic glutamate receptor 5 (mGluR5) has been identified as another possible target for reducing LID, for example by the mgluR5 antagonist AFQ056. Proof-of-concept clinical trials involving small numbers of patients have supported this hypothesis [40].

A larger, 13-week, randomized, double-blind, placebo-controlled, parallel-group study was performed at 42 sites in eight countries including Australia, Canada, Finland, France, Germany, Italy, Japan and Spain. Patients were required to have experienced LID for at least 3 months, have been receiving levodopa for at least 3 years and score at least 2 or greater on UPDRS items 32 and 33 (moderately disabling dyskinesias at least 26% of the day).

A total of 197 subjects were randomized, and 145 subjects completed this study. The subjects were randomized to AFQ056 50, 100, 150 or 200 mg/day or matching placebo. The primary efficacy measure was a reduction in the modified Abnormal Involuntary Movement Scale (AIMS) score from baseline to week 12, comparing each dose with placebo [41].

AFQ056 200 mg/day was observed to significantly reduce dyskinesias compared with placebo. In addition, based on achieved dose rather than assigned dose, there was a dose–response relationship. The most common reported adverse events included (AFQ056 200 mg/day vs placebo) dizziness (22.7 vs 0%), hallucinations (11.4 vs 1.6%), and fatigue (6.8 vs 3.2%).

However, as of November, 2013, Novartis reported that its development program for AFQ056 for LID had been discontinued based on a lack of efficacy in two phase 2 trials (NCT01385592 and NCT01491529). (http://www.ukmi.nhs.uk/applications/ndo/record_view_open.asp?newDrugID=5043; accessed May 29, 2014). No safety concerns were raised.

Disease-modifying treatments

Disease modification is the holy grail of treatments for neurodegenerative diseases including PD. In the last 25 years, numerous agents have been tested in well-designed, controlled clinical trials but without clear evidence of any agent significantly slowing progression of the underlying disease. Therefore, neurologists and neuroscientists around the globe are still searching for a medication or other type of therapy that could potentially arrest and/or slow the progression of PD. With new insights into the prion-like propagation of misfolded α-synuclein through the brain, therapies to slow or interrupt this process have become an intense area of focus for researchers. For the most part, these anti-synuclein therapies have not yet entered clinical trials, but we anticipate that they will in coming years. Here, we review several therapies that are being evaluated clinically for their ability to slow PD.

Calcium-channel antagonists: isradipine

Isradipine is a dihydropyridine calcium-channel antagonist that has demonstrated neuroprotective properties in animal models of PD. While the exact mechanism of this neuroprotection is unknown, it is possibly related to the prevention of calcium toxicity to the neuron. A phase 2 safety, tolerability, and dose selection study of isradipine as a potential disease-modifying intervention in early Parkinson's disease was undertaken in the STEADY-PD (Safety, Tolerability, and Efficacy Assessment of Isradipine for PD) trial to find a dosage that was well tolerated [42].

Patients with early PD were selected and randomized to four groups: isradipine controlled release 5, 10 or 20 mg or matching placebo once daily. There was no difference in change in UPDRS score among dosages over 52 weeks. The maximum tolerated dose was 10 mg [42]. A phase 3 trial is currently planned to study the effect of 10 mg isradipine as a disease-modifying agent in PD.

Uric acid precursor: inosine

A second novel but commercially available agent being investigated as a potential disease-modifying agent for the treatment of PD is inosine, a precursor to uric acid. Observational analyses of large clinical trials (PRECEPT [Parkinson Research Examination of CEP-1347 Trial] and DATATOP [Deprenyl And Tocopherol Antioxidant Treatment Of Parkinson's disease]) found that patients with higher urate levels experienced slower rates of clinical progression.

Inosine was then studied prospectively. Seventy-five patients with early PD were recruited into a study performed by the Parkinson Study Group [43]. Participants were randomized to one of three treatment arms: placebo or inosine titrated to produce mild or moderate serum urate elevation. Serious adverse events occurred at the same or lower rates in the inosine groups as in the placebo group, and none of the subjects developed gout. Overall, inosine was found to be generally safe, tolerable and effective in raising serum and cerebrospinal fluid urate levels. Secondary analyses demonstrated nonfutility of inosine treatment for slowing disability. These findings suggest that further evaluation of inosine as a potential disease-modifying medication for PD is warranted.

Conclusion

With long-acting oral levodopa medications and inhaled levodopa on the horizon, we will definitely be making progress toward minimizing or eliminating "off" episodes. For those who have motor complications that cannot be controlled with these medications, we will have the new (in the USA) option of LCIG infusion in addition to the current option of deep-brain stimulation.

It remains to be seen whether, by using more continuous levodopa delivery from early on, we can reduce the development of dyskinesias. However, it seems likely that even those who development dyskinesias will benefit from new levodopa formulations that deliver levodopa in a smoother fashion with less levodopa serum concentration variability. Nonetheless, it would still be helpful to have a very robust antidyskinetic medication. We can currently use amantadine IR in patients who can tolerate it, and it remains to be seen whether amantadine extended release will be better tolerated and useful in a larger population of patients. Although several antidyskinetic agents with new mechanisms of action have entered clinical development, most have struggled to demonstrate robust efficacy, and it remains to be seen whether they will reach the marketplace.

Our most pressing need is for a disease-modifying medication. Several are in clinical testing now, and results of informative trials are awaited. It seems that much hope for the future lies with interventions that can slow or disrupt the prion-like propagation of misfolded α-synuclein and the damage this process causes along the way. Clinicians anxiously await trials of such interventions.

References

1. Devos D. Patient profile, indications, efficacy and safety of duodenal levodopa infusion in advanced Parkinson's disease. *Mov Disord* 2009; **24**: 993–1000.
2. Nyholm D, Klangemo K, Johansson A. Levodopa/carbidopa intestinal gel infusion long-term therapy in advanced Parkinson's disease. *Eur J Neurol* 2012; **19**: 1079–85.
3. Zibetti M, Merola A, Artusi CA, et al. Levodopa/carbidopa intestinal gel infusion in advanced Parkinson's disease: a 7-year experience. *Eur J Neurol* 2014; **21**: 312–8.
4. Samanta J, Hauser RA. Duodenal levodopa infusion for the treatment of Parkinson's disease. *Expert Opin Pharmacother* 2007; **8**: 657–64.
5. Fernandez HH, Odin P. Levodopa-carbidopa intestinal gel for treatment of advanced Parkinson's disease. *Curr Med Res Opin*.2011; **27**: 907–19.
6. Nyholm D, Odin P, Johansson A, et al. Pharmacokinetics of levodopa, carbidopa, and 3-O-methyldopa following 16-hour jejunal infusion of levodopa-carbidopa intestinal gel in advanced Parkinson's disease patients. *AAPS J* 2013; **15**: 316–23.
7. Nyholm D, Askmark H, Gomes-Trolin C, et al. Optimizing levodopa pharmacokinetics: intestinal infusion versus oral sustained-release tablets. *Clin Neuropharmacol* 2003; **26**: 156–63.
8. Olanow CW, Kieburtz K, Odin P, et al. Continuous intrajejunal infusion of levodopa-carbidopa intestinal gel for patients with advanced Parkinson's disease: a randomised, controlled, double-blind, double-dummy study. *Lancet Neurol* 2014; **13**: 141–9.
9. Fernandez HH, Vanagunas A, Odin P, et al. Levodopa-carbidopa intestinal gel in advanced Parkinson's disease open-label study: interim results. *Parkinsonism Relat Disord* 2013; **19**: 339–45.
10. Espay AJ. Management of motor complications in Parkinson disease: current and emerging therapies. *Neurol Clin*. 2010; **28**: 913–25.
11. Hauser RA, Ellenbogen AL, Metman LV, et al. Crossover comparison of IPX066 and a standard levodopa formulation in advanced Parkinson's disease. *Mov Disord* 2011; **26**: 2246–52.
12. Hauser RA, Hsu A, Kell S, et al. Extended-release carbidopa-levodopa (IPX066) compared with immediate-release carbidopa-levodopa in patients with Parkinson's disease and motor fluctuations: a phase 3 randomised, double-blind trial. *Lancet Neurol* 2013; **12**: 346–56.
13. Pahwa R, Lyons KE, Hauser RA, et al. Randomized trial of IPX066, carbidopa/levodopa extended release, in early Parkinson's disease. *Parkinsonism Relat Disord* 2014; **20**: 142–8.
14. LeWitt PA, Huff FJ, Hauser RA, et al. Double-blind study of the actively transported levodopa prodrug XP21279 in Parkinson's disease. *Mov Disord* 2014; **29**: 75–82.
15. LeWitt PA, Friedman, H, Giladi, N, et al. Accordion pill carbidopa/levodopa for improved treatment of advanced Parkinson's disease symptoms [abstract]. 2013; **27** (Suppl. 1): S130–1.
16. Metman LV, Stover N, Cuiping C, Cowles VE, Sweeney M. Improved motor performance associated with smoother levodopa time-concentration profiles with DM-1992, a gastroretentive, extended-release carbidopa/levodopa tablet, in patients with advanced Parkinson's disease. *Neurology* 2014; **82**: poster 7.082.
17. *Depomed Announces Positive Results from Phase 2 Study of DM-1992 for Parkinson's Disease* [press release]. *PHARMABIZ.COM*, November 9, 2012.
18. Freed MF, Grosset D, Worth P, et al. Rapid levodopa augmentation following inhaled CVT-301 results in rapid improvement in motor response when administered to PD patients in the OFF state. *Neurology* 2014; **82**: S7.007.
19. Hauser RA, Schwarzschild MA. Adenosine A2A receptor antagonists for Parkinson's disease: rationale, therapeutic potential and clinical experience. *Drugs Aging* 2005; **22**: 471–82.
20. Kanda T, Jackson MJ, Smith LA, et al. Combined use of the adenosine A2A antagonist KW-6002 with l-DOPA or with selective D1 or D2 dopamine agonists increases antiparkinsonian activity but not dyskinesia in MPTP-treated monkeys. *Exp Neurol* 2000; **162**: 321–7.

21. Kase H, Aoyama S, Ichimura M, *et al.* Progress in pursuit of therapeutic A2A antagonists: the adenosine A2A receptor selective antagonist KW6002: research and development toward a novel nondopaminergic therapy for Parkinson's disease. *Neurology* 2003; **61** (Suppl. 6): S97–100.
22. Kalda A, Yu L, Oztas E, Chen JF. Novel neuroprotection by caffeine and adenosine A2A receptor antagonists in animal models of Parkinson's disease. *J Neurol Sci* 2006; **248**: 9–15.
23. Dungo R, Deeks ED. Istradefylline: first global approval. *Drugs* 2013; **73**: 875–82.
24. Hauser RA, Hubble JP, Truong DD, Istradefylline US-001 Study Group. Randomized trial of the adenosine A2A receptor antagonist istradefylline in advanced PD. *Neurology* 2003; **61**: 297–303.
25. LeWitt PA, Guttman M, Tetrud JW, *et al.* Adenosine A2A receptor antagonist istradefylline (KW-6002) reduces "off" time in Parkinson's disease: a double-blind, randomized, multicenter clinical trial (6002-US-005). *Ann Neurol* 2008; **63**: 295–302.
26. Stacy M, Silver D, Mendis T, *et al.* A 12-week, placebo-controlled study (6002-US-006) of istradefylline in Parkinson disease. *Neurology* 2008; **70**: 2233–40.
27. Hauser RA, Shulman LM, Trugman JM, *et al.* Study of istradefylline in patients with Parkinson's disease on levodopa with motor fluctuations. *Mov Disord* 2008; **23**: 2177–85.
28. Pourcher E, Fernandez HH, Stacy M, *et al.* Istradefylline for Parkinson's disease patients experiencing motor fluctuations: results of the KW-6002-US-018 study. *Parkinsonism Relat Disord* 2012; **18**: 178–84.
29. Hauser RA, Cantillon M, Pourcher E, *et al.* Preladenant in patients with Parkinson's disease and motor fluctuations: a phase 2, double-blind, randomised trial. *Lancet Neurol* 2011; **10**: 221–9.
30. Hauser R, Sticchi F, Rascol O, *et al.* Phase-3 Clinical Trials of Adjunctive Therapy with Preladenant, an Adenosine 2a Antagonist, in Patients with Parkinson's Disease. American Academy of Neurology Annual Meeting; 2014;
31. Black KJ CampBell CM, Dickerson W, *et al.*, eds. A randomized, double-blind, placebo-controlled crossover trial of the adenosine 2a antagonist SYN115 in Parkinson disease. *Neurology*; 2010; **82**: poster P7.087.
32. Hauser RA Olanow CW, Kieburtz KD, *et al.* A phase 2, placebo-controlled, double-blind trial of tozadenant (SYN-115) in patients with Parkinson's disease with wearing-off fluctuations on levodopa. *Mov Disord* 2013; **333** (Suppl. 1): e119.
33. Dall'Igna OP, Porciuncula LO, Souza DO, Cunha RA, Lara DR. Neuroprotection by caffeine and adenosine A2A receptor blockade of β-amyloid neurotoxicity. *Br J Pharmacol* 2003; **138**: 1207–9.
34. Stocchi F, Borgohain R, Onofrj M, *et al.* A randomized, double-blind, placebo-controlled trial of safinamide as add-on therapy in early Parkinson's disease patients. *Mov Disord* 2012; **27**: 106–12.
35. Stocchi F, Borgohain R, Onofrj M, *et al.* A randomized, double-blind, placebo-controlled trial of safinamide as add-on therapy in early Parkinson's disease patients. *Mov Disord* 2012; **27**: 106–12.
36. Gottwald MD, Aminoff MJ. Therapies for dopaminergic-induced dyskinesias in Parkinson disease. *Ann Neurol* 2011; **69**: 919–27.
37. Pahwa R, Tanner CM, Hauser RA, *et al.* Randomized trial of extended release amantadine in Parkinson's disease patients with levodopa-induced dyskinesia (EASED Study). *Mov Disord* 2013; **28** (Suppl. 1): 443.
38. Lewitt PA, Hauser RA, Lu M, *et al.* Randomized clinical trial of fipamezole for dyskinesia in Parkinson disease (FJORD study). *Neurology* 2012; **79**: 163–9.
39. Dimitrova T, Bara-Jimenez W, Savola JM, *et al.* Alpha-2 adrenergic antagonist effects in Parkinson's disease. *Mov Disord* 2009; **24** (Suppl. 1): S261.
40. Johnston TH, Fox SH, McIldowie MJ, Piggott MJ, Brotchie JM. Reduction of l-DOPA-induced dyskinesia by the selective metabotropic glutamate receptor 5 antagonist 3-[(2-methyl-1,3-thiazol-4-yl)ethynyl]pyridine in the 1-methyl-4-phenyl-1,2,3,6-tetrahydropyridine-lesioned macaque model of Parkinson's disease. *J Pharmacol Exp Ther* 2010; **333**: 865–73.
41. Stocchi F, Rascol O, Destée A, *et al.* AFQ056 in Parkinson patients with levodopa-induced dyskinesia: 13-week, randomized, dose-finding study. *Mov Disord* 2013; **28**: 1838–46.
42. Parkinson Study Group. Phase II safety, tolerability, and dose selection study of isradipine as a potential disease-modifying intervention in early Parkinson's disease (STEADY-PD). *Mov Disord* 2013; **28**: 1823–31.
43. Parkinson Study Group SURE-P Inbestigators, Schwarzschild MA, Ascherio A, *et al.* Inosine to increase serum and cerebrospinal fluid urate in Parkinson disease: a randomized clinical trial. *JAMA Neurol* 2014; **71**: 141–50.

Section II Management of Nonmotor Symptoms of Parkinson's Disease

Chapter 10

Management of autonomic dysfunction in Parkinson's disease

Shen-Yang Lim and Ai Huey Tan

Introduction

Autonomic dysfunction can occur many years before a diagnosis of Parkinson's disease (PD) is made [1], and symptoms are prevalent in patients with newly diagnosed, untreated PD [2]. Some studies reported that the most common nonmotor symptoms in PD are autonomic, and these correlate strongly with health-related quality of life [3]. Some of these symptoms, particularly persistent orthostatic hypotension, may also be a predictor of shorter survival [4]. Recognition of autonomic impairment is important, and physicians should actively investigate and treat these problems as an integral part of treating PD, since symptomatic treatment is frequently effective and may have an impact on the overall function and quality of life in PD (e.g. alleviating orthostatic hypotension could reduce the risk of falls).

Unlike the motor manifestations of PD, autonomic dysfunction is usually nonresponsive to dopaminergic medications. In fact, some autonomic problems, such as orthostatic hypotension, can be exacerbated by dopaminergic therapy. Physicians also need to bear in mind that drugs for autonomic problems may treat one symptom while potentially worsening another at the same time (e.g. anticholinergics for overactive bladder may aggravate constipation). Nonpharmacological measures should usually be administered in the first instance [5]. As for the management of other aspects of PD, an interdisciplinary approach can be of great benefit [6].

In this chapter, we review management strategies for the more common features of autonomic dysfunction. Less commonly recognized entities such as rhinorrhea or dry mouth will not be discussed. Details of epidemiology, assessment, pathophysiology and the impact of deep-brain stimulation surgery are also beyond the scope of this chapter and have been covered elsewhere [7–9]. It should be noted that in the recently published Movement Disorder Society Evidence-Based Medicine Review for the treatment of nonmotor symptoms in PD, which reviewed randomized controlled trials (RCTs) (i.e. level I studies), the only drugs for autonomic dysfunction receiving a designation of "efficacious" were botulinum toxin injections and glycopyrrolate (for sialorrhea) [10]. Macrogol and lubiprostone (for constipation) and domperidone (for anorexia, nausea and vomiting associated with dopaminergic therapy) were designated "likely efficacious" [10]. All other treatments for autonomic dysfunction in PD were designated as having "insufficient evidence," indicating that most of the management recommendations discussed below are based on a lower level of evidence.

Orthostatic hypotension

Orthostatic hypotension occurs in up to 58% of PD patients (but may be symptomatic in only 20%) [6, 7]. Orthostatic hypotension is defined as a reduction in systolic blood pressure of ≥20 mmHg or diastolic blood pressure ≥10 mmHg within 3 min of standing or head-up tilt to at least 60° on a tilt table (in some patients, however, 3 min of postural challenge may be insufficiently sensitive) [11]. Although the characteristic symptoms are light-headedness or syncope when upright, patients are frequently asymptomatic [11], or symptoms may be nonspecific (e.g. blurred vision, nausea, vertigo, disequilibrium, leg buckling, falls, impaired cognition, fatigue/tiredness, weakness or pain [e.g. in the head, posterior cervical or shoulder region]) [12–15]. Tilt-table testing or 24 h ambulatory

---

Parkinson's Disease: Current and Future Therapeutics and Clinical Trials, ed. Gálvez-Jiménez *et al.* Published by Cambridge University Press. © Cambridge University Press 2016.

blood pressure recording should be performed to confirm a diagnosis of suspected orthostatic hypotension when bedside sphygmomanometry is nondiagnostic [11, 16]. Nonneurogenic causes of orthostatic hypotension should also be considered, such as reduced cardiac output from aortic stenosis or cardiomyopathy [13, 17].

Orthostatic hypotension can be caused by antiparkinsonian medications (dopamine agonists, selegiline and amantadine more so than levodopa [L-DOPA]) [5, 7]. Antihypertensive (e.g. diuretics), antidepressant (e.g. tricyclics) and antipsychotic medications are other common causes of orthostatic hypotension [5, 18]. In one study, polypharmacy (defined as intake of five or more medicines) was an independent risk factor for orthostatic hypotension in PD patients, with an odds ratio of 3.6 [18]. Discontinuation, dose change or substitution of these drugs should be considered. Doses of antihypertensive medication, if needed, should be shifted to the afternoon or evening, as orthostatic hypotension is often worst in the morning. Patients should maintain a blood pressure diary to record measurements and note accompanying symptoms (e.g. sitting and standing up on awakening, before lunch and 1 h after lunch, and supine before retiring) [13, 14]. In individuals with advanced disease and disabling orthostatic symptoms, a pragmatic approach may need to be adopted, for instance, aiming for systolic blood pressure of >80 and <180 mmHg when supine, in conjunction with improvement of symptoms [14].

Nonpharmacological interventions

Nonpharmacological interventions should be the first line of therapy and are summarized in Table 10.1 [7, 13, 14, 19]. However, PD patients may also have difficulty adopting some of these measures (e.g. increasing fluid intake can worsen urinary symptoms), and in one study the overall compliance with nonpharmacological management was 78% over a 3-week period (patients were least compliant with compression stockings) [20].

Pharmacological interventions

Pharmacological interventions may be warranted if significant symptoms persist despite the above measures (Table 10.2). These are targeted at volume expansion and vasoconstriction. The drugs most commonly used are fludrocortisone and midodrine, either as monotherapy or combined. Droxidopa has recently received US Food and Drug Administration (FDA) approval for treatment of neurogenic orthostatic hypotension [21]. It is debatable whether patients with asymptomatic orthostatic hypotension should be treated pharmacologically [5]. Supine hypertension (see p. 97) can be caused or exacerbated by many of these agents.

Table 10.1 Nonpharmacological management of orthostatic hypotension

Ensure sufficient fluid intake (2–3 l/day). Intermittent water boluses (e.g. two glasses or 500 ml of water ingested rapidly) raises blood pressure within 5–15 min, for 1–2 h (e.g. this can be done in the morning, when orthostatic hypotension is usually worse)
Liberal addition of salt to the diet (up to 10 g/day)
Move from a lying to a standing position in gradual stages (e.g. sit on the side of the bed for 30 s before standing; wait for several seconds before starting to walk)
Avoid standing still for long periods
Avoid Valsalva maneuvers (straining). Constipation, urinary hesitancy or cough, if present, should be treated
Avoid large carbohydrate meals (instead, take small meals throughout the day)
Avoid alcohol consumption
Avoid exposure to hot environments (e.g. hot baths)
Avoid overly vigorous physical exercise (instead, exercise at a moderate level and/or in a recumbent or seated position)
Adopt physical countermaneuvers when symptoms occur (e.g. squatting, marching in place, toe raise [standing on tiptoes] or sitting with the legs crossed)
Wear tight waist-high stockings or a corset/abdominal binder
Raise the head of the bed while sleeping at night by 10–30°/10–30 cm

Fludrocortisone

Fludrocortisone (9-α-fluorohydrocortisone) is a synthetic mineralocorticoid. It increases plasma volume by promoting renal sodium retention and enhances the sensitivity of blood vessels to circulating catecholamines [13]. Fludrocortisone has a prolonged duration of action and the pressor effect requires several days to be apparent [13]. The starting dose is 0.05 or 0.1 mg, which can be uptitrated by 0.05 mg weekly according to response to 0.3 mg daily (although doses up to 1 mg daily have been used) [7, 13, 22]. This agent should be used cautiously in patients with heart disease because of the possibility of precipitating congestive heart failure. Peripheral edema, supine hypertension and headache are potential adverse effects; higher doses can

Table 10.2 Pharmacological agents commonly used to treat autonomic dysfunction in Parkinson's disease

Autonomic problem	Pharmacological agent, suggested doses and remarks
Orthostatic hypotension	Fludrocortisone (Florinef®): starting dose 0.05 or 0.1 mg, uptitrated by 0.05 mg weekly according to response to 0.3 mg daily (doses up to 1 mg daily have been used) Use cautiously in patients with heart disease (may precipitate heart failure)
	Midodrine (Amatine®, Gutron®): starting dose 2.5 mg bid or tid (before meals), and uptitrated according to response (e.g. by weekly increments of 2.5 mg) to 10 mg two to four times daily The last dose should be given no later than 4 h before recumbency/bedtime (e.g. at 5 or 6 pm)
	Domperidone (Motilium®): 10–20 mg orally tid (e.g. 30–60 min before dopamine agonist dosing)
	Droxidopa (Northera®): 100 mg orally tid, titrating in increments of 100 mg tid every 24–48 h (maximum dose, 600 mg tid)
Gastroparesis	Domperidone (Motilium®): 10–20 mg orally 30 min before meals
Constipation	Supplemental fiber/bulk-forming laxative: e.g. Psyllium (Fybogel® or Metamucil®, one sachet bid with breakfast and dinner)
	Osmotic laxative: e.g. Macrogol/polyethylene glycol (PEG) (Macrogol 3350/Movicol®, one sachet every 3 days to two sachets/day, or Macrogol 4000/Forlax®, one to two sachets/day) Lactulose (Duphalac® 10 ml/day, up to 40 ml bid)
	Stimulant laxative: e.g. Bisacodyl (Dulcolax®) 5–15 mg at bedtime
	Prokinetic agent: e.g. Prucalopride (Resolor®) 2 or 4 mg daily
	Rectal laxatives: e.g. Dulcolax® 10 mg, or glycerin, one suppository as needed
Sialorrhea	Glycopyrrolate (Robinul®, Cuvposa®): 1–2 mg tid
	Sublingual atropine: 1% ophthalmic drops, one drop (0.5 mg) bid
	The following are usually used for other primary indications, but may reduce sialorrhea as a side effect: Trihexyphenidyl (Artane®, Apo-Trihex®) Amitriptyline (e.g. Endep®, Elavil®) Amantadine (Symmetrel®, PK Merz®)

	Botulinum toxin injections
	Parotid gland (dose given for each side; each parotid injected in two sites):
	    Botox® 15–50 units
	    Dysport® 75–150 units
	    Neurobloc®/Myobloc® 500–4000 units
	Submandibular gland (dose given for each side; injected in one site):
	    Botox® 10–15 units
	    Dysport® 25–80 units
	    Neurobloc®/Myobloc® 250 units

"Irritative" urinary symptoms (urgency, frequency, nocturia)	Oxybutynin: immediate release (Ditropan®) 2.5–5 mg two to four times daily, or extended release (Gelnique®) 5–30 mg once daily, or patch (Oxytrol®) one application twice a week
	Tolterodine/detrusitol (Detrol®): immediate release 1 or 2 mg bid or tid, or extended release 2–4 mg once daily
	Trospium (Sanctura®, Spasmolyt®): 20 mg once daily or bid
	Solifenacin (Vesicare®): 5–10 mg once daily
Erectile dysfunction	Sildenafil (Viagra®): starting dose 50 mg, which can be titrated up to 100 mg (or down to 25 mg) as required Usually taken 1 h before sexual activity, but in some PD patients the onset of action may be delayed up to 4 h; efficacy is optimal when taken on an empty stomach Orthostatic hypotension may occur, and sildenafil is contraindicated if blood pressure is below 90/50 mmHg, or in patients receiving nitrate therapy (co-administration can produce life-threatening hypotension)

bid, Twice daily; tid, three times daily.

cause hypokalemia, and potassium supplementation may be necessary.

Midodrine

Midodrine is a prodrug with an active metabolite, desglymidodrine, that is an α_1-adrenoreceptor agonist that constricts arterioles and veins and increases total peripheral resistance. Midodrine should be started at 2.5 mg two or three times daily (before meals), and uptitrated according to response (e.g. by weekly increments of 2.5 mg) to 10 mg two to four times daily [12, 13, 23]. Most patients respond best to 10 mg [14]. The peak effect is at 1 h, and the duration of action of a single dose is approximately 4 h. Supine hypertension is a common side effect, but because midodrine has a short blood-pressure-raising effect, it can be withheld in the later part of the day (the last dose should be given no later than 4 h before recumbency/bedtime, e.g. at 5 or 6 pm) [12, 13]. Other potential side effects are piloerection (goosebumps), itch, paresthesias (especially of the scalp; these symptoms are due to its α-adrenergic effects on the skin and skin appendages) and urinary retention [12, 23]. It should be noted that the multicenter double-blinded placebo-controlled randomized studies reported by Jankovic et al. [23] and Low et al. [12] evaluating midodrine for neurogenic orthostatic hypotension ($n = 97$ and 171 subjects, respectively) included a total of only 41 PD patients. In the study by Jankovic et al. [23], the mean increase in standing blood pressure with midodrine (10 mg twice daily) was 22 mmHg for systolic and 15 mmHg for diastolic readings, and in the study by Low et al. [12] this was 19.5–22.4 mmHg for systolic and 11.1–13.3 mmHg for diastolic readings. These blood pressure changes were associated with improvement in orthostatic symptoms.

Domperidone

Domperidone is a peripheral dopamine D_2 receptor antagonist that does not cross the blood–brain barrier. Its mechanism of action has been proposed to be via inhibition of presynaptic dopamine receptors on sympathetic nerve endings, thereby enhancing norepinephrine release [20]. It is often used to treat and prevent orthostatic hypotension induced by dopamine agonist therapy [20, 24, 25]. The dosage is 10–20 mg 30–60 min orally before dopamine agonist dosing. In one small double-blinded crossover RCT ($n = 13$ PD patients with symptomatic orthostasis in the drug treatment phase) comparing domperidone 10 mg three times daily versus fludrocortisone 0.1 mg daily, both treatments resulted in improvement of orthostatic symptoms and a trend toward reduced orthostatic drop on tilt-table testing (with domperidone having a greater effect than fludrocortisone for the latter endpoint) [20]. In this study, all patients were on levodopa therapy and 24% received dopamine agonist treatment, suggesting that the efficacy of domperidone is not limited to patients on dopamine agonists (or only to orthostatic hypotension in PD, since efficacy has also been reported in diabetic orthostatic hypotension). The efficacy of domperidone for orthostatic hypotension in PD requires further study [19]. This agent does not appear to induce supine hypertension [20].

Droxidopa

Droxidopa (L-threo-3,4,-dihydroxyphenylserine or L-threo-DOPS or L-DOPS), a norepinephrine precursor, was tested in randomized placebo-controlled phase 3 clinical trial in PD and other patients with neurogenic orthostatic hypotension and showed that oral administration of droxidopa three times daily (study NOH301) increased blood pressure and improved symptoms of postural light-headedness [21]. Supine systolic BP of >180 mmHg was observed in 5% of droxidopa and 2.5% of placebo recipients, but no patients registered >200 mmHg. Interestingly, in a parallel study, droxidopa recipients reported fewer total falls than placebo recipients (79 vs 192) (50% fewer falls per patient in the droxidopa group; $P = 0.16$) [26], and this independent effect is being directly examined in further studies.

Treatments not commonly used currently in PD patients

Pyridostigmine, by inhibiting acetylcholinesterase, enhances sympathetic ganglionic neurotransmission (as preganglionic sympathetic neurons are cholinergic), primarily in the upright position. This agent is started at a dose of 30 mg twice daily, and increased gradually to the target dose of 60 mg three times daily [14, 27]. Singer et al. [28] reported in an RCT ($n = 58$, but none of the subjects had PD) that pyridostigmine 60 mg modestly reduced the fall in standing diastolic blood pressure (fall of 27.6 versus 34.0 mmHg with placebo; $P = 0.04$), with an improvement in orthostatic symptoms, without aggravating supine hypertension [13, 14]. However, in a recently published RCT (31 patients with severe orthostatic hypotension, including six patients with PD), pyridostigmine 60 mg did not increase standing diastolic blood pressure nor improve symptoms [29]. The difference observed between the two studies could be due to the greater severity of dysfunction in the cohort of Shibao et al. [29] (with a mean drop in standing systolic blood pressure of 67 mmHg). Potential adverse effects include excessive salivation, abdominal colic and diarrhea [13].

Indomethacin is a prostaglandin synthetase inhibitor and its effect may be due to an inhibition of vasodilatory prostaglandins [17]. Indomethacin improved orthostatic hypotension in a small, double-blinded placebo-controlled RCT involving 12 PD subjects. In this study, oral indomethacin reduced the fall in mean blood pressure on standing from 34.8 to 17.3 mmHg (while placebo had no noticeable effect), with a reduction in orthostatic symptoms. The dosage used is 25–50 mg three times daily [17, 19]. However, gastrointestinal toxicity is a limiting factor.

Desmopressin (DDAVP®) is a vasopressin analog that acts on the collecting ducts of renal tubules to reduce nocturnal diuresis [7, 13, 15, 19]. The usual dosage is 5–40 µg at bedtime by nasal spray [13]. However, in the only study involving patients with PD ($n = 8$, all with orthostatic hypotension), desmopressin produced no significant changes in blood pressure [30]. Water intoxication with hyponatremia is a potential side effect.

Erythropoietin increases the production of red blood cells and may also have may have direct or indirect effects on vascular walls [7, 13]. It was shown to increase upright blood pressure and improved postural symptoms in patients with neurogenic orthostatic hypotension; however, none of the published studies included patients with PD [13].

Octreotide is a somatostatin analog that inhibits the release of gastrointestinal peptides (some of which have vasodilatory properties) and causes splanchnic vasoconstriction [31]. This agent was shown in small studies to be effective for orthostatic and post-prandial hypotension, without causing supine hypertension; however, none of the published studies included PD patients [17, 31]. The method of administration (by daily subcutaneous injection) and expense limit more widespread use of this agent [17, 32].

Cardiac pacing to increase cardiac output by increasing heart rate was suggested in several case reports as a treatment for severe orthostatic hypotension, but in one RCT by Sahul et al. [33] involving six patients (two with PD) and tilt-table testing, dual chamber pacing at 90 and 110 beats/min did not produce any benefits.

Supine hypertension

Many patients with PD, particularly those with orthostatic hypotension, demonstrate nondipping (i.e. <10% blood pressure decrease during the night) or have supine hypertension, even before treatment of hypotension is initiated [16]. This raises concerns regarding hypertensive end-organ damage (such as cerebrovascular disease, cardiomyopathy, nephropathy and retinopathy), which has to be taken into consideration when treating orthostatic hypotension (although the incidence of these complications has not been studied prospectively in patients with neurogenic orthostatic hypotension) [13, 17]. During the day, patients should avoid the supine posture (e.g. should sit in a reclining chair with the feet on the floor), and at night the head of the bed should be raised 10–30° [13, 32]. Antihypotensive medications such as midodrine should be taken no later than 4 h before recumbency/bedtime, e.g. at 5 or 6 pm. Alternative antihypotensive agents that do not aggravate supine hypertension, such as pyridostigmine or octreotide, may be considered [17, 27]. Short-acting antihypertensive agents in the evening (so that their effects have waned by the next morning) may be considered in patients with severe sustained supine hypertension. These include nifedipine (30 mg), nitroglycerin transdermally (0.1–0.2 mg/h) and clonidine 0.1 mg [7, 13, 32]. Twenty-four-hour ambulatory blood pressure monitoring is recommended in this setting to evaluate therapeutic efficacy.

Gastroparesis

Gastroparesis is characterized by impaired gastric emptying in the absence of mechanical outlet obstruction, and can be associated with nausea, early satiety, bloating, heartburn, vomiting, abdominal pain ("dyspepsia" symptoms) and weight loss [6, 34, 35]. Gastroparesis occurs in untreated patients with early PD and is exacerbated by levodopa or dopamine agonist treatment [32, 36]. Gastroparesis can alter the bioavailability of levodopa (since levodopa must reach the small intestine to be absorbed) and contribute to the development of response fluctuations such as delayed "on" and even dose failures (due to gastric conversion of levodopa into dopamine, which prevents its absorption and transport to the brain) [6].

Patients should be encouraged to take small but frequent low-fat meals (fat empties from the stomach slowly) [32, 34, 35]. Dietitian referral may be beneficial to help correct malnutrition, if present. Domperidone is a peripheral dopamine D_2 receptor antagonist that is relatively impermeable to the blood–brain barrier [32, 35, 36]. It antagonizes dopamine's inhibitory effects on gastric motility and is the preferred prokinetic drug in PD [37, 38]. Domperidone also has antiemetic activity as a result of blockade of dopamine receptors in the chemoreceptor trigger zone, located outside the blood–brain barrier, and of gastric dopamine receptors [36]. The dosage is 10–20 mg, 30 min before meals as required. Some studies have used up to 120 mg daily in PD patients without adverse effects [36, 37, 39], but recently concerns have been raised about potential cardiotoxicity (prolongation of the QT interval and ventricular arrhythmias), especially at higher dosages (>30 mg daily), when combined with other QT-prolonging drugs (e.g. erythromycin, citalopram, escitalopram and tricyclic antidepressants), or in patients with cardiac disease [40]. Nevertheless, there is currently limited evidence relating drug-induced QT prolongation to morbidity and mortality specifically in PD patients [40]. Domperidone-induced worsening of parkinsonian symptoms is rare [36, 37, 39], but has been reported [37]. Metoclopramide, another D_2 receptor antagonist, also improves gastric emptying but is contraindicated in PD because it crosses the blood–brain barrier and worsens parkinsonism [36].

Treatments not commonly used currently in PD patients

Erythromycin (50–250 mg orally two or four times daily) is a potent prokinetic but has not been studied specifically in patients with PD (note that this antibiotic, like domperidone, also prolongs the QT interval) [32, 35].

The serotonergic 5-HT$_4$ agonists mosapride and prucalopride accelerate gastric emptying and colonic transit (activation of 5-HT$_4$ receptors on cholinergic nerve endings throughout the gastrointestinal tract enhances the release of acetylcholine from motor neurons, thereby stimulating gastrointestinal motility) [35, 41].

Mosapride prolonged "on" time in a small open-label study ($n = 5$ PD patients) by Asai et al. [42]; there are no studies as yet on prucalopride in PD patients. The nonselective 5-HT$_4$ agonists cisapride and tegaserod have been withdrawn from the market because of potential cardiovascular side effects [41].

Botulinum toxin injections into the pyloric sphincter (to reduce the resistance of the pyloric sphincter, thereby facilitating gastric emptying) improved gastric emptying in two PD patients, but further study is needed [6, 35]. This technique is invasive and endoscopic expertise is needed.

Gastric electrical stimulation (with electrodes surgically inserted into the stomach by laparotomy or laparoscopy, and the stimulator placed subcutaneously in the abdomen) is an emerging treatment for refractory gastroparesis but has not been studied specifically in PD [6, 35].

Constipation

Constipation, generally defined as fewer than three bowel movements per week, can be due to slow colonic transit or outlet obstruction (see below). Up to 80% of PD patients have slowed colonic transit [43]. However, a colonoscopy or barium enema to exclude organic obstruction by neoplasm or inflammatory disease should be performed in patients with a recent alteration in bowel habit if there is unexplained weight loss (although this is also common in patients with PD), rectal bleeding, anemia or a positive family history of colorectal or ovarian cancer [44].

Treatment should begin with simple measures (increasing fiber and fluid intake, and physical activity) [34, 43–45]. An open-label study of a high-fiber diet in 19 PD patients (mean daily fiber intake of 28 g/day) by Astarloa et al. [46] showed significant improvement of constipation severity in all patients (accompanied by improved levodopa bioavailability and motor function). It is thought that fiber increases stool bulk, distending the colon and promoting propulsive activity. Psyllium powder is obtained from the outer coat of the psyllium seed from the plant *Plantago ovata*. A small RCT by Ashraf et al. [47] ($n = 7$ PD patients) (three received 5.1 g of psyllium twice daily vs four receiving placebo) showed that stool frequency increased significantly after 8 weeks of treatment (on average, three additional bowel movements per week) [43]. One study in non-PD subjects found psyllium to be superior to different pharmacological agents such as lactulose in the treatment of constipation, with a lower incidence of adverse events [48]. Another study of frail elderly patients by Sturtzel et al. [49] reported that increased dietary fiber allowed discontinuation of laxatives in a majority of patients and, in contrast to laxative treatment, was not associated with weight loss. Bloating, abdominal pain and flatulence are potential side effects of increased fiber [45]. Regardless of the source (dietary vs supplemental), combining fiber with adequate fluid intake (e.g. 1.5–2 l/day) is important [45]. Medications that can exacerbate constipation should be replaced if possible (e.g. opioids, anticholinergics, tricyclic antidepressants, antihistamines, calcium-channel antagonists, diuretics and nonsteroidal anti-inflammatory drugs) [44, 45]. An association between dopaminergic medications and constipation remains debated [44, 50].

Osmotic laxatives

These agents produce an osmotic gradient and retain fluid in the colonic lumen, leading to softer stools and improved propulsion. A small open-label study of macrogol/polyethylene glycol (PEG) 3350 (PEG with a molecular mass of 3350) plus electrolytes (Movicol®) in severely constipated patients by Eichhorn et al. [51] ($n = 8$ PD and 2 multiple-system atrophy [MSA] patients) found this agent to be effective in improving stool frequency and ease of defecation in all patients studied (leading to the withdrawal of all concomitant laxatives). The maintenance dose ranged from two sachets daily to one sachet every 3 days. A larger RCT by Zangaglia et al. [52] (29 PD patients received PEG 7.3 g plus electrolytes, one to three sachets daily; 28 received placebo) provided level I evidence that PEG is effective and well-tolerated in the treatment of constipation in PD patients. One systematic review of drug trials for constipation concluded that PEG is modestly more effective than lactulose [48]. Adverse effects are few, but nausea, vomiting, diarrhea, flatulence and abdominal pain can occur [45, 48, 52]. Lactulose is commonly used, but there are no studies in patients with PD. Nausea, bloating, flatulence and loose stools are potential side effects [48]. Although lactulose is a nonabsorbable disaccharide, lactulose syrup may contain small amounts of absorbable sugars, and has rarely been reported to worsen glycemic control in diabetic patients, as reported by Kirkman et al. [53].

Stimulant/"irritant" laxatives

These agents simulate the colonic myenteric plexus. Bisacodyl and senna are commonly used examples. One study found these laxatives to be less effective than lactulose [48]. Tolerance may develop but appears to be uncommon [54]. The suggestion that chronic use of stimulant laxatives can damage intestinal smooth muscle or the myenteric plexus and cause "cathartic colon" is poorly documented. The prevailing opinion, supported by more recent investigations, is that stimulant laxatives used at the recommended doses are unlikely to be harmful to the colon [45, 48, 54].

Prokinetic agents

5-HT$_4$ agonists accelerate colonic transit by facilitating acetylcholine release from enteric cholinergic neurons. The nonselective 5-HT$_4$ agonists cisapride and tegaserod have been withdrawn from the market because of potential cardiovascular side effects [41]. A small open-label study by Liu et al. [55] ($n = 7$ patients with PD, 7 with MSA) showed that mosapride 15 mg daily augmented lower gastrointestinal tract motility with improvement in bowel frequency and difficult defecation. Prucalopride is a highly selective 5-HT$_4$ receptor agonist and has not been reported to be associated with cardiovascular side effects [41]. Camilleri et al. [56] randomized 620 subjects with severe idiopathic constipation to receive prucalopride 2 mg, prucalopride 4 mg or placebo once daily over 12 weeks. The proportion of patients with three or more spontaneous, complete bowel movements per week was higher in the prucalopride groups (2 mg, 30.9%; 4 mg, 28.4%) compared with placebo (12%, $P < 0.01$). Headache, nausea, abdominal pain and diarrhea are potential side effects [56]. Prucalopride has not been studied specifically in PD patients.

Stool softeners

The evidence for the effectiveness of these agents is weak [45]. Docusate has modest efficacy only [48]. Liquid paraffin has been associated with reduced absorption of fat-soluble vitamins, and lipoid pneumonia after aspiration [45].

Rectal laxatives

Glycerin (or glycerol) and bisacodyl suppositories are commonly used, with an onset of action occurring within minutes [45]. Anorectal irritation is a potential side effect.

Treatments not commonly used currently in PD patients

Probiotics have been suggested to have favorable effects on gastrointestinal function by suppressing the growth of pathogenic bacteria (which may contribute to gastrointestinal dysmotility), and they have become popular in treating a spectrum of gastrointestinal disorders. Cassani et al. [57] studied the use of *Lactobacillus casei* strain Shirota daily for 5 weeks in PD patients ($n = 40$) and found improvement in stool consistency and symptoms such as bloating, abdominal pain and the sensation of incomplete emptying.

Lubiprostone is a chloride channel activator that enhances fluid secretion into the intestinal lumen and intestinal motility, without altering serum concentrations of sodium and potassium [58]. Systemic absorption of the drug is negligible. In a 4-week double-blinded study, PD patients with significant constipation (n = 54) were randomly assigned to lubiprostone (uptitrated to 24 μg twice daily) or placebo [58]. A marked or very marked clinical global improvement was reported by 64% of subjects receiving lubiprostone versus 19% of the placebo group. The constipation rating scale, visual analog scale for change in constipation and number of daily stools by diary also improved significantly with lubiprostone. Adverse events were mild, most commonly intermittent loose stools, which did not result in study withdrawals. The agent was otherwise very well tolerated.

Sandyk et al. [59] reported that colchicine, frequently used for the treatment of gout, was effective in treating refractory constipation in three PD patients without adverse effects (0.3–0.6 mg). The mechanism of action is unclear, but the efficacy of colchicine (0.6 mg three times daily) was subsequently shown in a small 4-week, placebo-controlled RCT involving 16 patients with refractory idiopathic chronic constipation (0.6 mg three times daily) [45]. There was a mild increase in abdominal pain scores during treatment with colchicine, but this decreased by the fourth week of therapy.

An anecdotal report by Sadjadpour suggested that pyridostigmine, a cholinesterase inhibitor used in the treatment of myasthenia gravis, was effective in PD patients with refractory constipation (60 mg one to three times daily).

A small open-label study by Sakakibara et al. [60] (n = 6 PD patients, 4 MSA patients) suggested that Dai-Kenchu-To (a dietary herb extract) improved bowel movement frequency and difficult defecation, with no adverse effects. Objective measures of lower gastrointestinal tract motility also improved.

The efficacy of neutrophin-3 injections was reported by Pfeiffer et al. [61], but this agent has been abandoned.

In one study of 16 PD patients, magnetic stimulation (with the coil placed over the T9 and L3 spinal processes for 20 min twice daily, over 3 weeks) significantly improved colonic transit time and symptoms including frequency of bowel movement and stool consistency [62]. Treatment also improved pelvic floor descent and anorectal angle during defecation. The beneficial effects persisted at the 3-month follow-up [62].

Defecatory dysfunction

In one study, 13% of PD patients with chronic constipation had isolated or prominent outlet-type constipation [63]. This is caused by a failure of relaxation of the puborectalis muscles and the external anal sphincter during defecation [44]. Symptoms include anal pain with defecation, excessive straining and incomplete evacuation [64]. Anorectal manometry and fluoroscopic defecography are useful for evaluating anorectal dysfunction but may not always be readily available [64]. Treatment is often very challenging.

Albanese et al. [63] showed in a prospective study of ten PD patients that botulinum toxin injections into the puborectalis muscles resulted in objective improvements (reduced anorectal tone and increased anorectal angle, during straining); however, the effect on patients' symptoms was not reported. In another open-label study using a similar design (n = 18 PD patients, injected with 100 units of Botox® into the puborectalis under transrectal ultrasound guidance) [64], symptomatic improvement was noted at the 1- and 2-month follow-ups in eight (44%) and ten (56%) patients, respectively, accompanied by objective improvements similar to those reported by Albanese et al. [63]. The eight patients who did not respond to the initial treatment were retreated with 200 units of Botox®, resulting in symptomatic and objective improvements in four of them. No significant side effects were reported. There are anecdotal reports in a small number of PD patients that intermittent subcutaneous apomorphine injections can ameliorate symptoms of outlet constipation, with objective improvements documented by defecography and anorectal manometry [65, 66]. Biofeedback has been reported to benefit many patients with obstructed defecation, but no studies have been conducted in PD patients.

Sialorrhea

Sialorrhea (excessive build-up of saliva in the mouth) and drooling (involuntary spillage of saliva from the mouth) in PD are mainly due to dysphagia with decreased swallowing frequency or less efficient swallowing, and are often compounded by a tendency to keep the mouth open (facial hypomimia) and stooped posture. Although common in advanced PD, one recent study reported a high prevalence of increased saliva or drooling in patients with newly diagnosed and untreated PD (42 vs 6% of nonparkinsonian controls) [2]. Some drugs used frequently in advanced PD, such as clozapine and cholinesterase inhibitors, can increase salivary gland excretion. Sialorrhea can also be caused by factors other than PD (e.g. badly fitting dentures). Many patients experience only drooling on the pillow at night; however, in some patients, drooling causes social embarrassment and isolation, skin maceration, and speech and feeding may be disturbed.

Chewing gum or sucking on hard candy (preferably sugarless) may provide temporary improvement by serving as a cue to swallow more frequently [6]. In an acute experimental study, gum chewing increased swallow frequency and decreased the interval between swallows [67]. This may be an effective self-managed approach for saliva management without reducing salivary flow. In this study, patients performed gum chewing for only 5 min; therefore, the long-term efficacy of this approach requires further study. Behavior modification approaches, e.g. regular reminders to consciously swallow saliva using a beep-emitting brooch, may be effective in motivated patients but has been studied in only a small number of PD subjects ($n = 6$).

Better control of parkinsonian motor symptoms, including motor fluctuations (sialorrhea is more prominent during "off" periods) can improve sialorrhea; however, the response is usually only partial [68].

Salivation is mediated primarily through parasympathetic (cholinergic) innervation of the salivary glands, and anticholinergic agents are the first-line pharmacological therapy for sialorrhea [68]. Trihexyphenidyl is an anticholinergic commonly prescribed for tremor in PD. Dryness of the mouth is a very common side effect, but there has been no formal study of this agent as a treatment for sialorrhea in PD. Glycopyrrolate (glycopyrronium bromide) is an anticholinergic drug that does not cross the blood–brain barrier in considerable amounts and therefore exhibits minimal central side effects. One double-blinded RCT ($n = 23$ PD patients) showed that 39% of patients taking oral glycopyrrolate (1 mg three times daily) had a clinically relevant improvement (≥30% in mean sialorrhea score) versus only one patient (4%) in the placebo group ($P = 0.021$) [69]. The mean improvement in sialorrhea score with glycopyrrolate compared with placebo was 0.8 points (on a 9-point scale, $P = 0.011$). There were no significant adverse events with glycopyrrolate. The maximum recommended dose is 8 mg/day [69]. Sublingual atropine (1% ophthalmic drops; one drop [0.5 mg] twice daily) was effective in a small open-label study ($n = 6$ PD patients) by Hyson et al. [70], both in terms of self-reported drooling severity and objectively measured saliva production [56]. Although two patients experienced worsening of hallucinations in this study, this treatment appears to be relatively safe in clinical practice [71]. Sublingual application of ipratropium bromide spray (an anticholinergic that does not cross the blood–brain barrier; one to two sprays four times/day as needed [21 µg of ipratropium bromide per metered dose spray]) was evaluated by Thomsen et al. [72] in a double-blinded RCT ($n = 15$ patients completing the study). Treatment had no effect on the weight of saliva produced (the primary outcome measure), but there was a mild effect on subjective measures of sialorrhea. The treatment was well tolerated without any anticholinergic side effects. Amitriptyline (e.g. to treat depression, insomnia or pain) or amantadine (most often used for levodopa-induced dyskinesias) also have anticholinergic properties and may have the useful side effect of reducing sialorrhea [68].

Botulinum toxin blocks acetylcholine release at the cholinergic neurosecretory junction of the salivary glands, thereby reducing saliva production. Ninety percent of saliva production originates (in equal amounts) from the parotid and submandibular glands (the other salivary glands contributing the remaining 10%); these glands can be injected (bilaterally) using anatomical landmarks [68, 73]. Some authors reported superior efficacy with combined injections (of both the parotid and submandibular glands) or with ultrasound guidance, but there is no consensus on this issue [68]. Botulinum toxin type B may have a preferential action on autonomic neurons and could potentially be more effective for sialorrhea. However, one pilot study by Guidubaldi et al. [74] found no significant difference in the mean duration of benefit for botulinum toxin A (Dysport® 250 units) and botulinum toxin B (Neurobloc® 2500 units); this study was limited by a small sample size ($n = 7$ PD patients only completing the study). There is a risk of transiently exacerbating dysphagia and chewing difficulties, due to toxin diffusion into the pharyngeal, masseter and temporalis muscles. A large, multicenter, placebo-controlled trial with botulinum toxin type B (Myobloc® 2500 units) is ongoing in the USA (National Institutes of Health clinical trials registry [clinicaltrials.gov] NCT01994109).

Treatments not commonly used currently in PD patients

Tropicamide (slowly-dissolving, intraoral thin film) was evaluated in a pilot study ($n = 19$ PD patients) [5].

The primary efficacy outcome was negative, but some antisialorrhea effects were observed, without adverse events; a larger study of this agent is ongoing (clinicaltrials.gov identifier NCT01844648).

Other treatments that have been used for sialorrhea include clonidine, modafinil, and β-blockers, but there is only limited evidence currently to support their use in PD patients [5, 68].

Radiotherapy to the parotid and submandibular glands (dose of 12 gray) was shown in one study to be effective and safe in patients with parkinsonism ($n = 28$, 22 with PD) [75]. A treatment effect was seen within days in most patients, and lasted more than a year (with some patients still experiencing considerable improvement of drooling at the 5-year follow-up). One or more persistent adverse effects occurred in one-third of patients, including loss of taste, dry mouth and increased viscosity of saliva. Nevertheless, patients reported significantly improved quality of life, and clinical global impression scores at the final follow-up showed that 80% of patients were either satisfied or very satisfied. There can be up to a 40-fold increased risk of developing salivary gland tumors many years after radiotherapy, but patients with PD and severe drooling generally have advanced disease (and often also advanced age) with a limited life expectancy, which probably alters the risk:benefit ratio [68, 75].

Surgical treatments (e.g. submandibular duct relocation or neurectomy [sectioning the chorda tympani nerves]) are invasive and there are no published reports on these procedures in PD patients [68].

Urinary dysfunction

Overactive bladder (OAB) (or detrusor hyperreflexia) is the major cause of urinary symptoms associated with PD [36, 76, 77]. The resulting "irritative" (or "storage") symptoms include nocturia (the most common complaint), frequency, urgency and (particularly if poor mobility compounds the bladder disorder) urge incontinence [78]. Patients experience a sensation of bladder fullness and an urge to void before appropriate bladder filling has occurred.

Patients with urinary complaints should be screened and treated for urinary tract infection (UTI), and undergo behavioral evaluation of drinking and voiding habits and modification, if applicable (a voiding and intake diary is useful) [79]. Intake of caffeine and alcohol should be reduced as these cause polyuria [80, 81]. Drug treatments may need to be modified (e.g. frusemide exacerbating OAB symptoms) [80]. Constipation and fecal impaction can cause either irritation or obstruction in the lower urinary tract and should be treated [79]. Assessment of post-void residual urine volume (PVR) should be part of the initial workup [76, 78, 79].

Behavioral treatments can be highly effective to treat urge incontinence and other symptoms of OAB, without adverse effects [81]. Patients learn how to contract pelvic floor muscles selectively and quickly in response to urgency (Kegel exercises), which increases intra-urethral resistance and reduces or prevents urine loss; urinary frequency and nocturia often improve as well [81]. In one uncontrolled pilot study of exercise-based behavioral therapy to treat urinary incontinence in PD ($n = 17$ patients completing the study), patients learned pelvic floor muscle exercises and bladder control strategies including urge suppression [82]. At the 8-week evaluation, there was an 83% reduction in episodes of urinary incontinence (median weekly frequency reduced from nine to one). Symptom severity, symptom bother and quality of life related to OAB improved simultaneously. Computer-assisted anorectal or vaginal EMG biofeedback was used in this study, and whether similar results are achievable without this equipment is unknown. A larger randomized, double-blinded study involving PD patients is underway to further test the efficacy and safety of the intervention (clinicaltrials.gov NCT01520948). Behavioral treatment requires the active participation of a motivated patient, limiting its usefulness in patients with cognitive impairment or those who are not interested in exerting the effort required by a consistent daily regimen [81]. Depending on local practice settings, there may also be a lack of availability of practitioners (e.g. physical therapists) trained in these methods [80, 81]. Combining behavioral and drug treatment might enhance outcomes [81].

Dopaminergic therapy has unpredictable effects on urinary function [76, 77]. Since bladder contraction is mediated by cholinergic (muscarinic M3) parasympathetic receptors [38], anticholinergic medications such as oxybutynin (immediate release 2.5–5 mg two to four times daily, or extended release 5–30 mg once daily, or patch one application twice a week), tolterodine (also called detrusitol) (immediate release 1 or 2 mg two or three times daily, or extended release 2–4 mg once daily) or trospium (20 mg once or twice daily) are generally used as the first-line treatment for OAB [80, 83]. Potential side effects include altered mental status (confusion, hallucinations, drowsiness), dry mouth, blurred vision or aggravation of glaucoma (anticholinergics are contraindicated in patients with narrow-angle glaucoma), urinary retention, constipation and orthostasis [80, 83]. These agents should therefore be used with caution, particularly in elderly patients with cognitive impairment, and in patients with PVR >100–200 ml [76, 80]. Extended-release preparations may be associated with less dry mouth compared with the immediate-release formulations of oxybutynin or tolterodine, and are preferred [80, 83]. Trospium is less able to cross the blood–brain barrier due to its low lipid solubility and appears to be free of central nervous system adverse effects [6, 83]. Solifenacin (5–10 mg once daily) and darifenacin (7.5–15 mg once daily), newer agents that act specifically on the M3 muscarinic receptors present in the bladder, are also associated with less dry mouth and have no significant central nervous system or cardiac side effects [83]. Solifenacin 10 mg daily is currently being evaluated in PD patients with OAB in a double-blinded RCT (clinicaltrials.gov NCT01018264). The dosage of some of these agents may need to be reduced in patients with renal or hepatic disease [80]. Tricyclic antidepressants (e.g. imipramine) have been used to treat OAB, but high-quality evidence even in non-PD populations is lacking [80]. Mirabegron, a β_3-adrenergic receptor agonist, is a new agent for OAB and does not have antimuscarinic side effects [80], but there are no published data as yet in patients with PD.

"Obstructive" (or "voiding") symptoms such as straining to urinate or hesitancy, reduced urinary stream and incomplete emptying are due to obstruction or impaired bladder emptying without actual obstruction of urine outflow ("detrusor areflexia") [6, 76]. Overflow incontinence, due to bladder overfilling, may occur [71], and obstruction itself can cause detrusor overactivity [76, 79]. α-Blockers (e.g. alfuzosin, doxazosin, prazosin, terazosin and tamsulosin) targeting the α-adrenergic receptors of the urethra (which mediate urethral contraction) [38] have been used successfully, but postural hypotension can be a problem. Benign prostatic hypertrophy causing obstruction is common in this age group and may respond to 5α-reductase inhibitors (dutasteride and finasteride) [71]. In one small series of PD patients ($n = 23$), transurethral resection of the prostate was successful (i.e. obviating the need for catheterization, restoring continence or normalizing urinary frequency) in 70% of cases, without causing *de novo* urinary incontinence [84]. In patients with repeatedly high PVR (>100 ml) (in one study PVR was >100 ml in 15.6% of PD patients referred to a neurourology department, vs 67% of patients with MSA) [85]), intermittent self-catheterization is needed [76], or (in patients with advanced disease) an indwelling catheter can be placed. For intermittent self-catheterization, patients must be properly instructed on aseptic technique and appropriate handling. If infections are frequent, a suprapubic catheter may be preferable to a urethral catheter for chronic use [76].

Patients should be referred for evaluation by a urologist or neurourologist if the response to anticholinergics is unsatisfactory, if incontinence is a problem or when an indwelling catheter is needed [76]. Comprehensive urodynamic testing and/or endoscopic evaluation of the lower urinary tract can help to identify other causes of OAB or conditions that can coexist with OAB, including bladder outlet obstruction, other voiding-phase dysfunction, impaired bladder compliance or contractility, and bladder stones, ulcers, inflammation or tumor [78]. Imaging of the upper urinary tract may be needed in certain patients, including those with ominous urodynamic findings (e.g. high storage pressures) and those with incomplete emptying or hematuria [78].

In cases where incontinence is related to impaired cognition and/or mobility (e.g. interfering with the ability of the patient to manage clothing and hygiene when toileting), management must involve caregiver assistance. Timed voiding (e.g. once every 3–4 h during waking hours, even if there is no urge to urinate) may reduce incontinence episodes [80]. Use of diapers/absorbent pads or condom catheters (penile sheaths) may be appropriate [80]. Condom catheters are more comfortable and have a lower risk of UTI compared with indwelling catheters [80].

Treatments not commonly used currently in PD patients

Intranasal desmopressin (DDAVP) has been tried for PD patients with nocturnal polyuria ($n = 8$), but hyponatremia can be a side effect [5].

Botulinum toxin injections into the detrusor muscle, under cystoscopic guidance (either with sedation and local anesthesia, or general anesthesia), can be used to treat OAB [80]. In a study by Giannantoni *et al.* [86] ($n = 8$ [seven female, one male] PD patients with OAB refractory to anticholinergics), injection of 100 units of botulinum toxin type A (Botox®) resulted in improvement of irritative symptoms, quality of life and urodynamic findings in all patients, with the symptomatic benefit lasting for 6 months or more. The PVR increased transiently in most patients, and two patients required intermittent bladder catheterization. Kulaksizoglu et al. [87] used 500 units of botulinum toxin type A (Dysport®) in 16 patients (ten female, six male) and reported improvements in OAB symptoms, quality of life and urodynamic parameters for 12 months or more. Symptom improvement was seen in all patients, and caregiver burden was also reduced for 9 months post-procedure. No patient in this study required bladder catheterization after the procedure.

Repetitive transcranial magnetic stimulation (rTMS) has been studied in a small number of PD patients ($n = 8$), with transient benefit for up to 2 weeks in urinary function.

Neuromodulation of the sacral or pudendal nerve (and even of the posterior tibial nerve percutaneously) reduced OAB in small studies [5, 80].

Sexual dysfunction

Impaired sexual function in PD occurs in both men and women. Brown et al. [88] found that more male than female PD patients (68 vs 36%) reported having moderate to severe sexual problems. Erectile dysfunction (ED) (defined as the inability to attain or maintain penile erection sufficient for satisfactory sexual performance) develops in the majority of men with PD [6, 88, 89]. Sexual issues commonly experienced by women patients include reduced libido, and difficulties with arousal and in reaching orgasm (anorgasmia) [38, 88–90].

It should be noted that impaired sexual function in patients with PD may not arise solely from the neurodegenerative process affecting the autonomic nervous system. Psychological issues (lowered self-esteem, depression, anxiety, cognitive impairment, apathy, couple relationship problems), impaired mobility, fatigue and pain may contribute substantially to sexual dysfunction [88, 89, 91, 92]. Antiparkinsonian medications including dopamine agonists such as bromocriptine have been reported to reduce libido and induce ED in a dose-dependent manner [90]. In a case series by Cleeves et al. [93], ED improved when levodopa was substituted for bromocriptine. Antidepressant medications such as selective serotonin reuptake inhibitors (SSRIs) and tricyclics may be associated with ED or premature ejaculation [90, 94], whereas mirtazapine, bupropion and reboxetine are antidepressants with a low propensity to cause sexual dysfunction [89]. Antihypertensive medications such as thiazide diuretics and β-blockers may also contribute to ED [94]. The partner's reaction to the effects of the PD (e.g. loss of physical attractiveness due to changed appearance, drooling or excessive sweating) may be a compounding factor [88]. In line with this, management of sexual dysfunction often needs to be multifaceted and include the partner; referral to specialists (urologist, gynecologist, psychiatrist/psychologist, sex/couple therapist) should be considered (e.g. sex counseling may enable pleasure-oriented "outercourse" instead of goal/orgasmic-oriented intercourse) [88, 89, 91, 95]. Hypersexuality with distorted or aberrant sexual interest and activity is due, in the vast majority of cases, to the medications used to treat PD (especially dopamine agonists), rather than PD itself, and will not be discussed further in this review [91, 96]. No studies of treatment of sexual dysfunction in women with PD have been reported [6, 38]. Practical measures include lubricants for vaginal dryness or vibrator use for more intense stimulation to facilitate orgasms [89, 91, 95]. The following discussion is focused on the management of ED in male PD patients (the only sexual dysfunction in PD where evidence-based drug treatment is available) [97].

Dopamine agonists can induce erections in some patients with PD, thought to be mediated via dopamine D2-like (i.e. D2, D3 or D4) receptors in the paraventricular nucleus of the hypothalamus, although spinal and peripheral mechanisms have also been implicated [38, 92, 98]. Apomorphine (subcutaneous injections) and pergolide have been the best-studied dopamine agonists in terms of effect on erectile function, and apomorphine has also been used to treat ED in the general population [38]. Pergolide, like other ergot dopamine agonists, is associated with fibrotic valvular heart disease, and for this reason it has been removed from the market. O'sullivan and Hughes [99] first reported that some PD patients given subcutaneous injections of apomorphine to treat motor fluctuations started using the injections specifically for ED (erection result within 10 min and lasting up to 60 min). Although sublingual apomorphine (2 or 4 mg) has demonstrated efficacy and safety for ED in non-PD patients (but with sildenafil demonstrating superior efficacy), this agent has not been studied specifically as a treatment for ED in PD patients [5]. There are isolated case reports of oral DAs such as ropinirole regularly inducing erections in some patients [98].

The selective cyclic GMP phosphodiesterase type 5 inhibitors enhance nitric oxide mediated-relaxation of corpus cavernosum smooth muscle (with increased blood flow into cavernosal spaces), and are the first-line therapy for most men with ED. Sildenafil (Viagra®) is the most commonly used agent [92, 100]. One small RCT ($n = 10$ PD patients completing the study) demonstrated that sildenafil was efficacious in nine of the ten patients, with improvements in the ability to achieve and maintain erections and in the quality of sex life [101]. Similar improvements were reported in an open-label study by Zesiewicz et al. ($n = 10$) [102]. The starting dose is 50 mg, which can be titrated up to 100 mg (or down to 25 mg) depending on efficacy and tolerability (in the study by Hussain et al., 8/10 patients titrated up to 100 mg and one titrated down to 25 mg; in the study by Zesiewicz et al. 4/10 patients used 100 mg) [101, 102]. Other phosphodiesterase type 5 inhibitors such as tadalafil (Cialis®) and vardenafil (Levitra®) also seem to be effective, but these have not been evaluated specifically in PD [6, 97]. Sildenafil is usually taken 1 h before sexual activity, but in some PD patients the onset of action may be delayed up to 4 h, presumably due to slowed gastrointestinal motility [95]. Efficacy is optimal when taken on an empty stomach [100]. Sildenafil is usually well tolerated, with only minor and transient adverse effects, related to vasodilation, such as headache (the most frequent side effect, affecting approximately 10% of patients) and flushing [101, 102]. Transient visual symptoms, mainly disturbances of color vision, were reported predominantly at the 100 mg dose and is due to transient inhibition of phosphodiesterase in the retina [100]. Postural hypotension is a potential concern, but PD patients in the study by Hussain et al. [101] showed minimal change in blood pressure between active (sildenafil) and placebo medication (in contrast to a severe drop in postural blood pressure induced in patients with MSA). Supine and standing blood pressure measurements should be taken before prescribing sildenafil, and patients should be advised to seek medical advice if symptoms of orthostatic hypotension develop [6, 101]. Sildenafil is contraindicated if the blood pressure is below 90/50 mmHg [97], and in patients receiving nitrate therapy since their co-administration can produce life-threatening hypotension [103]. Coexistent heart disease is probably not a contraindication to treatment with phosphodiesterase type 5 inhibitors, and there is increasing evidence to suggest that these agents are safe and exert a variety of beneficial effects in patients with concomitant coronary artery disease or heart failure [97, 102, 103]. Nitrates can be safely administered 24 h after the last use of sildenafil or vardenafil, and 48 h after tadalafil (since this drug has a prolonged duration of action) [103].

An RCT of sildenafil for PD-related ED by Safarinejad and coworkers was positive, but this paper was retracted by the publisher. Curiously, in two studies from the group of Giammusso and Raffaele (reporting improved erections in 85% of PD patients), the results for the various ED and depression efficacy measures, at baseline and follow-up, were exactly the same, despite the fact that the cohorts would appear to be mutually exclusive (all patients in the report by Giammusso et al. [104] were stated to be on pramipexole but not levodopa treatment, whereas all patients in the report by Raffaele et al. [105] were receiving levodopa therapy but not dopamine agonists). The clinical characteristics of both cohorts (mean age 63.3 years, Hoehn and Yahr stage 2.1) were also identical. The findings of these studies should therefore be interpreted with caution.

Treatments not commonly used currently in PD patients

Testosterone replacement therapy (e.g. gel applied to the skin) may be considered in men with documented testosterone deficiency [6]. In one study, testosterone deficiency was present in 35% of men with PD and was more common with increasing age [106]. In a small case series ($n = 5$ PD patients receiving testosterone replacement therapy), Okun et al. [106] reported improvements in libido in four patients and erectile function in two patients, in addition to improvements in other nonmotor symptoms; similar results were seen in an open-label study involving ten patients (50 and 30% of patients had improved libido and erectile function, respectively, at 1 month) [107]. However, a subsequent blinded placebo-controlled RCT by the same authors showed no significant difference for these items on the St Louis Testosterone Deficiency Questionnaire (the primary outcome variable) [108]. One cross-sectional study by Ready et al. [109] also did not find a correlation between free testosterone levels and loss of interest in sex. Further study of the role of testosterone replacement in PD is required.

Local treatments include intracavernosal injections of vasodilators (prostaglandin E1) and vacuum constriction devices [91, 97]. Implantation of a penile prosthesis is a last resort.

Thermoregulatory dysfunction (excessive sweating, heat or cold intolerance)

Episodes of profuse sweating may occur as a wearing-off phenomenon or, conversely, during periods of severe dyskinesia [32, 110]. In such cases, treatment should be directed at the DOPA-related response complications. However, excessive sweating also commonly occurs randomly without correlation with the timing of medication intake (e.g. in 39% of consecutive PD patients in the study by Swinn *et al.* [111]). Propranolol or anticholinergics can be tried but it is unclear whether these are actually helpful. Patients avoid getting overheated. Witjas *et al.* [110] reported striking improvements in a range of nonmotor fluctuations, including drenching sweats, after subthalamic nucleus deep-brain stimulation. For focal hyperhidrosis (which appears to be uncommon in PD patients), botulinum toxin injections can be tried [19]. Other causes of excessive sweating may have to be considered, including menopause, hyperthyroidism, chronic infections and neoplasia.

Management of heat and cold intolerance primarily involves the common-sense instruction that patients avoid exposure to temperature extremes [6]. Patients with reduced sweating should also avoid anticholinergic medications, as these medicines may further reduce sweating and compromise heat dissipation [6].

Acknowledgements

We wish to thank Professor Sanjiv Mahadeva MD MRCP (Consultant Gastroenterologist) and Associate Professor Dr Tan Maw Pin MBBS BMedSci MD MRCP (Consultant Geriatrician with a special interest in syncope and falls) for their most helpful review and comments.

References

1. Postuma RB, Gagnon JF, Pelletier A, Montplaisir J. Prodromal autonomic symptoms and signs in Parkinson's disease and dementia with Lewy bodies. *Mov Disord* 2013; **28**: 597–604.
2. Muller B, Larsen JP, Wentzel-Larsen T, Skeie GO, Tysnes OB, Parkwest Study Group. Autonomic and sensory symptoms and signs in incident, untreated Parkinson's disease: frequent but mild. *Mov Disord* 2011; **26**: 65–72.
3. Gallagher DA, Lees AJ, Schrag A. What are the most important nonmotor symptoms in patients with Parkinson's disease and are we missing them? *Mov Disord* 2010; **25**: 2493–500.
4. Stubendorff K, Aarsland D, Minthon L, Londos E. The impact of autonomic dysfunction on survival in patients with dementia with Lewy bodies and Parkinson's disease with dementia. *PLoS One* 2012; **7**: e45451.
5. Perez-Lloret S, Rey MV, Pavy-Le Traon A, Rascol O. Emerging drugs for autonomic dysfunction in Parkinson's disease. *Expert Opin Emerging Drugs* 2013; **18**: 39–53.
6. Pfeiffer RF. Autonomic dysfunction in Parkinson's disease. *Expert Rev Neurother* 2012; **12**: 697–706.
7. Ziemssen T, Reichmann H. Cardiovascular autonomic dysfunction in Parkinson's disease. *J Neurol Sci* 2010; **289**: 74–80.
8. Asahina M, Vichayanrat E, Low DA, Iodice V, Mathias CJ. Autonomic dysfunction in parkinsonian disorders: Assessment and pathophysiology. *J Neurol Neurosurg Psychiatry* 2013; **84**: 674–80.
9. Lim SY, Moro E, Tan AH, Lang AE. Non-motor symptoms of Parkinson's disease and the effects of deep brain stimulation. In: Chaudhuri KR, Tolosa E, Schapira A, Poewe W, eds. *Non-Motor Symptoms of Parkinson's Disease*, 2nd edn. Oxford: Oxford University Press, 2014; 394–419.
10. Seppi K, Weintraub D, Coelho M, *et al.* The Movement Disorder Society evidence-based medicine review update: treatments for the non-motor symptoms of Parkinson's disease. *Mov Disord* 2011; **26** (Suppl. 3): S42–80.
11. Jamnadas-Khoda J, Koshy S, Mathias CJ, *et al.* Are current recommendations to diagnose orthostatic hypotension in Parkinson's disease satisfactory? *Mov Disord* 2009; **24**: 1747–51.
12. Low PA, Gilden JL, Freeman R, Sheng KN, McElligott MA. Efficacy of midodrine vs placebo in neurogenic orthostatic hypotension: a randomized, double-blind multicenter study. *JAMA* 1997; **277**: 1046–51.
13. Freeman R. Neurogenic orthostatic hypotension. *N Engl J Med* 2008; **358**: 615–24.
14. Low PA, Singer W. Management of neurogenic orthostatic hypotension: an update. *Lancet Neurol* 2008; **7**: 451–58.
15. Metzler M, Duerr S, Granata R, *et al.* Neurogenic orthostatic hypotension: Pathophysiology, evaluation, and management. *J Neurol* 2013; **260**: 2212–9.
16. Senard JM, Chamontin B, Rascol A, Montastruc JL. Ambulatory blood pressure in patients with

17. Maule S, Papotti G, Naso D, et al. Orthostatic hypotension: Evaluation and treatment. *Cardiovasc Haematol Disord Drug Targets* 2007; **7**: 63–70.
18. Perez-Lloret S, Rey MV, Fabre N, et al. Factors related to orthostatic hypotension in Parkinson's disease. *Parkinsonism Rel Disord* 2012; **18**: 501–5.
19. Mostile G, Jankovic J. Treatment of dysautonomia associated with Parkinson's disease. *Parkinsonism Related Disord* 2009; **15** (Suppl. 3): S224–32.
20. Schoffer KL, Henderson RD, O'Maley K, O'sullivan JD. Nonpharmacological treatment, fludrocortisone, and domperidone for orthostatic hypotension in Parkinson's disease. *Mov Disord* 2007; **22**: 1543–9.
21. Kaufmann H, Freeman R, Biaggioni I, et al. Droxidopa for neurogenic orthostatic hypotension: a randomized, placebo-controlled, phase 3 trial. *Neurology* 2014; **83**: 328–335
22. Hoehn MM. Levodopa-induced postural hypotension treatment with fludrocortisone. *Arch Neurol* 1975; **32**: 50–1.
23. Jankovic J, Gilden JL, Hiner BC, et al. Neurogenic orthostatic hypotension: A double-blind, placebo-controlled study with midodrine. *Am J Med* 1993; **95**: 38–48.
24. Corsini GU, Del Zompo M, Gessa GL, Mangoni A. Therapeutic efficacy of apomorphine combined with an extracerebral inhibitor of dopamine receptors in Parkinson's disease. *Lancet* 1979; **313**: 954–6.
25. Lang AE. Acute orthostatic hypotension when starting dopamine agonist therapy in Parkinson disease: the role of domperidone therapy. *Arch Neurol* 2001; **58**: 835.
26. Hauser RA, Hewitt LA, Isaacson S. Droxidopa in patients with neurogenic orthostatic hypotension associated with Parkinson's disease (NOH306A). *J Parkinsons Dis* 2013; **4**: 57–65.
27. Sandroni P, Opfer-Gehrking TL, Singer W, Low PA. Pyridostigmine for treatment of neurogenic orthostatic hypertension: a follow-up survey study. *Clin Auton Res* 2005; **15**: 51–3.
28. Singer W, Sandroni P, Opfer-Gehrking TL, et al. Pyridostigmine treatment trial in neurogenic orthostatic hypotension. *Arch Neurol* 2006; **63**: 513–18.
29. Shibao C, Okamoto LE, Gamboa A, et al. Comparative efficacy of yohimbine against pyridostigmine for the treatment of orthostatic hypotension in autonomic failure. *Hypertension* 2010; **56**: 847–51.
30. Suchowersky O, Furtado S, Rohs G. Beneficial effect of intranasal desmopressin for nocturnal polyuria in Parkinson's disease. *Mov Disord* 1995; **10**: 337–40.
31. Lahrmann H, Cortelli P, Hilz M, et al. EFNS guidelines on the diagnosis and management of orthostatic hypotension. *Eur J Neurol* 2006; **13**: 930–6.
32. Ziemssen T, Reichmann H. Treatment of dysautonomia in extrapyramidal disorders. *Ther Adv Neurol Disord* 2010; **3**: 53–67.
33. Sahul ZH, Trusty JM, Erickson M, Low PA, Shen WK. Pacing does not improve hypotension in patients with severe orthostatic hypotension – a prospective randomized cross-over pilot study. *Clin Auton Res* 2004; **14**: 255–8.
34. Salat-Foix D, Suchowersky O. The management of gastrointestinal symptoms in Parkinson's disease. *Expert Rev Neurother* 2012; **12**: 239–48.
35. Stevens JE, Jones KL, Rayner CK, Horowitz M. Pathophysiology and pharmacotherapy of gastroparesis: Current and future perspectives. *Expert Opin Pharmacother* 2013; **14**: 1171–86.
36. Parkes JD. Domperidone and Parkinson's disease. *Clin Neuropharmacol* 1986; **9**: 517–32.
37. Soykan I, Sarosiek I, Shifflett J, Wooten GF, McCallum RW. Effect of chronic oral domperidone therapy on gastrointestinal symptoms and gastric emptying in patients with Parkinson's disease. *Mov Disord* 1997; **12**: 952–7.
38. Sakakibara R, Kishi M, Ogawa E, et al. Bladder, bowel, and sexual dysfunction in Parkinson's disease. *Parkinson's Disease* 2011; 924605.
39. Critchley P, Langdon N, Parkes JD, et al. Domperidone. *Br Med J* 1985; **290**: 788.
40. Malek NM, Grosset KA, Stewart D, Macphee GJA, Grosset DG. Prescription of drugs with potential adverse effects on cardiac conduction in Parkinson's disease. *Parkinsonism Rel Disord* 2013; **19**: 586–9.
41. Tack J, Camilleri M, Chang L, et al. Systematic review: Cardiovascular safety profile of 5-HT4 agonists developed for gastrointestinal disorders. *Aliment Pharmacol Ther* 2012; **35**: 745–67.
42. Asai H, Udaka F, Hirano M, et al. Increased gastric motility during 5-HT4 agonist therapy reduces response fluctuations in Parkinson's disease. *Parkinsonism Relat Disord* 2005; **11**: 499–502.
43. Pfeiffer RF. Gastrointestinal dysfunction in Parkinson's disease. *Parkinsonism Rel Disord* 2011; **17**: 10–15.
44. Jost WH. Gastrointestinal dysfunction in Parkinson's disease. *J Neurol Sci* 2010; **289**: 69–73.
45. Bosshard W, Dreher R, Schnegg JF, Bula CJ. The treatment of chronic constipation in elderly people: An update. *Drugs Aging* 2004; **21**: 911–30.
46. Astarloa R, Mena MA, Sánchez V, de la Vega L, de Yébenes JG. Clinical and pharmacokinetic effects of a diet rich in insoluble fiber on Parkinson disease. *Clin Neuropharmacol.* 1992; **15**: 375–80.

47. Ashraf W, Pfeiffer RF, Park F, Lof J, Quigley EM. Constipation in Parkinson's disease: objective assessment and response to psyllium. *Mov Disord* 1997; **12**: 946–51.
48. Ramkumar D, Rao SS. Efficacy and safety of traditional medical therapies for chronic constipation: systematic review. *Am J Gastroenterol* 2005; **100**: 936–71.
49. Sturtzel B, Mikulits C, Gisinger C, Elmadfa I. Use of fiber instead of laxative treatment in a geriatric hospital to improve the wellbeing of seniors. *J Nutr Health Aging* 2009; **13**: 136–9.
50. Muller B, Assmus J, Larsen JP, et al. Autonomic symptoms and dopaminergic treatment in de novo Parkinson's disease. *Acta Neurol Scand* 2013; **127**: 290–4.
51. Eichhorn TE, Oertel WH. Macrogol 3350/electrolyte improves constipation in Parkinson's disease and multiple system atrophy. *Mov Disord* 2001; **16**: 1176–7.
52. Zangaglia R, Martignoni E, Glorioso M, et al. Macrogol for the treatment of constipation in Parkinson's disease. A randomized placebo-controlled study. *Mov Disord* 2007; **22**: 1239–44.
53. Kirkman MS, Zimmerman DR, Filippini SA. Marked deterioration in glycemic control with change in brand of lactulose syrup. *South Med J* 1995; **88**: 492–3.
54. Muller-Lissner SA1, Kamm MA, Scarpignato C, Wald A. Myths and misconceptions about chronic constipation. *Am J Gastroenterol* 2005; **100**: 232–42.
55. Liu Z, Sakakibara R, Odaka T, et al. Mosapride citrate, a novel 5-HT4 agonist and partial 5-HT3 antagonist, ameliorates constipation in parkinsonian patients. *Mov Disord* 2005; **20**: 680–6.
56. Camilleri M, Kerstens R, Rykx A, Vandeplassche L. A placebo-controlled trial of prucalopride for severe chronic constipation. *N Engl J Med* 2008; **358**: 2344–54.
57. Cassani E, Privitera G, Pezzoli G, et al. Use of probiotics for the treatment of constipation in Parkinson's disease patients. *Minerva Gastroenterol Dietol* 2011; **57**: 117–21.
58. Ondo WG, Kenney C, Sullivan K, et al. Placebo-controlled trial of lubiprostone for constipation associated with Parkinson disease. *Neurology* 2012; **78**: 1650–4.
59. Sandyk R, Gillman MA. Colchicine ameliorates constipation in Parkinson's disease. *J R Soc Med* 1984; **77**: 1066.
60. Sakakibara R, Odaka T, Lui Z, et al. Dietary herb extract dai-kenchu-to ameliorates constipation in parkinsonian patients (Parkinson's disease and multiple system atrophy). *Mov Disord* 2005; **20**: 261–2.
61. Pfeiffer RF, Markopoulou K, Quigley EM, Stambler N, Cedarbaum IM. Effect of NT-3 on bowel function in Parkinson's disease. *Mov Disord* 2002; **17**: 223–4.
62. Chiu CM, Wang CP, Sung WH, et al. Functional magnetic stimulation in constipation associated with Parkinson's disease. *J Rehabil Med* 2009; **41**: 1085–9.
63. Albanese A, Brisinda G, Bentivoglio AR, Maria G. Treatment of outlet obstruction constipation in Parkinson's disease with botulinum neurotoxin A. *Am J Gastroenterol* 2003; **98**: 1439–40.
64. Cadeddu F, Bentivoglio AR, Brandara F, et al. Outlet type constipation in Parkinson's disease: Results of botulinum toxin treatment. *Aliment Pharmacol Ther* 2005; **22**: 997–1003.
65. Mathers SE, Kempster PA, Law PJ, et al. Anal sphincter dysfunction in Parkinson's disease. *Arch Neurol* 1989; **46**: 1061–4.
66. Edwards LL, Quigley EM, Harned RK, Hofman R, Pfeiffer RF. Defecatory function in Parkinson's disease: Response to apomorphine. *Ann Neurol* 1993; **33**: 490–3.
67. South AR, Somers SM, Jog MS. Gum chewing improves swallow frequency and latency in Parkinson patients: a preliminary study. *Neurology* 2010; **74**: 1198–202.
68. Merello M. Sialorrhoea and drooling in patients with Parkinson's disease: epidemiology and management. *Drugs Aging* 2008; **25**: 1007–19.
69. Arbouw MEL, Movig KLL, Koopmann M, et al. Glycopyrrolate for sialorrhea in Parkinson disease: A randomized, double-blind, crossover trial. *Neurology* 2010; **74**: 1203–7.
70. Hyson HC, Johnson AM, Jog MS. Sublingual atropine for sialorrhea secondary to parkinsonism: a pilot study. *Mov Disord* 2002; **17**: 1318–20.
71. Pfeiffer RF. Gastrointestinal, urological, and sexual dysfunction in Parkinson's disease. *Mov Disord* 2010; **25** (Suppl. 1): S94–7.
72. Thomsen TR, Galpern WR, Asante A, Arenovich T, Fox SH. Ipratropium bromide spray as treatment for sialorrhea in Parkinson's disease. *Mov Disord* 2007; **22**: 2268–73.
73. Ondo WG, Hunter C, Moore W. A double-blind placebo-controlled trial of botulinum toxin B for sialorrhea in Parkinson's disease. *Neurology* 2004; **62**: 37–40.
74. Guidubaldi A, Fasano A, Ialongo T, et al. Botulinum toxin A versus B in sialorrhea: a prospective, randomized, double-blind, crossover pilot study in patients with amyotrophic lateral sclerosis or Parkinson's disease. *Mov Disord* 2011; **26**: 313–19.
75. Postma A-G, Heesters MAAM, van Laar T. Radiotherapy to the salivary glands as treatment of sialorrhea in patients with parkinsonism. *Mov Disord* 2007; **22**: 2430–5.

76. Winge K, Fowler CJ. Bladder dysfunction in parkinsonism: mechanisms, prevalence, symptoms, and management. *Mov Disord* 2006; **21**: 737–45.
77. Blackett H, Walker R, Wood B. Urinary dysfunction in Parkinson's disease: a review. *Parkinsonism Related Disord* 2009; **15**: 81–7.
78. Nitti V. Clinical testing for overactive bladder. *Can Urol Assoc J* 2011; **5** (Suppl.2): S137–8.
79. Ouslander JG. Geriatric considerations in the diagnosis and management of overactive bladder. *Urology* 2002; **60** (Suppl. 1): 50–5.
80. Cameron AP, Jimbo M, Heidelbaugh JJ. Diagnosis and office-based treatment of urinary incontinence in adults. Part two: treatment. *Ther Adv Urol* 2013; **5**: 189–200.
81. Burgio KL. Influence of behavior modification on overactive bladder. *Urology* 2002; **60** (Suppl. 1): 72–6.
82. Vaughan CP, Juncos JL, Burgio KL, et al. Behavioral therapy to treat urinary incontinence in Parkinson disease. *Neurology* 2011; **76**: 1631–4.
83. Appell RA. Pharmacotherapy for overactive bladder: an evidence-based approach to selecting an antimuscarinic agent. *Drugs* 2006; **66**: 1361–70.
84. Roth B, Studer UE, Fowler CJ, Kessler TM. Benign prostatic obstruction and Parkinson's disease: Should transurethral resection of the prostate be avoided? *J Urol* 2009; **181**: 2209–13.
85. Chandiramani VA, Palace J, Fowler CJ. How to recognize patients with parkinsonism who should not have urological surgery. *Br J Urol* 1997; **80**: 100–4.
86. Giannantoni A, Conte A, Proietti S, et al. Botulinum toxin type A in patients with Parkinson's disease and refractory overactive bladder. *J Urol* 2011; **186**: 960–4.
87. Kulaksizoglu H, Parman Y. Use of botulinum toxin-A for the treatment of overactive bladder symptoms in patients with Parkinson's disease. *Parkinsonism Rel Disord* 2010; **16**: 531–4.
88. Brown RG, Jahanshahi M, Quinn N, Marsden CD. Sexual function in patients with Parkinson's disease and their partners. *J Neurol Neurosurg Psychiatry* 1990; **53**: 480–86.
89. Bronner G. Sexual problems in Parkinson's disease: the multidimensional nature of the problem and of the intervention. *J Neurol Sci* 2011; **310**: 139–43.
90. Bronner G, Royter V, Korczyn AD, Giladi N. Sexual dysfunction in Parkinson's disease. *J Sex Marit Therapy* 2004; **30**: 95–105.
91. Basson R. Sexuality and Parkinson's disease. *Parkinsonism Rel Disord* 1996; **2**: 177–85.
92. Papatsoris AG, Deliveliotis C, Singer C, Papapetropoulos S. Erectile dysfunction in Parkinson's disease. *Urology* 2006; **67**: 447–51.
93. Cleeves L, Findley LJ. Bromocriptine induced impotence in Parkinson's disease. *Br Med J* 1987; **295**: 367–8.
94. Francis ME, Kusek JW, Nyberg LM, Eggers PW. The contribution of common medical conditions and drug exposures to erectile dysfunction in adult males. *J Urol* 2007; **178**: 591–6.
95. Bronner G. Practical strategies for the management of sexual problems in Parkinson's disease. *Parkinsonism Rel Disord* 2009; **15** (Suppl. 3): S96–100.
96. Lim SY, Evans AH, Miyasaki JM. Impulse control and related disorders in Parkinson's disease: review. *Ann N Y Acad Sci* 2008; **1142**: 85–107.
97. Bronner G, Vodusek DB. Management of sexual dysfunction in Parkinson's disease. *Ther Adv Neurol Disord* 2011; **4**: 375–83.
98. Fine J, Lang AE. Dose-induced penile erections in response to ropinirole therapy for Parkinson's disease. *Mov Disord* 1999; **14**: 701–3.
99. O'sullivan JD, Hughes AJ. Apomorphine-induced penile erections in Parkinson's disease. *Mov Disord* 1998; **13**: 536–9.
100. Briganti A, Salonia A, Gallina A. Drug insight: oral phosphodiesterase type 5 inhibitors for erectile dysfunction. *Nat Clin Pract Urol* 2005; **2**: 239–47.
101. Hussain IF, Brady CM, Swinn MJ, Mathias CJ, Fowler CJ. Treatment of erectile dysfunction with sildenafil citrate (Viagra) in parkinsonism due to Parkinson's disease or multiple system atrophy with observations on orthostatic hypotension. *J Neurol Neurosurg Psychiatry* 2001; **71**: 371–4.
102. Zesiewicz TA, Helal M, Hauser RA. Sildenafil citrate (Viagra) for the treatment of erectile dysfunction in men with Parkinson's disease. *Mov Disord* 2000; **15**: 305–8.
103. Chrysant SG. Effectiveness and safety of phosphodiesterase 5 inhibitors in patients with cardiovascular disease and hypertension. *Curr Hypertens Rep* 2013; **15**: 475–83.
104. Giammusso B, Raffaele R, Vecchio I, et al. Sildenafil in the treatment of erectile dysfunction in elderly depressed patients with idiopathic Parkinson's disease. *Arch Gerontol Geriatr Suppl* 2002; **8**: 157–63.
105. Raffaele R, Vecchio I, Giammusso B, et al. Efficacy and safety of fixed-dose oral sildenafil in the treatment of sexual dysfunction in depressed patients with idiopathic Parkinson's disease. *Eur Urol* 2002; **41**: 382–6.
106. Okun MS, McDonald WM, R. DeLong M. Refractory nonmotor symptoms in male patients with Parkinson disease due to testosterone deficiency: a common unrecognized comorbidity. *Arch Neurol* 2002; **59**: 807–11.
107. Okun MS, Walter BL, McDonald WM, et al. Beneficial effects of testosterone replacement for the nonmotor

symptoms of Parkinson disease. *Arch Neurol* 2002; **59**: 1750–3.

108. Okun MS, Fernandez HH, Rodriguez RL, *et al.* Testosterone therapy in men with Parkinson disease: results of the TEST-PD study. *Arch Neurol* 2006; **63**: 729–35.

109. Ready RE, Friedman J, Grace J, Fernandez H. Testosterone deficiency and apathy in Parkinson's disease: a pilot study. *J Neurol Neurosurg Psychiatry* 2004; **75**: 1323–6.

110. Witjas T, Kaphan E, Azulay JP, *et al.* Nonmotor fluctuations in Parkinson's disease: frequent and disabling. *Neurology* 2002; **59**: 408–13.

111. Swinn L, Schrag A, Viswanathan R, *et al.* Sweating dysfunction in Parkinson's disease. *Mov Disord* 2003; **18**: 1459–63.

Chapter 11

Management of cognitive impairment in Parkinson's disease

Dawn M. Schiehser, Eva Pirogovsky-Turk and Irene Litvan

Background on cognitive impairment in Parkinson's disease

Cognitive impairment is a very common problem in Parkinson's disease (PD). Parkinson's disease dementia (PDD) has a point prevalence estimated at about 40% [1], and prospective longitudinal studies find that up to 78% of PD patients can develop dementia over an 8-year period [2]. Parkinson's disease dementia can have a significant impact on the quality of life of both patients and caregivers, and is associated with greater risk of nursing home placement and mortality [3, 4]. Parkinson's disease patients also experience more subtle cognitive deficits not severe enough to warrant a diagnosis of dementia early in the course of the disease, with 25–30% of patients demonstrating some cognitive impairment even at the time of PD diagnosis [5]. Mild cognitive impairment in Parkinson's disease (PD-MCI), defined as mild cognitive decline that is not normal for age and with essentially normal functional activities, has been increasingly recognized as a distinct clinical entity that may represent a transitional state between normal cognition and PDD [6]. Approximately 20–50% of nondemented PD patients meet the criteria for PD-MCI [7].

The profile of cognitive impairment in PD-MCI is heterogeneous and often characterized as either amnestic (i.e. memory deficit) or nonamnestic (impaired cognition other than memory) and as single domain or multiple domain (i.e. impairments in more than one cognitive area). Nonamnestic single-domain MCI is the most common subtype, representing approximately 42–62% of all individuals with PD-MCI [8–10]. Of PD-MCI patients with nonamnestic domain MCI, approximately 13–26% exhibit executive dysfunction and 18% were found to have visuospatial deficits [9, 10]. Overall, 16–24% of PD-MCI patients are characterized as amnestic single-domain MCI, while 24–40% of individuals are characterized as multiple-domain MCI (19% amnestic multiple domain; 5% non-amnestic multiple domain) [8–10].

Executive dysfunction is the most common cognitive disturbance and is usually evident early in the course of PD as well as sometime being an early sign of incident PDD [11]. Studies suggest that executive function deficits in PD result from a disruption in frontostriatal circuitry, particularly the dorsolateral prefrontal circuit [12–14]. Executive function deficits found in PD include impaired complex attention, verbal fluency, cognitive set-shifting, abstract thinking and planning [15–18]. Although there can be heterogeneity in the memory performance of PD patients [19, 20], the memory profile in general can be characterized by mild retrieval deficits with relatively spared retention of information. Episodic memory deficits in PD are thought to be a result of frontostriatal dysfunction that leads to impairments in higher-level strategy or organization of information during encoding and retrieval [21, 22]. Visuospatial deficits found in PD include impairments in perception of line orientation, visuomotor construction, facial recognition and memory for spatial location [23, 24].

The cognitive deficits in PDD are generally qualitatively similar to those with PD-MCI but are more severe and pervasive, affecting subjects' functions [25]. The majority of individuals with PDD exhibit a subcortical profile, characterized by prominent executive dysfunction along with impaired attention, slowness of thought, and visuospatial and episodic memory deficits [26]. Compared with patients with Alzheimer's disease (AD), PDD patients show more severe impairments in executive function and visuospatial processes, and less severe deficits in learning and memory [27–29]. However, some individuals with PDD may present with a "cortical" profile, which is characterized by memory (impaired retention of information) and language impairments that are found in cortical dementias such as AD [9]. The extent to which this represents a mixed pathology is unknown.

Given the frequency and progressive nature of cognitive deficits in PD and the impact that cognitive impairment has on patients and their families, it is critically important to identify treatments for cognitive impairment. Treatments that could improve cognitive functioning or delay or stop progression from PD-MCI to PDD are vitally important for this population. The following sections review the research conducted examining pharmacological and nonpharmacological treatments for cognitive impairment in PD.

Pharmacological interventions

There are no standard pharmacological treatments for the cognitive impairment of patients with PD-MCI; however, there are good clinical practice guidelines that advocate the discontinuation of medications that have the potential of deteriorating cognition when the symptoms of cognitive disturbances start to manifest. Medications that can worsen cognition include anticholinergic agents (commonly used to treat tremor or urinary disturbances), amantadine; dopamine agonists and benzodiazepines (reviewed in [30]). Good clinical practice guidelines include ruling out metabolic disorders (e.g. thyroid or hepatic dysfunction), infections (e.g. usually urinary) and vitamin deficits (e.g. hypovitaminosis of vitamin D, hypovitaminosis D, B or folic acid B or folic acid).

Moreover, there have been no therapeutic trials to improve the cognitive aspects of patients with PD-MCI except for a pilot study with rasagiline, a monoamine oxidase B (MAO-B) inhibitor, which showed improvements in working memory and verbal fluency [31] [Table 11.1]. The results of this study have led to an ongoing 24-week, multicenter, double-blind, placebo-controlled study to determine whether 1 mg/day of rasagaline is more effective than placebo in improving the cognitive dysfunction of PD-MCI patients.

To improve the cognitive dysfunction of patients with PDD on the other hand, in addition to the above good clinical practice guidelines, the use of cholinesterase inhibitors such as rivastigmine, donepezil and galantamine provide modest benefit [34, 31]). There is good evidence (level A evidence) from a double-blind, randomized, placebo-controlled study that rivastigmine has moderate beneficial effects on cognition in PDD [32] (Table 11.1). One large and two small donepezil randomized, double-blind, placebo-controlled studies [33, 60, 61] also showed cognitive benefits (level A evidence) (Table 11.1). Despite these promising findings, cholinesterase inhibitors have side effects that include worsening of motor symptoms (tremor), nausea, vomiting, diarrhea and urinary disturbances.

Memantine, a N-methyl-D-aspartate (NMDA) receptor antagonist, which is also used in moderately advanced AD, does not or minimally benefits patients with PDD [34, 35] (Table 11.1), and it is at present not recommended. Neuroleptics are used to treat the neuropsychiatric disturbances (i.e. hallucinations, agitation, delusions), but do not influence cognition and may worsen the parkinsonism as well as leading to a neuroleptic malignant syndrome. Similarly, antidepressants useful for depression or anxiety do not appear to improve cognition in this population. Moreover, the use of serotoninergic antidepressants and selegiline in high doses may lead to a serotoninergic syndrome, which manifests with cognitive, somatic and autonomic disturbances.

Nonpharmacological interventions
Cognitive rehabilitation

One of the most promising nonpharmacological treatments for cognitive impairment in PD is cognitive rehabilitation. Cognitive rehabilitation is a structured intervention that aims to improve, maintain or delay the decline of cognitive skills with the ultimate goal of improving the person's ability to function in everyday life [62]. There are two main cognitive rehabilitation approaches: (i) restorative/remediative, which focuses on retraining with the goal of regaining specific cognitive skills lost due to trauma or disease; and (ii) compensatory, which provides alternative approaches to adapt to and "work around" cognitive weaknesses. Restorative methods frequently consist of computerized drills and/or practice worksheets aimed at remediating targeted cognitive deficit(s). Compensatory rehabilitation focuses on the teaching of specific strategies, such as mnemonics, time management and systematic problem solving, in order to improve functional cognitive skills in everyday life. Cognitive rehabilitation has been documented to be efficacious in nonprogressive conditions, such as traumatic brain

Table 11.1 Pharmacologic and nonpharmacological interventions for cognitive impairment in Parkinson's disease

Study	Sample/study design	Method	Intervention	Cognitive outcome	Results
Pharmacological interventions					
Emre et al. (2004) [32]: multicenter involving multiple countries	541 PDD patients (rivastigmine = 362, placebo = 179), 410 completed the study	24-weeks double-blind, placebo RCT	Rivastigmine 9–12 mg vs placebo	ADAS-Cog, ADCS-CGIC	ADAS-Cog, ADCS-CGIC improved significantly vs placebo
Dubois et al. (2012) [33]: multicenter involving multiple countries	550 PDD patients (5 mg = 195 patients, 10 mg = 182 patients, placebo = 173 patients), intention to treat analysis	24-weeks, double-blind, placebo RCT	Donepezil 5 or 10 mg vs placebo	ADAS-Cog, CGIC+	ADAS-Cog: not significant in intent to treat, but removing country interaction analysis improved significantly vs placebo at both doses; the CGIC improved significantly in the 10 mg group
Hanagasi et al. (2011) [31]: Turkey	55 PD-MCI: 48 patients completed the study (rasagaline = 23, placebo = 25), seven dropouts not included in the analyses	12-week double-blind, placebo RCT	Rasagaline 1 mg/day vs placebo	No primary endpoint (exploratory study)	WM (DS backward), VF and composite attention domain z-score improved significantly with rasagaline vs placebo
Emre et al. (2010) [34]: multicenter involving multiple countries	199 patients: 34 with DLB and 62 with PDD on memantine 20 mg/day and 41 with DLB and 58 with PDD on placebo	24-week double-blind, placebo RCT	Memantine 20 mg/day vs placebo	No primary endpoint	No significant differences were noted between the two treatments in patients with PDD
Aarsland et al. (2009) [35]: Norway, Sweden and UK	72 out of 75 patients (40 with PDD and 32 with DLB): 34 with memantine and 38 with placebo; 56 (78%) completed the study	24-week double-blind, placebo RCT	Memantine 20 mg/day vs placebo	Clinical global impression of change (CGIC)	Better CGIC scores
Cognitive rehabilitation					
Restorative					
Cerasa et al. (2014) [36]: Italy	Eight CR vs seven placebo (visuomotor task), ND PD with an attention, PS and/or EF deficit	Blind RCT	6 weeks of two 1 h computerized attention (RehaCom) trainings per week	Attention, PS, EF, VF, VS, and verbal and visual memory	PS (SDMT) and attention (DS forward) improved compared with controls; increased RS activity in parieto-prefrontal network
Disbrow et al. (2012) [37]: USA	14 pre-training task impaired vs 15 unimpaired ND PD	Non-RCT	10 days (h/day unclear) of computerized EF monitoring training (number sequencing)	Attention (DS), PS/EF (TMT), VF	Impaired group improved on EF motor training task; TMT B/TMT A improved in both groups
Mohlman et al. (2011) [38]: USA	14 ND PD with cognitive complaints	Non-RCT, within subject design	4 weeks of one 90 min attention process training (APT-II) per week	Attention (DS), PS/EF (TMT, CWIT), VF (COWAT)	VF (COWAT), WM (DS backward) EF (TMT B) and PS (CWIT color word trial) improved

(continued)

Table 11.1 (cont.)

Study	Sample/study design	Method	Intervention	Cognitive outcome	Results
París et al. (2011) [39]: Spain	16 CR vs 12 speech therapy ND PD	Double-blinded RCT	4 weeks of three 45 min computer + homework sessions per week	Attention, PS, EF, VS/VC, VF, visual and verbal learning and memory	Attention (DS), PS, EF (TMT B, TOL), VS/VC, category fluency, visual learning and memory improved
Sammer et al. (2006) [40]: Germany	14 CR vs 12 stc ND PD	RCT	Ten 30 min WM/EF training sessions	Attention, EF (BADS, TMT equivalent), face–name memory	EF (BADS) improved
Restorative+					
Sinforini et al. (2004) [41]: Italy	20 PD-MCI	Non-RCT, within subject design	6 weeks of two 1 h CT (TNP software) + motor rehab sessions	Attention (DS), VF (FAS), memory (Babcock's story), EF (Raven's Matrices; WCST, Stroop), MMSE	EF (Raven's matrices), VF (FAS) and story memory improved
Reuter et al. (2012) [42]: Germany	222 PD-MCI split into three CT groups	Double-blinded RCT	At least 14 1 h sessions: 71 CT (A) vs 75 CT+transfer (compensatory) (B) vs 76 CT+transfer+motor (C) training	ADAS-Cog, SCOPA-Cog, BADS, PASAT	All groups improved on all cognitive measures; group C did the best
Naismith et al. (2013) [43]: Australia	35 CR vs 15 waiting-list ND PD (62% PD-MCI)	Single-blinded RCT	7 weeks of 2 h sessions (1 h psychoeducation + 1 h computerized CT	EF/PS (TMT), VF (COWAT), learning/memory (LMT)	Episodic learning and memory (LMT) improved
Cognitive stimulation					
Nombela et al. (2012) [44]: Spain	Five puzzle vs five stc ND PD (MMSE >24)	Non-RCT	6 months of daily Sudoku exercises	MMSE, MDRS, modified Stroop	EF (Stroop) improved; reduced cortical activation (fMRI)
Pompeu et al. (2012) [45]: Brazil	16 Wii vs 16 balance exercise ND PD	Parallel, single-blinded RCT	7 weeks of two 1 h sessions	MoCA	Overall cognition (MoCA) improved in both groups pre- to post-intervention; no difference between groups
Physical exercise					
Cruise et al. (2011) [46]: Australia	15 PD vs 13 stc ND PD	Non-RCT	12 weeks of two 1 h aerobic and resistance training	MMSE, FAS and animal VF, Stockings of Cambridge, CANTAB-eclipse pattern recognition and spatial recognition memory, spatial working memory	Spatial WM, VF (FAS and animal) improved
Nocera et al. (2013) [47]: USA	15 PD vs 6 stc ND PD	Single-blinded RCT	16 weeks of three 1 h tai chi sessions	WM (DS backward test), FAS, Category Fluency, Stroop, TMT	No statistical improvement, but a trend ($P = 0.08$) trend toward improvement in WM (DS backward), associated with a large effect size of 0.89

(continued)

Table 11.1 (cont.)

Study	Sample/study design	Method	Intervention	Cognitive outcome	Results
Ridgel et al. (2011) [48]: USA	19 PD (cognitive status unknown)	Non-RCT, within subject design	Three sessions, over 3 weeks, of 30 min passive cycling	TMT A and B	EF (TMT B) improved
Tabak et al. (2013) [49]: USA	Two PDD patients (MoCA <22)	Non-RCT	24 1 h sessions cycling (three times a week for 8 weeks)	EF and processing speed, MoCA, Color Trails 1 and 2, Parkinson's Disease Cognitive Rating Scale	EF (all measures) improved
Tanaka et al. (2009) [50]: Brazil	10 PE vs 10 stc* ND PD	Non-RCT	Group exercise, mainly aerobic, 1 h sessions, three times a week for 6 months	EF (WCST) and PS (symbol search)	EF improved
Neural stimulation					
Boggio et al. (2005) [51]: Brazil	13 active rTMS and placebo drug treatment vs 12 sham rTMS and active drug treatment (fluoxetine, 20 mg/day) PD with major or minor depression	Double-blinded RCT	rTMS to left DLPFC for 10 sessions over 2-week period	EF (WCST, Stroop Color Word Interference test, TMT-B, FAS), visuospatial (HVOT), reasoning (Raven's Matrices), and WM (DS)	No difference between treatment groups; both groups improved in EF (WCST, Stroop) and VS (HVOT) at 2 weeks post-intervention; both groups improved on Hooper and WCST at 8 weeks post-intervention
Boggio et al. (2006) [52]: Brazil	18 ND PD	Non-RCT, within subject design	Single session tDCS to left DLPFC with two different intensities (1 mA and 2 mA) versus tDCS to primary motor cortex with two different intensities (1 mA and 2 mA) versus sham tDCS 20 min, each session 48 h apart	WM	WM improved with 2 mA to the left DLPFC
Epstein et al. (2007) [53]: USA	12 ND PD with moderate to severe depression	Non-RCT, open study	10 sessions over 2 weeks of rTMS to the left DLPFC	MMSE, RBANS, Brief Test of Attention, DRS	Overall cognition (DRS total score), EF (DRS Conceptualization) and memory (DRS Memory) improved
Pal et al. (2010) [54]: Hungary	12 rTMS vs 10 sham rTMS ND PD with mild to moderate depression	Double-blinded RCT	rTMS to the left DLPFC for 10 days	MMSE, EF (TMT, Stroop Color Word Test)	EF (Stroop) at 1 day and 30 days post-intervention improved
Sedlackova et al. (2009) [55]: Czech Republic	10 PD (cognitive status unknown)	Non-RCT, within subject design	One 30 min session rTMS to left dorsal premotor cortex and DLPFC and occipital cortex (control condition)	EF (WM, choice reaction time, VF, TMT)	No improvement

(continued)

Table 11.1 (cont.)

Study	Sample/study design	Method	Intervention	Cognitive outcome	Results
Srovnalova et al. (2011) [56]: Czech Republic	10 ND PD	Non-RCT, within subject design	One session of rTMS to left and right inferior frontal gyri in sequence vs sham rTMS	EF (Stroop Color Word test, Frontal Assessment Battery)	PS and EF (all conditions of the Stroop) improved
Srovnalova et al. (2012) [57]: Czech Republic	10 ND PD	Non-RCT, within subject design	Two sessions of rTMS to right and two sessions to left DLPFC vs sham rTMS	EF (Tower of London)	EF (Tower of London) after rTMS to right DLPFC improved
Furukawa et al. (2009) [58]: Japan	Six PD with impaired performance on WCST (≤ 4 categories) and MMSE ≤ 26	Non-RCT	Under EEG monitoring, rTMS to the frontal region (Fz) for 3 months, 1200 stimulations	TMT-B, WCST, WAIS-R	EF (WCST and TMT-B) improved
Fregni et al. (2004) [59]: USA and Brazil	21 rTMS and placebo drug treatment vs 21 sham rTMS and active drug treatment (fluoxetine 20 mg/day)	Double-blinded RCT	10 days of rTMS to left DLPFC	MMSE	Both groups improved on the MMSE, but the active rTMS group improved faster (showed more improvement at 2 weeks, but at 8 weeks no significant difference between groups)

PDD, Parkinson's disease dementia; DLB, dementia with Lewy bodies; ADAS-Cog, Alzheimer's Disease Assessment Scale – cognitive subscale; CIBIC+ (global function), Clinician's Interview-based Impression of Change plus caregiver input; PD-MCI, Individuals with Parkinson's disease and Mild Cognitive Impairment; WM, working memory; DS, digit span; VF, verbal fluency; CR, cognitive rehabilitation; ND, nondemented; PS, processing speed; EF, executive function; RCT, randomized controlled trial; VS, visuospatial; SDMT, Symbol Digit Modality Test; RS, resting-state fMRI; TMT, Trail Making Test; COWAT, Controlled Oral Word Association Test; CWIT, Color Word Interference Test; VC, visuoconstruction; TOL, Tower of London; stc, standard of care; BADS, Behavioural Assessment of the Dysexecutive Syndrome; Restorative+, restorative CR+ motor training and/or compensatory CR; CT, cognitive training; WCST, Wisconsin Card Sorting Test; MMSE, Mini Mental Status Examination; MDRS, Mattis Dementia Rating Scale; SCOPA-Cog, Scales for Outcome of Parkinson's Disease – Cognition; PASAT, Paced Auditory Serial Attention Task; LMT, Logical Memory Test; MoCA, Montreal Cognitive Assessment; PE, physical exercise intervention; CANTAB, Cambridge Neuropsychological Test Automated Battery; RBANS, Repeatable Battery for Assessment of Neuropsychological Status; HVOT, Hooper Visual Organization Test; WAIS-R, Wechsler Adult Intelligence Scale – Revised; DLPFC, dorsolateral prefrontal cortex; tDCS, transcranial direct current stimulation; rTMS, repetitive transcranial magnetic stimulation.

*Controls from a prior study.

---

injury and stroke [63], and there is a growing body of evidence of its efficacy with progressive conditions, such as mild AD [64] and amnestic MCI (reviewed in [65]).

Published data on the efficacy of cognitive rehabilitation in individuals with PD is sparse. To the best of our knowledge, only eight studies have evaluated cognition as an outcome following restorative and/or compensatory cognitive rehabilitation in PD, and only two of these studies were specific to PD-MCI (Table 11.1). Two additional studies [44, 45] used video or puzzle game practice as the primary treatment modality, which we have detailed in a separate section below (see 'Cognitive stimulation'). All of the studies detailed in Table 11.1 evaluated a restorative-based cognitive rehabilitation approach, which entailed 5–14 h of computer- and/or worksheet-based cognitive training based on analog versions of standard neuropsychological tests [37–43]. Two studies used aspects of compensatory strategy training and psychoeducation in addition to restorative training [42, 43], while one study conducted parallel motor training in addition to cognitive training [41]. Each study detailed in Table 11.1 revealed improvements in the respective cognitive domain in which the patients were trained, including improvements in executive function, memory and attention. With regard to the best approach, only one study to date has attempted to delineate which treatment strategy may be most efficacious. This study, conducted by Reuter et al. [42], compared a cognitive computer-based training program alone, with a compensatory (transfer) training program, and with both a compensatory and a motor training program in 222 nondemented PD patients. While all three interventions were deemed effective for improving cognition, the multimodal cognitive-psychomotor approach was found to be the most effective [42].

Taken together, there is evidence that cognitive rehabilitation improves cognition in nondemented PD. However, various treatment strategies and methodologies render interstudy comparisons and conclusions difficult. All studies to date have been limited by small sample sizes ($n = 6-35$), minimal use of control groups, mixed cognitively normal and MCI samples, and lack of use of a standard MCI diagnosis. Based on their review of studies on nonpharmacological interventions for PD conducted between 1985 and 2012, Hindle et al. [66] concluded that only one study, conducted by Paris et al. [39], was acceptable with regard to bias. In addition, there is limited information on the transfer of improvements to the everyday lives of individuals with PD and an impact on quality of life. The compensatory approach may be more beneficial to everyday, "real world" function and performance [67], but it has yet to be validated independently in PD. Finally, maintenance and long-term effects of treatment maintenance are virtually unknown, as only two studies conducted follow-up testing. These studies indicated that the effects of cognitive rehabilitation combined with motor training were maintained at the 6 months follow-up, yet a lack of control group comparisons in both studies limit drawing conclusions of efficacy [41, 42]. Future studies are critically needed to validate these intervention strategies and their long-term effects in PD-MCI.

To the best of our knowledge, no published literature exists on the efficacy of cognitive rehabilitation in individuals with PDD. However, there are several published studies on the efficacy of cognitive rehabilitation in AD. The findings in this population have been controversial, but there is evidence that cognitive training can improve and maintain cognition in mild to moderate AD, as well as improving their quality of life, mood and functional abilities [68]. Evidence further supports the use of a compensatory strategy approach (e.g. use of a memory notebook) compared with interactive computer games involving memory, concentration and problem-solving skills as superior in improving cognitive performance in AD [64]. Still, it is difficult to generalize these findings to individuals with PDD, as the neuropathological mechanisms and neuropsychological profiles of PDD are quite different from AD, especially in the early stages [69]. Efficacy studies are critically needed to determine the best cognitive intervention strategies for PDD.

Cognitive stimulation

There is increasing evidence that practicing puzzles or playing video games may increase cognitive function [44, 70]. While similar to a restorative approach, these interventions usually involve little to no guidance in practice or teaching of alternative strategies to the task, and thus we discuss them here. As detailed in Table 11.1, Pompeu et al. [45] demonstrated that after 14 30 min sessions of playing on a Wii (Nintendo Company, Kyoto, Japan), nondemented individuals with PD improved on a general cognitive screen (Montreal Cognitive Assessment [71]); however, these improvements were also noted in a physical therapy comparison group. In a small study that examined the neural and cognitive effects of 6 months of daily Sudoku puzzle practice, five nondemented PD participants demonstrated improved executive function and reduced cortical activation via functional MRI compared with control (no puzzle practice) PD patients. Although debated, a reduction in overall brain activation suggest improvements in brain functioning given that previous studies have linked cortical overactivation in PD to the neuropathological and neurochemical changes characteristic of this disease [72]. Further examination of this alternative treatment as an independent modality and/or adjunct to cognitive rehabilitation are needed.

Physical exercise

Studies examining various forms of physical exercise in healthy older adults without PD have shown improvements in cognition, particularly in executive function (e.g. [73]). However, surprisingly few studies have examined the effect of exercise on cognition in PD. A few small-sample studies have shown that exercise training and physical therapy programs can improve cognition, namely in the areas of executive function and attention in nondemented PD [46, 48, 74] (Table 11.1). Most studies evaluated the effects of aerobic or cycling exercise programs that ranged over a total of 4.5–72 h over 3–24 weeks, and, although promising, studies were limited by small ($n = 19-28$ total patients) and mixed patient samples, and lack of randomization and/or control groups, as well as undefined MCI patients. In an alternative approach,

Nocera et al. [47] examined the effects of a tai chi program in 15 nondememeted individuals with PD compared with six nondemented PD patients in a standard-of-care control group, revealing large (albeit nonsignificant at $P = 0.08$) effects on tests of attention.

With regard to PDD, only one study, to the best of our knowledge, has examined exercise as a treatment for dementia [49]. This case series study examined the effect of an 8-week program of aerobic exercise training on a stationary bicycle in two PDD patients and found improvements in global cognitive function and executive function [49]. However, the obvious limitation of this study was the very small sample size and lack of a control group. In summary, exercise as a treatment for cognitive impairment in PD is promising, but further studies are needed to prove if and which type of exercise is useful for the amelioration of cognitive deficits in this population.

Neural stimulation

As neural stimulation through deep-brain stimulation (DBS) has proved to be successful in ameliorating motor symptoms in PD, the use of neural stimulation techniques to improve cognition has been of recent interest. At the present time, no empirically based studies have shown that DBS is an effective treatment of cognition in PD, although one published case study ($n = 1$) observed improvements in cognition in an individual with PDD following implantation in the nucleus basalis of Meynert [75]. As there is limited research in this area due to a variety of technical and ethical concerns, it is yet to be seen whether DBS may be effective as an intervention for cognitive impairment in PD.

Noninvasive neural stimulation techniques such as repetitive transcranial magnetic stimulation (rTMS) and transcranial direct current stimulation (tDCS) have been studied in a handful of open trial studies with mixed results. Seven studies (of which only one was a randomized control trial [RCT]) demonstrated modest effects in executive functioning, working memory, processing speed and global cognitive function with rTMS or tDCS [53, 54, 56–59]), while two other studies, one of which was an RCT, showed no effects on cognition, or effects that were no different from a sham procedure [51, 55] [Table 11.1]. Therefore, these studies suggest that noninvasive neural stimulation techniques may improve cognition; however, larger samples and RCT designs are needed. Thus, while there is some evidence that this may be a promising treatment of cognitive impairment, further research needs to be done.

Summary and future directions

Clinical trials examining the efficacy of pharmacological and nonpharmacological interventions in PD are limited. Regarding pharmacological interventions for both PD-MCI and PDD, good clinical practice guidelines should be followed to identify medications and/or systemic conditions that could worsen cognition. In addition, in PDD, the use of cholinesterase inhibitors provides a modest improvement in cognition. Thus, in addition to searching for better therapies for PDD, it is clear that there is also a need for novel therapeutic approaches to improve the cognition of patients with PD-MCI. The most promising nonpharmacological intervention for cognitive impairment in PD is cognitive rehabilitation, with several studies showing improvements in some aspects of cognition. Other promising treatments include cognitive stimulation with video and/or puzzle game practice as well as physical exercise, while neural stimulation has yet to garner enough evidence to prove useful as an effective treatment. Despite the promising findings of most intervention studies, most are limited by several key factors, rendering it difficult to make judgments regarding specific programs or the abilities that may benefit from them. Future RCT studies are needed in order to address who can most benefit from these programs and what type of program is most efficacious.

References

1. Aarsland D, Zaccai J, Brayne C. A systematic review of prevalence studies of dementia in Parkinson's disease. *Mov Disord* 2005; **20**: 1255–63.
2. Aarsland D, Andersen K, Larsen JP, Lolk A, Kragh-Sorensen P. Prevalence and characteristics of dementia in Parkinson disease: an 8-year prospective study. *Arch Neurol* 2003; **60**: 387–92.
3. Aarsland, D, Karlsen, K. Neuropsychiatric aspects of Parkinson's disease. *Curr Psychiatry Rep* 1999; **1**: 61–8.
4. Hughes TA, Ross HF, Mindham RH, Spokes EG. Mortality in Parkinson's disease and its association with dementia and depression. *Acta Neurol Scand* 2004; **110**: 118–23.
5. Muslimovic D, Post B, Speelman JD, De Haan RJ, Schmand B. Cognitive decline in Parkinson's disease: a prospective longitudinal study. *J Int Neuropsychol Soc* 2009; **15**: 426–37.
6. Goldman JG, Litvan I. Mild cognitive impairment in Parkinson's disease. *Minerva Med* 2011; **102**: 441–59.
7. Litvan I, Aarsland D, Adler CH, et al. MDS Task Force on mild cognitive impairment in Parkinson's disease:

critical review of PD-MCI. *Mov Disord* 2011; **26**: 1814–24.

8. Aarsland D, Bronnick K, Williams-Gray C, et al. Mild cognitive impairment in Parkinson disease: a multicenter pooled analysis. *Neurology* 2010; **75**: 1062–9.

9. Janvin CC, Larsen JP, Aarsland D, Hugdahl K. Subtypes of mild cognitive impairment in Parkinson's disease: progression to dementia. *Mov Disord* 2006; **21**: 1343–9.

10. Mamikonyan E, Moberg PJ, Siderowf A, et al. Mild cognitive impairment is common in Parkinson's disease patients with normal Mini-Mental State Examination (MMSE) scores. *Parkinsonism Relat Disord* 2009; **15**: 226–31.

11. Woods SP, Tröster AI. Prodromal frontal/executive dysfunction predicts incident dementia in Parkinson's disease. *Journal of the International Neuropsychological Society* 2003; **9**: 17–24.

12. Owen AM. Cognitive dysfunction in Parkinson's disease: the role of frontostriatal circuitry. *Neuroscientist* 2004; **10**: 525–37.

13. Zgaljardic DJ, Borod JC, Foldi NS, Mattis P. A review of the cognitive and behavioral sequelae of Parkinson's disease: relationship to frontostriatal circuitry. *Cogn Behav Neurol* 2003; **16**: 193–210.

14. Zgaljardic DJ, Borod JC, Foldi NS, et al. An examination of executive dysfunction associated with frontostriatal circuitry in Parkinson's disease. *J Clin Exp Neuropsychol* 2006; **28**: 1127–44.

15. Filoteo JV, Maddox WT. Quantitative modeling of visual attention processes in patients with Parkinson's disease: effects of stimulus integrality on selective attention and dimensional integration. *Neuropsychology* 1999; **13**: 206–22.

16. Gabrieli JD, Singh J, Stebbins GT, Goetz CG. Reduced working memory span in Parkinson' disease: evidence for the role of a frontostriatal system in working and strategic memory. *Neuropsychology* 1996 **10**: 322–32.

17. Owen AM, Sahakian BJ, Hodges JR, Summers BA. Dopamine-dependent frontostriatal planning deficits in early Parkinson's disease. *Neuropsychology* 1995; **9**: 126–40.

18. Richards M, Cote LJ, Stern Y. Executive function in Parkinson's disease: set-shifting or set-maintenance? *J Clin Exp Neuropsychol* 1993; **15**: 266–79.

19. Filoteo JV, Rilling LM, Cole B, et al. Variable memory profiles in Parkinson's disease. *J Clin Exp Neuropsychol* 1997; **19**: 878–88.

20. Weintraub D, Moberg PJ, Culbertson WC, et al. Dimensions of executive function in Parkinson's disease. *Dement Geriatr Cogn Disord* 2005; **20**: 140–4.

21. Higginson CI, King DS, Levine D, et al. The relationship between executive function and verbal memory in Parkinson's disease. *Brain Cogn* 2003; **52**: 343–52.

22. Taylor AE, Saint-Cyr JA, Lang AE. Memory and learning in early Parkinson's disease: evidence for a "frontal lobe syndrome". *Brain Cogn* 1990; **13**: 211–32.

23. Levin BE, Llabre MM, Reisman S, et al. Visuospatial impairment in Parkinson's disease. *Neurology* 1991; **41**: 365–9.

24. Montse A, Pere V, Carme J, Francesc V, Eduardo T. Visuospatial deficits in Parkinson's disease assessed by judgment of line orientation test: error analyses and practice effects. *J Clin Exp Neuropsychol* 2001; **23**: 592–8.

25. Emre M. Dementia associated with Parkinson's disease. *Lancet Neurol* 2003; **2**: 229–37.

26. McPherson S, Cummings J. Neuropsychological aspects of Parkinson's disease and Parkinsonism. In Grant I, Adams KA, eds. *Neuropsychological Assessment of Neuropsychiatric and Neuromedical Disorders*. New York: Oxford University Press, 2009; 199–222.

27. Litvan I, Mohr E, Williams J, Gomez C, Chase TN. Differential memory and executive functions in demented patients with Parkinson's and Alzheimer's disease. *J Neurol Neurosurg Psychiatry* 1991; **54**: 25–9.

28. Pillon B, Dubois B, Ploska A, Agid Y. Severity and specificity of cognitive impairment in Alzheimer's, Huntington's, and Parkinson's diseases and progressive supranuclear palsy. *Neurology* 1991; **41**: 634–43.

29. Stern Y, Marder K, Tang MX, Mayeux R. Antecedent clinical features associated with dementia in Parkinson's disease. *Neurology* 1993; **43**: 1690–2.

30. Ferreira JJ, Katzenschlager R, Bloem BR, et al. Summary of the recommendations of the EFNS/MDS-ES review on therapeutic management of Parkinson's disease. *Eur J Neurol* 2013; **20**: 5–15.

31. Hanagasi HA, Gurvit H, Unsalan P, et al. The effects of rasagiline on cognitive deficits in Parkinson's disease patients without dementia: a randomized, double-blind, placebo-controlled, multicenter study. *Mov Disord* 2011; **26**: 1851–8.

32. Emre M, Aarsland D, Albanese A, et al. Rivastigmine for dementia associated with Parkinson's disease. *N Engl J Med* 2004; **351**: 2509–18.

33. Dubois B, Tolosa E, Katzenschlager R, et al. Donepezil in Parkinson's disease dementia: a randomized, double-blind efficacy and safety study. *Mov Disord* 2012; **27**: 1230–8.

34. Emre M, Tsolaki M, Bonuccelli U, et al. Memantine for patients with Parkinson's disease dementia or dementia with Lewy bodies: a randomised, double-blind, placebo-controlled trial. *Lancet Neurol* 2010; **9**: 969–77.

35. Aarsland D Ballard C, Walker Z, et al. Memantine in patients with Parkinson's disease dementia or dementia with Lewy bodies: a double-blind, placebo-controlled, multicentre trial. *Lancet Neurol* 2009; **8**: 613–18.

36. Cerasa A, Gioia MC, Salsone M, et al. Neurofunctional correlates of attention rehabilitation in Parkinson's disease: an explorative study. *Neurol Sci* 2014; **35**: 1173–80.

37. Disbrow EA, Russo KA, Higginson CI, et al. Efficacy of tailored computer-based neurorehabilitation for improvement of movement initiation in Parkinson's disease. *Brain Res* 2012; **1452**: 151–64.

38. Mohlman J, Chazin D, Georgescu B. Feasibility and acceptance of a nonpharmacological cognitive remediation intervention for patients with Parkinson disease. *J Geriatr Psychiatry Neurol* 2011; **24**: 91–7.

39. Paris AP, Saleta HG, de la Cruz Crespo Maraver M, et al. Blind randomized controlled study of the efficacy of cognitive training in Parkinson's disease. *Mov Disord* 2011; **26**: 1251–8.

40. Sammer G, Reuter I, Hullmann K, Kaps M, Vaitl D. Training of executive functions in Parkinson's disease. *J Neurol Sci* 2006; **248**: 115–19.

41. Sinforiani E, Banchieri L, Zucchella C, Pacchetti C, Sandrini G. Cognitive rehabilitation in Parkinson's disease. *Arch Gerontol Geriatr Suppl* 2004 (9): 387–91.

42. Reuter I, Mehnert S, Sammer G, Oechsner M, Engelhardt M. Efficacy of a multimodal cognitive rehabilitation including psychomotor and endurance training in Parkinson's disease. *J Aging Res* 2012; **2012**: 235765.

43. Naismith SL, Mowszowski L, Diamond K, Lewis SJ. Improving memory in Parkinson's disease: a healthy brain ageing cognitive training program. *Mov Disord* 2013; **28**: 1097–103.

44. Nombela C, Bustillo PJ, Castell PF, et al. Cognitive rehabilitation in Parkinson's disease: evidence from neuroimaging. *Front Neurol* 2011; **2**: 82.

45. Pompeu JE, Mendes FA, Silva KG, et al. Effect of Nintendo Wii-based motor and cognitive training on activities of daily living in patients with Parkinson's disease: a randomised clinical trial. *Physiotherapy* 2012; **98**: 196–204.

46. Cruise KE, Bucks RS, Loftus AM, et al. Exercise and Parkinson's: benefits for cognition and quality of life. *Acta Neurol Scand* 2011; **123**: 13–19.

47. Nocera JR, Amano S, Vallabhajosula S, Hass CJ. Tai Chi exercise to improve non-motor symptoms of Parkinson's disease. *J Yoga Phys Ther* 2013; **3**: 10.4172/2157-7595.1000137.

48. Ridgel AL, Muller MD, Kim CH, Fickes EJ, Mera TO. Acute effects of passive leg cycling on upper extremity tremor and bradykinesia in Parkinson's disease. *Phys Sportsmed* 2011; **39**: 83–93.

49. Tabak R, Aquije G, Fisher BE. Aerobic exercise to improve executive function in Parkinson disease: a case series. *J Neurol Phys Ther* 2013; **37**: 58–64.

50. Tanaka K, Quadros AC Jr, Santos RF, Stella F, Gobbi LT, Gobbi S. Benefits of physical exercise on executive functions in older people with Parkinson's disease. *Brain Cogn* 2009; **69**: 435–41.

51. Boggio PS, Fregni F, Bermpohl F, et al. Effect of repetitive TMS and fluoxetine on cognitive function in patients with Parkinson's disease and concurrent depression. *Mov Disord* 2005; **20**: 1178–84.

52. Boggio PS, Ferrucci R, Rigonatti SP, et al. Effects of transcranial direct current stimulation on working memory in patients with Parkinson's disease. *J Neurol Sci* 2006; **249**: 31–8.

53. Epstein CM, Evatt ML, Funk A, et al. An open study of repetitive transcranial magnetic stimulation in treatment-resistant depression with Parkinson's disease. *Clin Neurophysiol*, 2007; **118**: 2189–94.

54. Pal E, Nagy F, Aschermann Z, Balazs E, Kovacs N. The impact of left prefrontal repetitive transcranial magnetic stimulation on depression in Parkinson's disease: a randomized, double-blind, placebo-controlled study. *Mov Disord* 2010; **25**: 2311–17.

55. Sedlackova S, Rektorova I, Srovnalova H, Rektor I. Effect of high frequency repetitive transcranial magnetic stimulation on reaction time, clinical features and cognitive functions in patients with Parkinson's disease. *J Neural Transm* 2009; **116**: 1093–101.

56. Srovnalova H, Marecek R, Rektorova I. The role of the inferior frontal gyri in cognitive processing of patients with Parkinson's disease: a pilot rTMS study. *Mov Disord* 2011; **26**: 1545–8.

57. Srovnalova H, Marecek R, Kubikova R, Rektorova I. The role of the right dorsolateral prefrontal cortex in the Tower of London task performance: repetitive transcranial magnetic stimulation study in patients with Parkinson's disease. *Exp Brain Res* 2012; **223**: 251–7.

58. Furukawa T, Izumi S, Toyokura M, Masakado Y. Effects of low-frequency repetitive transcranial magnetic stimulation in Parkinson's disease. *Tokai J Exp Clin Med* 2009; **34**: 63–71.

59. Fregni F, Santos CM, Myczkowski ML, et al. Repetitive transcranial magnetic stimulation is as effective as fluoxetine in the treatment of depression in patients with Parkinson's disease. *J Neurol Neurosurg Psychiatry* 2004; **75**: 1171–4.

60. Leroi I, Brandt J, Reich SG, et al. Randomized placebo-controlled trial of donepezil in cognitive impairment in Parkinson's disease. *Int J Geriatr Psychiatry* 2004; **19**: 1–8.

61. Ravina B, Putt M, Siderowf A, et al. Donepezil for dementia in Parkinson's disease: a randomised, double blind, placebo controlled, crossover study. *J Neurol Neurosurg Psychiatry* 2005; **76**: 934–9.

62. Trail M, Protas EJ, Lai E (eds). *Neurorehabilitation in Parkinson's disease: An Evidence-based Treatment Model*. New Jersey: SLACK, Inc. 2008

63. Cicerone KD, Dahlberg C, Malec JF, et al. Evidence-based cognitive rehabilitation: updated review of the literature from 1998 through 2002. *Arch Phys Med Rehabil* 2005; **86**: 1681–92.
64. Loewenstein DA, Acevedo A, Czaja SJ, Duara R. Cognitive rehabilitation of mildly impaired Alzheimer disease patients on cholinesterase inhibitors. *Am J Geriatr Psychiatry* 2004; **12**: 395–402.
65. Jean L, Bergeron ME, Thivierge S, Simard M. Cognitive intervention programs for individuals with mild cognitive impairment: systematic review of the literature. *Am J Geriatr Psychiatry* 2010; **18**: 281–96.
66. Hindle JV, Petrelli A, Clare L, Kalbe E. Nonpharmacological enhancement of cognitive function in Parkinson's disease: a systematic review. *Mov Disord* 2013; **28**: 1034–49.
67. Twamley EW, Savla GN, Zurhellen CH, Heaton RK, Jeste DV. Development and pilot testing of a novel compensatory cognitive training intervention for people with psychosis. *Am J Psychiatr Rehabil* 2008; **11**: 144–63.
68. Olazaran J, Muniz R, Reisberg B, et al. Benefits of cognitive-motor intervention in MCI and mild to moderate Alzheimer disease. *Neurology* 2004; **63**: 2348–53.
69. Bronnick K, Emre M, Lane R, Tekin S, Aarsland D. Profile of cognitive impairment in dementia associated with Parkinson's disease compared with Alzheimer's disease. *J Neurol Neurosurg Psychiatry* 2007; **78**: 1064–8.
70. Achtman RL, Green CS, Bavelier D. Video games as a tool to train visual skills. *Restor Neurol Neurosci* 2008; **26**: 435–46.
71. Nasreddine ZS, Phillips NA, Bedirian V, et al. The Montreal Cognitive Assessment, MoCA: a brief screening tool for mild cognitive impairment. *J Am Geriatr Soc* 2005; **53**: 695–9.
72. Scatton B, Javoy-Agid F, Rouquier L, Dubois B, Agid Y. Reduction of cortical dopamine, noradrenaline, serotonin and their metabolites in Parkinson's disease. *Brain Res* 1983; **275**: 321–8.
73. Colcombe SJ, Erickson KI, Scalf PE, et al. Aerobic exercise training increases brain volume in aging humans. *J Gerontol A Biol Sci Med Sci* 2006; **61**: 1166–70.
74. Tanaka H, Koenig T, Pascual-Marqui RD, et al. Event-related potential and EEG measures in Parkinson's disease without and with dementia. *Dement Geriatr Cogn Disord* 2000; **11**: 39–45.
75. Barnikol TT, Barnikol UB, Kuhn J, Lenartz D, Tass PA. Changes in apraxia after deep brain stimulation of the nucleus basalis meynert in a patient With Parkinson dementia syndrome. *Mov Disord* 2010; **25**: 1519–20.

Chapter 12

A neurobehavioralist approach to the management of cognitive impairment in Parkinson's disease

Po-Heng Tsai

Introduction

Parkinson's disease (PD) is traditionally characterized by its motor symptoms of tremors, rigidity, bradykinesia and postural instability [1]. However, it has been increasingly recognized that nonmotor symptoms are frequently present in PD. Their onset sometimes predates the motor symptoms, and these nonmotor symptoms could lead to significant dysfunction [2, 3]. Cognitive impairment associated with PD is a common nonmotor symptom that should be recognized and managed appropriately to improve PD patients' quality of life.

Epidemiology

The spectrum of cognitive impairment in PD ranges from mild cognitive impairment (PD-MCI) to dementia (PDD). The term MCI is used to describe the intermediate stage between age-related cognitive changes and dementia. The main distinction between PD-MCI and PDD is that the deficits in PDD are severe enough to impair activities of daily living (ADLs). Instrumental ADLs such as management of finances, medication and transportation are usually affected before basic ADLs, which consist of self-care tasks such as eating, dressing, bathing and toileting.

The most frequently cited point prevalence of PDD is approximately 30%, with a cumulative prevalence of at least 75% for PD patients with a disease duration of more than 10 years. The incidence rate is such that approximately 10% of a PD population will develop dementia per year. The main risk factors for the development of PDD include higher age, more severe parkinsonism (in particular rigidity, postural instability and gait disturbance) and mild cognitive impairment at baseline [4].

Based on pooled data from various studies, the prevalence rate of PD-MCI is approximately 26–27%. The following features have been identified to be associated with the presence of MCI: older age at time of assessment and at disease onset, lower educational level, male gender, depression, advanced stage of PD and more severe motor symptoms [5, 6].

Recent efforts have been devoted to better defining PD-MCI because it may be the precursor to PDD, and early identification provides the opportunity to intervene before progression to dementia.

Cognitive profile and bedside assessment

The neuropsychological profile of PD has traditionally been viewed as being in a "frontal-subcortical" pattern (slow processing speed, impaired executive function and memory retrieval deficit) along with visuospatial dysfunction. Executive function difficulties, which include impairments in planning, initiating, sequencing, monitoring, set-shifting, adapting to novel situations and abstract reasoning, could be the earliest signs of impairment. However, studies have demonstrated variable patterns of impairments and the involvement of various cognitive domains [6, 7].

Mild cognitive impairment can be further divided into four subtypes according to a proposed classification: (i) amnestic single-domain MCI: only memory domain is impaired; (ii) amnestic multiple-domain MCI: memory plus one or more other domains are impaired; (iii) nonamnestic single-domain MCI: one nonmemory domain such as attention, executive function, visuospatial ability or language is impaired; and (iv) nonamnestic multiple-domain MCI: one or more nonmemory domains are impaired [8]. Based on this

Parkinson's Disease: Current and Future Therapeutics and Clinical Trials, ed. Gálvez-Jiménez et al. Published by Cambridge University Press. © Cambridge University Press 2016.

scheme, the majority of PD-MCI presents as nonamnestic single-domain MCI [6, 9].

Formal comprehensive neuropsychological assessment is considered the "gold standard" for the diagnosis of PD-MCI. However, sometimes obtaining a neuropsychological evaluation might not be feasible due to time demands, cost or the availability of a qualified neuropsychologist. Therefore, bedside cognitive screening tools have been recommended that can be administered quickly with relatively good sensitivity to detect PD-MCI. The Movement Disorder Society Task Force listed four such scales in their recent proposed diagnostic criteria for PD-MCI: the Montreal Cognitive Assessment (MoCA), the Parkinson's Disease Cognitive Rating Scale (PD-CRS), Scales of Outcomes of Parkinson's disease–Cognition (SCOPA-COG) and the Mattis Dementia Rating Scale (MDRS) [10]. MoCA appears to be one of the most recommended screening scales [11, 12]. It is freely available online at http://www.mocatest.org for clinical use for healthcare professionals and is available in multiple languages.

Pharmacological treatments

None of the current medications used for the treatment of cognitive impairments in PD have demonstrated effects in modifying the underling pathophysiology that leads to cell death. The available medications are considered symptomatic agents that aim to improve cognitive decline in patients with PD without modifying disease progression. Most of the agents focus on neurotransmitter systems that have been implicated to be altered in PD such as dopamine, norepinephrine, serotonin and acetylcholine.

Cholinesterase inhibitors

Rivastigmine, a cholinesterase inhibitor, is the only medication specifically approved by the US Food and Drug Administration (FDA) for the treatment of cognitive symptoms in PDD. The approval was based on a 24-week, randomized, placebo-controlled study that enrolled 541 patients and demonstrated moderate improvement in PDD but with higher rates of nausea, vomiting and tremor [13]. Cholinesterase inhibitors enhance cholinergic function through the reversible inhibition of acetylcholinesterase. The rationale of their use is based on biochemical and pathological studies that have demonstrated that cognitive impairment in PD is associated with cortical acetylcholine deficiency [14].

Besides rivastigmine, there are currently two other cholinesterase inhibitors available: donepezil and galantamine. In addition to inhibition of acetylcholinesterase, rivastigmine inhibits butyrylcholinesterase, whereas galantamine acts as an allosteric potentiating ligand of neuronal nicotinic receptors for acetylcholine. A recent Cochrane review of six clinical trials concluded that the use of cholinesterase inhibitors is beneficial in patients with PDD, with a positive impact on global assessment, cognitive function, behavioral disturbance and ADL rating scales [15].

Donepezil is available in tablets in three strengths (5, 10 and 23 mg) and in orally disintegrating tablets in two strengths (5 and 10 mg). Galantamine is available in extended-release capsules in three strengths (8, 16 and 24 mg) and as immediate-release tablets in three strengths (4, 8 and 12 mg). It is also available as a 4 mg/ml oral solution. Rivastigmine is available as a 24-h transdermal system ("patch") in three strengths (4.6, 9.5 and 13.3 mg), in capsules in four strengths (1.5, 3, 4.5 and 6 mg) and is available as a 2 mg/ml oral solution (Table 12.1). The most common adverse reactions of cholinesterase inhibitors are cholinergic-related gastrointestinal side effects, including nausea, vomiting and diarrhea. These side effects can be reduced by increasing the dose-titration duration, giving the medication with food or reducing the dose. Tremors may worsen but are usually mild and transient.

Memantine

Excitotoxicity has been hypothesized to be involved in neurodegenerative processes including PD. In this pathological process, neurons are damaged by excessive stimulation by excitatory neurotransmitters such as glutamate. This occurs when N-methyl-D-aspartate (NMDA) receptors are persistently activated. Memantine is a low- to moderate-affinity, noncompetitive NMDA receptor antagonist that binds preferentially to the NMDA receptor-operated cation channels and blocks excessive NDMA receptor activity [16]. Four placebo-controlled trials of memantine on cognition in PD have been reported, but the results were mixed, with only one study showing a significant effect on a predefined primary outcome of cognitive change [17].

Memantine is available in extended-release capsule formulation in four strengths (7, 14, 21 and 28 mg), in tablets in two strengths (5 and 10 mg) and as a 2 mg/ml oral solution (Table 12.2). The principal side effects of memantine are dizziness, headaches and somnolence.

Section II: Management of Nonmotor Symptoms of PD

Table 12.1 Administration, pharmacology and common adverse reactions of cholinesterase inhibitors

	Donepezil	Galantamine		Rivastigmine
Dosage and titration	Start at 5 mg daily and increase to 10 mg after 4–6 weeks. The dosage could then be increased to 23 mg daily after at least 3 months	Start at 4 mg twice daily (or 8 mg daily for extended-release [ER] formulation) and increase by 4 mg twice daily (or 8 mg ER daily) every 4 weeks at the minimum to maximum dosage of 12 mg twice daily (or 24 mg ER daily)	Oral formulation: start at 1.5 mg twice daily and increase by 1.5 mg twice daily every 2 weeks at the minimum to a maximum dosage of 6 mg twice daily	Transdermal system: start at 4.6 mg daily and increase to 9.5 mg after a minimum of 4 weeks. The dosage could then be increased to 13.3 mg after at least 4 weeks
Conversion between formulations	Not applicable	Conversion from immediate-release to extended-release formulation occurs on the same total daily dosage (e.g. 8 mg twice daily to 16 mg ER daily)	A total daily dose of <6 mg of oral rivastigmine can be switched to the 4.6 mg/24 h rivastigmine patch, and a total daily dose of 6–12 mg of oral rivastigmine can be switched to the 9.5 mg/24 h patch	
Elimination half-life	70 h	7 h	1.5 h	3 h (peripheral); 8 h in central nervous system; 24 h for patch formulation
Absorption	Can be given with or without food	Give with food	Give with food	Highest when applied to upper back, chest or upper arm
Most common adverse reactions	Nausea, diarrhea, insomnia, vomiting, muscle cramps, fatigue and anorexia	Nausea, vomiting, diarrhea, anorexia and weight decrease, and mild, transient increase in tremors	Nausea, vomiting, anorexia, dyspepsia and asthenia	Nausea, vomiting, diarrhea, depression, headache, anxiety, and application site reaction

Table 12.2 Administration, pharmacology and common adverse reactions of memantine

	Tablet and oral solution	Extended-release capsule formulation
Dosage and titration	Start at 5 mg once daily and increase by 5 mg daily every week at the minimum to a maximum dosage of 10 mg twice daily (5 mg daily, to 5 mg twice daily, to 5 and 10 mg separately, and 10 mg twice daily)	Start at 7 mg extended-release [ER] once daily and increase by 7 mg daily every week at the minimum to maximum dosage of 28 mg ER daily
Conversion between formulations	Patients taking 10 mg twice daily of memantine tablets could be converted to 28 mg ER formation once daily after the last tablet dose	
Elimination half-life	60–80 h	
Absorption	Can be given with or without food	
Most common adverse reactions	Dizziness, confusion, headache and constipation	Headache, diarrhea and dizziness

Atomoxetine

In addition to disturbances in the acetylcholine and glutamate neurotransmitter systems, cognitive changes in PD have been linked to norepinephrine deficiency. Atomoxetine is a selective norepinephrine reuptake inhibitor that has been approved by the FDA for the treatment of attention-deficit hyperactivity disorder. A pilot study of atomoxetine in 12 patients with PD and executive dysfunction demonstrated significant effects on both global change and cognition [18]. In addition, even though a study assessing the efficacy of atomoxetine for the treatment of clinically significant depressive symptoms in 55 PD subjects did not meet its primary outcome, atomoxetine was shown to significantly improve global cognition, as measured by the Mini Mental State Examination (MMSE) as part of the secondary outcomes [19]. A 12-week randomized, placebo-controlled phase II study of Atomoxetine Treatment for Cognitive Impairment in Parkinson's Disease (ATM-Cog) is actively recruiting patients.

Issues related to motor symptom treatments

Medications that are used to treat motor symptoms of PD have potential cognitive benefits. For example, levodopa (L-DOPA) can improve flexibility and working memory. Rasagiline, a monoamine oxidase type B inhibitor, has been shown in a small study to improve measures of attention and executive function in PD patients [20]. On the other hand, PD medications such as anticholinergics, high-dosage levodopa and dopamine agonists can impact cognition adversely, leading to confusion and hallucinations. In addition, negative cognitive outcomes have been observed in surgical treatment of PD with bilateral subthalamic nucleus deep-brain stimulation [21, 22].

Nonpharmacological treatments

Given the limited benefits of pharmacotherapies in treatment of cognitive impairment and dementia, there has been an increased interest in using nonpharmacological techniques such as physical activities, cognitive training and transcranial stimulation as therapy options. Proposed mechanisms of cognitive improvement include an increase in cognitive reserve and central nervous system plasticity via regular activation of various brain networks [23].

Most of the studies have been conducted in patients with Alzheimer's disease. With systematic reviews, nonpharmacological therapies have been found to be a useful approach to improve outcomes in patients with Alzheimer's disease. A recent systematic review that aimed to evaluate the effectiveness of nonpharmacological and noninvasive interventions in PD identified 18 studies with five studies of cognitive training, four with exercise and physical therapies, four using combined cognitive and physical interventions, and five of noninvasive brain-stimulation techniques such as transcranial direct current stimulation and repetitive transcranial magnetic stimulation [24]. Only one study, which focused on cognitive training, met the level of recommendation with randomized controlled design and low risk of bias. The authors concluded that current research on nonpharmacological therapies in cognitive dysfunction in PD is very limited in quantity and quality.

Summary

Cognitive impairment in PD is common and could significantly affect patients' functionality and quality of life. Current therapies focus on various neurotransmitter disturbances implicated in PD. Acetylcholinesterase inhibitors have the most evidence to support their use, with clinical trials demonstrating modest improvements in cognition, function and behavior. Nonpharmacological interventions have shown promise, but clinical trials supporting their use are lacking. Disease-modifying agents and new symptomatic agents are being developed and investigated.

References

1. Jankovic J. Parkinson's disease: clinical features and diagnosis. *J Neurol Neurosurg Psychiatry* 2007; **79**: 368–76.
2. Lim SY, Fox SH, Lang AE. Overview of the extranigral aspects of Parkinson disease. *Arch Neurol* 2009; **66**: 167–72.
3. Barone P, Antonini A, Colosimo C, *et al.* The PRIAMO study: A multicenter assessment of nonmotor symptoms and their impact on quality of life in Parkinson's disease. *Mov Disord* 2009; **24**: 1641–9.
4. Emre M, Aarsland D, Brown R, *et al.* Clinical diagnostic criteria for dementia associated with Parkinson's disease. *Mov Disord* 2007; **22**: 1689–707.
5. Aarsland D, Bronnick K, Williams-Gray C, *et al.* Mild cognitive impairment in Parkinson disease: a multicenter pooled analysis. *Neurology* 2010; **75**: 1062–9.
6. Litvan I, Aarsland D, Adler CH, *et al.* MDS Task Force on mild cognitive impairment in Parkinson's disease: critical review of PD-MCI. *Mov Disord* 2011; **26**: 1814–24.
7. Watson GS, Leverenz JB. Profile of cognitive impairment in Parkinson's disease. *Brain Pathol* 2010; **20**: 640–5.
8. Petersen RC. Mild cognitive impairment as a diagnostic entity. *J Intern Med* 2004; **256**: 183–194.
9. Aarsland D, Brønnick K, Larsen JP, Tysnes OB, Alves G. Cognitive impairment in incident, untreated Parkinson disease: the Norwegian ParkWest study. *Neurology* 2009; **72**: 1121–6.
10. Litvan I, Goldman JG, Tröster AI, *et al.* Diagnostic criteria for mild cognitive impairment in Parkinson's disease: Movement Disorder Society Task Force guidelines. *Mov Disord* 2012; **27**: 349–56.
11. Chou KL, Amick MM, Brandt J, *et al.* A recommended scale for cognitive screening in clinical trials of Parkinson's disease. *Mov Disord* 2010; **25**: 2501–7.
12. Dalrymple-Alford JC, MacAskill MR, Nakas CT, *et al.* The MoCA: well-suited screen for cognitive impairment in Parkinson disease. *Neurology* 2010; **75**: 1717–25.
13. Emre M, Aarsland D, Albanese A, *et al.* Rivastigmine for dementia associated with Parkinson's disease. *N Engl J Med* 2004; **351**: 2509–18.
14. Klein JC, Eggers C, Kalbe E, *et al.* Neurotransmitter changes in dementia with Lewy bodies and Parkinson disease dementia in vivo. *Neurology* 2010; **74**: 885–92.

15. Rolinski M, Fox C, Maidment I, McShane R. Cholinesterase inhibitors for dementia with Lewy bodies, Parkinson's disease dementia and cognitive impairment in Parkinson's disease. *Cochrane Database Syst Rev* 2012; **3**: CD006504.
16. Lipton SA. Paradigm shift in NMDA receptor antagonist drug development: molecular mechanism of uncompetitive inhibition by memantine in the treatment of Alzheimer's disease and other neurologic disorders. *J Alzheimers Dis* 2004; **6** (Suppl.): S61–74.
17. Svenningsson P, Westman E, Ballard C, Aarsland D. Cognitive impairment in patients with Parkinson's disease: diagnosis, biomarkers, and treatment. *Lancet Neurol* 2012; **11**: 697–707.
18. Marsh L, Biglan K, Gerstenhaber M, Williams JR. Atomoxetine for the treatment of executive dysfunction in Parkinson's disease: a pilot open-label study. *Mov Disord* 2009; **24**: 277–82.
19. Weintraub D, Mavandadi S, Mamikonyan E, *et al.* Atomoxetine for depression and other neuropsychiatric symptoms in Parkinson disease. *Neurology* 2010; **75**: 448–55.
20. Hanagasi HA, Gurvit H, Unsalan P, *et al.* The effects of rasagiline on cognitive deficits in Parkinson's disease patients without dementia: a randomized, double-blind, placebo-controlled, multicenter study. *Mov Disord* 2011; **26**: 1851–8.
21. Parsons TD, Rogers SA, Braaten AJ, Woods SP, Tröster AI. Cognitive sequelae of subthalamic nucleus deep brain stimulation in Parkinson's disease: a meta-analysis. *Lancet Neurol* 2006; **5**: 578–88.
22. Smeding HM, Speelman JD, Huizenga HM, Schuurman PR, Schmand B. Predictors of cognitive and psychosocial outcome after STN-DBS in Parkinson's Disease. *J Neurol Neurosurg Psychiatry* 2011; **82**: 754–60.
23. Buschert V, Bokde AL, Hampel H. Cognitive intervention in Alzheimer disease. *Nat Rev Neurol* 2010; **6**: 508–17.
24. Hindle JV, Petrelli A, Clare L, Kalbe E. Nonpharmacological enhancement of cognitive function in Parkinson's disease: a systematic review. *Mov Disord* 2013; **28**: 1034–49.

Chapter 13

Management of disease-related behavioral disturbances in Parkinson's disease

Joseph H. Friedman

Introduction

Although categorized as a movement disorder, Parkinson's disease (PD) is a neurobehavioral disorder [1] and the importance of the behavioral components should not be underestimated [2]. The nonmotor behavior symptoms in PD are the major determinants of health-related quality of life in most reports from all parts of the world [2, 3], reflecting the fact that these behavioral problems are not culturally based. Studies have shown that the greatest stress for caregivers arises from behavioral rather than motor problems, with the corollary observation that the most important precipitants for nursing home placement are behavioral problems, not motor [4]. Yet the vast majority of treatment trials have focused on the motor aspects. The increasing number of research studies on behavior in PD reflects the increasing recognition of the importance of these problems.

Behavioral problems in PD are particularly difficult to study, more so than behavior problems in psychiatric disorders because there are obvious interrelationships between the motor problems and the behavioral. It has been well known since the disease was described that tremor and other motor problems vary with anxiety. In addition, there are definite interrelationships among the various emotional states themselves, such as sleep, fatigue, depression and anxiety. Complicating the picture even further is the overlap among the various disorders. For example, fatigue is associated with depression, i.e. people with fatigue are more likely to be depressed than nonfatigued PD patients, yet many fatigued PD patients are not depressed. However, fatigue is one of the defining features for major depression, as defined in the *Diagnostic and Statistical Manual of Mental Disorders, 4th Edn, Text Revision* (DSM-IV-TR) [5], the standard catalogue for defining mental illnesses. Fatigue may be associated with sleep dysfunction and vice versa, but they may be occurring as separate but overlapping syndromes. Apathy and sleep disorders are symptoms of depression, yet these are also syndromes in PD that may be quite distinct from depression. Understanding these relationships is crucial not only for an understanding the individual patient's disorders but also for choosing treatment. Fatigue in the setting of depression may suggest the use of an antidepressant, whereas fatigue unrelated to a mood disorder may initiate the use of a stimulant medication. Patients have anxious, depressed, irritable or other unpleasant feelings when their motor condition is "off" but may also have these feelings when their motor condition is "on." These symptoms are often called "nonmotor off" and have an uncertain relationship with dopamine activity [6].

There are two important underlying aspects for understanding the many behavioral problems in PD. Aside from the complexity of the phenomenology and their interrelationships, the various behavioral problems in PD are mostly independent of dopamine. For many years, PD has been simplistically considered a dopamine deficiency disorder, and the vast majority of treatment trials have focused on improving dopaminergic stimulation in the brain, or compensating for decreased dopamine, by altering glutamate or acetylcholine transmission. While these interventions have improved motor control, they have not been helpful in treating behavioral problems. The second is that, unlike the motor problems, the behavioral problems are often not progressive. This suggests different disease processes than are usually considered for the neurodegenerative disorders.

Parkinson's Disease: Current and Future Therapeutics and Clinical Trials, ed. Gálvez-Jiménez et al. Published by Cambridge University Press. © Cambridge University Press 2016.

Personality

An intriguing but difficult question is whether there is a "Parkinson personality" [7] and, if so, which phenomena may be intrinsic to the disorder and which are due to the effects of the disease. There is a long but unknown duration of PD pathology present in the brain before the motor stigmata surface. The increasingly recognized "herald" symptom of rapid eye movement (REM) sleep behavior disorder being occasionally present for decades before motor symptoms makes it likely that some personality changes are part of the disease process. In addition, one of the most robust epidemiological associations for PD risk has been the inverse association with cigarette smoking [8]. Since cigarette smoking is likely one manifestation of personality, perhaps a measure of addiction potential, it is likely that this alone supports the existence of certain personality traits having an association with PD. Fatigue affects about one-third of patients by the time their PD is diagnosed [9], and both anxiety and depression are common. Olfactory impairment affects not only smell but also taste, thus perhaps reducing some enjoyable aspects of life, leading to subtle changes in habits and thus personality. Since these aspects of personality often appear before motor symptoms, and appear sufficiently often in the general population that they cannot be interpreted at the time as part of a disease process, they are seen as personality changes of aging. In the heyday of psychoanalysis, certain personality traits were thought to be risk factors for PD [10, 11], and some signs were interpreted as psychogenic rather than physiological.

Retrospective personality studies have shown differences between PD and non-PD, but these are obviously subject to recollection bias [12–14]. A large prospective general psychological study of patients in Minnesota followed almost 7000 patients for 40 years. Only anxiety present early was associated with later development of PD [15]. Depression and pessimism early on were *not* associated with an increased risk of PD. [15], and although several reports have described a reduction in novelty seeking in PD patients, a prospective study did not find this to be predictive of later development of PD [16].

Post-hoc studies of premorbid personality in PD patients have purported to find them more industrious, inflexible and cautious, with a low risk of impulsive decision making. Studies looking at contemporaneous personality differences between PD and controls generally found reduced novelty seeking, greater or equal levels of harm avoidance, and equal levels of reward dependence and perseverance [7]. Of note, however, is a small study of nine couples of monozygotic twins discordant for PD, which found no personality differences [17]. Poletti and Bonuccelli [7] concluded their review on the topic of personality in PD by noting that "empirical evidence does not robustly support the existence of a characteristic premorbid personality profile in PD patients."

However, given the inverse association of PD with cigarette smoking, the lengthy duration of REM sleep behavior disorder and the increased premorbid development of fatigue, anxiety and depression, it seems likely that personality differences have not been identified due to methodological limitations, depending on how long before the onset of motor changes the personality changes are looked for.

Apathy

Apathy is a behavioral state that has variable definitions. In common parlance, as defined in dictionaries, it is "a state of indifference or the suppression of emotions" (Wikipedia), "the lack of interest or concern: lack of emotion or feeling" (Free Online Dictionary) and "a complete lack of emotion or motivation" (Urban Dictionary), but in psychiatric literature it is considered both a syndrome [18–20] and a symptom. In the DSM-IV-TR [5], there are two categories of major depression, melancholic, in which patients feel sad, and anhedonic, in which patients are unable to feel pleasure. The latter condition could be considered an apathetic depression.

Apathy is generally considered a disorder of motivation, therefore having a relationship with fatigue, as well as depression. Apathy is common in dementing disorders such as Alzheimer's disease, dementia with Lewy bodies, PD and frontotemporal dementia, as well as in primary psychiatric disorders such as schizophrenia and major depression. Apathy is also a syndrome [20–22] (Box 13.1) Understanding the difference between a syndrome and a symptom is perhaps best appreciated by considering depression. One is thought to be depressed if sad; however, the syndrome of depression may involve several other symptoms such as fatigue, sleepiness, amotivation and irritability.

Data on apathy in PD has been inconsistent, presumably reflecting differences in assessment and populations. Prevalence rates in PD have been reported to be

> **Box 13.1 Apathy syndrome**
>
> The patient must meet the criteria for each of the following four symptom complexes [20, 22]:
> Abnormally decreased motivation
> Two of the following:
> - Loss of self-initiated behavior
> - Reduced responsiveness
> - Reduction in spontaneous emotion; blunted affect
> - Decreased emotional responses
>
> Clinically significant functional impairment
> The symptoms are not explained by a substance or a physical disability

between 7 and 70% [23]. Similarly discrepant overlap rates for apathy, dementia and depression have been published. One report from the USA found that 29% of 80 PD patients had abnormal Apathy Scale scores but normal depression scale scores [24]. In another country, 52 of 164 PD patients were deemed apathetic, of whom 35% were depressed but not demented, 8% demented but not depressed, and 48% had both dementia and depression. Only five patients suffered from apathy alone [25]. In France, 56% of 159 PD patients were apathetic but only 9% had apathy without depression or dementia [26]. Apathy correlated, in general, with cognitive dysfunction and not motor severity, suggesting a nondopaminergic neurochemical basis. In a Scandinavian study of 2323 PD patients, apathy was noted in 38% but most had cognitive dysfunction or were on medications for depression or psychosis [27].

Apathy has been associated with reduced quality of life, depression, dementia and fatigue [18]. Specific criteria for a diagnosis of apathy in PD have been proposed [28], requiring a reduction in motivation, reduced goal-directed cognitive activity and reduced emotional display, both spontaneous and evoked. It is interesting that these medical criteria sometimes minimize the more general perception of the meaning of apathy as expressed in dictionaries, which likely reflect the nonmedical understanding of the term, which is a lack of emotions. Apathy is primarily a self-reported symptom that is partly but not completely reflected by outside perception. A person who shows no emotion and has restricted capability for movement may seem apathetic yet may not be.

In clinical practice, the major differential in classifying apathy is with depression. Since the two syndromes include reduced motivation, the clinician often cannot be confident of the diagnosis. One of the unusual features of apathy in PD, since it so often co-exists with dementia, is that it sometimes provides emotional insulation from a very restricting condition. In many cases, the apathetic patient is far less emotionally disturbed by his condition than the family. The patient often does not appear to care about being unable to do things that formerly gave pleasure and appears content, or at least not disturbed by, a very restricted existence.

The natural course of apathy has not been studied. It is likely that apathy related to dementia is progressive, whereas apathy associated with depression may not be. This is, however, quite speculative.

Apathy as a response to acute dopaminergic withdrawal has been described [29], and therefore may respond to reintroduction of the discontinued medication. Apathy may also be a potential side effect of psychoactive medications, including antidepressants, antipsychotics and benzodiazepines, so medication reviews should be undertaken with this in mind.

Treatment for apathy, in general, is unknown. Anecdotal reports and theories suggest that dopaminergic agents and stimulants may be helpful, but no convincing data exists. Cholinesterase inhibitors are thought to produce mild benefits in apathy in demented patients, and since the majority of PD patients with apathy are demented, this should be entertained. When apathy is considered a problem for the patient and depression is considered a possible concomitant syndrome, a trial of an antidepressant seems reasonable. In clinical practice, it may be extremely helpful simply to provide counseling to the family, explaining that apathy is a common feature of PD, has no clear treatment and may, in fact, be protective.

Anxiety

Anxiety is a common problem in PD [30, 31], affecting over 40% [30] and generally is underappreciated [32]. This underappreciation is reflected both in movement disorder specialist evaluations and in research publication numbers. There are only rare reports of treatment trials [30]. An interesting study that should be of great interest to doctors who care for large numbers of PD patients found that anxiety was associated with an increased rate of telephone calls to the treating neurologist [33].

Anxiety is defined as excessive nervousness or fear. There are several subcategories of anxiety. The classification system has been significantly altered from DSM-IV-TR to DSM-V [34], and is likely not widely understood by neurologists. Anxiety is common in the general population but more so in PD. Its epidemiology is also different. In the general population, anxiety generally appears in young adults and is highly skewed toward women. In the PD population, it arises a few years before or after the onset of the motor symptoms and affects the genders equally. The published prevalence estimates for anxiety in PD vary from 4 to 40% [23, 31, 35].

Until the diagnostic categories changed in 2013 with the publication of DSM-V [34], the most common anxiety disorders affecting PD patients were generalized anxiety, panic disorder and social phobia. In the new nosology, generalized anxiety disorder, a condition in which people were excessively nervous in general, does not exist, as the long-term outcome of this disorder indicated that generalized anxiety was a transient condition that evolved into another disorder, most commonly depression with anxiety. Social phobias are excessive fears related to social interactions. Of course, in PD, many patients shun a variety of social interactions because they may have dysarthria, which makes them very self-conscious about participating in conversation, or they may be self-conscious because of drooling, dyskinesias or tremors. They may avoid crowds because of the risk of falling or a distaste for the commotion associated with a large group. Panic attacks refer to acute episodes, generally not provoked by identifiable precipitants, during which people feel chest pain, shortness of breath, a sensation of immanent death, tingling, and numbness or other somatic symptoms. Data on anxiety in PD available for this chapter was published before the classification system changed, so the data presented in this chapter will require re-interpretation within a few years. For the purpose of most treating physicians and family, recognition of anxiety, panic or phobia and their associations with PD are the important issues, not classification.

In a 1-year cross-sectional study performed in Europe, the USA and Australia, 34% of the 340 subjects attending university referral centers were classified as having at least one DSM-IV anxiety disorder, and 12% had more than one [30]. Multiple anxiety disorders were more prevalent than any single anxiety category. Generalized anxiety disorder was the most common, followed by agoraphobia without panic or social phobia. Twenty-six percent of those with anxiety disorders also suffered from major depression, while 13% suffered from dysthymia, a milder form of depression. Ponton *et al.* [36], using very different evaluations in an American population, found equal levels of social phobia and multiple anxiety disorders, but more panic. An Australian study [31] of 79 PD patients diagnosed one-quarter with anxiety disorders, half of whom also suffered from depression. These numbers are significantly higher than the prevalence in the age-matched general population. Although the Australian study found that anxiety prevalence was greater in the younger patients, and that there was no relationship with PD medication use, these associations have not been adequately studied. Whether there is any relationship between anxiety and the side of worse motor symptoms, as reported in one study [37], is unclear [31].

Although "nonmotor-off" symptoms have frequently been associated with the "off" motor state, Leentjens *et al.* [38] studied 250 PD patients of whom 118 had motor fluctuations. They found that the fluctuators were more likely to have generalized anxiety, but the majority with anxiety did not have fluctuations. Those who reported fluctuations in levels of anxiety generally were more anxious when "off," although some were more anxious when "on."

There are no medications approved by the US Food and Drug Administration (FDA) for the treatment of anxiety in PD. There have been few studies of anxiety in PD. In some studies of antidepressants in PD, anxiety was also evaluated, but these studies were underpowered, meaning that the design of the trial was not centered on anxiety, so that insufficient numbers of anxious subjects might have been recruited to make definitive statistical inferences on drug effect. In these studies, the antidepressants, which are approved by the FDA for treating anxiety as well as depression in the general population, were not beneficial for anxiety in PD. The medications used for treating anxiety in the general population are typically benzodiazepines, buspirone, trazodone and selective serotonin reuptake inhibitors (SSRIs). Benzodiazepines are considered relatively contraindicated in the elderly due to the risk of confusion and falls. On the other hand, the SSRIs need to be used for 2 weeks or more before antianxiety effects begin to take effect, and they cannot be used on an as-needed basis. They also have the possible advantage of not causing sedation. The benzodiazepines may be used on an as-needed basis and may be particularly useful for insomnia associated with anxiety. In addition, clonazepam is commonly used to treat REM sleep behavior disorder.

Psychotic symptoms

Psychosis has generally been understood as a disorder characterized by the loss of reality testing. This classical definition has been revised in favor of characterizing disorders by the nature of their psychotic symptoms, such as hallucinations and delusions. Parkinson's disease patients may develop these symptoms without medications, but typically they occur on medications for their motor problems. The relationship between medications and symptoms has been an area of interest because of the identical phenomenology seen in patients with dementia with Lewy bodies who are not taking anti-parkinsonism medications. In addition, in rare patients with long-standing PD that has never been treated, hallucinations have occurred [39]

Visual hallucinations affect approximately 20–30% of drug-treated patients; however, prevalence increases with the duration of follow-up [40]. In a study of 386 patients in Holland, 21% had hallucinations at baseline, but within 5 years, 45% of the ones who had not suffered hallucinations developed them [41]. Auditory hallucinations may occur as well but are generally about half as common, and usually occur in patients who are having visual hallucinations [40]. Unlike hallucinations that occur in primary psychiatric disorders such as schizophrenia, major depression or mania, the hallucinations are typically visual, whereas the primary psychiatric disorders are auditory, and, quite strikingly, mostly have no emotional import. Schizophrenic hallucinations are characterized by voices criticizing the patient, either directly or in the form of conversations about the patient. Parkinson's disease patients generally see people or animals, which are not threatening and usually ignore the patient. For example, they may see children playing in the living room, two adults watching television, marching bands outside in the yard or bugs on the wall. The hallucinations may be in color or black and white, vivid or somewhat obscured, and may last from seconds to minutes. The hallucinations tend to be stereotyped, the patient generally seeing the same people doing the same thing each time. The auditory hallucinations may be voices, music or mechanical sounds, and tend to be indistinct, like a radio playing in another room. Tactile, olfactory and gustatory hallucinations may occur but are considerably less common. Two unusual types of hallucinations are notable [42], "presence hallucinations" and "passage hallucinations." "Presence hallucinations" are not true hallucinations. They are a strong feeling that someone or something unseen is behind or to the side of the patient. These are not threatening. The patient feels that someone else, or possibly a pet, is in the room and turns to look. There are also "passage hallucinations," the visual perception of people, animals or shadows passing quickly in the peripheral field, which always disappear on direct inspection. Some patients will also report reflections off their eyeglasses although there is no light source.

Delusions are irrational beliefs. These are not based on data or they are grossly distorted interpretations of real events. Unfortunately, in PD, the delusions tend to be paranoid [43]. The most common delusions are "jealous" delusions, with patients believing that their spouses are having sexual affairs. Other delusions also tend to be paranoid in nature, such as thinking people are living in the home or that the patient is being spied upon. Institutionalized patients will complain privately of being manhandled by staff, or poisoned, or that a staff member is selling drugs, supplying sex or selling body parts.

In Holland, about 30% of hallucinators also had delusions [41]. A retrospective chart review of 1453 patients in one clinic found that psychotic symptoms increased in frequency with increasing duration of disease, so that the average was 27% but by 12 years of disease the prevalence was 34% [44]. Other reports have provided similar estimates.

Psychotic symptoms of PD are quite different from schizophrenic symptoms. Parkinson's disease patients do not experience delusions of grandeur. They do not believe themselves to be messengers of God. They do not hear voices commenting on them or believe that they are being controlled by aliens. In PD, the hallucinations have no emotional import, unlike the case with primary psychiatric disorders.

Several reports have mentioned conflicting risk factors for psychotic symptoms, but all agree that dementia is a risk factor, probably the most significant risk factor, and that the occurrence of visual hallucinations increases the risk of dementia developing within the next few years. Visual impairment is considered a risk factor for hallucinations [40]. A 2013 study reported many risk factors, including older age, depression, daytime sleepiness and others [41]. It must be noted that psychotic symptoms often develop without any change in medications or obvious change in medical status, so that a patient who had been stable and doing well for years may report new-onset hallucinations. This presumably reflects brain changes associated with disease progression, not a change in pharmacokinetics.

The evaluation of psychosis requires a review of all psychoactive medications to be certain that nonneurological medications, particularly anticholinergics for bladder control, are not contributors. Medical contributors such as occult infection and endocrine and metabolic disorders also need to be considered. When these have been excluded, then treatment requires a reduction, if possible, in PD medications, all of which may be contributory. There have been no studies comparing treatments for psychosis and no studies looking at dose reductions of PD medications. Double-blinded trials comparing levodopa (L-DOPA) and dopamine agonists have shown that dopamine agonists are more likely to cause hallucinations. It is therefore generally recommended that anticholinergics be tapered and stopped first, then amantadine and then dopamine agonists before levodopa. It is this author's belief that one medication should be tapered and stopped rather than having all medications reduced, the notion being that medication side effects may be synergistic.

After PD medications have been lowered to their lowest tolerable dose, then, if psychotic symptoms persist, an antipsychotic should be added. Clozapine, quetiapine, olanzapine and pimavanserin are the only medications that have been subject to double-blind, placebo-controlled trials [40]. Olanzapine was clearly shown to worsen motor function and *not* to be helpful for controlling the psychosis. Clozapine, in two multicentered, double-blind, placebo-controlled trials, was shown to be extremely helpful for the psychosis, without motor worsening, and even with significant improvement in tremor. Quetiapine failed to show efficacy in three double-blind, placebo-controlled trials, although open-label trials have been quite successful. However, all of the quetiapine trials have shown no worsening of motor function. The only successful double-blind, placebo-controlled trial was too small to be interpretable. The other atypical antipsychotics have had variable results in terms of worsening parkinsonism, with at least some reports of worsened motor function with all, including aripiprazole, a partial dopamine agonist. In some countries, clozapine has been accepted as a government-approved medication for PD psychosis but not in the USA. The American Academy of Neurology task force recommended consideration of both quetiapine and clozapine. The Movement Disorder Society Task Force on nonmotor symptoms recommended clozapine [45]

Clozapine requires a complete blood count weekly for 6 months, every other week for 6 months and then every month thereafter, due to the risk of agranulocytosis, which is believed to be 1% in young adults and possibly higher in older healthy adults. Since this risk is independent of dose, the low doses used do not ameliorate the risk. Clozapine is generally effective at doses between 6.25 and 50 mg/day. The time of greatest risk for agranulocytosis is the first 3 months.

Some experts have advocated the use of cholinesterase inhibitors to treat psychotic symptoms. In studies of PD dementia and dementia with Lewy bodies, these agents have been associated with a reduction in hallucinations; however, there have been no large studies of their effects when used directly to treat hallucinations or delusions. Their use is predicated on the association between dementia psychotic symptoms and the common observation that anticholinergics may induce psychotic symptoms in PD.

An entirely different pharmacological approach to treating psychosis was based in part on the observation that all of the second-generation antipsychotic drugs, in addition to blocking dopamine D2 receptors, also blocked the 5-HT2A serotonin receptor. Other observations have long linked serotonin to psychotic symptoms, so trials of pimavanserin, a 5-HT2A "inverse agonist" were undertaken. While the initial phase 3 and earlier phase 2 trials yielded results that were equivocal in terms of efficacy, all studies demonstrated that the drug was safe, without worsening of motor function, and had a side effect profile similar to placebo. Based on the initial trials, a very rigorous phase 3 trial was undertaken, with positive results [46]. At the time writing, the manufacturer is submitting data to the FDA for approval of this drug to specifically treat PD psychosis.

Depression

Depression is well known to be a common problem in PD, but the estimates for its prevalence vary significantly for a number of reasons. Primarily, the diagnosis of depression in the PD patient is a challenge. The markers generally used to recognize depression in the general population are facial expression, psychomotor retardation, soft voice, stooped posture and reduced gestures, all of which are intrinsic to the motor aspects of the disease. If one considers the requirements for the diagnosis of major depression in the general population using DSM-IV-TR criteria [5], fatigue, sleep disorders, psychomotor retardation and weight change, four of the required five symptoms, are already present in most PD patients, regardless of their mood.

The diagnosis of depression in PD rests primarily on mood, but useful symptoms include anxiety, which is, more often than not, associated with depression in PD, disability out of proportion to motor deficits [47], irritability and loss of interest in activities that should not be significantly compromised by motor dysfunction.

Depression is common in PD, regardless of the criteria used [48], with over 50% suffering from it in some form [49], with 17% having major depression and 35% having less severe problems [49]. Depression is associated with worse prognosis for both motor and cognitive function [50–52] and a greater effect on quality of life than motor dysfunction [53].

The course of depression is difficult to assess for many reasons. In a study that followed 413 early, mild, untreated PD patients who were participants in two observational (nontreatment) PD studies, 23% were rated as depressed on the Geriatric Depression Scale (GDS) at some point during the study [54]. Almost half were treated with antidepressants. Clinically significant depression remitted in half of the cases within 6 months. Those with mild depression were six times more likely to develop more severe depression than those who had not been depressed. Paradoxically, the use of antidepressants was associated with a reduced rate of remission of depression. In the general population, depression generally resolves spontaneously, although it may recur. It is unknown if this is true in PD.

The pathophysiology of depression remains unknown. For many years, the etiology of depression was debated, with one side advocating depression as a reaction to the diagnosis of PD, and the other maintaining that depression was an intrinsic disorder related to neurodegeneration in specific brain regions. Most authorities believe that depression occurs for both reasons. The reason for the opinion change was the discovery of the importance of basal ganglia structures in mood, uncovered by the results of the many deep-brain stimulation treatments for motor problems in PD. Abnormalities of serotonin and norepinephrine have been suggested but not confirmed [47]

Although depression is common in PD and had been the focus of discussions for many years, when a review article was published in 2013 [48], only six randomized controlled trials of antidepressants had been published, five of which involved placebo. This meta-analysis concluded that "antidepressant medications were not efficacious in depression in PD" [48]. This result supported a similar conclusion in 2005 [55], although the multicenter, placebo-controlled, three-arm study by Richard et al. [56] concluded that both venlafaxine and paroxetine were statistically more beneficial than placebo. However, the placebo response was so great in the study that the benefit of the active drug was diminished, as illustrated by the number needed to treat being 14 and 22 for the active drugs. None of the trials were longer than 12 weeks. A much larger double-blind, placebo-controlled study of pramipexole [57], a dopamine agonist used for treating the motor symptoms of PD, found a statistically significant but small antidepressant result, which, using the statistical technique of path analysis, was attributed to a direct antidepressant effect.

Although there are multiple statements in the literature decrying the undertreatment of depression in PD, it is unclear that treatment works well, and many patients treated long term with SSRI antidepressants remain depressed. There are no clear recommendations on treatment. The use of SSRI medications is generally preferred by authorities because of their more benign side-effect profile, but some data suggest that tricyclic antidepressants may work better. Most antidepressants have antianxiety properties so that the two often concurrent syndromes may be treated with a single agent. Often, the medication choice is dictated by the side-effect profile. Medications that cause sedation may be useful in the patient who sleeps poorly at night. Drugs that increase appetite and cause weight gain may be ideal if a patient is losing weight. Tricyclics generally have anticholinergic properties that may be useful in a patient with drooling or an overactive bladder. Antidepressants in other chemical families – noradrenergic, serotonergic reuptake inhibitors, bupropion (a dopamine reuptake inhibitor that does not enhance motor function), mirtazapine (a drug that increases noradrenergic and serotonergic transmission) – are also commonly used. Selective monoamine oxidase B (MAO-B) inhibitors approved for treating motor symptoms of PD do not have mood-altering properties unless used at high doses, which render the drugs nonselective. Nonselective MAO inhibitors are relatively contraindicated in PD because of the possibility of hypertensive crisis.

Electroconvulsive therapy has been reported in several small series to be helpful in treating refractory depression in PD [58] and has an added benefit of motor improvement, independent of improved mood.

In general, motor improvement precedes improvement in mood but, unfortunately, does not last. The motor improvement lasts from hours to weeks but not more than that. There are few reports on maintenance electroconvulsive therapy, in which treatments are given once every few weeks, but sustained motor improvement does not seem to be obtained (J. H. Friedman, personal observation).

Psychosocial interventions, including cognitive behavioral therapy, education and psychodrama, have been studied in PD [59] and, although producing improvement, involved small numbers of subjects. Cognitive behavioral therapy is the best studied and has produced results that rival medication. The advantage of psychosocial intervention is the absence of additional medication. The disadvantage is the time and expense.

Fatigue

Fatigue is a common problem in most disorders, both somatic and psychiatric. It is a particularly common problem in PD, affecting about half of the patients seen in specialty clinics around the world, independent of culture [60]. It is a term that has been defined differently in different settings. Physiological fatigue describes an objective, measurable decrease in strength with repeated muscle contractions. This occurs in normal people but occurs more quickly in PD [61] and is improved with levodopa. Central fatigue refers to a feeling or perception that has no identified physiological substrate or measure. It differs from sleepiness, although the term "tired" is often used to describe both fatigue and sleepiness, in that sleepiness is remedied by naps whereas fatigue is improved with rest without sleep. Fatigue in PD patients is, paradoxically, improved with exercise [62]. The subjective sensation of fatigue may be defined as "a sense of tiredness, lack of energy or total body give out" in the Fatigue Assessment Inventory [63], a commonly used instrument for measuring fatigue in several different disorders. Another fatigue questionnaire defined fatigue as a "feeling of abnormal and overwhelming tiredness and lack of energy, distinct both qualitatively and quantitatively from normal tiredness" [62]. Some dictionary definitions define fatigue as a response to work, whereas in medical conditions, fatigue exists before work and prevents a normal exertion. Early fatigue with exercise is generally considered poor endurance. Central fatigue can be categorized into two domains, physical and mental. The physical fatigue refers to a sense of physical exhaustion and low energy that prevents normal levels of physical exertion, whereas mental fatigue refers to cognitive impairments in attempting sustained concentration, as might be experienced after prolonged tasks involving concentration.

Parkinson's disease patients perceive their fatigue as different from what it was pre-morbidly and may use words like "heavy," "drained" and "exhaustion" to describe their condition [62]. One of the central difficulties in understanding fatigue is the confound introduced by sleepiness and other behavioral states. Although some authors [62] report that patients distinguish fatigue from sleepiness, this is not always the case, and many patients report that they suffer from both fatigue and excessive somnolence [64, 65]. However, fatigue occurs in syndromes of depression, anxiety, and apathy or amotivation, all of which are common in PD. There are no known markers to indicate whether fatigue in a patient with anxiety, depression or apathy is part of one syndrome or is distinct.

Fatigue affects 33–70% of PD patients and is more common than in the general population matched for age and gender [66]. In an early study of 100 consecutive PD patients at a movement disorders clinic, 58% rated fatigue as one of their three most disabling symptoms and one-third rated fatigue as their single most disabling symptom [67]. Similar figures from studies around the world support these surprisingly high numbers. In the ELLDOPA (Early versus Later Levodopa in Parkinson Disease) study [9], volunteers for a placebo-controlled trial in early, untreated PD, in which depression and dementia were exclusionary criteria, one-third were found to suffer from fatigue. In a Brazilian study 70% had fatigue; 42% of 461 consecutive Japanese patients were fatigued; 58% of Italian PD patients suffered from fatigue; a British study found that fatigue was the second most common nonmotor symptoms after autonomic dysfunction [60]. The long-term course of fatigue has not been so well studied. The ELLDOPA study found minor improvement on levodopa over a period of under 1 year. A 9-year study reported that initially fatigued patients tended to remain fatigued and that it worsened. Few patients developed fatigue. A Norwegian study found that fatigue became more common with duration and that some patients fell in or out of the fatigued category [65].

Fatigue, counterintuitively, does not correlate with motor severity and, in most but not all studies, has a positive association with depression. Yet fatigue is common in those who do not have depression [68] or excessive sleepiness [69]. It should be noted that some PD patients blame their depression on their fatigue. There is one report associating fatigue with apathy [70].

The pathophysiology of fatigue has not been well studied. One study compared fatigued and nonfatigued PD patients at a single clinic on exercise physiology [71]. The only physiological difference detected was a reduction in oxygen consumption during maximal exercise, indicating a reduced ability to exercise as hard. This correlated with self-report of fewer activities during the preceding week. A single study that reported abnormal serotonin binding in fatigued patients [72] requires confirmation. Serotonin reuptake inhibitors have not been reported to be helpful in treating fatigue in PD. It is likely that fatigue occurs for numerous reasons in PD, some psychological, with patients feeling fatigue as a mechanism for being unable to perform up to expectations, while other experience fatigue as a distinct physiological problem analogous to tremor or rigidity, and others experiencing fatigue as part of other behavioral syndromes such as depression, anxiety or sleep disorders. It is likely that their underlying mechanisms are different and that their treatments will be different as well. It should be noted that even when fatigue is present in the general, non-PD, depressed population, it often persists after the affective component of depression resolves. Thus, even in the non-PD population, fatigue often does not respond to antidepressants.

There are few data on treating fatigue. Certainly in patients who are also depressed or anxious, they should be treated with the hope that fatigue will also improve, but there are no data to support this hypothesis. Trials of modafinil for treating fatigue have not been positive, even when sleepiness improved. The only positive treatment trial was a double-blind, placebo-controlled trial of methylphenidate 15 mg three times daily involving 36 PD patients [73]. The two measures of fatigue used for ratings both showed benefit. There was no impact on motor symptoms and the side effects were very similar in the control and active arms. There is no reason, a priori, to believe that the benefit of methylphenidate is specific to this drug and not a class effect of stimulant medications. Amphetamine has been tried as a treatment for PD motor symptoms based on its pharmacological property of increasing catecholamine secretion. Stimulants have been used in similarly low doses by geriatric psychiatrists to enhance mood in non-PD patients. Thus, stimulants may be of value for fatigue, daytime somnolence and depression. The concerns are increased anxiety, restlessness, increased hypertension, aggravation of cardiac ischemia and weight loss due to loss of appetite.

Other disorders and therapeutic considerations

Rare psychiatric symptoms emerge from time to time in PD patients, usually with some degree of dementia. With rare syndromes, it is impossible to determine, without autopsy, whether an additional process such as concomitant Alzheimer's disease or vascular disease is present. Emotional incontinence is an occasional feature of PD, usually with patients crying rather than laughing. Delusional mis-identification syndromes are also rarely seen with patients, thinking that their spouse has been replaced by another lookalike, or that their home is not their real home but an exact copy. Patients may think they are dead. It is unclear how well these respond to either antidementia or antipsychotic drugs. Reducing psychoactive medications, including the anti-PD medications, is probably the best option, as these patients are almost always suffering from dementia.

Electroconvulsive therapy is mentioned briefly above as a potential treatment for refractory major depression in PD. However, there have been no controlled trials of its effects on PD patients, although many isolated case reports and small series have been reported. Electroconvulsive therapy has been reported to improve a wide spectrum of severe psychiatric problems in PD that were refractory to standard treatment, including anxiety, obsessive-compulsive disorder and psychosis, and often improving motor dysfunction as well. Electroconvulsive therapy induces a post-seizure delirium that usually lasts minutes to hours but may last for days, the latter making it unusable. When the electroconvulsive therapy improves the acute psychiatric problem, standard medication is then employed. There are few data on "maintenance electroconvulsive therapy," which is a delivery system in which one shock is induced every few weeks, rather than the standard treatment of two to three seizures per week.

Conclusions

Behavioral problems, even when excluding sleep disorders and cognitive dysfunction, are common in PD and are major determinants of quality of life. Apathy and psychosis probably worsen over time in relationship to the progression of dementia. Fatigue, depression and anxiety, on the other hand, do not necessarily worsen with duration of disease, suggesting that these syndromes may not correlate with brain cell loss.

The behavioral problems in PD dementia are identical to those seen in dementia with Lewy bodies, and many argue that these two conditions are, in fact, identical except in the order of the development of the impairments. Dementia with Lewy bodies begins with dementia and behavioral changes, with the motor features of parkinsonism developing later, whereas PD dementia begins with motor symptoms (criteria for the diagnosis of PD specifically makes dementia at the time of diagnosis exclusionary) and dementia develops later.

References

1. Weintraub D, Burn D. Parkinson's disease: the quintessential neuropsychiatric disorder. *Mov Disord* 2011; **26**: 1022–31.
2. Muller B, Assus J, Herlofson K, Larsen JP, Tysnes OB. Importance of motor vs non-motor symptoms for health-related quality of life in early Parkinson's disease. *Park Rel Disord* 2013; **19**: 1027–32.
3. Rana AQ, Athar A, Owlia A, et al. Impact of ethnicity on non-motor symptoms of Parkinson's disease. *J Park Dis* 2012; **2**: 281–5.
4. Aarsland D, Larsen JP, Tanberg E, Laake K. Predictors of nursing home placement in Parkinson's disease: a population-based, prospective study. *J Am Ger Soc* 2000; **48**: 938–42.
5. American Psychiatric Association. *Diagnostic and Statistical Manual of Mental Disorders, 4th edn, Text Revision*. Washington, DC: American Psychiatric Association Press, 1994.
6. Leentjens AF, Dujardin K, Marsh L, et al. Anxiety and motor fluctuations in Parkinson's disease: a cross sectional observational study. *Park Rel Disord* 2012; **18**: 1084–8.
7. Poletti M, Bonuccelli U. Personality traits in patients with Parkinson's disease: assessment and clinical implications. *J Neurol* 2012; **259**: 1029–38.
8. Noyce AJ, Bestwick JP, Silveira-Moriyama L, et al. Meta-analysis of early non-motor symptoms and risk factors for Parkinson's disease. *Ann Neurol* 2012; **72**: 893–901.
9. Schifitto G, Friedman JH, Oakes D, et al. Fatigue in levodopa-naive subjects with Parkinson's disease. *Neurology* 2008; **71**: 481–5.
10. Jeliffe SE. The parkinsonian body posture: some considerations on unconscious hostility. *Psychoanal Rev* 1940; **27**: 467–79.
11. Sands I. The type of personality susceptible to Parkinson's disease. *J Mt Sinai Hosp* 1942; **9**: 792–4.
12. Poewe W, Karamat E, Kemmler GW, Gerstenbrand F. The premorbid personality of patients with Parkinson's disease: a comparative study with healthy controls and patients with essential tremor. *Adv Neurol* 1990; **53**: 339–42.
13. Glosser G, Clark C, Freundlich B, et al. A controlled investigation of current and premorbid personality: characteristics of Parkinson's disease patients. *Mov Disord* 1995; **19**: 201–6.
14. Hubble JP, Venkatesh R, Hassanein RE, Gray C, Koller WC. Personality and depression in Parkinson's disease. *J Ner Ment Dis* 1993; **181**: 657–62.
15. Bower JH, Grossardt BR, Maraganore DM, et al. Anxious personality predicts an increased risk of Parkinson's disease. *Mov Disord* 2010; **25**: 2105–13.
16. Arabia G, Grossardt BR, Colligan RC, et al. Novelty seeking and introversion do not predict the long-term risk of Parkinson disease. *Neurology* 2010; **75**: 349–57.
17. Vieregge P, Hagenah J, Heberlein I, Klein C, Ludin HP. Parkinson's disease in twins: a follow up study. *Neurology* 1999; **53**: 566–72.
18. Starkstein SE. Apathy in Parkinson's disease: diagnostic and etiological dilemmas. *Mov Disord* 2012; **27**: 174–8.
19. Chase TN Apathy in neuropsychiatric diseases: diagnosis, pathophysiology and treatment. *Neurotox Res* 2011; **19**: 266–78.
20. Robert P, Onyike CU, Leentjens AF, et al. Proposed diagnostic criteria for apathy in Alzheimer's disease and other neuropsychiatric disorders. *Eur Psychiatry* 2009; **24**: 98–104.
21. Marin RS. Apathy: a neuropsychiatric syndrome. *J Neuropsychiatry Clin Neurosci* 1991; **3**: 243–54.
22. Drijgers RL, Dujardin K, Reijnders JS, Defebvre L, Leentjens AF. Validation of diagnostic criteria for apathy in Parkinson's disease. *Parkinson Rel Disord* 2010; **16**: 656–60.
23. Leentjens AF, Dujardin K, Marsh, L, et al. Anxiety rating scales in Parkinson's disease: critique and recomendations. *Mov Disord* 2008; **23**: 2105–25.
24. Kirsch-Darrow L, Fernandez HF, et al. Dissociating apathy and depression in Parkinson disease. *Neurology* 2006; **67**: 33–8.
25. Starkstein S, Merello M, Jorge R, et al. The syndromal validity and nosological position of apathy in Parkinson's disease. *Mov Disord* 2009; **15**: 1211–16.
26. Dujardin K, Sockeel P, Devos D, et al. Characteristics of apathy in Parkinson's disease. *Mov Disord* 2007; **22**: 778–84.
27. Pedersen KF, Larsen JP, Alves G, Aarsland D. Prevalence and clinical correlates of apathy in Parkinson's disease: a community-based study. *Park Rel Disord* 2009; **15**: 295–9.

28. Starkstein S, Leentjens AF. The nosological position of apathy in clinical practice. *J Neurol Neurosurg Psychiatry* 2008; **79**: 1088–92.
29. Nirenberg MJ. Dopamine agonist withdrawal syndrome: implications for patient care. *Drugs Aging* 2013; **30**: 587–92.
30. Leentjens AF, Dujardin K, Marsh L, et al. Anxiety rating scales in Parkinson's disease: a validation study of the Hamilton anxiety rating scale, the Beck anxiety inventory and the Hospital anxiety and depression rating scale. *Mov Disord* 2011; **26**: 407–15.
31. Dissanayaka NAD, Selbach A, Matheson S, et al. Anxiety disorders in Parkinson's disease: prevalence and risk factors. *Mov Disord* 2010; **25**: 838–45.
32. Shulman LM, Taback RL, Rabinstein AA, Weiner WJ. Non-recognition of depression and other non-motor symptoms in Parkinson's disease. *Park Rel Disord* 2002; **8**: 193–7.
33. Liu AA, Boxham CE, Klufas MA, et al. Clinical predictors of frequent patient telephone calls in Parkinson's disease. *Park Rel Disord* 2011; **17**: 95–9.
34. American Psychiatric Association. *Diagnostic and Statistical Manual V*. Washington, DC: American Psychiatric Press, 2013.
35. Walsh K, Bennet G. Parkinson's disease and anxiety. *Postgrad Med* 2001; **7**: 89–93.
36. Ponton GM, Williams JR, Anderson DE, et al. Prevalence of anxiety disorders and anxiety subtypes in patients with Parkinson's disease. *Mov Disord* 2009; **24**: 1333–8.
37. Fleminger S. Left sided Parkinson's disease is associated with greater anxiety and depression. *Psychol Med* 1991; **21**: 629–38.
38. Leentjens AF, Dujardin K, Marsh L, et al. Anxiety and motor fluctuations in Parkinson's disease: a cross sectional observational study. *Park Rel Disord* 2012; **18**: 1084–8.
39. Dotchin CL, Jusabani A, Walker RW. Non-motor symptoms in a prevalent population with Parkinson's disease in Tanzania. *Park Rel Disord* 2009; **15**: 457–60.
40. Friedman JH. Parkinson's disease psychosis: Update. *Behav Neurol* 2013; **27**: 469–77.
41. Zhu K, van Hilten JJ, Putter H, Marinus J. Risk factors for hallucinations in Parkinson's disease: results from a large prospective cohort study. *Mov Disord* 2013; **28**: 755–62.
42. Ravina B, Marder K, Fernandez HH, et al. Diagnostic criteria for psychosis in Parkinson's disease: report of an NINDS, NIMH work group. *Mov Disord* 2007; **22**: 1061–8.
43. Chou KL, Messing S, Oakes D, et al. Drug-induced psychosis in Parkinson's disease: phenomenology and correlations among psychiatric rating scales. *Clin Neuropharm* 2005; **28**: 215–9.
44. Yoritaka A, Shimo Y, Takanashi M, et al. Motor and non-motor symptoms of 1453 patients with Parkinson's disease: Prevalence and risks. *Park Rel Disord* 2013; **19**: 725–31.
45. Seppi K, Weintraub D, Coelho M, et al. The Movement Disorder Society Evidence-Based Medicine Review Update: treatments for the non-motor symptoms of Parkinson's disease. *Mov Disord* 2011; (Suppl. 3): S42–80.
46. Friedman JH. Pimavanserin in Parkinson's disease psychosis. *Expert Opin Pharmacother* 2013; **14**: 1969–75.
47. Chen JJ, Marsh L. Depression in Parkinson's disease: identification and management. *Pharmacotherapy* 2013; **33**: 972–83.
48. Rocha FL, Murad MGR, Stumpf BP, Hara C, Fuzikawa C. Antidepressants for depression in Parkinson's disease: systematic review and meta-analysis. *J Psychopharmacol* 2013; **27**: 417–23.
49. Reijnders JS, Ehrt U, Weber WE, Aarsland D, Leentjens AF. A systematic review of prevalence studies of depression in Parkinson's disease. *Mov Disord* 2008; **23**: 183–9.
50. Hughes TA, Ross HF, Mindham RH, Spokes EG. Mortality in Parkinson's disease and its association with dementia and depression. *Acta Neurol Scand* 2004; **110**: 118–23.
51. Ravina B, Camicioli R, Como PG, et al. The impact of depressive symptoms in early Parkinson disease. *Neurology* 2007; **69**: 342–7.
52. Schrag A, Hovris A, Morley D, Quinn N, Jahanshahi M. Caregiver burden in Parkinson's disease is closely associated with psychiatric symptoms, falls and disability. *Park Rel Dsord* 2005; **12**: 35–41.
53. Global Parkinson's Disease Survey Steering Committee. Factors impacting on quality of life in Parkinson's disease: results from an international survey. *Mov Disord* 2002; **17**: 60–7.
54. Ravina B, Elm J, Camicioli R, et al. The course of depressive symptoms in early Parkinson's disease. *Mov Disord* 2009; **24**: 1306–11.
55. Weintraub D, Morales KH, Moberg PJ, et al. Antidepressant studies in Parkinson's disease: a review and meta-analysis. *Mov Disord* 2005; **20**: 1161–9.
56. Richard IH, McDermott MP, Kurlan R, et al. A randomized, double-blind, placebo-controlled trial of antidepressants in Parkinson disease. *Neurology* 2012; **78**: 1229–36.
57. Barone P, Poewe W, Albrecht S, et al. Pramipexole for the treatment of depressive symptoms in patients with Parkinson's disease: a randomized double blind placebo controlled trial. *Lancet Neurol* 2010; **9**: 573–80.

58. Moellentine C, Rummans T, Ahlskog JE, *et al.* Effectiveness of ECT in patients with parkinsonism. *J Neuropsychiatr Clin Neurosci* 1998; **10**: 187–93.

59. Yang S, Sajatovic M, Walter BL. Psychosocial interventions for depression and anxiety in Parkinson's disease. *J Geratr Psychiatr Neurol* 2012; **25**: 113–21.

60. Friedman JH, Abrantes A, Sweet LH. Fatigue in Parkinson's disease. *Exp Opin Pharmacother* 2011; **12**: 1999–2007.

61. Lou JS, Kearns G, Benice T, *et al.* Levodopa improves physical fatigue in Parinson's disease: a double-blind placebo-controlled study. *Mov Disord* 2003; **18**: 1108–14.

62. Brown RG, Dittner A, Findley L, Wessely SC. The Parkinson fatigue scale. *Parkinson Rel Disord* 2005; **11**: 49–55.

63. Krupp LB, LaRocca NG, Muir-Nash J, Steinberg AD. The fatigue severity scale. Application to patients with multiple sclerosis and systemic lupus erythematosus. *Arch Neurol* 1989; **46**: 1121–3.

64. Valko PO, Waldvogel D, Weller M, *et al.* Fatigue and excessive daytime sleepiness in idiopathic Parkinson's disease differently correlate with motor symptoms, depression and dopaminergic treatment. *Eur J Neurol* 2010; **17**: 1428–36.

65. Alves G, Wentzel-Larsen T, Larsen JP. Is fatigue an independent and persistent symptom in patients with Parkinson's disease? *Neurol* 2004; **63**: 1908–11.

66. Friedman JH, Brown RG, Comella C, *et al.* Fatigue in Parkinson's disease: a review. *Mov Disord* 2007; **22**: 297–308.

67. Friedman J, Friedman H. Fatigue in Parkinson's disease. *Neurol* 1993; **43**: 2016–8.

68. Van Hilten JJ, Weggeman M, van der Velde EA, *et al.* Sleep, excessive daytime sleepiness and fatigue in Parkinson's disease. *J Neural Transm Park Dis Dement Secct* 1993; **5**: 235–44.

69. Karlsen K, Larsen JP, Tandberg E, Jørgensen K. Fatigue in patients with Parkinson's disease. *Mov Disord* 1999; **14**: 237–41.

70. Saez-Francas N, Hernandez-Vera J, Corominos Roso M, Alegre Martín J, Casas Brugué M. The association of apathy with central fatigue in patients with Parkinson's disease. *Behav Neurosci* 2013; **127**: 237–44.

71. Garber CE, Friedman JH. Effects of fatigue on physical activity and function in patients with Parkinson's disease. *Neurology* 2003; **60**: 1119–24.

72. Pavese N, Metta V, Bose SK, Chaudhuri KR, Brooks DJ. Fatigue in Parkinson's disease is linked to striatal and limbic serotonergic dysfunction. *Brain* 2010; **133**: 3434–43.

73. Mendonca DA, Menezes K, Jog MS. Methylphenidate improve fatigue scores in Parkinson's disease: a randomized controlled trial. *Mov Disord* 2007; **22**: 2070–6.

Chapter 14

Management of treatment-related behavioral disturbances in Parkinson's disease

Mayur Pandya, Dimitrios A. Nacopoulos and Naveed Khokhar

Introduction

Primum non nocere meaning "first, do no harm" is a fundamental ethical basis of medical practice. As conscientious physicians, we strive to provide our patients with safe and effective treatments free of permanent or even transient adverse effects. The management of Parkinson's disease (PD) may be complicated by unwanted behavioral effects of treatment with dopamine replacement therapy (DRT) and/or neurosurgery [1]. The decision to reduce or alter treatment may not always be a welcome one by the patient with PD for fear of losing motor benefits gained by the intervention. These psychiatric and behavioral disturbances pose significant morbidity and negatively impact the quality of life for patients with PD, as well as contributing to higher caregiver burden [2].

The treatment of PD has greatly advanced since George Cotzias' discovery of levodopa's seemingly miraculous benefits in PD. Since this discovery, dopamine (and, in turn, dopamine replacement) has naturally been at the center of the treatment approach. With time and further investigation, it is becoming clearer that nondopaminergic neurotransmitter systems and pathways may be vitally important in the pathogenesis of PD, particularly with regard to the production of psychiatric and behavioral manifestations [3]. This has been supported by pathological evidence of serotonin and norepinephrine degeneration in PD [1]. It has been suggested that a mesocorticolimbic variant of PD may exist that renders some patients more susceptible to adverse psychiatric and behavioral effects than others [4]. These disturbances are likely the effect of DRT exposure in the setting of frontal-subcortical dysfunction, coexisting conditions, environmental catalysts and individual personal factors (Figure 14.1). The need for vigilance in detecting these emerging behaviors is therefore essential.

Unfamiliarity with the delicate nuances of DRT can predispose patients to dramatic motor and nonmotor consequences when doses are purposefully or inadvertently adjusted. The extensive therapeutic options, sometimes in multiple delivery preparations, added to the seemingly infinite number of combinations, can create confusion for even the best medical providers. The options for management of motor symptoms in PD include: (i) levodopa (L-DOPA): in combination with carbidopa (available as standard-release [with or without entacapone] or controlled-release preparation, orally disintegrating tablet and intestinal gel); (ii) dopamine agonists: nonergot- and ergot-derivative tablets, transdermal patch and subcutaneous injection; (iii) catechol-O-methyltransferase (COMT) inhibitors; (iv) monoamine oxide type B (MAO-B) inhibitors: standard-release tablet, orally disintegrating tablet and transdermal patch; (v) glutamate antagonists; (vi) anticholinergics; and (vii) neurosurgical interventions (such as deep-brain stimulation [DBS], pallidotomy and thalamotomy).

Recommendations for effective treatments in managing treatment-related behavioral disturbances have lagged due to an unclear understanding of pathophysiology, the use of non-PD rating scales in many studies and a void of large, randomly controlled trials [5]. This chapter will focus on the discussion of four well-recognized behavioral manifestations that may arise directly from DRT in PD: (i) psychosis; (ii) impulse control disorders; (iii) dopamine dysregulation syndrome; and (iv) dopamine agonist withdrawal syndrome. The chapter will conclude with a review of behavioral effects that have been reported in the context of DBS surgery and programming.

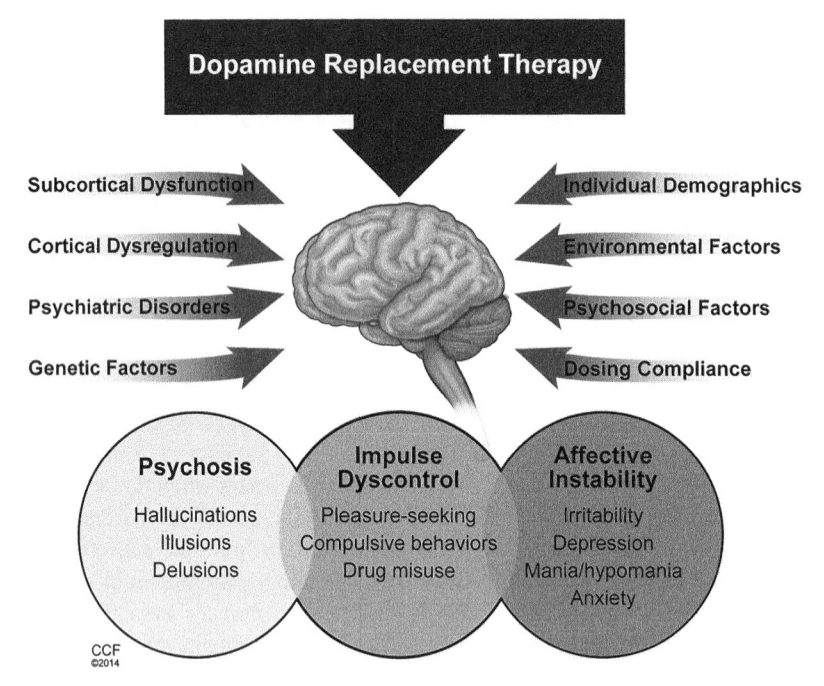

Figure 14.1 Outline of dopamine replacement therapy.
Reprinted with permission, Cleveland Clinic Center for Medical Art and Photography, 2014. All Rights Reserved.

Psychosis

Psychosis, as described in the previous chapter, is a departure from reality, is an unfortunate yet all too common side effect of PD management. Psychosis can be intrinsic to PD or drug induced, and therefore is discussed twice in this book. The presence of psychosis in those receiving PD treatment ranges from 5 to 30% [6]. Psychosis in PD may manifest as a range of perceptual disturbances and abnormal thought content. Hallucinations in PD most frequently present as visual hallucinations but may also present as auditory, olfactory, tactile or gustatory disturbances. Patients describe the presence of very vivid animals or people, and often retain insight into the artificial nature of these hallucinations, especially early in the disease process. Patients are typically not threatened by the hallucinations, in contrast to schizophrenia. In fact, unless educated proactively, patients may not volunteer this information out of embarrassment. They may also worry that divulging this information may lead to treatment being withheld or discontinued. Delusions, defined as fixed false beliefs, may surface and range from bizarre to subtle. False accusations by patients of spousal infidelity are frequently seen in PD and create significant distress for spouses and families.

Delusions may also be persecutory or somatic in nature. Illusions, the incorrect interpretation of an actual sensory stimulus, may also be reported in PD. Illusions in PD have been classified as "minor hallucinations" [7]. Other minor hallucinations may include reports of brief hallucinations in the peripheral vision or a feeling of someone or something nearby (without persecutory ideation). Because of the difficulties in capturing minor hallucinations that are mild and brief, the true prevalence of psychosis in PD has been difficult to quantify. A recent community-based study approximated that a quarter of nondemented patients with PD likely experience psychosis, with half of these experiences manifesting as minor hallucinations [8]. To improve detection and reporting accuracy, the National Institute of Neurological Disease and Stroke (NINDS)/ National Institute of Mental Health (NIMH) workgroup recently proposed a criterion set for psychosis in PD that encompasses any of the above manifestations of psychosis occurring for greater than 1 month [7]. Reported predictors of psychosis in PD include longer disease duration, visual dysfunction, higher use of DRT (particularly dopamine agonists), presence of rapid eye movement (REM) sleep behaviors, and cognitive dysfunction [6].

Disturbance in mesocorticolimbic dopaminergic neurotransmission has historically been thought to be largely responsible for psychosis in PD. This association in PD was generated primarily from the observation that dopamine replacement therapy has been associated with the development of psychosis, while dopamine antagonists have demonstrated efficacy in reducing psychotic phenomena in PD. The precise mechanism, however, has been poorly understood, as not all patients with PD develop psychosis in response to DRT. Recent evidence has suggested the contribution of other neurotransmitters in the generation of psychosis in PD. Psychosis in PD is often reported as a predictor of dementia in PD. As a result, acetylcholine deficiency has been implicated based on overlapping clinical features with Alzheimer's disease and evidence of degeneration of the nucleus basalis of Meynert in PD [9]. Moreover, cholinesterase inhibitors, whose mechanism is aimed at limiting the breakdown of acetylcholine, have shown some promise in the treatment of mild psychosis in PD [10], while anticholinergic agents are notorious for triggering hallucinations and altered mental states. Serotonin imbalance is another consideration in the pathophysiology of psychosis. Subtypes of serotonin receptors, particularly 5-HT2A, have been implicated in the generation of psychosis based on: (i) modulation of dopamine neurons in the ventral tegmental area by hyperstimulation of 5-HT2A [9]; (ii) awareness of agents that are known to act via 5-HT2A and produce psychosis, such as LSD (lysergic acid diethylamide); and (iii) evidence of atypical antipsychotics (which antagonize 5-HT2A) to successfully treat psychosis [11]. Particularly striking and supportive of 5-HT2A's prominent involvement in PD psychosis is the relatively low doses of atypical antipsychotics that can effectively treat psychotic phenomena in PD. These doses are often 10-fold lower compared with primary psychotic disorders [5], potentially suggesting a predominant serotonergic mechanism in PD. Studies examining visual hallucinations in PD have found clustering of 5-HT2A alterations in the temporal cortex and ventral visual pathway of patients with PD experiencing visual hallucinations, further supporting the contribution of serotonin to psychosis in PD [12].

The balancing act of providing optimal motor control without triggering psychosis is a common, yet sometimes challenging, dilemma in PD management. On the one hand, patients may require and/or request DRT to manage deteriorating motor symptoms while on the other hand experiencing vivid hallucinations that may predispose them to fear, confusion and/or falls. Prior to discontinuation of DRT, the first step in evaluating a patient with psychosis is to conduct a thorough evaluation to rule out any acute medical disturbances, such as infection, cerebrovascular event, respiratory insufficiency and/or metabolic derangements, which may predispose to confusion or delirium [13]. Delirium may differ from treatment-related psychosis in PD due to the presence of altered sensorium characterized by waxing and waning leves of consciousness, greater disorientation and no apparent association with DRT timing or dosing. Even in the setting of clear DRT-related psychosis, these should be investigated, since the underlying disturbance may have increased susceptibility to psychosis. Resolution of a systemic disturbance in some cases may then allow the patient to better tolerate DRT. Because of the frequent reports of hallucinations during the evening and upon awakening during the night (when visual acuity is lessened), the differential diagnosis should include consideration for Charles Bonnet syndrome, REM sleep behavior disorder, hypnogogic and hypnopompic hallucinations, and dementia [5]. Finally, evaluation of environmental, or extrinsic, factors should not be underestimated. In the setting of intrinsic vulnerabilities, patients may be prone to experience DRT-related psychosis in environments with ambiguous noise and poor lighting, particular if the setting is new or unfamiliar. Psychological support may confer some augmenting benefit for those with mild psychosis where insight is retained, but this has not been well studied.

Once the evaluation for metabolic abnormalities, coexisting medical and psychiatric conditions and environmental factors has not yielded any obvious contributing factors, the patient's PD medication regimen should be closely reviewed to eliminate any nonessential agents. Patients may, on occasion, still be taking medications that derive minimal motor benefit but contribute significantly to the emergence of psychosis. Dose reduction and discontinuation of these higher-risk agents (in the order anticholinergic agents, amantadine dopamine agonists and then COMT inhibitors, high risk to low risk) in a stepwise fashion [13] may be prudent as side effects multiply with increasing numbers of drugs [2]. Patients may ultimately be best managed with levodopa therapy alone.

Patients with significant or functionally disabling psychosis may require the addition of a psychotropic agent in order to treat DRT-related psychosis. Clozapine has demonstrated the best efficacy in PD psychosis [14] but remains grossly underutilized due to the burden of use (e.g. patient registry, coordination with pharmacy, frequent laboratory visits, side effects, warnings). Some patients may also express reservation due to knowledge of its reserved use in chronic or "severe" schizophrenia. Quetiapine is prescribed more frequently for PD psychosis due to ease of use, augmenting benefits (i.e. nighttime sedation) and favorable extrapyramidal risk profile. One retrospective study in a Veterans Affairs population found that quetiapine was prescribed in 66% of those with PD psychosis [15]. Unfortunately, there has been insufficient evidence in randomized controlled trials to recommend quetiapine in the treatment of psychosis in PD [14]. All other atypical antipsychotics have not demonstrated a clear benefit in controlled trials and are more likely to worsen motor symptoms in PD. Typical or conventional dopamine antagonists (such as haloperidol) should be avoided altogether due to the strong propensity to worsen parkinsonism. Pimavanserin, a selective 5-HT2A inverse agonist with minimal to no dopaminergic effects, is gaining attention. Its promise has been further strengthened by a recent successful randomized, placebo-controlled phase 3 trial in PD psychosis [16].

Impulse control disorders

According to the *Diagnostic and Statistical Manual of Mental Disorders, 4th Edn, Text Revision* (DSM-IV-TR), the category of impulse control disorders (ICDs) was characterized by a failure to resist an impulse, drive or temptation to perform an act that is harmful to the person or to others, with increased tension or arousal preceding the act, and pleasure or relief upon completing the act [17]. Pleasure-seeking impulse control behaviors seen in PD include pathological gambling, compulsive sexual behavior, compulsive buying, and compulsive or binge eating [18]. Impulse dyscontrol in PD commonly arises from DRT and may range from these pleasure-seeking behaviors to less purposeful behaviors, such as "punding" (compulsive fascination with and performance of repetitive, mechanical tasks, such as assembling and disassembling objects, collecting or sorting) or "walkabout" (unnecessary and aimless wandering). Patients rarely endorse intrusive egodystonic thoughts as a reason for their behavior, as typically seen in obsessive-compulsive disorder, and may not always have a conscious explanation for their actions. Impulse control disorders may occasionally present with elevated or expansive mood. Presence of clear hypomania and mania should prompt suspicion for dopamine dysregulation syndrome, or in some cases may also exist as its own distinct DRT-related entity [19]. The inconsistent presence of pleasurable (vs nonpleasurable) urges or drive may suggest the potential for differing mechanisms among the ICDs [20]. In the most recent edition of DSM-V [21], the simple category of ICDs has now been eliminated. Instead the prior ICDs have been reclassified into several different categories, comprising: (i) disruptive, impulse control and conduct disorders; (ii) obsessive-compulsive and related disorders (i.e. hoarding disorder); and (iii) substance-related and addictive disorders (i.e. gambling disorder). This presumably better reflects the heterogeneity in impulsive–compulsive conditions.

Similar to non-PD patients, pathological gambling may present in a variety of forms, including irresistible urges to purchase scratch-off tickets, participate in online gambling games or play slot machines at the casino. Gambling on items with delayed gratification (i.e. sports betting) is relatively uncommon. Hypersexuality presents as a maladaptive preoccupation with sex, ranging from compulsive masturbation and viewing of pornography to excessive requests for sex from a partner, extramarital affairs and habitual promiscuity. Compulsive shopping manifests as an intense preoccupation with buying or shopping above what can be afforded and/or is necessary. Compulsive or binge eating commonly includes cravings for sweets. Punding may represent its own distinct entity based on the purposeless nature. In some cases, punding may be referred to as "hobbyism" based on the intensification of an individual's already existing personal, professional and recreational interests [22]. Impulse control disorders and punding may also arise in the setting of excessive and/or compulsive use of DRT, referred to as dopamine dysregulation syndrome. Diagnostic criteria, including duration and functional impairment, have been proposed for each of these ICDs to improve detection and reporting [20], although it is possible to overlook subsyndromal cases that may still cause distress to patients and caregivers [23].

Observational studies have indicated that ICDs may occur at a higher frequency in PD than in the general population. An early retrospective database review identified a link between pathological gambling and dopamine agonists (DAs) in PD [24]. The largest epidemiological study (over 3000 patients) demonstrated that an ICD was identified in 13.6% of PD patients, and this was subdivided into gambling (5%), sexual behavior (3.5%), compulsive buying (5.7%) and binge-eating disorder (4.3%), with 4.9% of patients having two or more ICDs [25]. Dopamine agonists were strongly linked to an increased risk of ICDs in this cross-sectional study, and ICDs also appeared to be more frequent in men and associated with a greater mean daily DA dosage. Other independent variables associated are levodopa use, living in the USA, younger age, being unmarried, current cigarette smoking and a family history of gambling problems [25]. The degree of risk of ICDs among different DAs is believed to be similar, although recent evidence suggests a potential for lower risk with transdermal DA preparations [26].

Impulse control disorders involve alterations in neurotransmission and neural circuitry, particularly in reward pathways within the mesocorticolimbic pathways [18]. Dopamine agonists have a higher ratio of D3:D2 and D3:D1 striatal activation. D3 receptors are concentrated in limbic structures, and stimulation contributes to psychiatric and behavioral effects, compared with D1 and D2 receptors within the dorsal striatum [27]. The regions that appear most implicated include the ventromedial and orbitofrontal regions of the prefrontal cortex, and structures of the limbic system including the ventral striatum and amygdala [28]. These structures, particularly the nucleus accumbens within the ventral striatum, are associated with modulating motivated behaviors underlying engagement in risky behaviors, while the dorsal striatum is involved in motor habits [28]. Altered ventral striatum activation and dopamine transporter density, particularly in the right striatum, have been demonstrated in patients with ICD in PD [29, 30]. Moreover, patients receiving DRT, particularly DAs, are more sensitive to positive reinforcement, leading to impaired ability to avoid negative outcomes [18].

Practitioners should routinely obtain a careful history of preexisting symptoms or conditions (such as psychiatric or substance abuse) prior to starting DRT, most notably DA therapy. In addition, clinicians should educate patients on the risks prior to treatment, while monitoring for ICD behaviors during follow-up visits. Patients may withhold reporting these behaviors due to uncertainty about their relationship to DRT or embarrassment. There are no widely accepted or routinely utilized ICD screening instruments in PD. Although there are several general instruments available to screen for impulsivity (i.e. Minnesota Impulsive Disorders Interview), these instruments do not comprehensively screen for the spectrum of ICDs in PD. The Questionnaire for Impulsive–Compulsive Disorders in Parkinson's Disease – Rating Scale (QUIP-RS) may therefore be considered based on its intent for this purpose. The QUIP-RS is a rating scale designed to assist in the diagnosis and severity measurement of ICDs and related disorders in PD [31]. Routine use of this instrument may potentially serve a dual role: (i) to inform patients of the potential behaviors that may arise during the course of treatment (better vigilance); and (ii) to normalize the behaviors as a product of treatment when they do occur (better reporting).

Upon the discovery of an emerging or active ICD, patients should first be evaluated for any immediate safety concerns. Spouses and families may need to be alerted to damaging or serious consequences of the ICD behaviors, such as financial or sexual indiscretion that can quickly escalate. Management may also involve referral for inpatient psychiatric management if the behaviors cannot be de-escalated, or an acute threat to self or others is present. Ultimately, the management of an ICD in PD will entail an alteration in DRT. Studies have demonstrated recovery or improvement with discontinuing or significantly reducing DA treatment [32]. Discontinuation of DAs should be done gradually to minimize the risk of withdrawal symptoms. It may be necessary to implement additional specific strategies, such as preventing access to bank accounts or credit cards, while DRT is being lowered. Upon discontinuation of DAs, additional supplementation of DRT in the form of levodopa may be necessary to maintain motoric stability. Caution should be maintained for triggering compulsive behavior, particularly if higher doses of levodopa are needed. Intestinal levodopa infusion may potentially be a safer consideration [33]. The use of DBS, particularly subthalamic nucleus (STN)-DBS, may be a potential intervention due to the ability to reduce DRT postoperatively. These options are considered in the following three sections. Lastly, the utility of certain psychotropic agents, such as atypical antipsychotics and mood stabilizers, in alleviating impulsivity has been reported but not yet proven for use in treating ICDs [14].

Dopamine dysregulation syndrome

Dopamine dysregulation syndrome (DDS) refers to a severe behavioral condition that arises as a result of compulsive use of DRT in PD, commonly manifesting as hoarding, deceit, impulsivity, impatience, manipulation, aggression and poor insight [34]. As PD progresses, there is a need to escalate doses of DRT to gain better control of motor symptoms. A subset of predisposed patients may increase doses of DRT in excess of what is necessary for symptomatic control. Patients will often engage in escalation of DRT despite obvious disabling psychiatric and/or motoric consequences (i.e. dyskinesias). The compulsive aspects of DDS share some overlap with ICDs but appear to be a separate entity, driven by negative reinforcement, habit formation and/or incentive sensitization [34]. As a result, patients with DDS are motivated by a pathological "wanting" for DRT, rather than a "liking," similar to proposed addiction models [35]. Surreptitious use of DRT may therefore be undertaken to avoid the negative "off" effects (dysphoria) more so than to achieve euphoria or pleasure from "on" states. The potential for different subtypes (pleasure seeking versus dysphoria avoiding) has been suggested, but the exact pathophysiology still remains unclear [23]. Dramatic affective cycling and thought disturbances (such as hypomania, mania and psychosis) may be part of the clinical presentation. Dopamine dysregulation syndrome has synonymously been referred to as "hedonistic homeostatic dysregulation" in order to highlight the desperate, pathological, compulsive and behavioral disturbances of this condition [36].

Proposed diagnostic criteria for DDS include: (i) clinical diagnosis of levodopa-responsive PD; (ii) a need for increasing DRT in excess of what is necessary; (iii) pathological use despite psychiatric and motoric consequences; (iv) functional impairment; and (v) observed dopaminergic withdrawal state with dose reduction [36]. The exact prevalence of DDS is not well defined due to its overlap with ICD, limited reporting and lack of prospective studies but appears to be in the range of 4% [36]. There appears to be a higher association with levodopa and other short-acting DAs, such as apomorphine, suggesting that repeated pulsatile stimulation of shorter-acting oral agents may contribute to the emergence of DDS. Associated factors that have been reported include previous drug abuse, higher-sensation-seeking personalities, depression and creative professional backgrounds [34]. A recent retrospective longitudinal population-based cohort study identified 35 cases of DDS over a 6-year period of which 91% were associated with compulsive levodopa use and 9% due to DA addiction [37]. Patients with DDS had younger PD onset and more severe motor fluctuations, and DDS was also more likely to be associated with a history of depression, a family history of PD, and personal or family history of drug use.

Similar to ICD in PD, there are alterations in dopamine neurotransmission within limbic circuits during DDS [38], potentially representing a behavioral counterpart to levodopa-induced dyskinesias [39].

There is currently no evidence-based treatment for DDS, but the approach must be aimed at reducing the dopaminergic burden. All rescue or taken-as-needed DRT should be discontinued. This, however, can be difficult due to resistance from the patient with clear "dependency" for the DRT regimen. Similar to ICD, management of medication adjustment must be done with caution, as there may be increased anxiety or depression as doses are adjusted or decreased. Insight may be poor and assistance from caregivers to provide supervision is essential, as lack of monitoring is an associated trigger for relapse [37]. Caregivers should be alerted that aggression may surface when doses are not provided early or in excess as demanded by the patient craving DRT. Improvement may be possible with patients who successfully reduce doses of DRT; however, long-term outcome data is not available at this time. Some psychotropic agents investigated include treatment with antidepressants, mood stabilizers and atypical antipsychotics, which have shown a mixed response with no generalizable recommendations [34]. Cognitive-behavioral strategies aimed at disengaging negative somatic interpretations from the reactive need for additional DRT dosing has been reported as useful in supporting "off"-period distress in DDS [23]. Conversion to intestinal levodopa infusion or DBS implantation has been reported as a potentially helpful consideration in resolving DDS [40], while continuous apomorphine infusions appear much less favorable [37], although these recommendations need further investigation.

Dopamine agonist withdrawal syndrome

It is commonly recognized that substances with the propensity to trigger acute pleasurable states and reward-driven behavior (i.e. cocaine) have the potential for negative discontinuation effects. This may occur with abrupt or, in some cases, gradual cessation. Recently, a distinctive and stereotyped constellation of symptoms has been recognized with DA discontinuation, referred to as dopamine agonist withdrawal syndrome (DAWS) [4]. The syndrome is characterized by several key features, including: (i) the presence of psychological and physical disturbances with DA dose reduction or discontinuation; (ii) correlation of worsening symptoms with the extent of DA dose reduction; (iii) improvement of distress with resumption of the DA; (iv) lack of improvement with other dopaminergic agents (i.e. levodopa); and (v) significant psychosocial and functional impairment [4]. Similar to other disturbances discussed in this chapter, the reason for its occurrence in some patients and not others remains elusive. The symptoms of DAWS range from psychiatric and autonomic to generalized. Symptoms include anxiety (panic, restlessness and phobia), mood changes (irritability, dysphoria, depression and hopelessness), autonomic effects (diaphoresis, flushing and orthostasis) and generalized disturbance (agitation, pain, sleep difficulties and fatigue). The frequency of DAWS in PD ranges from 7.8 to 19% [41]. The syndrome may be difficult to identify in PD as many of the symptoms of DAWS may be confused with the sequelae of PD progression or the expected "wearing off" phenomena. Moreover, unlike other drug-withdrawal syndromes, there are no clear objective findings (e.g. vital sign changes, pupil reactivity, piloerection).

Several studies have noted a strong association (up to 100% of subjects) of DAWS occurring in those with a prior history of ICD [41]. As noted earlier, DAs have relative selectivity for D3 dopamine receptors, which are found disproportionately in limbic pathways and therefore frequently responsible for ICDs. Furthermore, drug cravings are often seen in both presentations, similar to other addictions. This raises the question of whether DAWS may be a manifestation along a continuum of behavioral disturbances in PD arising from the same etiological dysfunction as ICD and DDS [42]. In the initial published report of DAWS, the authors hypothesized the presence of a "mesocorticolimbic" variant of PD that is characterized by disproportionate dopaminergic dysfunction in the mesocorticolimbic connections, as opposed to nigrostriatal [4]. This hypothesis is supported by: (i) DAWS occurring in patients with less severe motor symptoms (Unified Parkinson's Disease Rating Scale [UPDRS] scores) than those who did not experience DAWS with DA taper [4]; and (ii) functional imaging evidence of mesolimbic dopaminergic denervation [43].

The discussion about management of DAWS must begin with strategies to avoid the occurrence of DAWS altogether. Dopamine agonist withdrawal syndrome has been associated with higher DA doses and longer DA exposure [44]. Subsequently, practitioners should be perpetually cognizant of this in the setting of longer-term management of PD. Providers should also be attentive of the risk in the context of postoperative management of DBS surgery (see below) when there may be pressure to reduce the dopaminergic burden. At present, there is no evidence of a difference in risk of DAWS between one DA over another or in the rate of DA taper [44], although conventional wisdom would likely favor a more gradual reduction. Once the symptoms of DAWS appear, the management of DAWS should first start with an investigation for other contributing factors, such as parallel systemic aberrations (e.g. infection, primary psychiatric disorder, other drug-withdrawal effects). If there is no clear contributing reason, and a recent reduction in DA dosage was conducted or found, there should be a high suspicion for DAWS.

There are no definitive evidence-based recommendations available for the treatment of DAWS. Frequent communication (via office visits and telephone communication with patients or caregivers) is essential for those at high risk for or actively experiencing DAWS. A milder, self-limiting form of DAWS may occur and resolve with supportive management (or without intervention) in a subset of patients [45]. However, for some, a more severe and debilitating form of DAWS will present. As noted above in the defining features of DAWS, the supplementation of other dopaminergic agents is not effective. Therefore, reintroduction of DAs may be the only consideration for palliation. The full reinstatement of DA dosage should be done with extreme caution, as reports have noted the recurrence of ICD in a chronic and debilitating fashion in these situations [4].

The lowest effective dosage is recommended when resuming or increasing DA dosage to alleviate DAWS. One report observed a necessary dose titration to a DA–levodopa-equivalent daily dose of 160 mg to treat DAWS in three patients [45]. It is also important to mention that, although other dopaminergic agents may be ineffective in managing DAWS, patients may inappropriately and unknowingly attempt to self-medicate their distress with compulsive or higher-than-prescribed doses of other DRT (i.e. levodopa), potentially exposing a vulnerability to DDS [4]. Therefore, patients should be informed in advance of this inappropriate consideration and approach in management. For those who ultimately are unable to cease DA use (due to triggering DAWS), close monitoring should be established and education of long-term risks must be discussed.

Deep-brain stimulation

Over the last decade, the potential benefits of DBS have been well established and globally recognized in the neurological community. The use of DBS for the management of PD has subsequently become commonplace, with over 70,000 patients having the procedure since approval in 2002 [46]. Similar to the discovery and use of levodopa, the primary (motor) benefits of DBS were appreciated early, but we have become increasingly aware of the possible adverse neuropsychiatric consequences of this technology with time and use [47]. Furthermore, DBS has recently been advertised to have *beneficial* effects in certain severe psychiatric disorders [48], which may inadvertently suggest minimal or absent risk of triggering behavioral disturbances.

Deep-brain stimulation in PD has been associated with a host of psychiatric disturbances, including depression, hypomania, mania, anxiety, aggression, impulsivity, psychosis, apathy and suicidal ideation, which can range from mild to life threatening [49, 50]. The incidence of neuropsychiatric symptoms varies widely in the literature based on the DBS target, specific symptom(s) investigated and/or behavioral rating methods/instruments utilized. The two most common targets for DBS implantation in PD are the subthalamic nucleus (STN) and globus pallidus internus (GPi), with both having similar motor outcomes [51]. The decision of which target to use may therefore be based on additional factors, such as the contribution of DRT to behavioral symptoms and the ability to keep or alter the DRT regimen. In addition, DBS itself may trigger psychiatric or behavioral effects. The mechanism has been proposed to be a result of unbalanced synergistic effects of DRT and neurostimulation early in the postoperative period [52]. Relative stimulation of more ventral contacts within STN appears to be associated with higher risk of psychiatric effects due to interconnections within limbic regions [53]. However, studies continue to challenge the notion of differing vulnerability to psychiatric effects between the two targets [54, 55]. Definitive conclusions about direct DBS-related effects have been difficult to confirm as a result of retrospective studies, limited sample sizes and/or a lack of control group in many reports [47]. Furthermore, the diversity in stimulation parameters can make comparisons between reports nearly impossible. In all likelihood, the behavioral disturbances following DBS are a combination of operative, stimulatory, biological, psychological and social (Table 14.1). The potential for and consequence of transformation in psychological identity should not be underestimated or ignored [56].

Table 14.1 Potential factors contributing to post-deep-brain stimulation (DBS) behavioral disturbances

Electrode insertion, including trajectory and microlesion effects
Site of implantation
Intra-/postoperative surgical complications
Area(s) of stimulation, including current spread
Stimulation parameters, including intensity, contact configurations and polarity
Synergistic effects of dopaminergic therapy and electrical stimulation
Adjustments in dopaminergic therapy, including specific agents, dose and degree
Emotional reaction(s) to extent of DBS-induced motor improvement
Psychological adaptation to DBS implantation
Psychosocial consequences of advanced Parkinson's disease
Psychiatric comorbidities
Underlying disease and degeneration

Routine and comprehensive screening for psychiatric and behavioral symptoms in all patients with PD *prior* to DBS implantation is highly encouraged [57]. Some patients may naturally escape detection preoperatively for a variety of reasons. Nevertheless, informing patients of potential adverse behavioral effects may lead to better reporting by patients and caregivers when disturbances arise. Preoperative discussion of goals and expectations of surgery is also vital to ensure realistic outcomes and minimize disappointment. Discussion of a possible anticipated reduction in DRT after DBS may expose those who are uncomfortable with such a plan and therefore psychologically "dependent" on DRT. This uneasiness may warn the clinician of a simmering behavioral disorder and/or risk for psychiatric withdrawal symptoms postoperatively. In the end, the decision to pursue DBS in those identified with a significant preoperative behavioral disturbance can be an uncomfortable one for many surgical teams. Although not absolute or a consensus, three conventional opinions regarding the selection of a DBS target in the setting of neuropsychiatric symptoms in PD are as follows:

- For those with DRT-induced behavioral effects preoperatively, STN-DBS may be preferred due to the ability to more easily wean DRT after DBS.

This, however, should be balanced with the potentially higher vulnerability (compared with GPi) for aberrant limbic stimulation.

- For those with a history of psychiatric disturbance unrelated to DRT (or of unclear etiology), GPi may be preferred as it is considered less prone to limbic effects (compared with STN-DBS).
- For those susceptible to DRT reduction or withdrawal effects (motor or psychiatric), GPi is preferred as it necessitates less DRT reduction postoperatively.

Postoperative surveillance by clinicians and caregivers is essential, especially during the first 6 months when most programming adjustments are conducted. There are no specific evidence-based recommendations for treating behavioral manifestations that occur in the context of DBS. The role of specific psychotropic agents (such as antidepressants, antipsychotics and mood stabilizers) to manage DBS-related psychiatric disturbances has not been well established. The general approach should entail investigation for potential etiologies, correction of modifiable factors and symptomatic management. Personal variations among patients make precise assignment of a behavioral disturbance to DBS alone quite challenging. This is supported by the heterogeneous and sometimes conflicting published reports, potentially suggesting that there may be both inhibitory and excitatory neuronal clusters being activated by DBS [58].

Behavioral "inhibition" (i.e. depression, apathy and suicidal ideation)

Depression and apathy after DBS may be related to DRT reduction or stimulation. If DRT reduction is necessary or desired postoperatively, this should be done in a manner to minimize the risk of DAWS (see above). In one study of 63 patients with PD after STN stimulation (and 82% reduction in dopaminergic therapy), apathy presented in 54% of patients, with depression being a common comorbidity of apathy [43]. Resumption of dopaminergic therapy may therefore be a reasonable attempt to treat suspected hypodopaminergic effects, although this intervention has shown individual variability, lending further support to a multifactorial etiology. Apathy does not appear to be related to DBS laterality or target [59], while mood may improve more from left, than right, DBS [60]. Patients should be screened for suicide due to the higher-than-expected frequency of completed suicide reported among those undergoing STN-DBS [61]. Seventy-five percent of suicide attempts in a retrospective study occurred in the first 17 months and were associated with postoperative depression, being single and a history of ICDs [61]. A recent randomized study of both STN-BDS and GPi-DBS found no elevation of suicidality within the 6-month postoperative period [62]. The contribution of poor impulse control (not just mood deterioration) to attempted suicide should always be considered [63]. Regardless of the situation, if severe depression and/or suicidal ideation are elicited, particularly with an endorsement of intent or plan, an emergent and thorough psychiatric assessment should be obtained.

Behavioral "excitation" (i.e. hypomania, mania, impulsivity and compulsivity)

Hypomania following DBS has been reported as an acute and early effect after surgery [50]. Aggressive stimulation titration at ventral contacts should be avoided during a single visit. Dramatic acute mood improvement may pose of risk for escalation to hypomania during stimulation of the ventral striatum in non-PD subjects [64]. Therefore, it may be prudent to monitor any significant mood changes during programming with a "wait time" (i.e. 30–45 min), ideally with the caregiver, to confirm improvement or stability prior to the patient leaving the office [64]. Evidence of clear manic symptoms (such as euphoria, disinhibition, aggression, psychomotor agitation and/or thought disorganization, especially with psychosis) should prompt consideration for immediate psychiatric stabilization and/or programming adjustment to minimize further mood and behavioral escalation. Stimulation adjustments alone may not always mitigate mania [65]. New cases of ICD and DDS have been reported to emerge after DBS [66], although prospective studies are needed to confirm this observation. The prevalence of preoperative compulsive dopamine use may be as high as 16% of patients undergoing STN-DBS [67]. This is not surprising considering that dopamine misuse is common in young patients with high levodopa-equivalent daily dose, advanced motor complications and a higher propensity for risk taking, similar to characteristics of individuals undergoing DBS [68]. One study reported complete resolution of compulsive dopamine misuse in 15 of 18 patients within 1 year following STN-DBS implantation [67]. Furthermore, there were also no new occurrences in those without preoperative dopamine misuse ($n = 92$), suggesting STN-DBS may be a therapeutic intervention strategy to reduce DRT, although these preliminary findings need to be reproduced.

Conclusion

The range of psychiatric and behavioral disturbances arising from treatment in PD is diverse. Psychosis, ICDs, DDS and DAWS are four conditions that are frequently a source of great distress for providers, patients and caregivers. The underlying pathophysiology is not well understood and the clinical presentations may vary. Behavioral disturbances in the setting of DBS introduce another set of unique challenges in the diagnosis and management of such presentations. Thus, DBS may be considered a substitution for DRT in those with DRT-related behavioral complications but, in turn, may trigger a host of other behavioral complications from the ensuing DRT-deficient state and aberrant stimulation. Well-designed studies with reproducible outcomes are unfortunately lacking. The approach to these disturbances should therefore always start with proactive education about the risks prior to treatment, followed by routine monitoring for the occurrence, investigation for the etiology of the disturbance once manifested and, ultimately, sound management of the behavioral disturbance, taking into consideration the potential for adverse motor consequences. In the spirit of nonmaleficence, definitive recommendations are urgently needed for the prevention and management of treatment-related disturbances in PD.

References

1. Tang J, Strafella AP. The frontostriatal circuitry and behavioral complications in PD. *Parkinsonism Relat Disord* 2012; **18** (Suppl. 1): S104–6.
2. Aarons S, Peisah C, Wijeratne C. Neuropsychiatric effects of Parkinson's disease treatment. *Australas J Ageing* 2012; **31**: 198–202.
3. Huot P, Fox SH. The serotonergic system in motor and non-motor manifestations of Parkinson's disease. *Exp Brain Res* 2013; **230**: 463–76.
4. Rabinak CA, Nirenberg MJ. Dopamine agonist withdrawal syndrome in Parkinson disease. *Arch Neurol* 2010; **67**: 58–63.
5. Connolly BS, Fox SH. Drug treatments for the neuropsychiatric complications of Parkinson's disease. *Expert Rev Neurother* 2012; **12**: 1439–49.
6. Friedman JH. Parkinson disease psychosis: update. *Behav Neurol* 2013; **27**: 469–77.
7. Ravina B, Marder K, Fernandez HH, et al. Diagnostic criteria for psychosis in Parkinson's disease: report of an NINDS, NIMH work group. *Mov Disord* 2007; Jun 15; **22**: 1061–8.
8. Mack J, Rabins P, Anderson K, et al. Prevalence of psychotic symptoms in a community-based Parkinson disease sample. *Am J Geriatr Psychiatry* 2012; **20**: 123–32.
9. Goldman JG. New thoughts on thought disorders in Parkinson's disease: review of current research strategies and challenges. *Parkinsons Dis* 2011; **2011**: 675630.
10. Emre M, Aarsland D, Albanese A, et al. Rivastigmine for dementia associated with Parkinson's disease. *N Engl J Med* 2004; **351**: 2509–18.
11. Meltzer HY, Massey BW. The role of serotonin receptors in the action of atypical antipsychotic drugs. *Curr Opin Pharmacol* 2011; **11**: 59–67.
12. Ballanger B, Strafella AP, van Eimeren T, et al. Serotonin 2A receptors and visual hallucinations in Parkinson disease. *Arch Neurol* 2010; **67**: 416–21.
13. Hindle JV. The practical management of cognitive impairment and psychosis in the older Parkinson's disease patient. *J Neural Transm* 2013; **120**: 649–53.
14. Seppi K, Weintraub D, Coelho M, et al. The Movement Disorder Society evidence-based medicine review update: treatments for the non-motor symptoms of Parkinson's disease. *Mov Disord* 2011; **26**: 42–78.
15. Weintraub D, Chen P, Ignacio RV, Mamikonyan E, Kales HC. Patterns and trends in antipsychotic prescribing for Parkinson disease psychosis. *Arch Neurol* 2011; **68**: 899–904.
16. Cummings J, Isaacson S, Mills R, et al. Pimavanserin for patients with Parkinson's disease psychosis: a randomised, placebo-controlled phase 3 trial. *Lancet* 2014; **383**: 533–40.
17. American Psychiatric Association. *Diagnostic and Statistical Manual of Mental Disorders*, 4th edn, Text Revision. Washington, DC: American Psychiatric Association Press, 1994.
18. Evans AH, Strafella AP, Weintraub D, Stacy M. Impulsive and compulsive behaviors in Parkinson's disease. *Mov Disord* 2009; **24**: 1561–70.
19. Maier F, Merkl J, Ellereit AL, et al. Hypomania and mania related to dopamine replacement therapy in Parkinson's disease. *Parkinsonism Relat Disord* 2014; **20**: 421–7.
20. Voon V, Fox SH. Medication-related impulse control and repetitive behaviors in Parkinson disease. *Arch Neurol* 2007; **64**: 1089–96.
21. American Psychiatric Association. *Diagnostic and Statistical Manual of Mental Disorders*, 5th edn. Washington, DC: American Psychiatric Publishing, 2013.

22. Evans AH, Katzenschlager R, Paviour D, et al. Punding in Parkinson's disease: its relation to the dopamine dysregulation syndrome. *Mov Disord* 2004; **19**: 397–405.

23. Okai D, Samuel M, Askey-Jones S, David AS, Brown RG. Impulse control disorders and dopamine dysregulation in Parkinson's disease: a broader conceptual framework. *Eur J Neurol* 2011; **18**: 1379–83.

24. Driver-Dunckley E, Samanta J, Stacy M. Pathological gambling associated with dopamine agonist therapy in Parkinson's disease. *Neurology* 2003; **61**: 422–3.

25. Weintraub D, Koester J, Potenza MN, et al. Impulse control disorders in Parkinson disease: a cross-sectional study of 3090 patients. *Arch Neurol* 2010; **67**: 589–95.

26. Garcia-Ruiz PJ, Martinez Castrillo JC, Alonso-Canovas A, et al. Impulse control disorder in patients with Parkinson's disease under dopamine agonist therapy: a multicentre study. *J Neurol Neurosurg Psychiatry* 2014; **85**: 840–4.

27. Gerlach M, Double K, Arzberger T, et al. Dopamine receptor agonists in current clinical use: comparative dopamine receptor binding profiles defined in the human striatum. *J Neural Transm* 2003; **110**: 1119–27.

28. Yin HH, Knowlton BJ. The role of the basal ganglia in habit formation. *Nat Rev Neurosci* 2006; **7**: 464–76.

29. Rao H, Mamikonyan E, Detre JA, et al. Decreased ventral striatal activity with impulse control disorders in Parkinson's disease. *Mov Disord* 2010; **25**: 1660–9.

30. Voon V, Rizos A, Chakravartty R, et al. Impulse control disorders in Parkinson's disease: decreased striatal dopamine transporter levels. *J Neurol Neurosurg Psychiatry* 2014; **85**: 148–52.

31. Weintraub D, Mamikonyan E, Papay K, et al. Questionnaire for impulsive-compulsive disorders in Parkinson's disease – rating scale. *Mov Disord* 2012; **27**: 242–7.

32. Sohtaoğlu M, Demiray DY, Kenangil G, Ozekmekçi S, Erginöz E. Long term follow-up of Parkinson's disease patients with impulse control disorders. *Parkinsonism Relat Disord* 2010; **16**: 334–7.

33. Catalán MJ, de Pablo-Fernández E, Villanueva C, et al. Levodopa infusion improves impulsivity and dopamine dysregulation syndrome in Parkinson's disease. *Mov Disord* 2013; **28**: 2007–10.

34. Katzenschlager R. Dopamine dysregulation syndrome in Parkinson's disease. *J Neurol Sci* 2011; **310**: 271–5.

35. Kringelbach ML, Berridge KC. Towards a functional neuroanatomy of pleasure and happiness. *Trends Cogn Sci*. 2009; **13**: 479–87.

36. Giovannoni G, O'sullivan JD, Turner K, Manson AJ, Lees AJ. Hedonistic homeostatic dysregulation in patients with Parkinson's disease on dopamine replacement therapies. *J Neurol Neurosurg Psychiatry* 2000; **68**: 423–8.

37. Cilia R, Siri C, Canesi M, et al. Dopamine dysregulation syndrome in Parkinson's disease: from clinical and neuropsychological characterisation to management and long-term outcome. *J Neurol Neurosurg Psychiatry* 2014; **85**: 311–8.

38. Evans AH, Pavese N, Lawrence AD, et al. Compulsive drug use linked to sensitized ventral striatal dopamine transmission. *Ann Neurol* 2006; **59**: 852–8.

39. Linazasoro G. Dopamine dysregulation syndrome and levodopa-induced dyskinesias in Parkinson disease: common consequences of anomalous forms of neural plasticity. *Clin Neuropharmacol* 2009; **32**: 22–7.

40. Okun MS, Weintraub D. Should impulse control disorders and dopamine dysregulation syndrome be indications for deep brain stimulation and intestinal levodopa? *Mov Disord* 2013; **28**: 1915–9.

41. Pondal M, Marras C, Miyasaki J, et al. Clinical features of dopamine agonist withdrawal syndrome in a movement disorders clinic. *J Neurol Neurosurg Psychiatry* 2013; **84**: 130–5.

42. Limotai N, Oyama G, Go C, et al. Addiction-like manifestations and Parkinson's disease: a large single center 9-year experience. *Int J Neurosci* 2012; **122**: 145–53.

43. Thobois S, Ardouin C, Lhommée E, et al. Non-motor dopamine withdrawal syndrome after surgery for Parkinson's disease: predictors and underlying mesolimbic denervation. *Brain* 2010; **133**: 1111–27.

44. Nirenberg MJ. Dopamine agonist withdrawal syndrome: implications for patient care. *Drugs Aging* 2013; **30**: 587–92.

45. Cunnington AL, White L, Hood K. Identification of possible risk factors for the development of dopamine agonist withdrawal syndrome in Parkinson's disease. *Parkinsonism Relat Disord* 2012; **18**: 1051–2.

46. Bronstein JM, Tagliati M, Alterman RL, et al. Deep brain stimulation for Parkinson disease: an expert consensus and review of key issues. *Arch Neurol* 2011; **68**: 165.

47. Voon V, Kubu C, Krack P, Houeto JL, Tröster AI. Deep brain stimulation: neuropsychological and neuropsychiatric issues. *Mov Disord* 2006; **21** (Suppl. 14): S305–27.

48. Greenberg BD, Gabriels LA, Malone DA Jr, et al. Deep brain stimulation of the ventral internal capsule/ventral striatum for obsessive-compulsive disorder: worldwide experience. *Mol Psychiatry*. 2010; **15**: 64–79.

49. Temel Y, Kessels A, Tan S, et al. Behavioural changes after bilateral subthalamic stimulation in advanced Parkinson disease: a systematic review. *Parkinsonism Relat Disord* 2006; **12**: 265–72.

50. Funkiewiez A, Ardouin C, Krack P, *et al*. Acute psychotropic effects of bilateral subthalamic nucleus stimulation and levodopa in Parkinson's disease. *Mov Disord* 2003; **18**: 524–30.
51. Follett KA, Weaver FM, Stern M, *et al*. Pallidal versus subthalamic deep-brain stimulation for Parkinson's disease. *N Engl J Med* 2010; **362**: 2077–91.
52. Witt K, Daniels C, Volkmann J. Factors associated with neuropsychiatric side effects after STN-DBS in Parkinson's disease. *Parkinsonism Relat Disord* 2012; **18**(Suppl. 1): S168–70.
53. Temel Y. Limbic effects of high-frequency stimulation of the subthalamic nucleus. *Vitam Horm* 2010; **82**: 47–63.
54. Okun MS, Fernandez HH, Wu SS, *et al*. Cognition and mood in Parkinson's disease in subthalamic nucleus versus globus pallidus interna deep brain stimulation: the COMPARE trial. *Ann Neurol* 2009; **65**: 586–95.
55. Odekerken VJ, van Laar T, Staal MJ, *et al*. Subthalamic nucleus versus globus pallidus bilateral deep brain stimulation for advanced Parkinson's disease (NSTAPS study): a randomised controlled trial. *Lancet Neurol* 2013; **12**: 37–44.
56. Klaming L, Haselager P. Did my brain implant make me do it? Questions raised by DBS regarding psychological continuity, responsibility for action and mental competence. *Neuroethics* 2013; **6**: 527–39.
57. Rodriguez RL, Fernandez HH, Haq I, Okun MS. Pearls in patient selection for deep brain stimulation. *Neurologist*. 2007; **13**: 253–60.
58. Broen M, Duits A, Visser-Vandewalle V, Temel Y, Winogrodzka A. Impulse control and related disorders in Parkinson's disease patients treated with bilateral subthalamic nucleus stimulation: a review. *Parkinsonism Relat Disord* 2011; **17**: 413–7.
59. Kirsch-Darrow L, Zahodne LB, Marsiske M, *et al*. The trajectory of apathy after deep brain stimulation: from pre-surgery to 6 months post-surgery in Parkinson's disease. *Parkinsonism Relat Disord* 2011; **17**: 182–8.
60. Campbell MC, Black KJ, Weaver PM, *et al*. Mood response to deep brain stimulation of the subthalamic nucleus in Parkinson's disease. *J Neuropsychiatry Clin Neurosci*. 2012; **24**: 28–36.
61. Voon V, Krack P, Lang AE, *et al*. A multicentre study on suicide outcomes following subthalamic stimulation for Parkinson's disease. *Brain* 2008; **131**: 2720–8.
62. Weintraub D, Duda JE, Carlson K, *et al*. Suicide ideation and behaviours after STN and GPi DBS surgery for Parkinson's disease: results from a randomised, controlled trial. *J Neurol Neurosurg Psychiatry* 2013; **84**: 1113–18.
63. Struhal W, Guger M, Hödl S, *et al*. Attempted suicide under high dose dopaminergic therapy including apomorphine. *Wien Klin Wochenschr* 2012; **124**: 461–3.
64. Pandya M, Machado A, Malone, D. Depression in humans: the ventral capsule/ventral striatum. In: Denys D, Feenstra E, Schuurman R, eds. *Deep Brain Stimulation: A New Frontier in Psychiatry*; 2012; 95–102.
65. Saleh C. How to treat DBS-induced mania? *J Neurol Sci* 2011; **301**: 116.
66. Moum SJ, Price CC, Limotai N, *et al*. Effects of STN and GPi deep brain stimulation on impulse control disorders and dopamine dysregulation syndrome. *PLoS One* 2012; **7**: e29768.
67. Eusebio A, Witjas T, Cohen J, *et al*. Subthalamic nucleus stimulation and compulsive use of dopaminergic medication in Parkinson's disease. *J Neurol Neurosurg Psychiatry* 2013; **84**: 868–74.
68. Shotbolt P, Moriarty J, Costello A, *et al*. Relationships between deep brain stimulation and impulse control disorders in Parkinson's disease, with a literature review. *Parkinsonism Relat Disord* 2012; **18**: 10–16.

Chapter 15: Management of sleep disorders in Parkinson's disease

Daniela Calandrella and Alberto Albanese

Introduction

Parkinson's disease (PD) is a progressive neurodegenerative disease and its pathological hallmarks are neuronal loss and Lewy bodies in the substantia nigra and other vulnerable structures [1]. Parkinson's disease has long been considered a purely motor disorder, and research has mainly focused on motor features. However, PD patients also present with other symptoms, such as sleep disorders, psychiatric and cognitive features, loss of olfaction, pain and dysautonomia [2].

Sleep disorders are the most common nonmotor symptoms and an important cause of disability in PD. Sleep disorders appear either before or after the motor appearance of parkinsonian signs. They may precede the onset of the cardinal motor features in the so-called premotor PD stage [3]. In particular, hypersomnia and rapid eye movement (REM) sleep behavior disorder (RBD) can be part of the premotor phase of PD and can predate the later development of motor PD [2, 4].

Between 67 and 98% of PD patients experience sleep disorders at night or on waking [5, 6]. The incidence of sleep disorders increases with disease progression and is positively related to older age, male gender, higher dopaminergic treatment, cognitive impairment and hallucinations [7].

A number of sleep disorders are observed in PD. They may be classified into two broad categories: disorders of nocturnal sleep and a reduction of daytime alertness. Nighttime sleep disorders include insomnia, RBD, sleep-disordered breathing (obstructive sleep apnea [OSA]), restless legs syndrome (RLS), and periodic limb movement disorder (PLMD) [8]. Daytime symptoms include a reduction of daytime alertness, also referred to as excessive daytime sleepiness (EDS) and sleep attacks, defined as the sudden onset of sleep without warning.

Dopaminergic drugs can have an opposite effect on sleep architecture. In patients who have insufficient motor control at night, due to discontinuation of oral medication, dopaminergic treatment may be beneficial to nocturnal sleep. On the other hand, dopaminergic medications may cause aggravation of excessive daytime sleepiness. The main pharmacological effect of dopaminergic drugs is to promote slow-wave and REM sleep and induce somnolence at low doses, whereas at higher doses they reduce slow-wave and REM sleep and increase alertness [9].

Nighttime sleep disorders in PD

Insomnia

Insomnia is the most common sleep disorder in PD patients. Sleep fragmentation remains the most prevalent problem, affecting up to 74–88% of patients [10], and is associated with decreased total sleep time and an increased number of awakenings and wakefulness after sleep onset.

The etiology of insomnia is multifactorial but is mainly related to the nocturnal reappearance of PD motor symptoms including akinesia, rigidity and reduced mobility or dystonia, and tremor, all of which interfere with sleep maintenance. Sleep quality also may be affected by nonmotor symptoms, such as nocturia, cramps, pain and depression [11]. Another common cause of fragmented sleep in PD is the presence of hallucinations, which affect almost 20% of patients [11].

Motor and nonmotor symptoms may also develop early in the morning, resulting in early awakenings and reduced sleep time [12]. Other sleep-related disorders, such as OSA, RLS and PMLD, may additionally contribute to poor or diminished sleep [7]. Finally, drugs used for PD treatment, such as selegiline or rasagiline, and co-occurring diseases may affect sleep [13].

REM sleep behavior disorder

The parasomnia RBD is characterized by the presence of muscle activity enabling dream enactment during REM sleep [14]. Patients may present complex, vigorous, and sometimes violent behaviors [15].

Definite diagnosis requires a positive clinical history and polysomnographic evaluation showing signs of loss of muscle atonia during REM sleep, such as excessive sustained or intermittent muscle activity on electromyography, or excessive phasic twitching on chin or limb electromyography [16]. Differential diagnoses include normal dream-enacting behaviors, non-REM parasomnias, such as night terrors and sleepwalking, frequent in the young population [17], and confused arousals with disorientation, amnesia and confused behavior following arousal from sleep. Involuntary movements that occur during sleep, but are not related to sleep content, namely nocturnal myoclonus and periodic leg movements, should also be differentiated from RBD.

Around 25–50% of PD patients have RBD [18] and it may precede the onset of motor symptoms of parkinsonism by several years [19]. Longitudinal studies reported the development of PD or atypical parkinsonism (PD, Lewy body dementia and multiple-system atrophy) in 50–80% of patients with idiopathic RBD, suggesting that RBD could be a prodromal sign of PD heralding the onset of motor features. Indeed, signs of dopaminergic pathway degeneration, in particular decreased nigrostriatal dopamine transporter activity [20] and increased midbrain hyperechogenicity [21], have been reported in patients with RBD without parkinsonism. Therefore, RBD has been considered a potential early biomarker for neurodegeneration and a target for the administration of new neuroprotective therapies [22].

Restless legs syndrome and periodic limb movement disorder

Restless legs syndrome is defined as an irresistible urge to move the legs, accompanied by unpleasant sensations, with worsening in the evening hours and with inactivity, that improves with movement and significantly interferes with sleep [23]. The symptoms usually appear in lower extremities, but some patients refer symptoms in the upper limbs. The estimated prevalence of RLS in the general population is 2.5–10% [24]. The prevalence of RLS in the PD population ranges between 8 and 50% [11].

Initially described as nocturnal myoclonus [25], PLMD is manifested by involuntary, periodic leg and hip flexion movements, coexisting with RLS, or occurring independently, and is present in 30–80% of PD patients [26].

The diagnosis of RLS is based on clinical criteria [23]; polysomnography is not needed for the confirmation of RLS, but it can establish the presence of PLMD. Secondary causes of RLS, such as renal failure, iron deficiency, hormonal alterations and neuropathies, should be considered [11].

Recently, an "RLS-like syndrome" was described [27]. This is a psychiatric disease that satisfies the International Restless Legs Syndrome Study Group criteria but is unresponsive to dopamine agonist treatment.

Obstructive sleep apnea

Obstructive sleep apnea is the most common type of breathing disorder during sleep and is characterized by repeated episodes of obstruction of the upper airway and oxygen desaturation of the arterial hemoglobin. Recent studies suggest a high prevalence of sleep-disordered breathing in patients with PD, ranging from 20 to 60% [28]. Parkinson's disease may predispose patients to airway and lung function abnormalities that could increase risk for OSA.

Several studies reported a higher prevalence of OSA in PD patients than in the general population [29, 30]; however, recent studies reported similar rates of OSA in the PD population relative to controls, suggesting that OSA may not be specifically associated with PD [30, 31].

A detailed medical and sleep history obtained from the patient and from the bed partner and an overnight polysomnogram are useful for a correct diagnosis of OSA.

Daytime sleep disorders in PD
Excessive daytime sleepiness

Excessive daytime sleepiness is characterized by the inability to stay awake during the day, resulting in undesirable lapses into sleep. In PD, it is a common phenomenon and may lead to social problems and car accidents and may have a high impact on quality of life. It is manifested as a persistent hypersomnolence or as episodes of sudden onset of sleep, namely "sleep attacks." There is a variability in the frequency of daytime sleepiness depending on the population investigated and the instrument used [32]. Using the Epworth

Sleepiness Scale to define daytime somnolence, the frequency reaches 33% of patients compared with 11–16% in non-PD controls [33].

Excessive daytime sleepiness may be triggered by a number of factors, including dopaminergic therapy, dementia, parkinsonism severity and duration, hallucinations, sleep–wake cycle disruption, nocturnal sleep quantity and quality, OSA, depression and genetic susceptibility [2], although no clear relationships have been demonstrated between nocturnal sleep disorders and the severity of daytime sleepiness [34].

Sleep attacks

Sudden-onset sleep episodes ("sleep attacks") were originally described as "sudden, irresistible, and overwhelming sleepiness without awareness of falling asleep." The percentage of PD patients complaining of sleep episodes varies greatly in different reports ranging between 3.8 and 20.8% [35].

Sleep attacks were first described in PD patients after treatment with pramipexole or ropinirole [36]. Levodopa (L-DOPA) monotherapy is associated with a low risk of sleep attacks, whereas the combination of levodopa and dopamine agonists increases the risk by two- or threefold [37].

Pathophysiology of sleep disorders in Parkinson's disease

The role of dopamine in the pathophysiology processes leading to development of motor deficits in PD is well established, whereas the processes responsible for the development of sleep disturbances are much less understood [38]. Dopamine is thought to be involved in promoting wakefulness and arousal.

Different dopaminergic areas, such as the pars compacta of the substantia nigra and the ventral tegmental area, have reciprocal projections with brain regions involved in the regulation of sleep–wake states including brainstem, and hypothalamic, thalamic and cortical areas [39, 40]. The loss of cells in the substantia nigra and the ventral tegmental area may disrupt these reciprocal pathways, which are normally in charge of maintaining the sleep–wake cycle [41]. Moreover, the locus subcoeruleus in the brainstem is involved into the abolition of muscle tone during REM sleep and can be damaged in PD [42]. Another dopaminergic nucleus, the ventrolateral region of the periaqueductal gray in the midbrain, is connected with the reticular activating system, and also is involved in the sleep–wake cycle [43].

Neurons in this region are active during waking, less active during slow-wave sleep and silent during REM sleep. In patients with PD, degeneration of this area has been reported to precede the degeneration in the substantia nigra [44].

The involvement of dopaminergic pathways in the regulation of sleep is supported by several lines of evidence. Happe *et al.* [45] observed a significant inverse correlation between the Epworth Sleepiness Scale score and dopamine transporter binding in the striatum, putamen and caudate nucleus of patients with PD and daytime sleepiness. Furthermore, worsening of daytime sleepiness with dopamine agonists is an indirect indicator of dopaminergic involvement. Finally, dopaminergic neurotransmission is involved in circadian control systems [11, 46], in particular in expression of melanopsin, a photopigment of intrinsically photosensitive retinal cells implicated in the circadian cycle [47].

Findings from animal studies have suggested that lesions or dysfunction in REM sleep and motor control circuitry in the pontomedullary structures cause RBDs, and converging evidence supports a similar pathogenesis in humans [4]. Histopathology studies reported accumulation of Lewy bodies and Lewy neurites in the substantia nigra, locus coeruleus and central raphe [48], whereas diffusion tension imagery studies showed abnormal fractional anisotropy in the tegmentum of the midbrain and rostral pons [49].

In addition to a direct involvement of dopaminergic transmission in the control of sleep and wakefulness, several other factors may interfere with physiological sleep in PD patients. Sleep disorders may be caused by nocturnal akinesia (causing insufficient turning in bed caused by nighttime fluctuation and wearing off), by dysautonomia (nocturia and hypotension) and by drug side effects. For example, selegiline may cause insomnia as it leads to the production of its metabolites, methamphetamine and amphetamine. There may also be other factors, unrelated to PD, such as age-related sleep disturbances, cardiac diseases (heart insufficiency, nocturnal hypertension), pulmonary diseases (sleep apnea and asthma), depression and anxiety [50].

Diagnosis

A correct diagnosis of sleep disorders in PD is the prerequisite for a specific treatment [5]. An accurate clinical interview remains the most important diagnostic instrument. Although sleep disorders are common in PD, they are not always mentioned spontaneously by patients [51]. In particular, a systematic assessment of sleepiness is mandatory in PD patients since EDS and sleep attacks are associated with increased risk of driving accidents, potentially leading to car accidents or injury at work.

Sleep questionnaires help in collecting standardized data, although they are no substitute for a clinical interview of the patient and the caregiver [5]. A variety of scales have been developed and applied to the evaluation of PD sleep-related issues, but only a small number have been assessed for clinimetric properties in the PD population. Four scales were found to meet the criteria for recommendation by the Sleep Scale Task Force [52]. The PD Sleep Scale and the Pittsburgh Sleep Quality Index are recommended for rating overall sleep problems, to screen and to measure severity; the SCOPA-Sleep Scale is recommended for rating overall sleep problems, either to screen or to measure severity, and for rating daytime sleepiness; and the Epworth Sleepiness Scale is recommended for rating daytime sleepiness, to screen and measure severity.

Polysomnography used in clinical practice for the assessment of sleep architecture and the detection of nocturnal sleep disorders should always be used in combination with a clinical interview and a sleep scale.

Management

There are numerous publications on the treatment of sleep disorders in PD. However, the evidence collected is not very strong. There are no class I data to support management of sleep-related issues. Figure 15.1

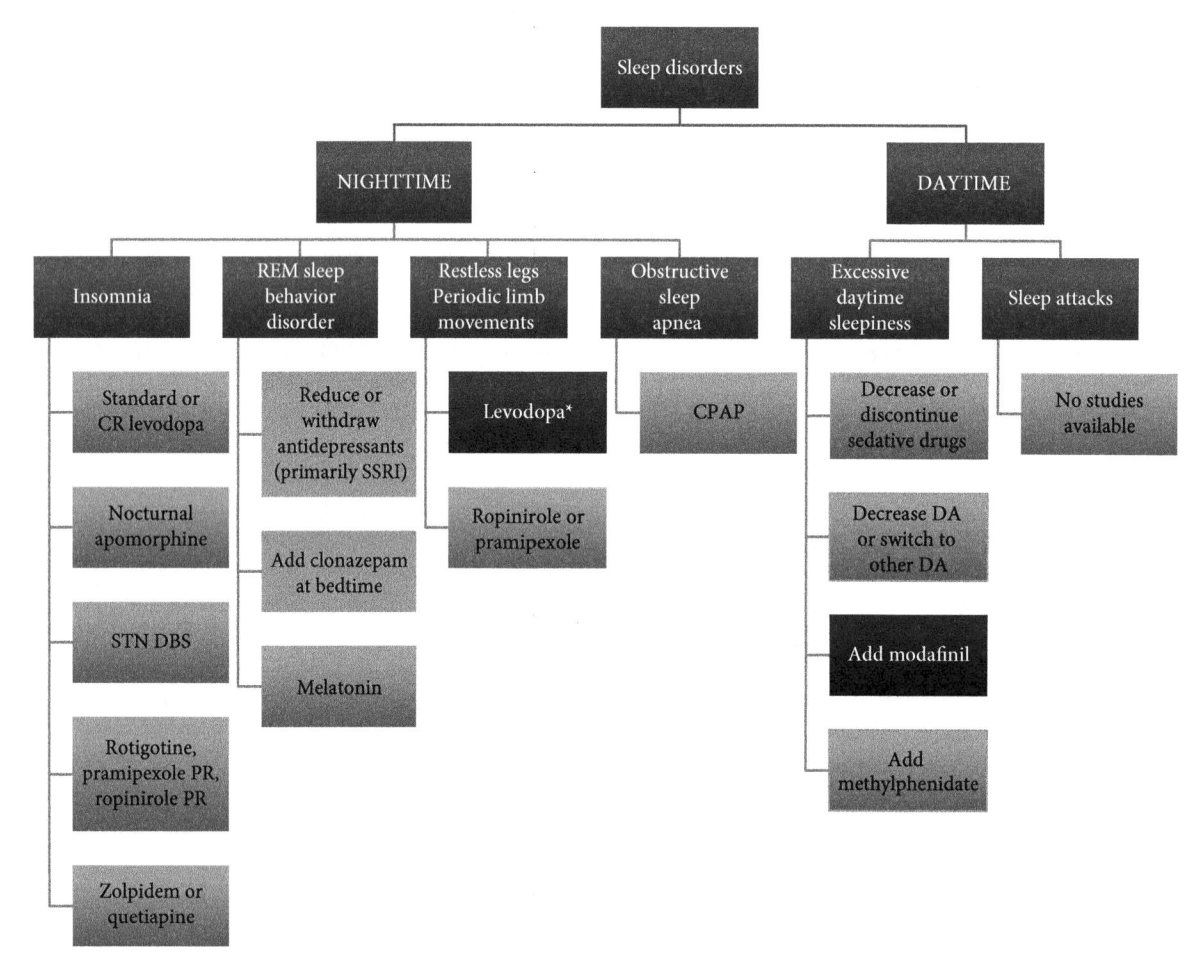

Figure 15.1 Summary flowchart for the treatment of sleep disorders in Parkinson's disease resulting from evidence-based data. Levels of recommendation are based on the American Academy of Neurology practice parameters [53]: level A recommendations are in red, level B recommendations are in violet; level U recommendations are in green. CPAP, continuous positive airway pressure; DA, dopamine agonist; DBS, deep-brain stimulation; PR, prolonged release; SSRI, selective serotonin reuptake inhibitor; STN, subthalamic nucleus. *This option refers only to periodic limb movement disorder. (A black and white version of this figure will appear in some formats. For the color version, please refer to the plate section.)

summarizes the levels of evidence for different sleep disorders.

Despite the importance of identifying and treating sleep disorders in PD, we still lack evidence-based guidelines, meta-analyses and review articles concerning the treatment of sleep disorders in PD due to the lack of large-scale, randomized controlled trials.

The American Academy of Neurology (AAN) practice parameters for the treatment of nonmotor symptoms in PD [53] reported no level A recommendations for the treatment of sleep disorders. The European Federation of Neurological Societies (EFNS) and the Movement Disorder Society (MDS) European Section recently produced evidence-based recommendations for the management of PD [54]. According to these guidelines, management of sleep-related issues has a low level of evidence often rated as a Good Practice Point.

The hypothesis of several studies was that the improvement of nocturnal motor symptoms in PD abates sleep dysfunction in PD; these studies have shown improvement of nocturnal akinesia and other motor or nonmotor dopamine-dependent symptoms, as well as several subjective sleep parameters [55]. Continuous dopaminergic stimulation appears to be the best option, and use of slow-release levodopa or long-acting dopamine agonists has been recommended [50].

Medical management

Insomnia

Two placebo-controlled trials showed that standard or controlled-release levodopa at bedtime may improve sleeping time [56, 57]. A placebo-controlled trial demonstrated that pergolide worsened sleep efficiency and fragmentation [58]. A small open-label trial showed that nocturnal apomorphine infusion [59] reduced awakenings. Rotigotine, pramipexole and ropinirole prolonged-release formulations improved sleep quality [60, 61]. Two small open-label studies [62, 63] reported improvements in sleep quality but aggravation of sleep fragmentation with cabergoline at bedtime.

Specifically designed studies primarily aimed at evaluating the effect of long-acting dopamine agonists on sleep disorders have been carried out only for rotigotine [64]. This double-blind, placebo-controlled trial showed improvement of PD Sleep Scale domain scores (disturbed sleep, motor symptoms at night and PD symptoms at night) and Non-Motor Symptoms Scale scores. However, no significant change was found in PD Sleep Scale scores in an open-label study of an extended-release tablet formulation of pramipexole [65].

Improved sleep was reported in two class II placebo-controlled studies [66, 67] with melatonin (ranging from 3 to 50 mg), without appreciable adverse events. A case series with zolpidem [68], a short-acting hypnotic drug, and quetiapine [69] reported an improvement of insomnia. Low-dose clozapine improved nocturnal akathisia and tremor [70].

An MDS evidence-based review on the treatment of PD nonmotor symptoms reported the results of five randomized controlled trials assessed the efficacy of the controlled-release formulations of levodopa/carbidopa, pergolide, eszopiclone (a γ-aminobutyric acid A receptor agonist approved for short-term treatment of primary insomnia in older adults) and melatonin at bedtime to treat insomnia in PD [71]. The review concluded that there was insufficient evidence on the efficacy of these drugs administered at bedtime for the treatment of insomnia in PD.

Recommendations from the AAN and the EFNS/MDS guidelines can be integrated as follows.
- Standard or controlled-release levodopa/carbidopa improves nocturnal motor symptoms that may contribute to insomnia, although data demonstrating an improvement in objective sleep parameters or sleep satisfaction are insufficient [53, 54].
- Based on the reported melatonin studies, there is insufficient evidence to conclude on the efficacy of melatonin at doses of 3–5 and 50 mg for the treatment of insomnia in PD. However, melatonin is established as effective in improving the perception of sleep quality, although clinical data are conflicting with polysomnographic data [53]. Melatonin (3 and 50 mg) improved sleep without relevant adverse events (placebo-controlled studies) [54].
- Pergolide worsens sleep efficiency and fragmentation [54].
- Nocturnal apomorphine infusion reduces awakenings and improves nocturia and akinesia [54].
- Rotigotine, pramipexole and ropinirole prolonged-release formulations improves sleep quality [54].
- Zolpidem and quetiapine are suggested to improve insomnia [54].

Other clinical trials have been performed. As reported by the National Institutes of Health clinical trials registry (clinicaltrials.gov), the randomized double-blinded study of ramelteon (NCT00462254) for the treatment of sleep disturbances in PD has been terminated recently. Ramelteon is a selective melatonin-1 and melatonin-2 receptor agonist currently approved in the USA and Japan for the treatment of insomnia. Two studies are underway to evaluate the effects of rasagiline on sleep disturbances in PD (open-label NCT01032486 and placebo-controlled NCT01178047).

In addition or alternatively to pharmacotherapy, several nonpharmacological options to treat insomnia should be considered in clinical practice [72]: stimulus control therapy, relaxation training, sleep restriction, paradoxical intention, biofeedback, cognitive behavioral therapy [73] and multicomponent therapy have been recommended by the American Academy of Sleep Medicine as effective therapies for insomnia [74], but for these therapies, no evidence of efficacy in PD exists. Recently, a pilot study [73] compared nonpharmacological treatment (cognitive behavioral therapy with bright-light therapy) with doxepin (10 mg at bedtime) to treat insomnia, with randomized, but not blinded, treatment allocation. Doxepin is interesting because it has a high affinity for the H1 receptor, making it a selective H1 antagonist at low doses, and it has been shown to display sedating properties. The study showed a significant benefit of doxepin in both primary outcomes (the Insomnia Severity Index and the Scales for Outcomes in Parkinson's Disease – night scale) at 6 weeks.

RBD

There are no controlled trials that have specifically addressed the treatment of RBD in PD.

The EFNS/MDS guidelines [54] reported two case series [75, 76] suggesting that clonazepam (0.5–2 mg) is efficacious. Clonazepam may lead to sedation, exacerbated obstructive breathing and increased risk of falling. Two open-label studies [77, 78] reported conflicting results with pramipexole for RBD in PD. Most antidepressants, especially selective serotonin reuptake inhibitors (SSRIs) and mirtazapine, may worsen RBD [79]. The AAN Practice parameter [53] concludes that data on the treatment of RBD in PD are insufficient and in a clinical practice clonazepam and melatonin are often used to treat RBD in the general population.

Recommendations from the AAN and EFNS/MDS are as follows.

- Take protective measures to prevent sleep-related injuries (safeguard the bedroom environment) [54].
- Reduce or withdraw antidepressants, primarily SSRIs [54].
- Add clonazepam at bedtime (0.5–2 mg) [54] or melatonine [53].

Recently, Kunz and Mahlberg [80] conducted a double-blind, placebo-controlled, crossover trial of melatonin in eight patients with RBD, one of whom had PD. A significant improvement in global scores was reported after 4 weeks of 3 mg melatonin daily, with a complete resolution of behaviors in four of the eight patients and no reported adverse events.

A randomized, double-blind, crossover trial of rivastigmine in 10 patients with PD and RBD [22], and without response to melatonin and clonazepam, supported the hypothesis that an impairment of cholinergic pathways has been implicated in the development of RBD [81]. The authors showed that the use of rivastigmine (transdermal patch 4.6 mg/24 h) resulted in a significant decrease in bed partner-reported RBD episodes compared with placebo.

The use of ramelteon to treat two Japanese patients with PD and multiple-system atrophy, and RBD [82] was also reported. These patients improved symptomatically and had a decrease in the proportion of REM sleep without atonia at polysomnography.

Nonpharmacological therapy includes safety measures, for example the use of padded bed rails [83] or customized bed alarms that play messages from a familiar person, triggered by patient movement [84], and the removal of potentially dangerous objects from near the bed.

RLS and PLMS

Ropinirole and pramipexole are approved by the US Food and Drug Administration to treat RLS in the general population, but there are no controlled trials in patients with PD and RLS. An open-label study of 15 patients with PD and PLMS [63] who were treated with cabergoline found an increased number of awakenings and stage shifts but a reduction of PLMS. Another study found that levodopa/carbidopa administered at bedtime decreased the frequency of spontaneous movements in bed [56]. When RLS and PD coexist, the RLS symptoms may theoretically be treated with the dopaminergic therapy used for PD, as dopamine agonists are effective for treatment of RLS.

With specific regard to the occurrence of such symptoms in PD patients, however, the AAN Practice parameter [53] report that levodopa/carbidopa probably decreases the frequency of spontaneous nighttime leg movements, and data regarding the use of nonergot dopamine agonists to treat RLS and PLMS specifically in patients with PD are insufficient.

Obstructive sleep apnea

Studies on the treatment of OSA in PD patients are virtually nonexistent [85]. Treatment is typically with continuous positive airway pressure (CPAP) and is effective in reducing the symptoms of sleepiness and improving quality-of-life measures in people with moderate and severe OSA [86].

Clinical experience suggests that individual PD patients may have an improvement in daytime sleepiness when using CPAP [83].

EDS

Two small placebo-controlled trials with modafinil [87–89] and an open-label study with methylphenidate [90] found improvements in EDS in PD patients. Modafinil is an orally administered wake-promoting agent, indicated to improve wakefulness in adults with excessive sleepiness associated with OSA, shift work disorder and narcolepsy.

Recommendations from the AAN and EFNS/MDS-ES are based on the following approach:

- Optimize improvement of nocturnal sleep by reducing disturbing factors, such as akinesia, tremor, urinary frequency, etc. [54].
- Recommend that the patient stops driving [54].
- Decrease the dosage or discontinue sedative drugs prescribed for other medical conditions [54].
- Decrease the dose of dopaminergic drugs (mainly dopamine agonists) because all dopaminergic drugs may induce daytime somnolence [54].
- Try switching to another dopamine agonist [54].
- Add modafinil [53, 54] or other wake-promoting agents such as methylphenidate [54].

Recently, a 6-week randomly controlled trial of caffeine was conducted in PD patients to assess effects upon daytime somnolence, motor severity and other nonmotor features [91]. Patients with PD and daytime somnolence (Epworth Sleepiness Scale [ESS] >10) were given caffeine 100 mg twice daily for 3 weeks and then 200 mg twice daily for 3 weeks, or matching placebo. On the ESS (primary endpoint), there was no significant improvement with caffeine at either dose; however, somnolence improved significantly with caffeine for the secondary outcome on the Clinical Global Impression of Change.

Other clinical trials have been performed. As reported by the National Institutes of Health clinical trials registry (clinicaltrials.gov), an open-label study (NCT00641186) to evaluate the sodium oxybate for the treatment of excessive daytime sleepiness and nocturnal sleep disturbance in patients with mild to moderate PD has been completed.

Dopaminergic drugs may play a significant role in daytime alertness of PD. Treatment with dopamine agonists, including the ergot agonists pergolide and bromocriptine and the nonergot agonists pramipexole and ropinirole, increases the incidence of EDS in patients with PD [92]. Moreover, there is a strong relationship between the dosages of dopaminergic medications and EDS. A recent study found that higher doses of levodopa (≥1000 mg) and use of dopamine agonist (vs nonuse) were both predictors of higher ESS scores indicative of more severe EDS [93], although no differences in sleep latency were identified between the different types of dopamine agonists.

Sleep attacks

There are no studies that have specifically addressed the treatment or prevention of sudden-onset sleep in PD.

Recommendations from the AAN and EFNS/MDS are similar to those proposed for excessive daytime somnolence. Levodopa monotherapy is associated with a low risk of sleep attacks, whereas the combination of levodopa and dopamine agonists increases the risk by two- or threefold [37]. Systematic assessment of sleepiness is mandatory in PD patients, since sleep attacks are associated with increased risk of driving accidents and injuries at work.

Management is based mainly on simplification and reduction of the antiparkinsonian drug regimen when possible.

Deep-brain stimulation

Bilateral DBS of the subthalamic nucleus (STN) improves motor function and decreases motor fluctuations in patients with moderate to advanced PD with evidence of improvement in nonmotor symptoms after the procedure [94].

The AAN Practice Parameter [53] reported three class III studies demonstrating improvement of sleep quality following STN-DBS [95–97]. In one, the total sleep time improved by 28% (from a mean of 281 min before DBS to a mean of 360 min after DBS) [95]. The other two showed a significant decrease in the arousal index (the total number of arousals scored per hour of sleep) [96] and total sleep efficiency increased by a mean of 36% [97].

The EFNS/MDS guidelines [54] reported two class III studies [98, 99] showing that STN-DBS improves sleep duration and reduces akinesia and sleep fragmentation.

Combined recommendations from the AAN and EFNS/MDS can be summarized as follows:
- STN-DBS possibly improves sleep quality in patients with advanced PD, although it is not currently used to treat sleep disorders [53].
- DBS improves sleep quality in advanced PD patients except for the nocturnal motor phenomena of sleep disorders [54].

Improvement in RLS severity has been reported in PD patients after STN-DBS, even though dopaminergic medications had been reduced [100, 101]. By contrast, development of new RLS symptoms were noted in 11 of 195 implanted patients in another study [102].

Other clinical trials have been performed. As reported by the National Institutes of Health clinical trials registry (clinicaltrials.gov), there are two ongoing studies on the effects of DBS on sleep architecture in PD patients (NCT01169324 and NCT01769690). The first is designed to determine primary changes in sleep efficiency in a cohort of subjects who have undergone DBS; the second is designed to measure differences in sleep efficiency with different DBS stimulation parameters to address the hypothesis that low-frequency parameters are more effective than conventional parameters at improving sleep.

References

1. Dickson DW, Fujishiro H, Orr C, et al. Neuropathology of non-motor features of Parkinson disease. *Parkinsonism Relat Disord* 2009; **15** (Suppl. 3): S1–5.
2. Iranzo A. Parkinson disease and sleep: sleep–wake changes in the premotor stage of Parkinson disease; impaired olfaction and other prodromal features. *Curr Neurol Neurosci Rep* 2013; **13**: 373.
3. Tolosa E, Gaig C, Santamaria J, Compta Y. Diagnosis and the premotor phase of Parkinson disease. *Neurology* 2009; **72** (Suppl.): S12–20.
4. Boeve BF. Idiopathic REM sleep behaviour disorder in the development of Parkinson's disease. *Lancet Neurol* 2013; **12**: 469–82.
5. Louter M, Aarden WC, Lion J, Bloem BR, Overeem S. Recognition and diagnosis of sleep disorders in Parkinson's disease. *J Neurol* 2012; **259**: 2031–40.
6. Lees AJ, Blackburn NA, Campbell VL. The nighttime problems of Parkinson's disease. *Clin Neuropharmacol* 1988; **11**: 512–9.
7. Zoccolella S, Savarese M, Lamberti P, et al. Sleep disorders and the natural history of Parkinson's disease: the contribution of epidemiological studies. *Sleep Med Rev* 2011; **15**: 41–50.
8. Comella CL. Sleep disorders in Parkinson's disease: an overview. *Mov Disord* 2007; **22** (Suppl. 17): S367–73.
9. Chaudhuri KR, Logishetty K. Dopamine receptor agonists and sleep disturbances in Parkinson's disease. *Parkinsonism Relat Disord* 2009; **15** (Suppl. 4): S101–4.
10. Oerlemans WG, de Weerd AW. The prevalence of sleep disorders in patients with Parkinson's disease. A self-reported, community-based survey. *Sleep Med* 2002; **3**: 147–9.
11. Videnovic A, Golombek D. Circadian and sleep disorders in Parkinson's disease. *Exp Neurol* 2013; **243**: 45–56.
12. Iranzo A. Sleep–wake changes in the premotor stage of Parkinson disease. *J Neurol Sci* 2011; **310**: 283–5.
13. Menza M, Dobkin RD, Marin H, Bienfait K. Sleep disturbances in Parkinson's disease. *Mov Disord* 2010; **25** (Suppl. 1): S117–22.
14. Schenck CH, Bundlie SR, Ettinger MG, Mahowald MW. Chronic behavioral disorders of human REM sleep: a new category of parasomnia. *Sleep* 1986; **9**: 293–308.
15. Comella CL, Nardine TM, Diederich NJ, Stebbins GT. Sleep-related violence, injury, and REM sleep behavior disorder in Parkinson's disease. *Neurology* 1998; **51**: 526–9.
16. Montplaisir J, Gagnon JF, Fantini ML, et al. Polysomnographic diagnosis of idiopathic REM sleep behavior disorder. *Mov Disord* 2010; **25**: 2044–51.
17. Nielsen T, Svob C, Kuiken D. Dream-enacting behaviors in a normal population. *Sleep* 2009; **32**: 1629–36.
18. Gagnon JF, Bedard MA, Fantini ML, et al. REM sleep behavior disorder and REM sleep without atonia in Parkinson's disease. *Neurology* 2002; **59**: 585–9.
19. Iranzo A, Molinuevo JL, Santamaria J, et al. Rapid-eye-movement sleep behaviour disorder as an early marker for a neurodegenerative disorder: a descriptive study. *Lancet Neurol* 2006; **5**: 572–7.
20. Iranzo A, Valldeoriola F, Lomena F, et al. Serial dopamine transporter imaging of nigrostriatal function in patients with idiopathic rapid-eye-movement sleep behaviour disorder: a prospective study. *Lancet Neurol* 2011; **10**: 797–805.
21. Stockner H, Iranzo A, Seppi K, et al. Midbrain hyperechogenicity in idiopathic REM sleep behavior disorder. *Mov Disord* 2009; **24**: 1906–9.

22. McCarter SJ, Boswell CL, St Louis EK, et al. Treatment outcomes in REM sleep behavior disorder. *Sleep Med* 2013; **14**: 237–42.
23. Allen RP, Picchietti D, Hening WA, et al. Restless legs syndrome: diagnostic criteria, special considerations, and epidemiology. A report from the restless legs syndrome diagnosis and epidemiology workshop at the National Institutes of Health. *Sleep Med* 2003; **4**: 101–19.
24. Garcia-Borreguero D, Egatz R, Winkelmann J, Berger K. Epidemiology of restless legs syndrome: the current status. *Sleep Med Rev* 2006; **10**: 153–67.
25. Lugaresi E, Coccagna G, Gambi D, Berti CG, Poppi M. Symonds' nocturnal myoclonus. *Electroencephalogr Clin Neurophysiol* 1967; **23**: 289.
26. Poewe W, Högl B. Akathisia, restless legs and periodic limb movements in sleep in Parkinson's disease. *Neurology* 2004; **63** (Suppl. 3): S12–16.
27. Baumann CR, Marti I, Bassetti CL. Restless legs symptoms without periodic limb movements in sleep and without response to dopaminergic agents: a restless legs-like syndrome? *Eur J Neurol* 2007; **14**: 1369–72.
28. Chotinaiwattarakul W, Dayalu P, Chervin RD, Albin RL. Risk of sleep-disordered breathing in Parkinson's disease. *Sleep Breath* 2011; **15**: 471–8.
29. Arnulf I, Konofal E, Merino-Andreu M, et al. Parkinson's disease and sleepiness: an integral part of PD. *Neurology* 2002; **58**: 1019–24.
30. Cochen de Cock V, Abouda M, Leu S, et al. Is obstructive sleep apnea a problem in Parkinson's disease? *Sleep Med* 2010; **11**: 247–52.
31. Trotti LM, Bliwise DL. No increased risk of obstructive sleep apnea in Parkinson's disease. *Mov Disord* 2010; **25**: 2246–9.
32. Tandberg E, Larsen JP, Karlsen K. Excessive daytime sleepiness and sleep benefit in Parkinson's disease: a community-based study. *Mov Disord* 1999; **14**: 922–7.
33. Tan EK, Lum SY, Fook-Chong SM, et al. Evaluation of somnolence in Parkinson's disease: comparison with age- and sex-matched controls. *Neurology* 2002; **58**: 465–8.
34. Razmy A, Lang AE, Shapiro CM. Predictors of impaired daytime sleep and wakefulness in patients with Parkinson disease treated with older (ergot) vs newer (nonergot) dopamine agonists. *Arch Neurol* 2004; **61**: 97–102.
35. Ondo WG, Dat VK, Khan H, et al. Daytime sleepiness and other sleep disorders in Parkinson's disease. *Neurology* 2001; **57**: 1392–6.
36. Frucht S, Rogers JD, Greene PE, Gordon MF, Fahn S. Falling asleep at the wheel: motor vehicle mishaps in persons taking pramipexole and ropinirole. *Neurology* 1999; **52**: 1908–10.
37. Paus S, Brecht HM, Koster J, et al. Sleep attacks, daytime sleepiness, and dopamine agonists in Parkinson's disease. *Mov Disord* 2003; **18**: 659–67.
38. Chaudhuri KR. The dopaminergic basis of sleep dysfunction and non motor symptoms of Parkinson's disease: evidence from functional imaging. *Exp Neurol* 2009; **216**: 247–8.
39. Monti JM, Jantos H. The roles of dopamine and serotonin, and of their receptors, in regulating sleep and waking. *Prog Brain Res* 2008; **172**: 625–46.
40. Grinberg LT, Rueb U, Alho AT, Heinsen H. Brainstem pathology and non-motor symptoms in PD. *J Neurol Sci* 2010; **289**: 81–8.
41. Monti JM, Monti D. The involvement of dopamine in the modulation of sleep and waking. *Sleep Med Rev* 2007; **11**: 113–33.
42. Garcia-Lorenzo D, Longo-Dos SC, Ewenczyk C, et al. The coeruleus/subcoeruleus complex in rapid eye movement sleep behaviour disorders in Parkinson's disease. *Brain* 2013; **136**): 2120–9.
43. Lu J, Jhou TC, Saper CB. Identification of wake-active dopaminergic neurons in the ventral periaqueductal gray matter. *J Neurosci* 2006; **26**: 193–202.
44. Suzuki K, Miyamoto M, Miyamoto T, Iwanami M, Hirata K. Sleep disturbances associated with Parkinson's disease. *Parkinsons Dis* 2011; **2011**: 219056.
45. Happe S, Baier PC, Helmschmied K, et al. Association of daytime sleepiness with nigrostriatal dopaminergic degeneration in early Parkinson's disease. *J Neurol* 2007; **254**: 1037–43.
46. Iranzo A, Lomena F, Stockner H, et al. Decreased striatal dopamine transporter uptake and substantia nigra hyperechogenicity as risk markers of synucleinopathy in patients with idiopathic rapid-eye-movement sleep behaviour disorder: a prospective study [corrected]. *Lancet Neurol* 2010; **9**: 1070–7.
47. Witkovsky P. Dopamine and retinal function. *Doc Ophthalmol* 2004; **108**: 17–40.
48. Boeve BF, Silber MH, Saper CB, et al. Pathophysiology of REM sleep behaviour disorder and relevance to neurodegenerative disease. *Brain* 2007; **130**: 2770–88.
49. Scherfler C, Frauscher B, Schocke M, et al. White and gray matter abnormalities in idiopathic rapid eye movement sleep behavior disorder: a diffusion-tensor imaging and voxel-based morphometry study. *Ann Neurol* 2011; **69**: 400–7.
50. Diederich NJ, McIntyre DJ. Sleep disorders in Parkinson's disease: many causes, few therapeutic options. *J Neurol Sci* 2012; **314**: 12–9.
51. Chaudhuri KR, Prieto-Jurcynska C, Naidu Y, et al. The nondeclaration of nonmotor symptoms of Parkinson's disease to health care professionals: an international

52. Högl B, Arnulf I, Comella C, et al. Scales to assess sleep impairment in Parkinson's disease: critique and recommendations. *Mov Disord* 2010; **25**: 2704–16.
53. Zesiewicz TA, Sullivan KL, Arnulf I, et al. Practice parameter: treatment of nonmotor symptoms of Parkinson disease: report of the Quality Standards Subcommittee of the American Academy of Neurology *Neurology* 2010; **74**: 924–31.
54. Ferreira JJ, Katzenschlager R, Bloem BR, et al. Summary of the recommendations of the EFNS/MDS-ES review on therapeutic management of Parkinson's disease. *Eur J Neurol* 2013; **20**: 5–15.
55. Chaudhuri KR, Schapira AH. Non-motor symptoms of Parkinson's disease: dopaminergic pathophysiology and treatment. *Lancet Neurol* 2009; **8**: 464–74.
56. Leeman AL, O'Neill CJ, Nicholson PW, et al. Parkinson's disease in the elderly: response to and optimal spacing of night time dosing with levodopa. *Br J Clin Pharmacol* 1987; **24**: 637–43.
57. Stocchi F, Barbato L, Nordera G, Berardelli A, Ruggieri S. Sleep disorders in Parkinson's disease. *J Neurol* 1998; **245** (Suppl. 1): S15–18.
58. Comella CL, Morrissey M, Janko K. Nocturnal activity with nighttime pergolide in Parkinson disease: a controlled study using actigraphy. *Neurology* 2005; **64**: 1450–1.
59. Reuter I, Ellis CM, Ray CK. Nocturnal subcutaneous apomorphine infusion in Parkinson's disease and restless legs syndrome. *Acta Neurol Scand* 1999; **100**: 163–7.
60. Poewe WH, Rascol O, Quinn N, et al. Efficacy of pramipexole and transdermal rotigotine in advanced Parkinson's disease: a double-blind, double-dummy, randomised controlled trial. *Lancet Neurol* 2007; **6**: 513–20.
61. Pahwa R, Stacy MA, Factor SA, et al. Ropinirole 24-hour prolonged release: randomized, controlled study in advanced Parkinson disease. *Neurology* 2007; **68**: 1108–15.
62. Romigi A, Stanzione P, Marciani MG, et al. Effect of cabergoline added to levodopa treatment on sleep–wake cycle in idiopathic Parkinson's disease: an open label 24-hour polysomnographic study. *J Neural Transm* 2006; **113**: 1909–13.
63. Högl B, Rothdach A, Wetter TC, Trenkwalder C. The effect of cabergoline on sleep, periodic leg movements in sleep, and early morning motor function in patients with Parkinson's disease. *Neuropsychopharmacology* 2003; **28**: 1866–70.
64. Trenkwalder C, Kies B, Rudzinska M, et al. Rotigotine effects on early morning motor function and sleep in Parkinson's disease: a double-blind, randomized, placebo-controlled study (RECOVER). *Mov Disord* 2011; **26**: 90–9.
65. Takanashi M, Shimo Y, Hatano T, Oyama G, Hattori N. Efficacy and safety of a once-daily extended-release formulation of pramipexole switched from an immediate-release formulation in patients with advanced Parkinson's disease: results from an open-label study. *Drug Res (Stuttg)* 2013; **63**: 639–43.
66. Dowling GA, Mastick J, Colling E, et al. Melatonin for sleep disturbances in Parkinson's disease. *Sleep Med* 2005; **6**: 459–66.
67. Medeiros CA, Carvalhedo de Bruin PF, Lopes LA, et al. Effect of exogenous melatonin on sleep and motor dysfunction in Parkinson's disease. A randomized, double blind, placebo-controlled study. *J Neurol* 2007; **254**: 459–64.
68. Abe K, Hikita T, Sakoda S. [A hypnotic drug for sleep disturbances in patients with Parkinson's disease]. *No To Shinkei* 2005; **57**: 301–5 (in Japanese).
69. Juri C, Chana P, Tapia J, Kunstmann C, Parrao T. Quetiapine for insomnia in Parkinson disease: results from an open-label trial. *Clin Neuropharmacol* 2005; **28**: 185–7.
70. Linazasoro G, Marti Masso JF, Suarez JA. Nocturnal akathisia in Parkinson's disease: treatment with clozapine. *Mov Disord* 1993; **8**: 171–4.
71. Seppi K, Weintraub D, Coelho M, et al. The Movement Disorder Society evidence-based medicine review update: treatments for the non-motor symptoms of Parkinson's disease. *Mov Disord* 2011; **26** (Suppl. 3): S42–80.
72. Dresler M, Spoormaker VI, Beitinger P, et al. Neuroscience-driven discovery and development of sleep therapeutics. *Pharmacol Ther* 2013; **141**: 300–4.
73. Rios RS, Creti L, Fichten C, et al. Doxepin and cognitive behavioural therapy for insomnia in patients with Parkinson's disease – a randomized study. *Parkinsonism Relat Disord* 2013; **19**: 670–5.
74. Morgenthaler T, Kramer M, Alessi C, et al. Practice parameters for the psychological and behavioral treatment of insomnia: an update. An American Academy of Sleep Medicine Report. *Sleep* 2006; **29**: 1415–19.
75. Iranzo A, Santamaria J, Rye DB, et al. Characteristics of idiopathic REM sleep behavior disorder and that associated with MSA and PD. *Neurology* 2005; **65**: 247–52.
76. Olson EJ, Boeve BF, Silber MH. Rapid eye movement sleep behaviour disorder: demographic, clinical and laboratory findings in 93 cases. *Brain* 2000; **123**: 331–9.
77. Schmidt MH, Koshal VB, Schmidt HS. Use of pramipexole in REM sleep behavior disorder: results from a case series. *Sleep Med* 2006; **7**: 418–23.

78. Kumru H, Iranzo A, Carrasco E, et al. Lack of effects of pramipexole on REM sleep behavior disorder in Parkinson disease. *Sleep* 2008; **31**: 1418–21.

79. Antonini A, Tesei S, Zecchinelli A, et al. Randomized study of sertraline and low-dose amitriptyline in patients with Parkinson's disease and depression: effect on quality of life. *Mov Disord* 2006; **21**: 1119–22.

80. Kunz D, Mahlberg R. A two-part, double-blind, placebo-controlled trial of exogenous melatonin in REM sleep behaviour disorder. *J Sleep Res* 2010; **19**: 591–6.

81. Kotagal V, Albin RL, Muller ML, et al. Symptoms of rapid eye movement sleep behavior disorder are associated with cholinergic denervation in Parkinson disease. *Ann Neurol* 2012; **71**: 560–8.

82. Nomura T, Kawase S, Watanabe Y, Nakashima K. Use of ramelteon for the treatment of secondary REM sleep behavior disorder. *Intern Med* 2013; **52**: 2123–6.

83. Trotti LM, Bliwise DL. Treatment of the sleep disorders associated with Parkinson's disease. *Neurotherapeutics* 2013; **11**: 68–77.

84. Howell MJ, Arneson PA, Schenck CH. A novel therapy for REM sleep behavior disorder (RBD). *J Clin Sleep Med* 2011; **7**: 639–644A.

85. Bruin VM, Bittencourt LR, Tufik S. Sleep–wake disturbances in Parkinson's disease: current evidence regarding diagnostic and therapeutic decisions. *Eur Neurol* 2012; **67**: 257–67.

86. Giles TL, Lasserson TJ, Smith BH, et al. Continuous positive airways pressure for obstructive sleep apnoea in adults. *Cochrane Database Syst Rev* 2006; CD001106.

87. Högl B, Saletu M, Brandauer E, et al. Modafinil for the treatment of daytime sleepiness in Parkinson's disease: a double-blind, randomized, crossover, placebo-controlled polygraphic trial. *Sleep* 2002; **25**: 905–9.

88. Adler CH, Caviness JN, Hentz JG, Lind M, Tiede J. Randomized trial of modafinil for treating subjective daytime sleepiness in patients with Parkinson's disease. *Mov Disord* 2003; **18**: 287–93.

89. Ondo WG, Fayle R, Atassi F, Jankovic J. Modafinil for daytime somnolence in Parkinson's disease: double blind, placebo controlled parallel trial. *J Neurol Neurosurg Psychiatry* 2005; **76**: 1636–9.

90. Devos D, Krystkowiak P, Clement F, et al. Improvement of gait by chronic, high doses of methylphenidate in patients with advanced Parkinson's disease. *J Neurol Neurosurg Psychiatry* 2007; **78**: 470–5.

91. Postuma RB, Lang AE, Munhoz RP, et al. Caffeine for treatment of Parkinson disease: a randomized controlled trial. *Neurology* 2012; **79**: 651–8.

92. O'suilleabhain PE, Dewey RB, Jr. Contributions of dopaminergic drugs and disease severity to daytime sleepiness in Parkinson disease. *Arch Neurol* 2002; **59**: 986–9.

93. Breen DP, Williams-Gray CH, Mason SL, Foltynie T, Barker RA. Excessive daytime sleepiness and its risk factors in incident Parkinson's disease. *J Neurol Neurosurg Psychiatry* 2013; **84**: 233–4.

94. Fasano A, Daniele A, Albanese A. Treatment of motor and non-motor features of Parkinson's disease with deep brain stimulation. *Lancet Neurol* 2012; **11**: 429–42.

95. Monaca C, Ozsancak C, Jacquesson JM, et al. Effects of bilateral subthalamic stimulation on sleep in Parkinson's disease. *J Neurol* 2004; **251**: 214–8.

96. Iranzo A, Valldeoriola F, Santamaria J, Tolosa E, Rumia J. Sleep symptoms and polysomnographic architecture in advanced Parkinson's disease after chronic bilateral subthalamic stimulation. *J Neurol Neurosurg Psychiatry* 2002; **72**: 661–4.

97. Arnulf I, Bejjani BP, Garma L, et al. Improvement of sleep architecture in PD with subthalamic nucleus stimulation. *Neurology* 2000; **55**: 1732–4.

98. Hjort N, Ostergaard K, Dupont E. Improvement of sleep quality in patients with advanced Parkinson's disease treated with deep brain stimulation of the subthalamic nucleus. *Mov Disord* 2004; **19**: 196–9.

99. Lyons KE, Pahwa R. Effects of bilateral subthalamic nucleus stimulation on sleep, daytime sleepiness, and early morning dystonia in patients with Parkinson disease. *J Neurosurg* 2006; **104**: 502–5.

100. Chahine LM, Ahmed A, Sun Z. Effects of STN DBS for Parkinson's disease on restless legs syndrome and other sleep-related measures. *Parkinsonism Relat Disord* 2011; **17**: 208–11.

101. Driver-Dunckley E, Evidente VG, Adler CH, et al. Restless legs syndrome in Parkinson's disease patients may improve with subthalamic stimulation. *Mov Disord* 2006; **21**: 1287–9.

102. Kedia S, Moro E, Tagliati M, Lang AE, Kumar R. Emergence of restless legs syndrome during subthalamic stimulation for Parkinson disease. *Neurology* 2004; **63**: 2410–12.

Chapter 16

Management of pain and neuromuscular complications in Parkinson's disease

John A. Morren

Introduction

James Parkinson acknowledged the comorbidity of pain in Parkinson's disease (PD) in his original 1817 paper [1]. Although this was also recognized in other early descriptions of PD [2, 3], pain generally garnered little attention among researchers and clinicians over the years. Data shows that about 50% of PD patients with pain do not receive any analgesic treatment [4]. It has been speculated that such underuse may be related to pain underreporting; however, this may reflect the reality that empirically prescribed analgesics are often ineffective for certain pain types in PD.

Based on the projected increase in the prevalence of PD and current rates of nontreatment, it is estimated that by 2030 that there will be 3.7 million PD patients with pain that will remain untreated [5]. Rather recently, pain in PD patients has been recognized as a significant quality-of-life determinant, obligating more attention as it pertains to early recognition and appropriate management.

Although neuromuscular complications with PD seem to be expected, the literature has been deficient in details about the prevalence, risk factors and characteristics of this important group of comorbidities that would also benefit from timely diagnosis and targeted management.

Pain in Parkinson's disease

Pathophysiology

Studies show that pain may represent significant comorbidity in up to 85% of PD patients [4, 6]. Due to several challenges including inconsistencies in methodology, it has been difficult to ascertain whether pain in these studies is definitely related to PD versus other etiologies. It has been proposed that PD-related pain would start after PD diagnosis, respond to antiparkinsonian treatment, be more prominent on the side that is maximally affected by PD and/or represent pain that does not have any reasonable alternative cause [6, 7]. In many studies, it is not clear whether the onset of pain occurred after the diagnosis of PD. However, it has been demonstrated that pain may precede significant motor symptoms and may be the presenting feature, occurring ipsilateral to the side of the body with the first or most severe motor impairments [8].

There is a growing body of evidence implicating a role of the basal ganglia in somatosensory and pain modulation. This confers a function in discriminative, behavioral and cognitive facets of nociceptive processing [9–11]. This has also been the presumed basis for improvement in pain associated with PD in patients after pallidotomy [12] and deep-brain stimulation (DBS) [13]. Greater comprehension of the putative pathophysiological cascade involved in aberrant nociception is gleaned from appraising the role of two distinct pain pathways: the medial and lateral pain systems (see Figure 16.1) [14].

Paleospinothalamic, spinomesencephalic, spinoreticular, spinoparabrachial hypothalamic and spinothalamic tract fibers comprise the medial system. This system participates in the cognitive–evaluative and affective aspects of pain, pain memory and autonomic responses. Even in the presymptomatic stage of PD, before substantia nigra pars compacta neuronal degeneration is appreciable, several structures within the medial pain pathway are the site of neuronal loss and Lewy body development [16].

The neospinothalamic, neotrigeminothalamic, cervical bundle and beam of the dorsal horn comprise the lateral system, which functions in the sensory discriminative component of pain, informing pain localization and duration [16, 17].

Parkinson's Disease: Current and Future Therapeutics and Clinical Trials, ed. Gálvez-Jiménez et al. Published by Cambridge University Press. © Cambridge University Press 2016.

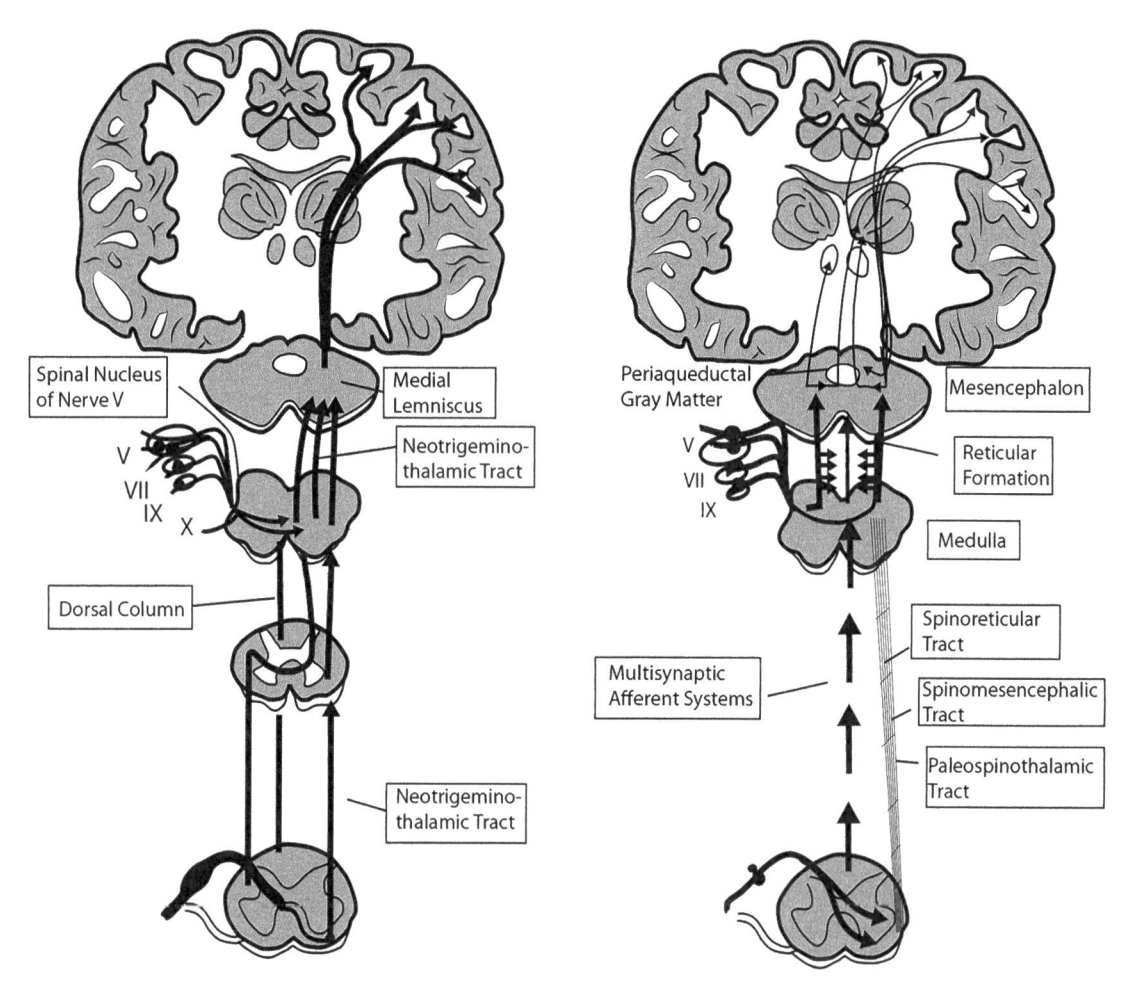

Figure 16.1 Central pain pathways in Parkinson's disease. Left: The lateral system is formed by the neospinothalamic, the neotrigeminothalamic, the cervical bundle and the beam of the dorsal horn whose fibers terminate in the lateral thalamus, the primary and secondary somatosensory areas, the parietal operculum and the insula. Right: The medial system is constituted mainly by the paleospinothalamic, spinomesencephalic, spinoreticular, spinoparabrachial hypothalamic and spinothalamic tract fibers, which terminate in the parabrachial nucleus, the locus coeruleus, the peri-aqueductal gray substance, intralaminar and medial thalamic nuclei, thalamic ventral caudal parvocellular nucleus and ventral caudal portae, the insula, parietal operculum, the secondary somatosensory cortex, the amygdala and the hippocampus.
From Fil et al. [15], by permission from Elsevier.

In PD patients, significant dropout of free nerve endings and Meissner's corpuscle has been demonstrated, independent of age or disease duration [18]. It is postulated that these changes, which comprise a component of deafferentation, contribute to significant sensory dysfunction in PD.

Degenerative changes occurring in the spinal cord, particularly in lamina I of the dorsal horn, have been described early in PD pathogenesis [19]. The serotonergic (including raphe nuclei), noradrenergic (including locus coeruleus) and dopaminergic descending pathway networks originating in the cerebral and brain stem structures participate in the modulation and integration of pain signals processed in the dorsal horn. There is also evidence for glutaminergic and GABAergic involvement [20]. Collectively, these networks up- or downregulate pain gain thresholds [21].

Conceivably, the multifocal neurodegenerative processes in PD may cause damage to many of these pertinent structures participating in nociceptive information relay, modulation, reception and interpretation anywhere along the continuum from peripheral receptors to cerebral centers.

Other data demonstrate that nigrostriatal denervation results in the inhibition of the lateral thalamic region, with consequential reduction in the sensory discriminative dimensions of pain and the potential development of a central pain syndrome [17]. Evidence also suggests that striatum involvement in PD produces disturbance in the emotional registration of pain, as well as the perception of pain intensity [22]. It has been shown that pain occurs more frequently in untreated patient's during their "off" periods, which correlates with low dopaminergic activity in the striatum [22]. Accordingly, dopamine appears to confer an analgesic role through mechanisms in multiple supraspinal structures including the basal ganglia, insula, anterior cingulate cortex, thalamus and periaqueductal gray matter [23]. Not surprisingly, lowered pain thresholds were shown to be normalized after administration of levodopa (L-DOPA), with findings corroborated by positron emission tomography imaging [24]. Of note, other studies have produced less supportive and sometimes conflicting evidence for the effects of dopaminergic activity on pain [25, 26].

Risk factors for pain in Parkinson's disease

Age
This is a somewhat controversial area but there is emerging data suggesting that PD-related pain (especially dystonic pain) is associated with a younger age of onset [7, 27, 28]. Other data suggest no significant association between these two variables [4, 6, 29].

Gender
Studies indicate that mechanical sensitivity is higher in women with PD [30], who may have a predilection to musculoskeletal pain, including neck and lower back pain [4, 31]. Other data appear to dispel significant gender differences [7, 27–29, 32].

Disease severity and duration
Some data have supported a significant relationship between PD disease duration, severity (often reflected by motor symptoms) and the presence of pain [28, 29, 33]. Such findings have not been disclosed by other studies [4, 7, 32].

Depression
In one study that evaluated depression in PD patients with and without pain, the incidence of depression was the same but there was a correlation between pain intensity and the presence of depression [34]. Depression was also more severe in PD patients with pain, compared with those without. Similar correlations have also been seen in a few other studies, but have not been definitely demonstrated in others [29, 32]. The recognition of depression in PD has practical implications since the mood disorder negatively impacts on pain processing and other experiential dimensions but is generally amenable to treatment.

Preexisting comorbidities
The notion that at least some pain in PD is due to non-neurological, age-related changes has been supported in the literature [4, 7] This may be explained in large part by the natural progression of preexisting degenerative musculoskeletal conditions such as osteoarthritis (both appendicular and axial joints), as well as other chronic painful conditions often associated with advancing age (e.g. peripheral neuropathy).

Pain classification and treatment
Pain in PD has been categorized in several ways; however, grouping of sensory and pain symptoms into "primary" (germane to the nervous system) and "secondary" (for all etiologies extrinsic to the nervous system) represents a basic approach [35]. Nociceptive pain can be regarded as pain arising from actual or potential injury to nonneural tissue and is a result of activation of nociceptors [5]. In the PD patient population, neuropathic pain may be defined as pain caused by lesions of the central or peripheral somatosensory system leading to central or peripheral neuropathic pain, respectively. In this scenario, symptoms are thought to arise, at least in part, from altered pain processing [5].

Similarly, pain and sensory symptoms may be broadly attributable to PD (directly) or non-PD causes. There is growing acceptance of a more practical classification scheme that identifies the following categories: musculoskeletal pain, radicular/neuropathic pain, dystonia-related pain, akathitic discomfort/pain and central parkinsonian pain [27, 36]. Pain management options can be usefully arranged according to these groupings (see Table 16.1). For many PD patients, pain symptoms may fall into more than one category [4, 37].

Musculoskeletal pain
Musculoskeletal pain is reported among one-half to two-thirds of PD patients [28, 39]. Symptoms are referable to muscular, truncal and appendicular articular/periarticular discomfort including aching and

Table 16.1 Etiological classification of principal pain syndromes in Parkinson's disease and their practical management

Etiological category	Painful syndromes	Management
Primary pain	Central pain	Dopaminergic therapy (levodopa, dopamine agonists) Anti-inflammatory agents, opioids, antiepileptics, tricyclic, antidepressants and atypical neuroleptics
Secondary pain	Musculoskeletal pain	Musculoskeletal examination, eventually rheumatological/orthopedic evaluation Physical therapy and occupational therapy Medical therapy: dopaminergic therapy (for parkinsonian rigidity and akinesia); anti-inflammatory and analgesic drugs (for rheumatological and orthopedic conditions) Surgical therapy: orthopedic joint surgery if indicated
	Radicular/neuropathic pain	Neurological examination, eventually electrophysiological and imaging investigations Physical and occupational therapy Medical therapy: antidepressants, anticonvulsants, opioid analgesics, non-steroidal anti-inflammatory drugs, also in combination Surgical therapy: decompressive surgery if indicated
	Dystonia-related pain	Evaluation of painful dystonia and its relationship to dopaminergic medication: provide more continuous dopaminergic stimulation Additional medical therapy: anticholinergics, amantadine, injections of botulinum toxin, baclofen
	Pain related to akathisia	Dopaminergic therapy (levodopa, dopamine agonists), opioids, clozapine
	Pain related to restless legs syndrome	Lifestyle changes and activities: decreased use of caffeine, alcohol and tobacco Eventual supplements to correct deficiencies in iron, folate and magnesium A program of moderate exercise and massaging the legs Dopaminergic therapy (dopamine agonists, levodopa); benzodiazepines, opioids, anticonvulsants

From Del Sorbo et al. [38], by permission from Elsevier.

cramping sensations, occurring in the conspicuous absence of definite dystonia. There may be manifestations of preexisting or coexisting rheumatological and orthopedic conditions, such as osteoarthritis or spinal degenerative disease [28]. Pathophysiological biomechanics in PD including rigidity and reduced joint/limb mobility, as well as abnormal posture and gait, have been regarded as major contributing factors [38, 40, 41]. Joints commonly affected by pain include the shoulders, hips, knees and ankles, whereas muscle tightness and cramps are typical complaints in the arm, calf, neck and paraspinal muscles [27].

Musculoskeletal pain treatment is dictated by the specific underlying cause. In instances where parkinsonian rigidity predominates, dopaminergic pharmacotherapy, physical therapy and a customized physical exercise regimen are beneficial. There may be distinct benefits from a passive range of motion exercises aimed at reducing the risk of contractures seen with decreased mobility [36].

Orthopedic and rheumatological comorbidity, which may be exacerbated by uncontrolled PD motor symptoms, is often best managed with the input of the appropriate specialist. There is often a role for analgesics in conjunction with physical therapy – these drugs include nonsteroidal anti-inflammatory agents, acetaminophen and low-potency opioids [42]. There may also be a role for serotonergic and noradrenergic antidepressant medications.

When more conservative measures produce suboptimal results, intra-articular corticosteroid injections, nerve blocks and possibly surgical intervention may be exploited.

Dystonic pain

This pain subtype is seen in up to 70% of PD patients [7, 29], and may be among the most painful symptoms a PD patient may experience. The culprit dystonia may be due to PD itself, or may be the adverse effects of therapy with dopaminergic agents or DBS. Dystonia in this context is often focal or regional. The foot is often involved in early-onset PD, with prominent toe cramping, usually early in the morning [43]. With many patients, exacerbations tend also to occur late in the dosing interval when dopaminergic effects are wearing off. Conversely, about one-third of patients on long-term levodopa therapy may have significant dystonia during their "on" periods [44].

For dystonia that is attributable to a decrement in dopaminergic drug effects, several approaches to reduce the "off" period may be beneficial. These include earlier or preemptive dosing of levodopa, using controlled-release formulations, or employing longer-acting dopamine agonists [45]. The severity of early-morning dystonia in some cases may warrant the use of subcutaneous apomorphine, which confers a rapid therapeutic effect. Other dopaminergic strategies to avoid these untoward effects during the "off" periods have utilized continuous infusion of duodenal levodopa [46], intranasal or subcutaneous apomorphine [47], transdermal rotigotine [48] and lisuride infusion [49]. Other pharmacological agents that are not primarily dopaminergic but may be used empirically for "off"-period dystonia include benzodiazepines, baclofen and lithium. Focal dystonia may also be amenable to botulinum toxin injections [50, 51], and further uses in PD patients are being explored in clinical trials.

The nonpharmacological treatment of pain associated with focal dystonia includes DBS of the subthalamic nucleus (STN) [52–54] or globus pallidus internus (GPi) [13] targets. Repetitive transcranial magnetic stimulation is a promising modality in development that is further discussed below.

Peak-dose dystonia requires a different strategy, often necessitating a reduction of the levodopa/dopaminergic agent dose. Dystonic dyskinesias may respond to amantadine [55, 56] or low-dose clozapine [57], and a therapeutic trial of these agents may be worth considering.

Radicular/neuropathic pain

This type of pain is localized to a spinal root or peripheral nerve territory. This pattern of nerve injury may be seen in up to 25% of PD patients with pain [7, 38]. The literature espouses that median neuropathy at the wrist (carpal tunnel syndrome) is seen more commonly in PD patients [58]. A predilection to other entrapment or compression syndromes in PD, such as that involving the radial nerve, has been less robustly supported through case series [59, 60]. In some patients, these neuropathies may represent chronic sequelae of limb immobility and arrested positions while being wheelchair- or bed-bound. The repeated trauma conceivable from the repetitive movement of tremor may be another contributory mechanism. The adverse motor milieu in PD (including rigidity, tremor, akinesia/bradykinesia, dystonia, camptocormia, and festination) is believed to promote structural stresses and maladaptations affecting the spine and appendicular musculoskeletal system that places nerve roots and peripheral nerves at increased risk for compression and/or entrapment. Evaluation of pertinent symptoms should prompt a workup that may include electromyography (EMG) and/or neuromuscular ultrasound, as well as other neuroimaging, which may demonstrate lesions amenable to release/decompression surgery.

Back pain with or without radicular pain is more prevalent in PD patients compared with controls [41]. Data also suggest that radicular pain is more prevalent in PD patients (14–35%) [61] compared with the general population (10%) [41]. Accompanying radicular symptoms may also necessitate electrodiagnostic and neuroimaging evaluation, and findings may inform a decision about spine surgery.

It has been shown that peripheral neuropathy is seen more commonly in PD patients, and various associations/risk factors have been implicated, including the use of amantadine [62], cumulative dose effects of levodopa and low vitamin B12 levels [63, 64].

If pain appears to correlate strongly with "off" periods, then a trial of dopaminergic therapy would be a reasonable endeavor. The pharmacological approaches to management of radicular or neuropathic pain in PD is not very different from that in other patients. Agents include tricyclic antidepressants (e.g. amitriptyline, nortriptyline, desipramine), serotonin and norepinephrine reuptake inhibitors (e.g. venlafaxine, duloxetine), calcium-channel $\alpha 2\delta$ ligands (e.g. gabapentin and pregabalin), topical lidocaine and opioids (sparingly).

Akathitic discomfort/pain

Akathisia is characterized by a subjective restlessness and uncomfortable urge or impulse to move persistently, producing an intolerance of remaining still. This usually responds to levodopa and other dopaminergic treatments, especially when it occurs prominently in the "off" period [36]. Clozapine may be additionally helpful [65]. Restless legs syndrome (RLS) may also be present in PD patients and potentially represents another source of discomfort. Symptoms tend more commonly to involve the lower limbs and are generally worse at night. Restless legs syndrome appears to be more prevalent among PD patients, at 8–20% [66, 67] compared with 1% [66] in the general population. Treatment for RLS in this context would typically comprise levodopa and/or a dopamine agonist. The use of pramipexole and ropinirole in this context has not been studied in a controlled trial, although they are approved for the treatment of RLS in the general population.

Central pain

Central pain occurs when there is a primary lesion or dysfunction in the central nervous system. It has been reported in 10–12% of PD patients [4, 32]. The poorly localizable pain is typically severe and often has a quality of tingling, burning or itching, or it may have an autonomic or visceral character that usually prompts uninformative investigations. It may be the basis for several bizarre pain manifestations that can be seen in PD involving the face/head, mouth/throat, chest, abdomen, pelvis and genitalia [68].

This pain type is relatively uncommon and, although is not thought to be due to dystonia or rigidity, it tends to coincide with motor fluctuations, being more prominent in "off" periods. On this basis, it is thought to be a consequence of dysfunction in dopaminergic autonomic centers, which may also play a role in pain control [69].

Treatment with dopaminergic agents is usually beneficial. In cases with a poor response to this first-line approach, conventional analgesics, atypical antipsychotics (e.g. clozapine), tricyclic antidepressants and opioids may be beneficial. Opioid use in PD patients should always be exercised with fair caution, given the potential to exacerbate parkinsonism, especially at higher doses. There may be pain improvement utilizing STN-DBS; however, the available evidence on this is sometimes conflicting [54, 70].

Due to interplay between chronic pain and depression, the treatment of any comorbid depression (seen in about 40–50% of PD patients) [71] is quite important in a pain management strategy. Antidepressants with overlap indication for the particular subtype of the pain (e.g. neuropathic) should be used if possible. Psychotherapy may also constitute part of the multimodal therapy that is beneficial in the management of both depression and pain.

Duloxetine, a serotonin and norepinephrine reuptake inhibitor known to exhibit both antidepressant and analgesic properties, was evaluated in an open-label study recruiting PD patients having pain excluding that associated with dystonia, limb rigidity, nocturnal muscle spasm or lumbago, as well as non-PD-related pain (e.g. post-stroke central pain) [72]. Duloxetine 60 mg daily for 6 weeks was used, and pain relief was seen in 65% of patients. Interestingly, the pain threshold, depression and quality-of-life measures were not significantly affected. More robustly designed future trials would be helpful in better defining the potential benefits of duloxetine for pain in PD patients.

Choosing an analgesic medication with pleiotropic effects may increase the chance of improving health-related quality of life, as opposed to choosing a pain medication without other actions.

Nonpharmacological management

To more comprehensively address pain in PD, a multidisciplinary approach employing medications as well as nonpharmacological management modalities is required.

Physical therapy and exercise programs that may be beneficial include aerobic exercises, systematic stretching, and strength and balance training. Relevant cautionary measures should be taken, given the inherently increased fall risk in the PD patient population. Exercise in this context has been shown to improve physical functioning, leg strength, balance, gait and overall health-related quality-of-life measures [73]. There is also data that purport a pain improvement benefit, especially with musculoskeletal type pain [74].

Complementary and alternative medicine modalities for pain in PD patients include homeopathy, "traditional medicine," acupuncture and massage. These options are usually sought when the response to more conventional approaches is suboptimal [75]. Data indicate an effective reduction of stiffness and pain in PD patients receiving massage therapy [76] and acupuncture [77, 78].

The effects of DBS and other stereotactic brain surgeries on the various PD pain subtypes have been evaluated in a few studies [12, 53, 79]. Investigators have shown a significant reduction in musculoskeletal and dystonic-type pain with DBS targeting the bilateral STNs [53, 79]. However, this treatment appeared to be associated with increased risk for postoperative deterioration in radicular/peripheral neuropathic pain and spine disease-related back pain [53]. There have also been reports of significantly reduced PD-related pain in patients receiving unilateral pallidotomy [12].

Prospective analgesic therapies

Repetitive transcranial magnetic stimulation (rTMS) is an emerging modality that has been producing promising results [80, 81]. The precise mechanism of action of rTMS is not fully understood, but data show that, when applied over the primary motor cortex, there is modulation of the activity in pain-processing areas including the thalamus, the insular cortex and the anterior cingulate cortex [82]. There may be downstream involvement of the endogenous opioid system [83].

Cranial electrotherapy stimulation is another non-invasive modality that involves the application of a small electrical current through the head utilizing ear-clip electrodes. Cranial electrotherapy stimulation was shown to produce significant analgesic effects in a randomized, double-blind, placebo-controlled, non-PD sample [84]. The therapy was also investigated in a sample of 13 PD patients with pain [85]. Pain among those enrolled was not necessarily PD related. In this double-blinded study, participants were randomized to either an active or sham device, which they used for 40 min daily over 6 weeks. Although patients assigned to the active-treatment arm had higher PD motor impairment scores and a longer disease duration, they obtained significantly greater pain reduction compared with the sham group. No serious study-related adverse events were reported. Cranial electrotherapy stimulation may represent another nonpharmacological option that confers particular advantage to this patient population, which is already at risk for polypharmacy.

Other neuromuscular complications in Parkinson's disease

As previously alluded to, various mechanical stressors seen in PD may place patients at significantly increased risk for various peripheral nerve injuries. These stressors include repetitive involuntary motion, increased appendicular and axial tone, relative immobility and contractures. Peripheral nerve injuries may also result from injuries sustained with falls, to which PD patients are particularly susceptible.

There are data describing peripheral nerve injuries in other movement disorders. For example, secondary cervical radiculopathy has been found in up to 32% of patients with cervical dystonia [86]. However, the literature is quite deficient in the description of peripheral nerve injuries among PD patients.

In a study of 1087 PD patients, a diagnosis consistent with peripheral nerve injuries was found in 4.8% [87]. Among those with electrodiagnostic confirmation (42%), radiculopathies, mononeuropathies and peripheral polyneuropathy were seen in equal proportions (41% for each). Most commonly seen were L5–S1 radiculopathies and peripheral polyneuropathy with evidence of active/ongoing denervation, as well as severe median neuropathies at or distal to the wrist (carpal tunnel syndrome).

Entrapment mononeuropathies may be an initiating factor in the development of limb deformities in patients with late-stage parkinsonism [59]. This was illustrated in a case series of four patients with advanced PD demonstrating radial compression neuropathy and flexion deformity of the wrist and hand [59]. The common contributing factor appeared to be advance chronic motor disability with wheelchair or bed confinement. In this scenario, preventative measures include frequent position changes and avoidance of sleeping in wheelchairs. To help prevent the development of a fixed flexion wrist deformity, the use of a wrist splint is also recommended.

More recently, it has been shown that neuropathy is more prevalent in PD patients, and prolonged levodopa therapy as well as vitamin B12 deficiency may be further implicated [64, 88]. One study disclosed peripheral neuropathy in 55% of PD patients and described a correlation between cumulative levodopa exposure and neuropathy severity [64].

Rajabally and Martey found neuropathy in 37.8% of PD patients versus 8.1% in age- and gender-matched controls [63]. Cumulative levodopa exposure correlated with the duration of PD and vitamin B12 levels in PD patients with neuropathy. The precise pathophysiological details have not yet been elucidated, but it is believed that genetically predisposed PD patients may develop levodopa-induced vitamin B12 deficiency with consequential neurotoxic accumulation of methylmalonic acid [Figure 16.2]. On the basis of their findings, the investigators advised that vitamin B12 monitoring and supplementation, as well as serial clinical assessments for neuropathy be conducted in PD patients [89].

Several case reports of peripheral neuropathy have also been described in association with continuous intraduodenal infusion of levodopa/carbidopa intestinal gel (LCIG) [91, 92]. These were often associated with vitamin B12 [90, 91, 93, 94] and/or B6 deficiency, and less commonly folate deficiency [90, 93, 94]. Peripheral

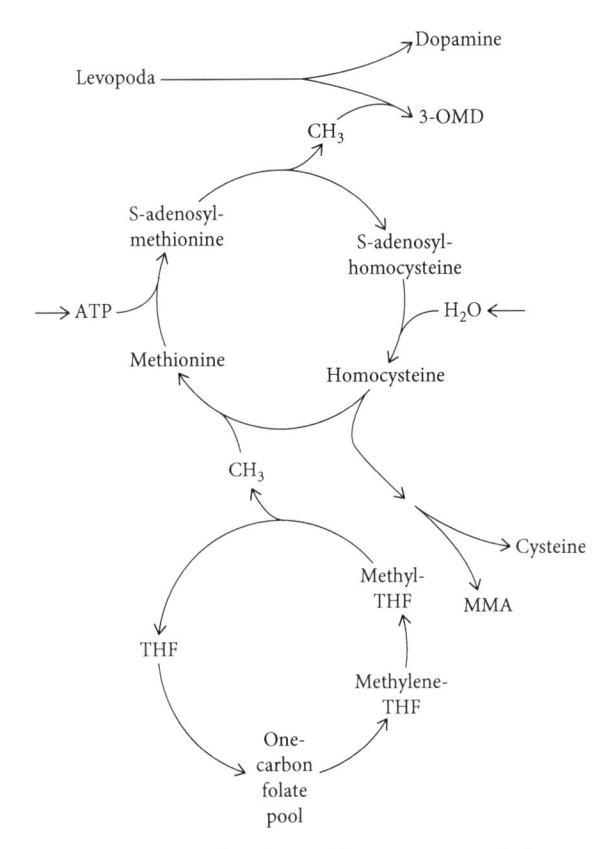

Figure 16.2 Facets of levodopa and homocysteine metabolism hypothesized to be relevant to peripheral neuropathy in patients with Parkinson's disease. Conversion of levodopa into 3-*O*-methyldopa (3-OMD) depletes methyl-group (CH$_3$) reserves and leads to homocysteine production. Subsequent homocysteine remethylation (into methionine) requires vitamin B12 (cobalamin) as a cofactor and obtains its CH$_3$ from the one-carbon folate pool. Involvement of methylenetetrahydrofolate (methylene-THF) in supplying the CH$_3$ makes polymorphism in methylene-THF reductase an important determinant of plasma homocysteine level. Homocysteine *trans*-sulfuration (into cysteine) requires vitamin B6 (pyridoxine). A pathway leading to methylmalonic acid (MMA) makes MMA as well as homocysteine a marker of functional vitamin B12 deficiency. ATP, adenosine triphosphate.
From Müller *et al.* [90], by permission from Elsevier.

neuropathy onset may occur from a few weeks to up to 3 years after LCIG is initiated [89]. Nerve conduction studies disclosed both axon loss and demyelinating features, and a Guillain–Barré-like phenotype is possible [89]. Generally, there is symptomatic improvement after discontinuation or dose modification of LCIG, vitamin B supplementation or both [90, 93, 94].

There is also some evidence to suggest that other PD medications like amantadine may contribute to peripheral neuropathy [62].

Identification of peripheral nerve injuries in PD patients is necessary for appropriate and timely workup and management. With the proper index of suspicion, detection of radiculopathies, mononeuropathies and peripheral neuropathies can be made earlier when appropriate medication changes, orthotics (including splints and bracing), customized physical therapy and/or decompressive surgery may be implemented.

Conclusion

Although there has been some recent increase in the literature relating to pain in PD, treatment recommendations are often based on anecdotal evidence and expert opinion. This is a major reason for the general lack of consensus in this area. Apart from the under-recognition of pain itself as a common nonmotor PD symptom, there is also poor appreciation of the various pain subtypes. Classifying pain is useful in choosing the appropriate workup and management options (both pharmacological and nonpharmacological) that are most likely to be successful. With the approach to pain subtype recognition as discussed, the clinician can be mindful in selecting treatment along the lines of anti-parkinsonism, antinociceptive and antineuropathic options.

The data demonstrate a correlation between pain, sleep disturbance and depression in PD patients [34, 95]. These determinants tend to feed into a positive feedback loop and auger poorly for quality-of-life measures [96, 97]. When both early and late PD duration groups were studied to determine their subjective experience of problems in order of importance, both cohorts indicated pain as one of their top nonmotor complaints [98]. Better pain control goes beyond analgesia, since benefits are likely to accrue in other spheres of well-being that ultimately improve health-related quality of life.

In many cases, pain symptoms are best managed in a multidisciplinary context, obtaining input from physical therapists and other specialties including orthopedics, spine medicine, rheumatology, neurosurgery and pain management. The patient's primary care physician also has a role with other aspects of health promotion and, when indicated, the treatment of depression. Depression management may also require the involvement of a psychiatrist and psychologist.

As we move toward unveiling more details in the pathophysiological cascade of pain in PD, it is hopeful that future treatments will be more targeted and more effective therapies emerge. Prospective nonpharmacological modalities such as rTMS and cranial electrotherapy stimulation, as well as new applications of

DBS, may offer pain treatment without further increasing the pill burden on patients.

The progress in this field may come about with appropriate improvements in research study design and methodologies including multicenter involvement with similar or standardized protocols. For future trials, useful standardized core outcome measures may include pain subtype, rated pain intensity, physical functioning, emotional functioning, safety and health-related quality-of-life measures, as well as metrics for capturing patients' overall impression of treatment effects [5].

The early identification and timely management of neuromuscular complications in PD patients may positively impact on the burden of illness, mitigate disability and ultimately also lead to improved quality-of-life measures in this particularly vulnerable population.

References

1. Parkinson J. *An Essay on the Shaking Palsy*. London: Whittingham and Rowland. 1817.
2. Charcot J. *Lectures on Diseases of the Nervous System*. London: The New Sydenham Society. 1877.
3. Gowers W. *A Manual of Disease of the Nervous System*. Philadelphia: Blakiston. 1888.
4. Beiske AG, Loge JH, Rønningen A, Svensson E. Pain in Parkinson's disease: prevalence and characteristics. *Pain* 2009; **141**: 173–7.
5. Perez-Lloret S, Rey MV, Dellapina E, et al. Emerging analgesic drugs for Parkinson's disease. *Expert Opin Emerg Drugs* 2012; **17**: 157–71.
6. Lee MA, Walker RW, Hildreth TJ, Prentice WM. A survey of pain in idiopathic Parkinson's disease. *J Pain Symptom Manage* 2006; **32**: 462–9.
7. Defazio G, Berardelli A, Fabbrini G, et al. Pain as a nonmotor symptom of Parkinson disease: evidence from a case–control study. *Arch Neurol* 2008; **65**: 1191–4.
8. O'sullivan SS, Williams DR, Gallagher DA, et al. Nonmotor symptoms as presenting complaints in Parkinson's disease: a clinicopathological study. *Mov Disord* 2008; **23**: 101–6.
9. Burkey AR, Carstens E, Jasmin L. Dopamine reuptake inhibition in the rostral agranular insular cortex produces antinociception. *J Neurosci* 1999; **19**: 4169–79.
10. Barnes CD, Fung SJ, Adams WL. Inhibitory effects of substantia nigra on impulse transmission from nociceptors. *Pain* 1979; **6**: 207–15.
11. Chudler EH, Dong WK. The role of the basal ganglia in nociception and pain. *Pain* 1995; **60**: 3–38.
12. Honey CR, Stoessl AJ, Tsui JK, Schulzer M, Calne DB. Unilateral pallidotomy for reduction of parkinsonian pain. *J Neurosurg* 1999; **91**: 198–201.
13. Loher TJ, Burgunder JM, Weber S, Sommerhalder R, Krauss JK. Effect of chronic pallidal deep brain stimulation on off period dystonia and sensory symptoms in advanced Parkinson's disease. *J Neurol Neurosurg Psychiatry* 2002; **73**: 395–9.
14. Fil A, Cano-de-la-Cuerda R, Muñoz-Hellín E, et al. Pain in Parkinson disease: a review of the literature. *Parkinsonism Relat Disord* 2013; **19**: 285–94; discussion 285.
15. Willis WD, Westlund KN. Neuroanatomy of the pain system and of the pathways that modulate pain. *J Clin Neurophysiol* 1997; **14**: 2–31.
16. Braak H, Del Tredici K, Rüb U, et al. Staging of brain pathology related to sporadic Parkinson's disease. *Neurobiol Aging* 24: 197–211.
17. Scherder E, Wolters E, Polman C, Sergeant J, Swaab D. Pain in Parkinson's disease and multiple sclerosis: its relation to the medial and lateral pain systems. *Neurosci Biobehav Rev* 2005; **29**: 1047–56.
18. Nolano M, Provitera V, Estraneo A, et al. Sensory deficit in Parkinson's disease: evidence of a cutaneous denervation. *Brain* 2008; **131**: 1903–11.
19. Braak H, Sastre M, Bohl JRE, de Vos RAI, Del Tredici K. Parkinson's disease: lesions in dorsal horn layer I, involvement of parasympathetic and sympathetic pre- and postganglionic neurons. *Acta Neuropathol* 2007; **113**: 421–9.
20. Barone P. Neurotransmission in Parkinson's disease: beyond dopamine. *Eur J Neurol* 2010; **17**: 364–76.
21. Millan MJ. The induction of pain: an integrative review. *Prog Neurobiol* 1999; **57**: 1–164.
22. Juri C, Rodriguez-Oroz M, Obeso JA. The pathophysiological basis of sensory disturbances in Parkinson's disease. *J Neurolog Sci* 2010; **289**: 60–5.
23. Wood PB. Role of central dopamine in pain and analgesia. *Expert Rev Neurother* 2008; **8**: 781–97.
24. Brefel-Courbon C, Payoux P, Thalamas C, et al. Effect of levodopa on pain threshold in Parkinson's disease: a clinical and positron emission tomography study. *Mov Disord* 2005; **20**: 1557–63.
25. Djaldetti R, Shifrin A, Rogowski Z, et al. Quantitative measurement of pain sensation in patients with Parkinson disease. *Neurology* 2004; **62**: 2171–5.
26. Dellapina E, Gerdelat-Mas A, Ory-Magne F, et al. Apomorphine effect on pain threshold in Parkinson's disease: a clinical and positron emission tomography study. *Mov Disord* 2011; **26**: 153–7.
27. Goetz CG, Tanner CM, Levy M, Wilson RS, Garron DC. Pain in Parkinson's disease. *Mov Disord* 1986; **1**: 45–9.

28. Nègre-Pagès L, Regragui W, Bouhassira D, Grandjean H, Rascol O. Chronic pain in Parkinson's disease: the cross-sectional French DoPaMiP survey. *Mov Disord* 2008; **23**: 1361–9.

29. Tinazzi M, Del Vesco C, Fincati E, et al. Pain and motor complications in Parkinson's disease. *J Neurol Neurosurg Psychiatry* 2006; **77**: 822–5.

30. Rollman GB, Lautenbacher S. Sex differences in musculoskeletal pain. *Clin J Pain* 2001; **17**: 20–4.

31. Scott B, Borgman A, Engler H, Johnels B, Aquilonius SM. Gender differences in Parkinson's disease symptom profile. *Acta Neurol Scand* 2000; **102**: 37–43.

32. Hanagasi HA, Akat S, Gurvit H, Yazici J, Emre M. Pain is common in Parkinson's disease. *Clin Neurol Neurosurg* 2011; **113**: 11–13.

33. Ehrt U, Larsen JP, Aarsland D. Pain and its relationship to depression in Parkinson disease. *Am J Geriatr Psychiatry* 2009; **17**: 269–75.

34. Goetz CG, Wilson RS, Tanner CM, Garron DC. Relationships among pain, depression, and sleep alterations in Parkinson's disease. *Adv Neurol* 1987; **45**: 345–7.

35. Snider SR, Fahn S, Isgreen WP, Cote LJ. Primary sensory symptoms in parkinsonism. *Neurology* 1976; **26**: 423–9.

36. Ford B. Pain in Parkinson's disease. *Mov Disord* 2010; **25**(Suppl. 1): S98–103.

37. Del Sorbo F, Albanese A. Clinical management of pain and fatigue in Parkinson's disease. *Parkinsonism Relat Disord* 2012; **18** (Suppl. 1): S233–6.

38. Bissonnette B. Pseudorheumatoid deformity of the feet associated with parkinsonism. *J Rheumatol* 1986; **13**: 825–6.

39. Santos-García D, Abella-Corral J, Aneiros-Díaz Á, et al. [Pain in Parkinson's disease: prevalence, characteristics, associated factors, and relation with other non motor symptoms, quality of life, autonomy, and caregiver burden]. *Rev Neurol* 2011; **52**: 385–93 (in Spanish).

40. Duvoisin RC, Marsden CD. Note on the scoliosis of Parkinsonism. *J Neurol Neurosurg Psychiatry* 1975; **38**: 787–93.

41. Broetz D, Eichner M, Gasser T, Weller M, Steinbach JP. Radicular and nonradicular back pain in Parkinson's disease: a controlled study. *Mov Disord* 2007; **22**: 853–6.

42. Schnitzer TJ. Update on guidelines for the treatment of chronic musculoskeletal pain. *Clin Rheumatol* 2006; **25** (Suppl. 1): S22–9.

43. Tolosa E, Compta Y. Dystonia in Parkinson's disease. *J Neurol* 2006; **253** (Suppl. VII): 7–13.

44. Kidron D, Melamed E. Forms of dystonia in patients with Parkinson's disease. *Neurology* 1987; **37**: 1009–11.

45. Sophie M, Ford B. Management of pain in Parkinson's disease. *CNS Drugs* 2012; **26**: 937–48.

46. Karlsborg M, Korbo L, Regeur L, Glad A. Duodopa pump treatment in patients with advanced Parkinson's disease. *Dan Med Bull* 2010; **57**: A4155.

47. Lees AJ. Dopamine agonists in Parkinson's disease: a look at apomorphine. *Fundam Clin Pharmacol* 1993; **7**: 121–8.

48. Sanford M, Scott LJ. Rotigotine transdermal patch: a review of its use in the treatment of Parkinson's disease. *CNS Drugs* 2011; **25**: 699–719.

49. Stocchi F, Ruggieri S, Antonini A, et al. Subcutaneous lisuride infusion in Parkinson's disease: clinical results using different modes of administration. *J Neural Transm Suppl* 1988; **27**: 27–33.

50. Cordivari C, Misra VP, Catania S, Lees AJ. Treatment of dystonic clenched fist with botulinum toxin. *Mov Disord* 2001; **16**: 907–13.

51. Pacchetti C, Albani G, Martignoni E, et al. "Off" painful dystonia in Parkinson's disease treated with botulinum toxin. *Mov Disord* 1995; **10**: 333–6.

52. Kim HJ, Jeon BS, Paek SH. Effect of deep brain stimulation on pain in Parkinson disease. *J Neurolog Sci* 2011; **310**: 251–5.

53. Oshima H, Katayama Y, Morishita T, et al. Subthalamic nucleus stimulation for attenuation of pain related to Parkinson disease. *J Neurosurg* 2012; **116**: 99–106.

54. Witjas T, Kaphan E, Régis J, et al. Effects of chronic subthalamic stimulation on nonmotor fluctuations in Parkinson's disease. *Mov Disord* 2007; **22**: 1729–34.

55. Thomas A, Iacono D, Luciano AL, et al. Duration of amantadine benefit on dyskinesia of severe Parkinson's disease. *J Neurol Neurosurg Psychiatry* 2004; **75**: 141–3.

56. Metman LV, Del Dotto P, LePoole K, et al. Amantadine for levodopa-induced dyskinesias: a 1-year follow-up study. *Arch Neurol* 1999; **56**: 1383–6.

57. Durif F. Foot dystonia treatment by botulinum toxin injections in Parkinson disease: efficiency of injections made in extrinsic muscle (flexor digitorum longus muscle) compared to intrinsic muscle (flexor digitorum brevis or quadratus plantae muscles) (RBHP 2008). *ClinicalTrials.gov*, 2009; NCT00909883. Available from: http://clinicaltrials.gov/ct2/show/NCT00909883?term=botulinum+pain+parkinson's&rank=1.

58. Yucel A, Yilmaz O, Babaoglu S, Acar M, Degirmenci B. Sonographic findings of the median nerve and prevalence of carpal tunnel syndrome in patients with Parkinson's disease. *Eur J Radiol* 2008; **67**: 546–50.

59. Preston DN, Grimes JD. Radial compression neuropathy in advanced Parkinson's disease. *Arch Neurol* 1985; **42**: 695–6.

60. Kurlan R, Baker P, Miller C, Shoulson I. Severe compression neuropathy following sudden onset of parkinsonian immobility. *Arch Neurol* 1985; **42**: 720.

61. Wasner G, Deuschl G. Pains in Parkinson disease – many syndromes under one umbrella. *Nature reviews. Neurology* 2012; **8**: 284–94.
62. Shulman LM, Minagar A, Sharma K, Weiner WJ. Amantadine-induced peripheral neuropathy. *Neurology* 1999; **53**: 1862–5.
63. Rajabally YA, Martey J. Neuropathy in Parkinson disease: prevalence and determinants. *Neurology* 2011; **77**: 1947–50.
64. Toth C, Breithaupt K, Ge S, et al. Levodopa, methylmalonic acid, and neuropathy in idiopathic Parkinson disease. *Ann Neurol* 2010; **68**: 28–36.
65. Comella CL, Goetz CG. Akathisia in Parkinson's disease. *Mov Disord* 1994; **9**: 545–9.
66. Krishnan PR, Bhatia M, Behari M. Restless legs syndrome in Parkinson's disease: a case-controlled study. *Mov Disord* 2003; **18**: 181–5.
67. Ondo WG, Vuong KD, Jankovic J. Exploring the relationship between Parkinson disease and restless legs syndrome. *Arch Neurol* 2002; **59**: 421–4.
68. Ford B, Louis ED, Greene P, Fahn S. Oral and genital pain syndromes in Parkinson's disease. *Mov Disord* 1996; **11**: 421–6.
69. Schestatsky P, Kumru H, Valls-Solé J, et al. Neurophysiologic study of central pain in patients with Parkinson disease. *Neurology* 2007; **69**: 2162–9.
70. Gierthmühlen J, Arning P, Binder A, et al. Influence of deep brain stimulation and levodopa on sensory signs in Parkinson's disease. *Mov Disord* 2010; **25**: 1195–202.
71. Allain H, Schuck S, Mauduit N. Depression in Parkinson's disease. *BMJ* 2000; **320**: 1287–8.
72. Djaldetti R, Yust-Katz S, Kolianov V, Melamed E, Dabby R. The effect of duloxetine on primary pain symptoms in Parkinson disease. *Clin Neuropharmacol* **30**: 201–5.
73. Goodwin VA, Richards SH, Taylor RS, Taylor AH, Campbell JL. The effectiveness of exercise interventions for people with Parkinson's disease: a systematic review and meta-analysis. *Mov Disord* 2008; **23**: 631–40.
74. Reuter I, Mehnert S, Leone P, et al. Effects of a flexibility and relaxation programme, walking, and nordic walking on Parkinson's disease. *J Aging Res* 2011; **2011**: 232473.
75. Ferry P, Johnson M, Wallis P. Use of complementary therapies and non-prescribed medication in patients with Parkinson's disease. *Postgrad Med J* 2002; **78**: 612–4.
76. Kim SR, Lee TY, Kim MS, Lee MC, Chung SJ. Use of complementary and alternative medicine by Korean patients with Parkinson's disease. *Clin Neurol Neurosurg* 2009; **111**: 156–60.
77. Cristian A, Katz M, Cutrone E, Walker RH. Evaluation of acupuncture in the treatment of Parkinson's disease: a double-blind pilot study. *Mov Disord* 2005; **20**: 1185–8.
78. Shulman LM, Wen X, Weiner WJ, et al. Acupuncture therapy for the symptoms of Parkinson's disease. *Mov Disord* 2002; **17**: 799–802.
79. Kim HJ, Paek SH, Kim JY, et al. Chronic subthalamic deep brain stimulation improves pain in Parkinson disease. *J Neurol* 2008; **255**: 1889–94.
80. Lomarev MP, Kanchana S, Bara-Jimenez W, et al. Placebo-controlled study of rTMS for the treatment of Parkinson's disease. *Mov Disord* 2006; **21**: 325–31.
81. Kodama M, Kasahara T, Hyodo M, et al. Effect of low-frequency repetitive transcranial magnetic stimulation combined with physical therapy on L-dopa-induced painful off-period dystonia in Parkinson's disease. *Am J Phys Med Rehabil* 2011; **90**: 150–5.
82. Bestmann S, Baudewig J, Siebner HR, Rothwell JC, Frahm J. Functional MRI of the immediate impact of transcranial magnetic stimulation on cortical and subcortical motor circuits. *Eur J Neurosci* 2004; **19**: 1950–62.
83. Maarrawi J, Peyron R, Mertens P, et al. Motor cortex stimulation for pain control induces changes in the endogenous opioid system. *Neurology* 2007; **69**: 827–34.
84. Gabis L, Shklar B, Baruch YK, et al. Pain reduction using transcranial electrostimulation: a double blind "active placebo" controlled trial. *J Rehabil Med* 2009; **41**: 256–61.
85. Rintala DH, Tan G, Willson P, Bryant MS, Lai ECH. Feasibility of using cranial electrotherapy stimulation for pain in persons with Parkinson's disease. *Parkinsons Dis* 2010; **2010**: 569154.
86. Jankovic J, Leder S, Warner D, Schwartz K. Cervical dystonia: clinical findings and associated movement disorders. *Neurology* 1991; **41**: 1088–91.
87. Morren JA, Lugo R, Gálvez-jiménez N. EMG findings in Parkinson's disease patients with peripheral nerve injuries. In: The Movement Disorder Society's 15th International Congress of Parkinson's Disease and Movement Disorders, Toronto, Abstact 809, 2011.
88. Toth C, Brown MS, Furtado S, Suchowersky O, Zochodne D. Neuropathy as a potential complication of levodopa use in Parkinson's disease. *Mov Disord* 2008; **23**: 1850–9.
89. Müller T, van Laar T, Cornblath DR, et al. Peripheral neuropathy in Parkinson's disease: levodopa exposure and implications for duodenal delivery. *Parkinsonism Relat Disord* 2013; **19**: 501–7; discussion 501.
90. Urban PP, Wellach I, Faiss S, et al. Subacute axonal neuropathy in Parkinson's disease with cobalamin and vitamin B6 deficiency under duodopa therapy. *Mov Disord* 2010; **25**: 1748–52.
91. Manca D, Cossu G, Murgia D, et al. Reversible encephalopathy and axonal neuropathy in Parkinson's disease during duodopa therapy. *Mov Disord* 2009; **24**: 2293–4.

92. Antonini A, Isaias IU, Canesi M, *et al.* Duodenal levodopa infusion for advanced Parkinson's disease: 12-month treatment outcome. *Mov Disord* 2007; **22**: 1145–9.

93. Klostermann F, Jugel C, Müller T, Marzinzik F. Malnutritional neuropathy under intestinal levodopa infusion. *J Neural Transm* 2012; **119**: 369–72.

94. Meppelink AM, Nyman R, van Laar T, *et al.* Transcutaneous port for continuous duodenal levodopa/carbidopa administration in Parkinson's disease. *Mov Disord* 2011; **26**: 331–4.

95. van Hilten JJ, Weggeman M, van der Velde EA, *et al.* Sleep, excessive daytime sleepiness and fatigue in Parkinson's disease. *J Neural Transm* 1993; **5**: 235–44.

96. Quittenbaum BH, Grahn B. Quality of life and pain in Parkinson's disease: a controlled cross-sectional study. *Parkinsonism Relat Disord* 2004; **10**: 129–36.

97. Caap-Ahlgren M, Dehlin O. Insomnia and depressive symptoms in patients with Parkinson's disease. Relationship to health-related quality of life. An interview study of patients living at home. *Arch Gerontol Geriatr* 2001; **32**: 23–33.

98. Politis M, Wu K, Molloy S, *et al.* Parkinson's disease symptoms: the patient's perspective. *Mov Disord* 2010; **25**: 1646–51.

Section III Surgical Management of Parkinson's Disease

Chapter 17

Thalamotomy, pallidotomy and subthalamotomy in the management of Parkinson's disease

Malco Rossi, Daniel Cerquetti, Jorge Mandolesi and Marcelo Merello

Introduction

Surgery for movement disorders, especially for "athetosis" and parkinsonism, was introduced mainly by Leriche, Foerster, Putnam, Meyers and Bucy at the end of the 19th century and beginning of the 20th. They included posterior rhizotomy, cortical resection of the premotor area, pedunculotomy, cordotomy, anterior choroidal artery ligation and ablation of subcortical areas, such as the caudate and oral parts of the putamen and globus pallidus. Clinical benefits on tremor and rigidity were observed in approximately half of the patients, but aphasia, focal epilepsy, transient hemiparesis and permanent hemiplegia were frequent side effects, reaching a mean morbidity and mortality of 50 and 15%, respectively, which was excessively high for an elective surgery. These open functional procedures were soon abandoned or limited to severe cases [1].

In 1947, Spiegel and Wycis carried out the first effective stereotactic surgery for intractable pain, psychiatric disorders and epilepsy. In 1953, they published a series of cases of pallidal and ansa lenticularis lesions, known as "pallidoansotomy," in 50 parkinsonian patients, improving tremor in 78% but inducing permanent hemiplegia in 4% of patients and with a mortality of 3% [2]. Posteroventral pallidotomy was introduced and replicated extensively afterwards by Leksell's group, who found better outcomes with lesions in the posteroventral portion of the globus pallidus, relieving tremor and rigidity in up to 90% of the cases, with minimal neurological deficits and mortality [3].

At the same time, ventrolateral thalamotomy was introduced by Hassler and Riechert, and Cooper extended this procedure with chemical lesions [4, 5]. Thalamotomy became rapidly the preferred surgical strategy for Parkinson's disease (PD), because of a higher effectiveness for tremor and an equal response to rigidity, with fewer complications than pallidotomy [6]. However, bradykinesia relief received little attention at that time. Lesions in the posterior part of the ventrolateral thalamus (ventral oral posterior [VOP] and ventral intermediate nucleus [VIM]) were effective for tremor, and lesions in the anterior part (ventro oralis anterior [VOA]) were better for rigidity and levodopa (L-DOPA)-induced dyskinesias. Lesions in the subthalamic region (Forel's field H and zona incerta) were published a few years later than pallidotomy and thalamotomy, with comparable results, but were then abandoned for a long time [7].

In the late 1960s and early 1970s, standard ablative procedures were cataclysmically relegated by the introduction of levodopa as an efficient and easily administered dopamine replacement therapy for motor features of PD. Thalamotomy for severe and levodopa-refractory tremor was still performed occasionally for medication-refractory tremor. By that time, more than 37,000 stereotactic procedures had been achieved, mostly for PD and with a marked decline in morbidity and mortality (approximately 10 and 1–5%, respectively) in comparison with open functional procedures. Surgical therapy for PD was clearly refined [1].

However, some circumstances led ablative procedures by lesioning to regain their place in the treatment of motor symptoms of PD. The most important one was the development of disabling motor fluctuations and dyskinesias after 5–10 years of chronic levodopa use. Furthermore, there have been important advances in the understanding of basal ganglia pathophysiology and the mechanisms underlying the causes of parkinsonism, in addition to improvements in stereotactic techniques with CT and MRI imaging and

Parkinson's Disease: Current and Future Therapeutics and Clinical Trials, ed. Gálvez-Jiménez et al. Published by Cambridge University Press. © Cambridge University Press 2016.

the refinement of neurophysiological mapping with microelectrode recordings. Finally, modifications in the pallidum target to the medial posteroventral portion (globus pallidus internus [GPi]) led to a significant effect on bradykinesia. The pioneering work of Laitinen revitalized pallidotomy [8]. In the 1990s, unilateral posteroventral pallidotomy was the most common surgical procedure for PD and was soon followed by experimental results on subthalamotomy [9], which led to the development of deep-brain stimulation (DBS).

Since bilateral lesions were associated with a higher incidence of side effects, such as speech problems, dysphagia and cognitive impairment [10], the development of DBS pioneered by the French group of Grenoble replaced ablative procedures at most of the centers, due to its reversibility, adjustability and lower side effects in bilateral procedures [11]. However, DBS is not exempt from complications, such as electrode misplacement, infection, hardware failures and improper device programming, and in many cases, ablative procedures are still a valid option as an alternative to DBS therapy. In this chapter, we will discuss the advantages and disadvantages of ablative procedures and the rationale for still considering them as a useful therapeutic tool within the surgical armamentarium for treatment of movement disorders.

Indications

Stereotactic functional neurosurgery is mostly indicated for PD patients with medication-induced complications despite best medical treatment. As mentioned above, DBS has become the preferred surgical treatment due to several advantages over ablative surgery, such as programmability and reversibility.

Despite the usefulness of DBS, ablative surgery for PD treatment should not become underestimated, since there remain several situations where thalamotomy, pallidotomy or subthalamotomy may provide an alternative option to. Low financial position or absence of health insurance able to cover the cost of devices, inability or distant access to frequent follow-up care and programming, poor commitment to DBS programming by the patient and family, allergic reactions to or rejection of implanted materials, infection or scarring caused by system parts, immunocompromised status that increases risk of infections (e.g CD4 counts below 200/μl or high human immunodeficiency virus load) and lack of expertise in DBS management at small centers are some of the situations where ablative surgery might be preferred over DBS [12]. Ablative surgery may also be chosen after failure of DBS therapy due to misplacement of electrodes, electric malfunctioning, defective contacts, wiring fractures, damaged insulation, mechanic aggression to system parts during or after surgery, improper implant setting, anchoring problems, loose contact screws, current leakage due to blood, fluids or debris in connectors, lead overheating after MRI, lack of tolerance to stimulation or inadmissible side effects, and loss of efficacy of DBS [13, 14]. In addition, some particular indications and novel techniques for noninvasive ablative procedures on certain targets (gamma knife radiosurgery and high-intensity focused ultrasound) may enlarge the possibilities of the standard radiofrequency thermolesion, although they remain at an experimental level [15–17].

As a rescue option in certain DBS therapy-failure cases, a limited thermolesion could also be performed through the DBS electrodes before explanting them [18]. However, this indication should be carefully evaluated, as DBS electrodes are not designed to be able to transport radiofrequency power, or to tolerate overheating. Special care should be taken, and intervention of a multidisciplinary professional team is advised. As DBS electrodes do not have a temperature sensor, it is not possible to directly measure tip overheating, and temperature at the lesion site during radiofrequency power injection should be estimated very carefully. Serious injuries to the patient might be caused using these nonstandardized and nonapproved techniques.

The usefulness of thalamotomy for medically intractable tremor or tremor-predominant PD has been well established [19]. However, as will be further described in detail, the subthalamic nucleus (STN) or globus pallidus are usually preferred as the target because of offering additional improvements in bradykinesia and rigidity.

Surgery should be indicated by a specialist in movement disorders, discussed and consented properly with a multidisciplinary team about the benefits, risks, type of surgery and target, and performed in specialized centers after a realistic discussion with the patient and his or her family to avoid or minimize false expectations.

Patient selection

One of the most critical factors for a favorable outcome is appropriate patient selection. The vast experience accumulated over the past years has permitted the development of clinical inclusion and exclusion criteria to select the most adequate patients to undergo surgery. A detailed description will be found in other chapters of this book.

A comprehensive and standardized assessment should follow a battery of timed motor and neuropsychological tests named The Core Assessment Program for Surgical Interventional Therapies in Parkinson's disease (CAPSIT-PD) recommendations, which includes "on" and "off" evaluation of Unified Parkinson's Disease Rating Scale (UPDRS) scores, dyskinesias types, severity and duration, an "on"/"off" home diary, quality-of-life scales and a neuropsychological evaluation for cognition and mood [20]. Nonmotor symptoms should also be addressed.

In brief, the ideal PD candidate would be one with at least 5 years of disease duration, with an excellent response to levodopa but marked bradykinesia; severe "off" states; troublesome medication-resistant tremor or disabling dyskinesias during the "on" state, despite best medical treatment; no or minimal axial compromise, dysarthria or nonmotor features, specially cognition and behavior; preferably younger than 75 years old; no comorbidities; a normal MRI; and a supportive family. Such an ideal profile is hard to find, and most patients do not fit all of these criteria. Currently, the mean disease duration of those patients undergoing surgery is 12 years, but recent studies suggest that surgery could be used at early stages of the disease, during the first 3 years after the development of motor fluctuations [21, 22].

Surgical procedure

Patient preparation

Although the approach may differ between centers, in most cases ablative procedures are performed with the patient being awake. To prevent the development of drug-induced dyskinesias and allow parkinsonian motor signs to be maximized during intraoperative procedure and neurological assessments, all parkinsonian medication should be stopped the previous night.

Target planification

CT- and MRI-based stereotactic techniques have become the standard techniques for target planning. They determine stereotactic coordinates according to target definitions, trajectory planning, anatomic landmarks, safety regions and other surgical concerns [23, 24]. Specific software performs image fusion and tridimensional reconstruction.

Target confirmation

Some techniques are commonly used to confirm anatomical structures and functional regions, such as microelectrode recording (MER), which is widely used and is employed to register extracellular activity. This is very useful in helping to determine the somatosensory regions of the target and confirm the boundaries of the explored areas [25, 26]. By means of single or multiunit recognition of the registered neuronal activity, it is possible to determine with high accuracy the optimal region of the target to be operated on. One group reported that MER led to targeting changes in 98% of 132 consecutive pallidotomies, and in 12% of these cases, the MER-refined target was more than 4 mm from the original, MRI-guided site [27]. Other advantages of MER are decreased lesion size and side effects, which together enhance the results of surgery [26]. Additionally, MER allows neuronal discharge recording for research purposes. Nonetheless, a critical review of the literature in 1999 found a higher rate of severe complications, such as hemorrhage and mortality, when microelectrodes were used, in both lesion and DBS surgeries, without increasing the accuracy of target localization and lesion size, or improving clinical outcome, which was also found in two meta-analysis [28, 29]. Another meta-analysis showed that intracranial hemorrhage risk increased from 0.25 ± 0.2 without MER to 1.3 ± 0.4 when MER was used, and this might be explained by an increased number of electrode trajectories and/or by injuries caused by the sharper tip of the microelectrodes [30]. However, 85% of the pallidotomies conducted in a large study were performed with only one or two trajectories, which minimized this risk [27]. Randomized trials may be necessary to clarify these issues.

Despite the benefits offered by MER, there are some controversies concerning the use of this technique [29, 31]. Other centers prefer macroelectrode-based mapping. According to the electrode characteristics, different methods may be employed. While some groups rely only on neuroimaging techniques combined with electrical macrostimulation of the target area [32, 33], others use macro-electrodes for impedance recording to differentiate between gray matter, white matter and cerebrospinal fluid (CSF) space. In addition, macrostimulation and lesioning may be carried out with the same macroelectrode. Additionally, local field potential (LFP) recording can be helpful as an additional tool to map the trajectory toward the optimal target region [34]. Sometimes, specific LFP recording electrodes are used, but it is very common to use DBS electrodes to register these potentials [35]. However, these last devices are not used during ablative procedures.

The development of other techniques that provide additional clinical information to the electrophysiological recording may also help in improving the outcome of patients undergoing ablative surgery, such as the intraoperative apomorphine test to check lesion efficacy on dyskinesias [36].

Lesioning technique

Radiofrequency thermolesion is the preferred method for the ablative procedure. Electrical macrostimulation through the lesion electrode tip is generally applied at various frequency rates and intensities (usually 2, 50, 150 and 300 Hz with pulse durations ranging from 100 to 300 ms and currents from 0.5 to 10 mA or voltages from 0.5 to 5 V, depending on the electrode specifications), while looking for either beneficial or deleterious effects. Once macrostimulation has been applied and the target finally approved to undergo a lesion procedure, a transient and reversible intervention is usually performed before delivering the radiofrequency energy necessary to overheat the electrode tip and produce a permanent tissue lesion. This temporary lesion is commonly implemented by controlling the tip temperature not to exceed 41–42 °C for 30–60 s and allows a realistic simulation of what the ablation will perform in that place. Afterwards, neurological and functional assessments are carried out and, if the patient response was satisfactory, the permanent lesion protocol is executed. The electrode tip temperature is then raised and electronically controlled up to 75–80 °C for 60–90 s, and by using different tip configurations (usually 0.7–2.1 mm diameter and 2–10 mm tip exposure), lesions of various extensions and volumes are produced in the surrounding tissue. The size and shape of the lesion volume will be directly related to the tip temperature, elapsed time during energy injection and tip configuration. Different groups use their own lesion protocol in order to "shape" the desired ablated volume. According to the surgical plan, it is common practice to perform several lesions in the mapped area, thus enlarging single lesion volumes produced by each procedure up to the desired ablative therapy. Several lesions can be done throughout a single tract, or single lesions in different tracts, or a combination of both.

While producing the lesion, potential side effects such as neurological and clinical manifestations are carefully examined. The feasibility of performing an additional lesion, if needed, will greatly depend on the clinical response to the previous lesion. Bilateral ablations can be conducted during the same surgical procedure or in two stages, after a few days, weeks or months, according to the experience of different centers. Some centers submit patients to control CT scans and/or MRI imaging right after surgery for safety purposes (e.g. hemorrhages, CSF loss, pneumocephalus, lesion misplacement) Alternatively, between 48 h and 3 months postoperatively, MRI can be performed to confirm lesion placement and volume [10, 37].

Outcomes

Standardization of surgical procedures and clinical evaluations prior to and after surgery are necessary in order to compare outcomes across different surgical targets and techniques, such as lesions or DBS. Unfortunately, only a few studies have been methodologically comparable or were controlled and randomized, and comparable efficacy within ablative procedures and between them and DBS is still a matter of debate.

Thalamotomy

Thalamotomy produces improvements in PD patients with drug-resistant tremor when VIM is used as the target and has also an antidyskinetic effect by lesioning VOA and VOP. In some cases, it reduces rigidity, but it has no (or depreciable) effect on bradykinesia or postural instability and gait disability [38, 39]. A retrospective study analyzed the outcome of 42 PD patients (of whom two underwent bilateral surgery) with a mean follow-up of 52 months and found that 86% of the patients had resolution of or moderate-to-marked improvement in their contralateral tremor, with a concomitant improvement in function. None experienced tremor recurrence. The mean daily dose of levodopa was slightly reduced by approximately 138 mg at a mean of 53.4 months after thalamotomy. Five patients experienced preoperative levodopa-induced dyskinesias, which were considerably improved independently of the reduction in levodopa intake [19]. This positive effect on dyskinesias was reported previously in all 13 PD patients operated on in one study, especially those with Vo-complex lesions [39]. A summary of a large series reported improvement of tremor in 80–90% of the patients and functional improvement in 30–50%. Tremor amplitude normalizes after thalamotomy, from an average of 10 mm pre-surgery to less than 0.5 mm after the surgical procedure, but tremor characteristics in the frequency domain do not regain normal values [40, 41].

In addition to motor symptoms, unilateral thalamotomy improves quality of life according to the 36-Item Short Form Health Survey (SF-36) and 39-item Parkinson's Disease Questionnaire (PDQ-39) in general areas and also in ones specific to PD, such as self-ratings of stigma and bodily discomfort [42].

A second thalamotomy, contralateral to the initial side, has been indicated after a mean interval of 56 months because of deterioration of activities of daily living (ADLs) due to the progression of the symptoms on the nontreated side. In a study, five out of nine patients benefitted from this staged bilateral procedure. However, as will be mentioned below, bilateral thalamotomy results in a prohibitively high rate of cognitive and speech problems, preventing its use in PD patients [19, 38, 43].

A randomized study compared the efficacy of unilateral thalamotomy (23 PD patients) versus unilateral or bilateral thalamic DBS (22 PD patients) for the treatment of drug-resistant tremor [44]. The primary outcome measure was the change in functional abilities as measured by the Frenchay Activities Index, which assesses 15 ADLs, such as domestic tasks, leisure or work-related activities, and other activities. An increase of 4 points in the score indicates an improvement in the patient's ability to perform at least two of these activities and an increase of 5 points indicates a clinically relevant improvement in the ability to perform ADLs. Secondary outcome measures were the severity of tremor, the number of adverse effects and patients' assessment of the outcome. The difference between groups in the Frenchay Activities Index at 6 months was 4.7 points (95% confidence interval [CI]: 1.2–8.0; $P < 0.05$) in favor of DBS and 7.0 points (95% CI: 2.4–11.6; $P < 0.05$) after 5 years. Tremor suppression was achieved irrespective of age, disease duration and baseline disease severity. In those patients with bilateral tremor who underwent contralateral electrode implantation after 6 months, functional outcome was better at long-term follow-up than in those who did not undergo contralateral surgery but was not quite as good as in those who underwent bilateral stimulation. Absolute values of the functional score in both treatment groups declined after 5 years, back to baseline in the stimulation group and below baseline in the thalamotomy group, in concurrence with disease progression. However, most patients in both groups still experienced satisfactory tremor suppression at 5 years.

Studies comparing the clinical outcome of thalamotomy with that of pallidotomy are scarce [45].

Pallidotomy

A randomized rater-blinded study of unilateral posteroventral medial pallidotomy in 14 advanced PD patients reported that motor scores in the "off" state and drug-induced dyskinesias were improved by 30 and 92%, respectively, after 6 months postsurgery. Gait and postural instability improved less (<25%). Rigidity, bradykinesia and tremor were improved mainly on the contralateral side but also ipsilaterally, although to a lesser extent [46]. This study was extended to 39 patients, with 27 of them examined at 1 year and 11 at 2 years. The positive effects on dyskinesias and the total scores for "off"-period parkinsonism, contralateral bradykinesia and rigidity were sustained in the 11 patients examined at 2 years. The improvement in ipsilateral dyskinesias was lost after 1 year, and the improvements in postural stability and gait lasted only 3–6 months [47].

The Sweden group of Hariz, Bergenhein and Laitinen followed Lars Leksell's technique introduced in the 1950s and reported a 10-year follow-up review of 13 PD patients who were part of a large series of 38 patients who received posteroventral pallidotomy (11 unilateral and two staged bilateral procedures) between 1985 and 1990 [8]. There was an important alleviation of rigidity and bradykinesia in almost all of the patients. Contralateral tremor, if it was initially controlled by surgery, remained improved, although additional surgeries were needed in some patients. Most patients exhibited a gradual recurrence of akinesia and an increase in gait freezing. Dyskinesias were successfully abolished without recurrence or induction of them contralateral to the pallidotomy, despite increases in dopaminergic medication due to disease progression. The lack of availability of comprehensive validated rating scales at that time made critical assessment of the results difficult [48].

Schuurman and Speelman evaluated the effect of unilateral pallidotomy in 19 patients enrolled in a randomized, single-blinded, multicenter trial comprising 37 patients who had, despite optimum pharmacological treatment, at least one of the following symptoms: severe response fluctuations, dyskinesias, painful dystonia or bradykinesia. Nineteen patients underwent unilateral pallidotomy and the rest were postponed for 6 months. They found that the median UPDRS motor subscore during the "off" period improved by 31% following surgery. During the "on" phase, the dyskinesia rating scale improved by 50%

in patients who underwent pallidotomy compared with no change in those who did not. Because patients were aware of the treatment allocation, a part of the measured effect could be explained by the placebo effect. This study was extended to 32 patients and to 1-year follow-up for the original 19 patients operated. The positive effects of unilateral pallidotomy on contralateral rigidity, bradykinesia and tremor, as well as on dyskinesias, were maintained, and functioning in ADLs and quality of life were improved after the 1-year follow-up [49].

We conducted a prospective case–control study in which we followed over 1 year 10 PD patients with indication for pallidotomy who did not undergo surgery because of lack of financial support and 10 PD patients who did undergo pallidotomy. A significant reduction in ADL scores and UPDRS motor scores, and in the subsets addressing rigidity, bradykinesia and tremor, as well as dyskinesias, was found in the group who were operated on [37].

Vitek et al. [50] performed the first randomized trial comparing unilateral pallidotomy with medical treatment in 18 PD patients in each group. At the 6 month follow-up, patients receiving pallidotomy had a statistically significant reduction of 32% in the total UPDRS score compared with those randomized to medical therapy (5% increase). They also showed improvement in tremor (abolished in 70% of the patients), rigidity (an average of 55% improvement in 88% of the cases) and bradykinesia (average 40% of improvement). Gait and balance improvement of 32 and 34%, respectively, at the 1-year follow-up was no longer observed at 2 years. A significant improvement in both drug-induced dyskinesias (improved in all and completely relieved in 70%) and motor fluctuations after pallidotomy was found at 6 months and maintained for 2 years. An ipsilateral improvement was observed also for bradykinesia, rigidity and dyskinesias. No significant levodopa dosage reductions were achieved following surgery. Surprisingly, no significant differences in ADL subscores were found in the two treatment groups.

A long-term follow-up study (3.5–5.5 years) of a cohort of 20 patients who had undergone unilateral posteroventral pallidotomy found a sustained improvement in "off" state contralateral motor signs and contralateral dyskinesias during "on" but not in other "on"-state parkinsonian signs [51].

Regarding ADLs, in 2001, a meta-analysis of 12 studies reporting ADL outcome found that unilateral pallidotomy successfully enhanced functional outcome in PD patients [52], which was also found in our meta-analysis [28].

Merello et al. [53] prospectively randomized a group of 13 PD patients to receive a unilateral thermolesion or DBS on the posteroventral GPi to compare the efficacy and safety of both procedures. Patients improved in the "off" stage on average by 29% of the motor UPDRS score contralateral to the side of either type of surgery. Tremor, rigidity and bradykinesia also improved significantly, regardless of the procedure type. The safety of both techniques was comparable.

Esselink et al. [54] reported 1- and 4-year outcomes of a randomized, multicenter, observer-blind comparison of unilateral pallidotomy ($n = 14$) versus bilateral STN-DBS ($n = 20$) in advanced PD patients. They showed a significant long-term superiority in the efficacy of bilateral STN-DBS over pallidotomy with respect to motor UPDRS score during the "off" state (46 vs 27%, respectively). However, no significant differences between the two procedures were found regarding ADL score, drug-induced dyskinesias severity or levodopa dosage, possibly due to the small sample size included.

Fewer results have been published for bilateral pallidotomy. One study found a 53% improvement in UPDRS scores after bilateral pallidotomy ($n = 8$) compared with a 27% improvement after a unilateral procedure ($n = 12$), but at the expense of a greater deterioration in verbal fluency, dysarthria and sialorrhea. The role of bilateral pallidotomy remains uncertain, and when possible, a combined procedure including unilateral pallidotomy and contralateral DBS might be preferred when bilateral DBS is not possible [33, 55, 56].

An interesting finding is the appearance of transient abnormal involuntary movements such as hemichorea or hemiballism during macrostimulation or thermolesion and may predict a better motor outcome following pallidotomy [57].

In summary, pallidotomy exerts its main effect on limb dyskinesias and "off"-state dystonia, and also shows a good response for rigidity, bradykinesia and tremor. Although one meta-analysis including 17 studies with unilateral pallidotomy found improvement of axial symptoms, such as postural instability and gait disability during "on" and "off" periods [58], the beneficial effect usually waned beyond 1 year of follow-up [51]. Pallidotomy also has almost no positive effect on speech and nonmotor symptoms. Almost always, those clinical features that responded better were those responsive to levodopa. The benefits were sustained in a mean follow-up of 10 years. Motor scores may worsen over time, possibly due to disease progression, but loss of surgical benefit cannot be ruled out. Lesions that involved the caudal portion of the GPi are more effective in providing long-term improvement in tremor, rigidity and bradykinesia than lesions that only partially involve this territory or involve the globus pallidus externus (GPe).

Subthalamotomy

There is less experience with subthalamotomy in comparison with the abovementioned procedures, in part because of the potential risk of intractable hemiballism. However, subthalamotomy was explored in more depth after success of STN-DBS for PD and the need to offer less expensive alternatives to DBS in some countries or to offer an option for patients living at large distances from the implantation center or having an underlying general condition precluding DBS. No randomized controlled trials have been conducted, but several case series have been reported.

Su et al. [59] showed in 12 patients with unilateral dorsolateral subthalamotomy extending to the pallidofugal fibers, and followed up after 1 year, a 38% improvement in UPDRS-ADL and motor scores during the "on" state, including rigidity (79%), tremor (66%) and bradykinesia (40%). A daily dopaminergic medication dosage reduction of 42% was accomplished. Axial motor features, gait, postural stability, "off"-state tremor and motor fluctuation improved at 6 and 12 months but showed a decline in benefits at 18 months. It should be noted that five out of 12 patients had STN-DBS surgery 1–3 months before subthalamotomy and two simultaneously. However, none of them had DBS implanted after subthalamotomy and while in the off-stimulation and off-medication state, their UPDRS scores were not significantly different from the presurgical scores.

Recently, the effects of unilateral subthalamotomy were reported in 89 PD patients, of which 25 were followed for up to 3 years [60]. A marked improvement in contralateral parkinsonian features was obtained during both "on" and "off" states, with an average of 20–50% reduction. Axial and ipsilateral to the lesion, features were not modified and progressed steadily. The levodopa daily dosage was reduced by 45, 36 and 28% at 12, 24 and 36 months after surgery, respectively. Despite this reduction, which also occurs after STN-DBS, levodopa-induced dyskinesias were not significantly decreased in comparison with the stimulation procedure, but at least they were not increased contralateral to the lesion, while they continued to worsen in the nonoperated side. Fourteen patients (15%) developed postoperative hemichorea or hemiballism, which required pallidotomy in eight. Interestingly, these 14 patients had significantly higher levodopa-induced dyskinesia scores before surgery than the rest of the patients. There was no evidence of cognitive impairment resulting from surgery.

Bilateral subthalamotomy was reported in 18 advanced PD patients, with reductions in the UPDRS motor scores during "off" and "on" states by means of 50 and 35%, respectively [61]. Not only did rigidity, tremor and bradykinesia improve markedly but also ADL scores. Levodopa daily doses were reduced by 47%, which in turn decreased levodopa-induced dyskinesias by 50%. This finding contrasts with those obtained after unilateral procedures. The motor benefit persisted for a follow-up of 3–6 years.

Another study evaluated the effect of unilateral subthalamotomy in 17 asymmetrical tremor-dominant PD patients and unilateral subthalamotomy plus contralateral STN-DBS in four PD patients with bilateral features. All patients were at an advanced stage of the disease. Ninety percent of the lesions extended beyond the STN to involve pallidofugal fibers (H2 field of Forel) and the zona incerta. All patients were followed up at least for 1 year. Tremor, bradykinesia and rigidity improved markedly. Dopaminergic medication dosage was reduced to approximately half, together with a significant reduction in dyskinesias and motor fluctuations. Cognition was mostly unaffected [62].

Merello et al. [10] compared the efficacy and safety of different surgical approaches to STN in a prospective randomized study involving 16 patients who underwent bilateral STN-DBS, bilateral subthalamotomy or unilateral subthalamotomy plus contralateral STN-DBS and were followed for 1 year after surgery. Total and motor UPDRS scores, as well as drug-induced dyskinesias, improved significantly at the 1-year follow-up, regardless of the procedure administered and without statistically significant differences between treatment modalities. Dopaminergic medication dosage dropped to a similar degree after surgery in all groups.

A recent prospective, randomized, double-blinded pilot study compared unilateral pallidotomy and unilateral subthalamotomy in six and four advanced PD patients, respectively. Both approaches were equally safe and effective regarding motor and ADL measures. Levodopa-equivalent daily intake was significantly reduced in the subthalamotomy group [63].

Table 17.1 Effects of thalamotomy, pallidotomy and subthalamotomy on Parkinson's disease clinical features, dopaminergic medication and side effects

Clinical features	Thalamotomy Unilateral	Thalamotomy Bilateral	Pallidotomy Unilateral	Pallidotomy Bilateral	Subthalamotomy Unilateral	Subthalamotomy Bilateral
Clinical features						
Bradykinesia	−	−	++	++	++	++
Rigidity	+	+	+++	+++	+++	+++
Tremor	+++	+++	+++	+++	+++	+++
Postural stability/gait[a]	−	−	−	−	−	−
Motor fluctuations	+	+	+++	+++	++	+++
Dyskinesias	+	+	+++	+++	++	+++
"Off" dystonia	−	−	+++	+++	++	+++
LDED reduction	−	−	−	−	++	++
Side effects	+	+++	+	++	+	++

LDED, Levodopa daily equivalent dose.
[a]Transient effects on postural stability and gait may occur after surgery but are usually not sustained beyond 1 year.

In conclusion, subthalamotomy improves bradykinesia, rigidity and tremor, and allows reductions of levodopa dosage. The beneficial effects are comparable to those of pallidotomy or STN and GPi stimulation. Although the risk of hemiballism is a concern, its frequency is not as high as previously expected. The role of bilateral subthalamotomy in patients unable to receive DBS merits further exploration in large, randomized controlled trials with longer follow-up periods.

The Movement Disorder Society Evidence-based Medicine Review Update in 2011 for the motor symptoms treatments of PD concluded that unilateral pallidotomy is efficacious and clinically useful as a symptomatic adjunct to levodopa and in the treatment of motor fluctuations and dyskinesias, whereas thalamotomy is likely efficacious and possibly useful as a symptomatic adjunct to levodopa therapy. There is insufficient evidence for subthalamotomy as a treatment for motor fluctuations and dyskinesia or as a symptomatic adjunct to levodopa therapy [64]. Unfortunately, the diverse combinations of procedures for PD patients and the lack of standardized outcome measures and side effects reported, in addition to scarcely controlled randomized and long-term studies, preclude low qualifications by evidence-based reviews. However, these reviews hardly mirror the reality of the clinical setting. As an example, the lack of double-blind, controlled randomized trials of thalamotomy or thalamic DBS for essential tremor mean that these procedures are classified as "Level C, possibly effective" according to the recent evidence-based guideline update of the American Academy of Neurology [65], which does not reflect properly the great efficacy of these techniques in clinical practice.

The clinical effects of thalamotomy, pallidotomy and subthalamotomy are shown in Table 17.1.

Safety and side effects

The frequency of side effects varies largely across series but is usually around 30%, most of them being transient. The most common, serious and potentially devastating complications of surgery are infections and hemorrhage. Ablative procedures were not associated with an increased risk in comparison with DBS according to a recent literature systematic review. The overall incidence for intracranial hemorrhage in patients undergoing movement disorders surgery is 5% but varies considerably across different series. Asymptomatic hemorrhage occurred in 1.9% of patients, symptomatic hemorrhage in 2.1% and hemorrhage resulting in permanent deficit or death in 1.1%. Older age, hypertension, the use of microelectrode recording, number of microelectrode recording penetrations, and sulcal or ventricular incursion are possible factors associated with an increased risk of hemorrhage [66, 67]. Surgical target is a controversial risk factor for hemorrhage. A study that used DBS found a risk of hemorrhage of 7.0% associated with pallidal DBS compared with 2.2%

with subthalamic nucleus DBS and 1.2% with thalamic DBS. The authors theorized that the lenticulostriate vascular supply arising from the anterior circulation might be more sensitive to surgical trauma, such as hypertension-induced changes, than the posterior circulation perforators [68]. Other uncommon complications of PD surgery and hospitalization are seizures, aspiration pneumonia, pulmonary embolism and infections, although the latter are less frequent than with DBS.

Surgery for PD, the most common indication for movement disorder surgery, appears to carry an increased risk of hemorrhage or stroke and in-hospital complications when compared with essential tremor and dystonia [69]. In 2011, the Movement Disorder Society Evidence-based Medicine Review Update for the motor symptoms treatments of Parkinson's disease concluded that thalamotomy, pallidotomy and subthalamotomy have an acceptable risk with specialized monitoring [64]. The major disadvantage of ablative surgeries is that, unlike stimulation procedures, some side effects are permanent and not passive of modulation.

Motor side effects

The most frequent motor side effects are: hypophonia, dysarthria, anarthria, dysphagia, facial weakness, postural instability and gait disturbances, hemiparesis and worsening of handwriting [28, 70]. Bilateral procedures more often have side effects than unilateral procedures, but fortunately they are usually transient. Staged bilateral surgeries are preferred in many centers, but simultaneous procedures are also performed frequently, without an apparent increased frequency of side effects in comparison with the former procedure. However, it is possible that authors of those reports on bilateral procedures without motor side effects may have performed smaller lesions than usual. Longer follow-up of these patients is necessary.

Limb ataxia can be observed following thalamotomy and usually lasts up to 21 days post-surgery [71].

The development of involuntary choreo-ballistic movements is the main concern after subthalamotomy, either unilateral or bilateral. The frequency is around 5–50% and the effect usually resolves rapidly, lasting from a few hours to 5 days [10, 61]. It might be reduced if lesions are extended to the pallidofugal fibers (H_2 field of Forel) and the zona incerta. When hemiballism remains persistent, it may require ulterior posteroventral pallidotomy or pallidal stimulation, as well as thalamotomy or thalamic stimulation for complete resolution. Choreo-ballistic movements induced by subthalamotomy are unresponsive to amantadine in patients who achieved improvement with amantadine for levodopa-induced dyskinesias prior to surgery. Possible explanations for this observation might be: (i) that amantadine probably exerts its antidyskinetic effect by acting on the "indirect" pathway; (ii) that the physiopathological mechanisms of subthalamotomy-induced dyskinesias may differ from those involved in levodopa-induced dyskinesias; or (iii) that dyskinesias induced by STN surgery resolve spontaneously as compensatory mechanisms develop [72].

Nonmotor side effects

Surgical targets, such as GPi and STN, have a cognitive, limbic and somatosensory part and are in close proximity to widespread connections involved in nonmotor function. The most common nonmotor side effects are acute confusion or somnolence, changes in personality or behavior other than psychosis, such as depression or apathy, sialorrhea, weight gain and urinary incontinence. Some suicide commitments have also been reported. Transient visual-field defects due to optic tract lesions can be found after pallidotomy in 2.1% of cases, and in 0.2% they are permanent [66]. Worsening of cognitive decline, mainly a transient reduction in verbal fluency, can be observed after pallidotomy and thalamotomy but to a lesser extend following subthalamotomy [10, 28, 42, 55, 70, 73]. However, a study of 10 PD patients undergoing subthalamothomy found no significant cognitive decline after 2 years of follow-up [74]. Both thalamotomy and thalamic stimulation are associated with a similar and minimal overall risk of cognitive deterioration [75]. Paresthesias are rarely encountered after thalamotomy. The frequency of the side effects of thalamotomy, pallidotomy and subthalamotomy are shown in Table 17.1.

Conclusions

In the last few decades, there has been a revival of ablative and stimulation surgeries because of the shortcomings of levodopa and other dopaminergic agents. Surgery is the only treatment available for PD that can improve some of the parkinsonian motor features, such as bradykinesia, rigidity and tremor, and at the same time it abolishes or significantly reduces drug-induced intractable dyskinesias.

Thalamic DBS is preferable to thalamotomy as a means of improving function with fewer adverse effects. Bilateral thalamotomy is not recommended due to the high incidence of adverse effects. Pallidotomy or GPi-DBS, as well as subthalamotomy and STN-DBS, suppress tremor adequately and have positive effects on bradykinesia and rigidity, making them preferable to thalamotomy or thalamic DBS in PD patients. Using the STN as a surgical target has the advantage of allowing levodopa dosage reductions; however, more research is needed to confirm its safety and efficacy.

Although DBS is currently preferred over ablative surgery, there is still a role for the latter in some circumstances as explained above. Patient and family commitment and problems of availability are important factors in the decision to forgo DBS in favor of ablative surgery. Therefore, ablative therapy should not be totally replaced by DBS, as it may be the only or best option in some circumstances. The indication should be discussed on an individual basis with a multidisciplinary team.

References

1. Speelman JD, Bosch DA. Resurgence of functional neurosurgery for Parkinson's disease: a historical perspective. *Mov Disord* 1998; **13**: 582–8.
2. Spiegel EA, Wycis HT. Ansotomy in paralysis agitans. *AMA Arch Neurol Psychiatry* 1953; **69**: 652–3.
3. Svennilson E, Torvik A, Lowe R, Leksell L. Treatment of parkinsonism by stereotatic thermolesions in the pallidal region. A clinical evaluation of 81 cases. *Acta Psychiatr Scand* 1960; **35**: 358–77.
4. Cooper IS, Bravo GJ. Implications of a five-year study of 700 basal ganglia operations. *Neurology* 1958; **8**: 701–7.
5. Hassler R, Riechert T, Mundinger F, Umbach W, Ganglberger JA. Physiological observations in stereotaxic operations in extrapyramidal motor disturbances. *Brain* 1960; **83**: 337–50.
6. Krayenbuhl H, Wyss OA, Yasargil MG. Bilateral thalamotomy and pallidotomy as treatment for bilateral Parkinsonism. *J Neurosurg* 1961; **18**: 429–44.
7. Andy OJ, Jurko MF, Sias FR, Jr. Subthalamotomy in treatment of Parkinsonian tremor. *J Neurosurg* 1963; **20**: 860–70.
8. Laitinen LV, Bergenheim AT, Hariz MI. Leksell's posteroventral pallidotomy in the treatment of Parkinson's disease. *J Neurosurg* 1992; **76**: 53–61.
9. Alvarez L, Macias R, Guridi J, et al. Dorsal subthalamotomy for Parkinson's disease. *Mov Disord* 2001; **16**: 72–8.
10. Merello M, Tenca E, Perez Lloret S, et al. Prospective randomized 1-year follow-up comparison of bilateral subthalamotomy versus bilateral subthalamic stimulation and the combination of both in Parkinson's disease patients: a pilot study. *British J Neurosurg* 2008; **22**: 415–22.
11. Benabid AL, Pollak P, Gross C, et al. Acute and long-term effects of subthalamic nucleus stimulation in Parkinson's disease. *Stereotact Funct Neurosurg* 1994; **62**: 76–84.
12. Hooper AK, Okun MS, Foote KD, et al. Clinical cases where lesion therapy was chosen over deep brain stimulation. *Stereotact Funct Neurosurg* 2008; **86**: 147–52.
13. Bahgat D, Magill ST, Berk C, McCartney S, Burchiel KJ. Thalamotomy as a treatment option for tremor after ineffective deep brain stimulation. *Stereotact Funct Neurosurg* 2013; **91**: 18–23.
14. Bulluss KJ, Pereira EA, Joint C, Aziz TZ. Pallidotomy after chronic deep brain stimulation. *Neurosurg Focus* 2013; **35**: E5.
15. Elias WJ, Huss D, Voss T, et al. A pilot study of focused ultrasound thalamotomy for essential tremor. *N Engl J Med* 2013; **369**: 640–8.
16. Lipsman N, Schwartz ML, Huang Y, et al. MR-guided focused ultrasound thalamotomy for essential tremor: a proof-of-concept study. *Lancet Neurol* 2013; **12**: 462–8.
17. Young RF, Shumway-Cook A, Vermeulen SS, et al. Gamma knife radiosurgery as a lesioning technique in movement disorder surgery. *J Neurosurg* 1998; **89**: 183–93.
18. Deligny C, Drapier S, Verin M, et al. Bilateral subthalamotomy through DBS electrodes: A rescue option for device-related infection. *Neurology* 2009; **73**: 1243–4.
19. Jankovic J, Cardoso F, Grossman RG, Hamilton WJ. Outcome after stereotactic thalamotomy for parkinsonian, essential, and other types of tremor. *Neurosurgery* 1995; **37**: 680–6; discussion 6–7.
20. Defer GL, Widner H, Marie RM, Remy P, Levivier M. Core assessment program for surgical interventional therapies in Parkinson's disease (CAPSIT-PD). *Mov Disord* 1999; **14**: 572–84.
21. deSouza RM, Moro E, Lang AE, Schapira AH. Timing of deep brain stimulation in Parkinson disease: a need for reappraisal? *Ann Neurol* 2013; **73**: 565–75.
22. Schuepbach WM, Rau J, Knudsen K, et al. Neurostimulation for Parkinson's disease with early motor complications. *N Engl J Med* 2013; **368**: 610–22.
23. Hirabayashi H, Tengvar M, Hariz MI. Stereotactic imaging of the pallidal target. *Mov Disord* 2002; **17** (Suppl. 3): S130–4.
24. Starr PA, Vitek JL, DeLong M, Bakay RA. Magnetic resonance imaging-based stereotactic localization of the globus pallidus and subthalamic nucleus. *Neurosurgery* 1999; **44**: 303–13; discussion 13–4.

25. Lozano AM, Hutchison WD, Dostrovsky JO. Microelectrode monitoring of cortical and subcortical structures during stereotactic surgery. *Acta Neurochir Suppl* 1995; **64**: 30–4.

26. Vitek JL, Bakay RA, Hashimoto T, et al. Microelectrode-guided pallidotomy: technical approach and its application in medically intractable Parkinson's disease. *J Neurosurg* 1998; **88**: 1027–43.

27. Alterman RL, Sterio D, Beric A, Kelly PJ. Microelectrode recording during posteroventral pallidotomy: impact on target selection and complications. *Neurosurgery* 1999; **44**: 315–21; discussion 21–3.

28. Boucai L, Cerquetti D, Merello M. Functional surgery for Parkinson's disease treatment: a structured analysis of a decade of published literature. *British J Neurosurg* 2004; **18**: 213–22.

29. Hariz MI, Fodstad H. Do microelectrode techniques increase accuracy or decrease risks in pallidotomy and deep brain stimulation? A critical review of the literature. *Stereotact Funct Neurosurg* 1999; **72**: 157–69.

30. Palur RS, Berk C, Schulzer M, Honey CR. A metaanalysis comparing the results of pallidotomy performed using microelectrode recording or macroelectrode stimulation. *J Neurosurg* 2002; **96**: 1058–62.

31. Hariz MI, Bergenheim AT, Fodstad H. Crusade for microelectrode guidance in pallidotomy. *J Neurosurg* 1999; **90**: 175–9.

32. Giller CA, Dewey RB, Ginsburg MI, Mendelsohn DB, Berk AM. Stereotactic pallidotomy and thalamotomy using individual variations of anatomic landmarks for localization. *Neurosurgery* 1998; **42**: 56–62; discussion 62–5.

33. Scott R, Gregory R, Hines N, et al. Neuropsychological, neurological and functional outcome following pallidotomy for Parkinson's disease. A consecutive series of eight simultaneous bilateral and twelve unilateral procedures. *Brain* 1998; **121**: 659–75.

34. Tan H, Pogosyan A, Anzak A, et al. Frequency specific activity in subthalamic nucleus correlates with hand bradykinesia in Parkinson's disease. *Exp Neurol* 2013; **240**: 122–9.

35. Pogosyan A, Yoshida F, Chen CC, et al. Parkinsonian impairment correlates with spatially extensive subthalamic oscillatory synchronization. *Neuroscience* 2010; **171**: 245–57.

36. Merello M, Cammarota A, Nouzeilles MI, Betti O, Leiguarda R. Confirmation of the antidyskinetic effect of posteroventral pallidotomy by means of an intraoperative apomorphine test. *Mov Disord* 1998; **13**: 533–5.

37. Merello M, Nouzeilles MI, Cammarota A, Betti O, Leiguarda R. Comparison of 1-year follow-up evaluations of patients with indication for pallidotomy who did not undergo surgery versus patients with Parkinson's disease who did undergo pallidotomy: a case control study. *Neurosurgery* 1999; **44**: 461–7; discussion 7–8.

38. Moriyama E, Beck H, Miyamoto T. Long-term results of ventrolateral thalamotomy for patients with Parkinson's disease. *Neurol Med Chir (Tokyo)* 1999; **39**: 350–6; discussion 6–7.

39. Narabayashi H, Yokochi F, Nakajima Y. Levodopa-induced dyskinesia and thalamotomy. *J Neurol Neurosurg Psychiatry* 1984; **47**: 831–9.

40. Duval C, Strafella AP, Sadikot AF. The impact of ventrolateral thalamotomy on high-frequency components of tremor. *Clin Neurophysiol.* 2005; **116**: 1391–9.

41. Speelman JD, Schuurman PR, de Bie RM, Bosch DA. Thalamic surgery and tremor. Movement disorders: official journal of the Movement Disorder *Society*. 1998; **13** (Suppl. 3): 103–6.

42. Nijhawan SR, Banks SJ, Aziz TZ, et al. Changes in cognition and health-related quality of life with unilateral thalamotomy for Parkinsonian tremor. *J Clin Neurosci* 2009; **16**: 44–50.

43. Walter BL, Vitek JL. Surgical treatment for Parkinson's disease. *Lancet Neurol* 2004; **3**: 719–28.

44. Schuurman PR, Bosch DA, Merkus MP, Speelman JD. Long-term follow-up of thalamic stimulation versus thalamotomy for tremor suppression. *Mov Disord* 2008; **23**: 1146–53.

45. Hariz MI, Hirabayashi H. Is there a relationship between size and site of the stereotactic lesion and symptomatic results of pallidotomy and thalamotomy? *Stereotact Funct Neurosurg* 1997; **69**: 28–45.

46. Lozano AM, Lang AE, Gálvez-jiménez N, et al. Effect of GPi pallidotomy on motor function in Parkinson's disease. *Lancet* 1995; **346**: 1383–7.

47. Lang AE, Lozano AM, Montgomery E, et al. Posteroventral medial pallidotomy in advanced Parkinson's disease. *N Engl J Med* 1997; **337**: 1036–42.

48. Hariz MI, Bergenheim AT. A 10-year follow-up review of patients who underwent Leksell's posteroventral pallidotomy for Parkinson disease. *J Neurosurg* 2001; **94**: 552–8.

49. de Bie RM, de Haan RJ, Nijssen PC, et al. Unilateral pallidotomy in Parkinson's disease: a randomised, single-blind, multicentre trial. *Lancet* 1999; **354**: 1665–9.

50. Vitek JL, Bakay RA, Freeman A, et al. Randomized trial of pallidotomy versus medical therapy for Parkinson's disease. *Ann Neurol* 2003; **53**: 558–69.

51. Fine J, Duff J, Chen R, et al. Long-term follow-up of unilateral pallidotomy in advanced Parkinson's disease. *N Engl J Med* 2000; **342**: 1708–14.

52. Ahmad SO, Mu K, Scott SA. Meta-analysis of functional outcome in Parkinson patients treated with unilateral pallidotomy. *Neurosc Lett* 2001; **312**: 153–6.

53. Merello M, Nouzeilles MI, Kuzis G, et al. Unilateral radiofrequency lesion versus electrostimulation of posteroventral pallidum: a prospective randomized comparison. *Mov Disord* 1999; **14**: 50–6.
54. Esselink RA, de Bie RM, de Haan RJ, et al. Long-term superiority of subthalamic nucleus stimulation over pallidotomy in Parkinson disease. *Neurology* 2009; **73**: 151–3.
55. Lang AE, Duff J, Saint-Cyr JA, et al. Posteroventral medial pallidotomy in Parkinson's disease. *J Neurol* 1999; **246** (Suppl. 2): II28–41.
56. Schuurman PR, de Bie RM, Speelman JD, Bosch DA. Bilateral posteroventral pallidotomy in advanced Parkinson's disease in three patients. *Mov Disord* 1997; **12**: 752–5.
57. Merello M, Cammarota A, Betti O, et al. Involuntary movements during thermolesion predict a better outcome after microelectrode guided posteroventral pallidotomy. *J Neurol Neurosurg Psychiatry* 1997; **63**: 210–3.
58. Bakker M, Esselink RA, Munneke M, et al. Effects of stereotactic neurosurgery on postural instability and gait in Parkinson's disease. *Mov Disord* 2004; **19**: 1092–9.
59. Su PC, Tseng HM, Liou HH. Postural asymmetries following unilateral subthalomotomy for advanced Parkinson's disease. *Mov Disord* 2002; **17**: 191–4.
60. Alvarez L, Macias R, Pavon N, et al. Therapeutic efficacy of unilateral subthalamotomy in Parkinson's disease: results in 89 patients followed for up to 36 months. *J Neurol Neurosurg Psychiatry* 2009; **80**: 979–85.
61. Alvarez L, Macias R, Lopez G, et al. Bilateral subthalamotomy in Parkinson's disease: initial and long-term response. *Brain* 2005; **128**: 570–83.
62. Patel NK, Heywood P, O'sullivan K, et al. Unilateral subthalamotomy in the treatment of Parkinson's disease. *Brain* 2003; **126**: 1136–45.
63. Coban A, Hanagasi HA, Karamursel S, Barlas O. Comparison of unilateral pallidotomy and subthalamotomy findings in advanced idiopathic Parkinson's disease. *British J Neurosurg* 2009; **23**: 23–9.
64. Fox SH, Katzenschlager R, Lim SY, et al. The Movement Disorder Society Evidence-Based Medicine Review Update: treatments for the motor symptoms of Parkinson's disease. *Mov Disord* 2011; **26** (Suppl. 3): S2–41.
65. Zesiewicz TA, Elble RJ, Louis ED, et al. Evidence-based guideline update: treatment of essential tremor: report of the Quality Standards subcommittee of the American Academy of Neurology. *Neurology* 2011; **77**: 1752–5.
66. Higuchi Y, Iacono RP. Surgical complications in patients with Parkinson's disease after posteroventral pallidotomy. *Neurosurgery* 2003; **52**: 558–71; discussion 68–71.
67. Zrinzo L, Foltynie T, Limousin P, Hariz MI. Reducing hemorrhagic complications in functional neurosurgery: a large case series and systematic literature review. *J Neurosurg* 2012; **116**: 84–94.
68. Binder DK, Rau GM, Starr PA. Risk factors for hemorrhage during microelectrode-guided deep brain stimulator implantation for movement disorders. *Neurosurgery* 2005; **56**: 722–32.
69. Rughani AI, Hodaie M, Lozano AM. Acute complications of movement disorders surgery: effects of age and comorbidities. *Mov Disord* 2013; **28**: 1661–7.
70. de Bie RM, de Haan RJ, Schuurman PR, et al. Morbidity and mortality following pallidotomy in Parkinson's disease: a systematic review. *Neurology* 2002; **58**: 1008–12.
71. Kimber TE, Brophy BP, Thompson PD. Ataxic arm movements after thalamotomy for Parkinsonian tremor. *J Neurol Neurosurg Psychiatry* 2003; **74**: 258–9.
72. Merello M, Perez-Lloret S, Antico J, Obeso JA. Dyskinesias induced by subthalamotomy in Parkinson's disease are unresponsive to amantadine. *J Neurol Neurosurg Psychiatry* 2006; **77**: 172–4.
73. Green J, McDonald WM, Vitek JL, et al. Neuropsychological and psychiatric sequelae of pallidotomy for PD: clinical trial findings. *Neurology* 2002; **58**: 858–65.
74. Bickel S, Alvarez L, Macias R, et al. Cognitive and neuropsychiatric effects of subthalamotomy for Parkinson's disease. *Parkinsonism Relat Disord* 2010; **16**: 535–9.
75. Schuurman PR, Bruins J, Merkus MP, Bosch DA, Speelman JD. A comparison of neuropsychological effects of thalamotomy and thalamic stimulation. *Neurology* 2002; **59**: 1232–9.

Chapter 18

Deep-brain stimulation of the globus pallidus internus in the management of Parkinson's disease

Lilia C. Lovera, Alberto J. Espay and Andrew P. Duker

Introduction and history

Since James Parkinson's first description in 1817, the treatment of the disease that bears his name has evolved considerably. The poor results from early oral therapies (e.g. atropine and other anticholinergics) led to the development of surgical procedures such as posterior cervical rhizotomies [1], performed in an attempt to improve rigidity and tremor, or transections of the pyramidal tracts [2]. In the 1950s, Cooper, while performing a pedunculotomy on a patient with Parkinson's disease (PD), ligated the anterior choroidal artery to treat accidental bleeding and noticed the serendipitous improvement in tremor and rigidity following the surgery. This made the inner segment of the globus pallidus internus (GPi) and ansa lenticularis the common target for functional neurosurgery in the treatment of PD. Pallidotomy became a popular treatment for PD in the 1960s before the introduction of levodopa (L-DOPA) [3]. The remarkable therapeutic benefit brought on by levodopa was associated with a decline in the prevalence of surgical therapies. However, surgical interventions regained popularity in the 1990s, when it was recognized that pharmacological therapies were associated with motor complications of their own and that chronic treatment with levodopa led to motor fluctuations, dyskinesias and psychiatric complications [4].

Unilateral pallidotomy improved contralateral parkinsonism and levodopa-induced dyskinesias [5]. However, levodopa-resistant symptoms were not affected. In addition, the surgical procedure itself entailed a risk of complications including hemiparesis or visual-field deficits during the final step of electrocoagulation [6]. Bilateral pallidotomy was more likely to cause speech and bulbar side effects [7]. For this reason, this procedure was generally performed unilaterally, which kept intolerable dyskinesias and parkinsonian deficits unabated on the side ipsilateral to the lesion.

In 1994, Siegfried and colleagues were the first to report results of deep-brain stimulation (DBS) of the GPi in three patients. They noted improvements in all motor manifestations, motor fluctuations and levodopa-induced dyskinesias [8]. Deep-brain stimulation allowed the stimulation of bilateral GPi targets and improved "off" medication symptoms and dyskinesias [9]. The use of GPi-DBS became favored over lesional surgeries due to the lower risk of adverse events, and the fact that side effects could be reduced by adjusting the stimulation parameters [10]. Bilateral DBS was found to be associated with decreased morbidity compared with bilateral lesional procedures [11]. Despite the advantages of GPi-DBS, there may still be a role for unilateral pallidotomy. This is especially true in patients who live a long distance from specialized centers, lack the ability or the support to cooperate in extended evaluations and programming, or lack the time necessary to optimize stimulation [9]. This option may also be considered as a palliative intervention in those with refractory levodopa-induced dyskinesias but with contraindications to DBS, including the logistical difficulties listed above.

Why the globus pallidus internus? The mechanism of deep-brain stimulation

After the serendipitous discovery of motor function improvement after ligation of the anterior choroidal artery, further experimentation supported targeting of the GPi in neurosurgical procedures to ameliorate the symptoms of PD. The segregated-circuit hypothesis, the idea that the basal ganglia and associated areas of cortex

---

Parkinson's Disease: Current and Future Therapeutics and Clinical Trials, ed. Gálvez-Jiménez *et al*. Published by Cambridge University Press. © Cambridge University Press 2016.

and thalamus could be divided into separate functional areas, was introduced in 1986 by Alexander *et al.* [12]. In 1989, Albin *et al.* [13] proposed that specific types of basal ganglia disorders were associated with changes in the function of subpopulations of striatal projection neurons. It was postulated that, in PD, excessive excitatory drive from the subthalamic nucleus (STN) caused excessive inhibitory output from the GPi and substantia nigra reticulata (SNr). This in turn reduced thalamic activation of the primary motor cortex, premotor cortex, and supplementary motor area [14]. Therefore, the goal of lesioning or stimulation of the GPi or STN was thought to disrupt the abnormal neural activity of these nuclei, reduce the inhibitory effect of the basal ganglia on the thalamus and subsequently cortex, and improve parkinsonian symptoms [15].

It later became evident that, despite similar efficacy profiles, DBS did not inhibit firing in the same way as ablative surgery. Measurement of firing rates of downstream neurons instead showed increased firing rates [16]. Although the cell bodies of the stimulated deep nuclei are indirectly inhibited, DBS directly activates their axons [17]. In 2001, Brown *et al.* [18] observed marked changes in the oscillatory activity within the GPi and STN in treated and untreated patients with PD. When off levodopa, local potentials in both nuclei were dominated by synchronized low-frequency activity in the "beta band" (between 6 and 20 Hz). With levodopa-induced improvement in parkinsonism, the low-frequency synchronization was replaced by a higher frequency synchronization of about 70 Hz. Later experimentation revealed that the beta-band synchronization is also attenuated by high-frequency DBS [19]. Current theories as to the mechanisms of DBS now postulate that DBS increases high-frequency output of the stimulated nucleus, preventing transmission of the presumed pathological bursting and oscillatory activity [20].

Patient selection

The success of DBS depends largely on proper patient selection and reconciliation between potential improvements and patient expectations. Patients should only be considered after adequate trials of dopaminergic medications have not reached an appropriate risk:benefit ratio. It is important to note that, with rare exceptions, only an excellent response to levodopa predicts optimal results. Eligibility is made clear when that response is dampened by impaired tolerability or development of psychiatric or motor complications, most notably dyskinesias. If the response to levodopa remains suboptimal despite doses beyond 1600 mg/day, it is unlikely that any other drug class (dopamine agonists, monoamine oxidase inhibitors or catechol-O-methyltransferase inhibitors) would alter the assessment of treatment response and, with it, GPi-DBS eligibility. Thus, it is technically not mandatory that all surgical candidates must have tried all medication classes prior to consideration for GPi-DBS [21]. The diagnosis, cognitive and psychiatric status, access to care and patient expectations are also key features in the selection process [22]. Levodopa-responsive symptoms, tremor, "on"/"off" fluctuations and dyskinesias are the features most likely to improve with GPi-DBS. A multidisciplinary screening process including a neurologist, neurosurgeon, neuropsychologist and other health professionals should evaluate the patient to address suitability for GPi-DBS and whether alternative treatment approaches may be warranted.

Technique

Once the patient has been selected for GPi-DBS, detailed CT or MRI is performed prior to the procedure to delineate the target. Specialized computer software is applied to assist with target localization in relation to the stereotactic frame or, in some cases, fiducial markers placed on the patient's skull. All PD-related medications are withheld 12 h before the procedure. In most cases, the patient remains awake during the surgery to assess physiological recordings and behavioral responses. A burr hole is created in the skull for insertion of a quadripolar DBS electrode and microelectrodes. The depth of the target is determined based on characteristic electrophysiological recordings from the microelectrodes (Figure 18.1). The optic tract is located 1–2 mm deep to the ventral pallidum, and light shone at the pupils will produce an evoked discharge that can be heard on the recording [23]. Once the target is identified, the stimulating macroelectrode is placed at the ventral border of the GPi and tested intraoperatively to assess thresholds necessary to evoke side effects. Low-frequency stimulation, if too close to the internal capsule, can evoke rhythmic muscle contractions of certain muscle groups, such as the craniofacial musculature or tongue. Higher-frequency stimulation can evoke phosphenes in the contralateral visual field if too close to the optic tract. The macroelectrode is then secured and the contralateral target is approached in cases of bilateral procedures. A separate procedure is performed to implant the pulse generator.

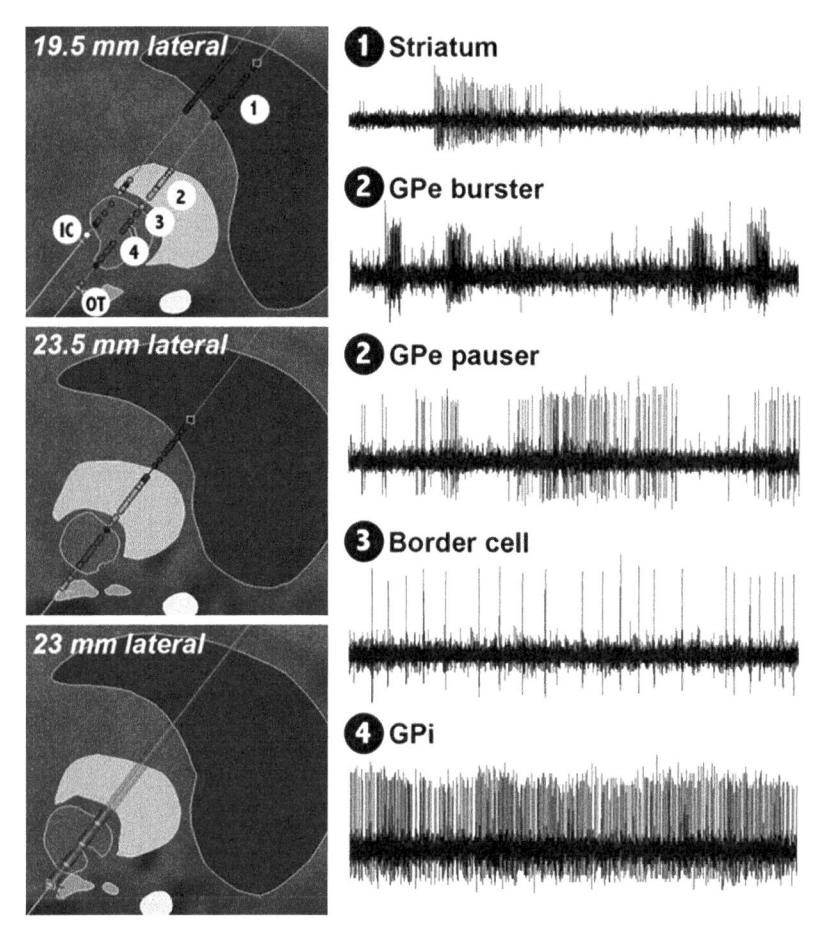

Figure 18.1 Microelectrode mapping of the globus pallidus. Characteristic firing patterns seen in the striatum (1), globus pallidus externus (GPe) (2), border cells (3) and globus pallidus internus (GPi) (4).
Reproduced with permission from Gross *et al.* Electrophysiological mapping for the implantation of deep brain stimulators for Parkinson's disease and tremor. Reproduced with permission from *Mov Disord* 2006 Jun; 21 Suppl. 1: S259–83 [23].

The presence of an immediate response following electrode implantation into the GPi does tend to correlate with future benefit observed once the stimulation is turned on in the postoperative period [24].

Initial programming occurs several weeks after implantation, in order to give time for resolution of any postoperative "lesion effect," which can result in improved symptoms (and therefore more difficult initial programming) for 1–2 weeks after the macroelectode is placed. Stimulation is started at a low amplitude and increased gradually over time. There are four contacts on the electrode, and stimulation can be delivered in a monopolar or bipolar fashion. The most effective contact configuration and frequency settings provide the greatest benefit with the least number of side effects due to the spread of current to surrounding structures.

Generally, programming may require multiple programming sessions and can take up to 4–6 months before full optimization of function is reached [25].

Globus pallidus internus deep-brain stimulation outcomes

The use of GPi-DBS produces a significant improvement in the off-medication Unified Parkinson's Disease Rating Scale (UPDRS) III scores with respect to baseline, by about 40%. It also improves cardinal features and activities of daily living (ADLs) while prolonging the "on" time with good mobility and without dyskinesias [26]. There is improvement in the ADL score of about 40%, and 66% improvement in levodopa-induced dyskinesias [9, 27]. In advanced

PD, pallidal DBS can also ameliorate "off"-period dystonia, cramps and sensory symptoms [28]. The duration of benefit from GPi-DBS is sustained, with retention of beneficial effects demonstrated in long-term follow-up [26, 29].

The effect of GPi-DBS is predominantly stimulation related. However, in addition to the aforementioned "lesion effect" that can last for 1–2 weeks after macroelectrode implantation, there are some benefits found when off stimulation even after this time, with some studies reporting an improvement in levodopa-induced dyskinesias at the 6-month follow-up during on-medication periods despite the stimulator being turned off [9].

Comparing subthalamic nucleus and globus pallidus internus deep-brain stimulation

Multiple studies have compared the outcomes of GPi and STN stimulation to determine which stimulation target is more effective for the treatment of PD symptoms. The first double-blinded crossover study comparing GPi-DBS and STN-DBS for PD was published in 2001. The results showed an improvement in dyskinesias in both STN-DBS and GPi-DBS of 58 and 66%, respectively, with an improvement in motor function of 49 and 37%, respectively, and an improvement in "on" time [30]. Daily levodopa dose equivalents were significantly reduced in the STN group (from 1218.8 mg at baseline to 764.0 mg at 6 months), and were unchanged in the GPi group (1090.9 mg at baseline and 1120 mg at 6 months). With DBS at either target, there is an increase in "on" time of about 4.6 h a day [31]. In 2005, Anderson et al. [32] found that there was insufficient evidence to support the superiority of one target over the other. Twelve months of stimulation at either location improved baseline rigidity, bradykinesia, tremor and axial symptoms (speech, gait, posture and postural stability), along with ADLs. In 2010, the Veterans Affairs Cooperative Studies Program (CSP 468) – a multicenter, randomized, blinded study – found similar improvements in motor function, quality of life and adverse events in both groups [33]. Another comparative trial in 2013 found that, during the on-medication state, there was a greater antidyskinetic effect in the GPi group, whereas in the STN group there were better off-medication motor symptoms and improvements in disability [34]. However, the results of this trial may have been confounded by some of the methods. The on-medication dosages were similar in both the GPi and STN groups, which may have increased the dyskinesia burden in the STN group. In addition, the DBS programmers were not blinded to subject assignment and could have differentially managed the settings and medications. Table 18.1 looks at seven randomized controlled trials comparing STN-DBS and GPi-DBS to date.

Dyskinesias improve significantly in both STN-DBS and GPi-DBS. This occurs by a direct dyskinesia suppression effect of GPi stimulation [39] or a reduction in levodopa dosage by STN stimulation. Levodopa and levodopa-equivalent dosages in general are significantly reduced after STN-DBS but not after GPi-DBS. The improvements in motor function after GPi-DBS have been shown to be sustained for up to 5–6 years after surgery [40].

Some studies endorse a trend toward increased improvement in bradykinesia and rigidity with STN-DBS compared with GPi-DBS [3, 32, 36]. However, GPi-DBS may be more effective against axial deficits resistant to levodopa [41]. The higher DBS settings required to obtain optimal benefit at the GPi may lead to more frequent replacements of pulse generators [33, 34]. However, GPi-DBS may be associated with a greater reduction in nonmotor features, including an improvement in depression [42].

Alternatively, unilateral GPi-DBS can be an effective option for PD patients with baseline asymmetry in symptoms. In a study with a 3.5 year follow-up, patients implanted with unilateral GPi-DBS were less likely to require a future second lead implantation than patients with unilateral STN-DBS [43]. The most likely cause for implantation in the contralateral side was insufficient relief of motor symptoms. The odds of proceeding to bilateral DBS were 5.2 times higher in the STN-DBS group than in the GPi-DBS group [43].

Complications

Complications from GPi-DBS include perioperative infection, hardware fracture and premature battery failure [9]. Transient adverse effects include paresthesias and tonic muscle contractions contralateral to the side of stimulation. Dysarthria can also be observed, likely due to stimulation of the internal capsule. Stimulation fields too close to the optic tract (ventrally) can cause photopsias or nausea. These adverse effects are relieved upon turning off the stimulation and can be managed in the long term by reducing the voltage or considering an alternative stimulating electrode to

Table 18.1 Blinded, randomized controlled trials comparing globus pallidus internus (GPi) and subthalamic nucleus (STN) deep-brain stimulation (DBS)

Author (country of origin)	Year	No. in sample (GPi/STN)	Primary outcome measure(s)	Primary outcomes	Other outcomes
Anderson et al. [32] (USA)	2005	11/12	Change in off-medication UPDRS-III	*Bilateral:* GPi = STN	Trend toward greater improvement in bradykinesia in STN
Rothlind et al. [35] (USA)	2007	23/19	Neuropsychological testing	*Unilateral and bilateral:* WAIS-R digit symbol GPi > STN; backward digit span GPi < STN; otherwise GPi = STN	Decrease in verbal fluency and working memory for both GPi and STN; trend toward decline in arithmetic and Stroop with STN
Okun et al. [36] (USA)	2009	23/22	Visual Analog Mood Scale; verbal fluency	*Unilateral:* GPi = STN in optimal DBS state	Motor UPDRS GPi = STN; Adverse mood effects with ventral stimulation both targets; worsening of verbal fluency in "off" STN-DBS
Zahodne et al. [37] (USA)	2009	22/20	Quality of life, measured by PDQ-39 summary index	*Unilateral:* GPi > STN	STN group: reduction in letter fluency
Follett et al. [33] (USA)	2010	152/147	Change in motor function measured by UPDRS-III	*Bilateral:* GPi = STN	STN required lower dopaminergic medication; visuomotor processing speed declined more after STN; depression worsened after STN and improved after GPi
Rocchi et al. [38] (Italy)	2012	14/15; 22 of the 29 patients were part of the VA Coop study Follett [33]	Step initiation measured by APAs, first-step length and velocity	*Bilateral:* postoperative APA same for GPi and STN; first-step velocity worsened in STN but not GPi	Although equal, APA for both GPi and STN were worse than non-DBS PD controls
Odekerken et al. [34] (The Netherlands)	2013	65/63	Functional health as measured by the weighted ALDS; composite score for cognitive, mood and behavioral effects	Bilateral GPi = STN	STN associated with more improvement in "off"-phase motor disability

ALDS, Academic Medical Center Linear Disability Scale, a functional health measure comparing time spent in the "off" phase compared with the "on" phase; PDQ-39, Parkinson's Disease Questionnaire; APA, Anticipatory postural adjustments – feed-forward postural preparation preceding voluntary step initiation; UPDRS, Unified Parkinson's Disease Rating Scale.

maintain the antiparkinsonian benefit with minimal side effects [9].

Cognitive changes following GPi-DBS, if present, appear to be mild, limited to specific areas and of debatable clinical significance. Early research suggested that older patients may be at a higher risk for significant cognitive or behavioral decline after bilateral STN-DBS, while GPi-DBS was thought to be safer [44]. More recent comparative trials have shown that the cognitive side effects are actually similar between the two groups. Subscores of neurocognitive function in the VA Cooperative study revealed similar slight decrements in all measures for both targets, except for a greater decline in visuomotor processing speed after STN-DBS [33]. Declines in letter verbal fluency, a consistent finding after STN-DBS, are present to a lesser extent with GPi-DBS [36]. Compared with best medical therapy, GPi-DBS was associated with lower performance on one measure of learning and memory that requires mental control and cognitive flexibility [45].

Regarding behavioral complications, postoperative delirium and perioperative anxiety may also be less common with GPi-DBS when compared with

Table 18.2 Decision making: patient characteristics and goals favoring globus pallidus internus (GPi) and subthalamic nucleus (STN) deep-brain stimulation

Clinical features/targets	GPi	STN
Troublesome levodopa-induced dyskinesias	x	x
Mild cognitive impairment	x (consider unilateral)	
Dose-limiting side effects limiting ability to increase levodopa		x
Levodopa-resistant axial motor signs	x	
Prominent bradykinesia		x
Preoperative depression	x	
Physician preference	x	x

STN-DBS [32]. As noted above, GPi-DBS may result in a slight improvement in depressive symptoms compared with a decline following STN-DBS, although the difference is small and the clinical meaningfulness is debatable [33].

Impulse control disorders may improve following medication reduction after DBS surgery; however, there is emerging evidence that impulse control disorders could also be precipitated by DBS [41]. It does not appear that the target (STN vs GPi) influences the extent to which this complication may occur, but the numbers studied so far are small.

Conclusion

The use of GPi-DBS is an effective treatment option for the management of PD-related motor fluctuations and dyskinesias. Selection of the optimal surgical target must take into account the full spectrum of both motor and nonmotor symptoms that affect quality of life in individual patients. The evidence suggests an overall similar efficacy for both STN-DBS and GPi-DBS but with differential cognitive side effect profiles, although these are of uncertain clinical relevance. Individual factors may make one target more attractive. Table 18.2 summarizes the various characteristics that may lead to the decision to choose STN over GPi as the stimulation target. Ultimately, the decision between targets also depends on the neurosurgeon's preference and expertise.

References

1. Leriche R. Über Chirurgischen Eingriff bei Parkinson'scher Krankheit. *Neurologische Zeitblaetter* 1912; **13**: 1093–6.
2. Putnam T. Relief from unilateral paralysis agitans by section of the pyramidal tract. *Arch Neurol* 1938; **40**: 1049–50.
3. Krack P, Pollak P, Limousin P, et al. Subthalamic nucleus or internal pallidal stimulation in young onset Parkinson's disease. *Brain* 1998; **121**: 451–7.
4. Marsden C, Parkes, JD, Quinn, N. Fluctuations of disability in Parkinson's disease: clinical aspects. In: Marsden CD, Fahn S, eds. *Movement Disorders*. London: Butterworths; 1982; 96–122.
5. Laitinen LV, Bergenheim AT, Hariz MI. Ventroposterolateral pallidotomy can abolish all parkinsonian symptoms. *Stereotact Funct Neurosurg* 1992; **58**: 14–21.
6. Shannon KM, Penn RD, Kroin JS, et al. Stereotactic pallidotomy for the treatment of Parkinson's disease. Efficacy and adverse effects at 6 months in 26 patients. *Neurology* 1998; **50**: 434–8.
7. Intemann PM, Masterman D, Subramanian I, et al. Staged bilateral pallidotomy for treatment of Parkinson disease. *J Neurosurg* 2001; **94**: 437–44.
8. Siegfried J, Lippitz B. Bilateral chronic electrostimulation of ventroposterolateral pallidum: a new therapeutic approach for alleviating all parkinsonian symptoms. *Neurosurgery* 1994; **35**: 1126–9; discussion 1129–30.
9. Kumar R, Lang AE, Rodriguez-Oroz MC, et al. Deep brain stimulation of the globus pallidus pars interna in advanced Parkinson's disease. *Neurology* 2000; **55** (Suppl. 6): S34–9.
10. Dostrovsky JO, Hutchison WD, Lozano AM. The globus pallidus, deep brain stimulation, and Parkinson's disease. *Neuroscientist* 2002; **8**: 284–90.
11. Merello M, Starkstein S, Nouzeilles MI, Kuzis G, Leiguarda R. Bilateral pallidotomy for treatment of Parkinson's disease induced corticobulbar syndrome and psychic akinesia avoidable by globus pallidus lesion combined with contralateral stimulation. *J Neurol Neurosurg Psychiatry* 2001; **71**: 611–4.
12. Alexander GE, DeLong MR, Strick PL. Parallel organization of functionally segregated circuits linking basal ganglia and cortex. *Annu Rev Neurosci* 1986; **9**: 357–81.
13. Albin RL, Young AB, Penney JB. The functional anatomy of basal ganglia disorders. *Trends Neurosci* 1989; **12**: 366–75.
14. Alexander GE, Crutcher MD, DeLong MR. Basal ganglia-thalamocortical circuits: parallel substrates for motor, oculomotor, "prefrontal" and "limbic" functions. *Prog Brain Res* 1990; **85**: 119–46.
15. Grafton ST, DeLong M. Tracing the brain's circuitry with functional imaging. *Nat Med* 1997; **3**: 602–3.
16. Anderson ME, Postupna N, Ruffo M. Effects of high-frequency stimulation in the internal globus pallidus

on the activity of thalamic neurons in the awake monkey. *J Neurophysiol* 2003; **89**: 1150–60.
17. McIntyre CC, Savasta M, Kerkerian-Le Goff L, Vitek JL. Uncovering the mechanism(s) of action of deep brain stimulation: activation, inhibition, or both. *Clin Neurophysiol* 2004; **115**: 1239–48.
18. Brown P, Oliviero A, Mazzone P, et al. Dopamine dependency of oscillations between subthalamic nucleus and pallidum in Parkinson's disease. *J Neurosci* 2001; **21**: 1033–8.
19. Brown P, Mazzone P, Oliviero A, et al. Effects of stimulation of the subthalamic area on oscillatory pallidal activity in Parkinson's disease. *Exp Neurol* 2004; **188**: 480–90.
20. Miocinovic S, Somayajula S, Chitnis S, Vitek JL. History, applications, and mechanisms of deep brain stimulation. *JAMA Neurol* 2013; **70**: 163–71.
21. Okun MS. Deep-brain stimulation for Parkinson's disease. *N Engl J Med* 2012; **367**: 1529–38.
22. Rodriguez RL, Fernandez HH, Haq I, Okun MS. Pearls in patient selection for deep brain stimulation. *Neurologist* 2007; **13**: 253–60.
23. Gross RE, Krack P, Rodriguez-Oroz MC, Rezai AR, Benabid AL. Electrophysiological mapping for the implantation of deep brain stimulators for Parkinson's disease and tremor. *Mov Disord* 2006; **21** (Suppl. 14): S259–83.
24. Cersosimo MG, Raina GB, Benarroch EE, et al. Micro lesion effect of the globus pallidus internus and outcome with deep brain stimulation in patients with Parkinson disease and dystonia. *Mov Disord* 2009; **24**: 1488–93.
25. Duker AP, Espay AJ. Surgical treatment of Parkinson disease: past, present, and future. *Neurol Clin* 2013; **31**: 799–808.
26. Rodriguez-Oroz MC, Obeso JA, Lang AE, et al. Bilateral deep brain stimulation in Parkinson's disease: a multicentre study with 4 years follow-up. *Brain* 2005; **128**: 2240–9.
27. Rodrigues JP, Walters SE, Watson P, Stell R, Mastaglia FL. Globus pallidus stimulation improves both motor and nonmotor aspects of quality of life in advanced Parkinson's disease. *Mov Disord* 2007; **22**: 1866–70.
28. Loher TJ, Burgunder JM, Weber S, Sommerhalder R, Krauss JK. Effect of chronic pallidal deep brain stimulation on off period dystonia and sensory symptoms in advanced Parkinson's disease. *J Neurol Neurosurg Psychiatry* 2002; **73**: 395–9.
29. Weaver FM, Follett KA, Stern M, et al. Randomized trial of deep brain stimulation for Parkinson disease: thirty-six-month outcomes. *Neurology* 2012; **79**: 55–65.
30. Deep-Brain Stimulation for Parkinson's Disease Study Group. Deep-brain stimulation of the subthalamic nucleus or the pars interna of the globus pallidus in Parkinson's disease. *N Engl J Med* 2001; **345**: 956–63.
31. Weaver FM, Follett K, Stern M, et al. Bilateral deep brain stimulation vs best medical therapy for patients with advanced Parkinson disease: a randomized controlled trial. *JAMA* 2009; **301**: 63–73.
32. Anderson VC, Burchiel KJ, Hogarth P, Favre J, Hammerstad JP. Pallidal vs subthalamic nucleus deep brain stimulation in Parkinson disease. *Arch Neurol* 2005; **62**: 554–60.
33. Follett KA, Weaver FM, Stern M, et al. Pallidal versus subthalamic deep-brain stimulation for Parkinson's disease. *N Engl J Med* 2010; **362**: 2077–91.
34. Odekerken VJ, van Laar T, Staal MJ, et al. Subthalamic nucleus versus globus pallidus bilateral deep brain stimulation for advanced Parkinson's disease (NSTAPS study): a randomised controlled trial. *Lancet Neurol* 2013; **12**: 37–44.
35. Rothlind JC, Cockshott RW, Starr PA, Marks WJ, Jr. Neuropsychological performance following staged bilateral pallidal or subthalamic nucleus deep brain stimulation for Parkinson's disease. *J Int Neuropsychol Soc* 2007; **13**: 68–79.
36. Okun MS, Fernandez HH, Wu SS, et al. Cognition and mood in Parkinson's disease in subthalamic nucleus versus globus pallidus interna deep brain stimulation: the COMPARE trial. *Ann Neurol* 2009; **65**: 586–95.
37. Zahodne LB, Okun MS, Foote KD, et al. Greater improvement in quality of life following unilateral deep brain stimulation surgery in the globus pallidus as compared to the subthalamic nucleus. *J Neurol* 2009; **256**: 1321–9.
38. Rocchi L, Carlson-Kuhta P, Chiari L, et al. Effects of deep brain stimulation in the subthalamic nucleus or globus pallidus internus on step initiation in Parkinson disease: laboratory investigation. *J Neurosurg* 2012; **117**: 1141–9.
39. Oyama G, Foote KD, Jacobson CE, 4th, et al. GPi and STN deep brain stimulation can suppress dyskinesia in Parkinson's disease. *Parkinsonism Relat Disord* 2012; **18**: 814–18.
40. Moro E, Lozano AM, Pollak P, et al. Long-term results of a multicenter study on subthalamic and pallidal stimulation in Parkinson's disease. *Movement Dis* 2010; **25**: 578–86.
41. Rouaud T, Dondaine T, Drapier S, et al. Pallidal stimulation in advanced Parkinson's patients with contraindications for subthalamic stimulation. *Mov Disord* 2010; **25**: 1839–46.

42. Liu Y, Li W, Tan C, *et al*. Meta-analysis comparing deep brain stimulation of the globus pallidus and subthalamic nucleus to treat advanced Parkinson disease. *J Neurosurg* 2014; **121**: 709–18.
43. Taba HA, Wu SS, Foote KD, *et al*. A closer look at unilateral versus bilateral deep brain stimulation: results of the National Institutes of Health COMPARE cohort. *J Neurosurg* 2010; **113**: 1224–9.
44. Trepanier LL, Kumar R, Lozano AM, Lang AE, Saint-Cyr JA. Neuropsychological outcome of GPi pallidotomy and GPi or STN deep brain stimulation in Parkinson's disease. *Brain Cogn* 2000; **42**: 324–47.
45. Rothlind JC, York MK, Carlson K, *et al*. Neuropsychological changes following deep brain stimulation surgery for Parkinson's disease: comparisons of treatment at pallidal and subthalamic targets versus best medical therapy. *J Neurol Neurosurg Psychiatry* 2014; **86**: 622–9.

Chapter 19

Deep-brain stimulation of the subthalamic nucleus in the management of Parkinson's disease

David A. Schmerler, Alberto J. Espay and Andrew P. Duker

Introduction

The use of deep-brain stimulation (DBS) for the surgical treatment of Parkinson's disease (PD) was born out of the observation that high-frequency stimulation used for localization during lesional neurosurgery could itself have an effect on PD symptoms. While intraoperative [1] and chronic [2] stimulation of the deep structures of the brain were performed previously, the modern era of DBS was ushered in with the work of Benabid and colleagues, targeting first the ventral intermediate (VIM) nucleus of the thalamus [3]. As the functional connectivity of the basal ganglia became better understood [4], the utility of targeting the subthalamic nucleus (STN) for the amelioration of parkinsonism was tested, first in animal models [5] and then in humans [6]. Since then, a number of other DBS targets have been examined, including the globus pallidus internus (GPi) and pedunculopontine nucleus (PPN). This chapter will focus on the indications, technique, mechanism and efficacy of STN-DBS for patients with PD.

Indications and patient selection

Parkinson's disease is a disabling chronic neurological condition that causes significant deterioration in the quality of life [7]. Despite the marked benefits of oral levodopa (L-DOPA) therapy, patients develop medication-associated motor complications including shortened duration of benefit and dyskinesias. These motor fluctuations are theorized to arise from the effect of rising and falling plasma levodopa levels, which induce pulsatile or phasic stimulation of striatal dopamine receptors, contrary to the tonic stimulation in physiological conditions [8]. While adjunctive medications such as dopamine agonists, catechol-O-methyltransferase inhibitors, monoamine oxidase type B inhibitors and amantadine can improve motor symptoms or (only in the case of amantadine) reduce dyskinesias, they tend to exhibit declining tolerability with disease progression [9, 10]. The technique of STN-DBS has been shown to excel in this respect, with demonstrated improvements in motor fluctuations, dyskinesia severity and appendicular motor features, such as tremor, rigidity and bradykinesia [11–13]. In general, the response to STN stimulation matches the best response to levodopa, but with overall enhancement of motor function, a reduction in "off" time and an increase in "on" time without dyskinesias.

For this reason, optimal candidates for consideration of STN-DBS are those with PD with an excellent levodopa response but experiencing a severe "off"-related disability, which may not be amenable to pharmacotherapeutic optimization due to concurrent, and often prominent, levodopa-induced dyskinesias [14]. Evaluation for DBS candidacy is typically performed in the context of a multidisciplinary team including a neurologist, neurosurgeon, neuropsychologist and, if needed, a psychiatrist. In an attempt to standardize the patient selection, originally to guide patient selection for a program on intracerebral transplantation of fetal dopamine neurons, the Core Assessment Program for Intracerebral Transplantations (CAPIT) protocol [15] was developed in 1992, later adapted into a Core Assessment Program for Surgical Interventional

Parkinson's Disease: Current and Future Therapeutics and Clinical Trials, ed. Gálvez-Jiménez *et al*. Published by Cambridge University Press. © Cambridge University Press 2016.

Therapies (CAPSIT) [16]. The CAPSIT protocol remains the most comprehensive and stringent guide to assist in the selection of patients most likely to benefit from ablative and neurostimulation procedures, ensuring that suitable patients are ideal from a cognitive, emotional and social standpoint for DBS [17]. The CAPSIT protocol has been modified and individualized by many centers, but its basic decision nodes remain unchanged (Figure 19.1).

Given that DBS benefits those symptoms that are predominately levodopa responsive, improvement from levodopa is a fundamental criteria for selection, and a 33% decrease in Unified Parkinson's Disease Rating Scale (UPDRS)-III motor score between the off-medication and on-medication states is widely considered the threshold for predicting a good outcome from DBS. This is tested by performing an evaluation of the motor response to levodopa whereby a patient undergoes an assessment in the practically defined "off" period, i.e. following a 12 h washout from any dopaminergic medication, and again in the "on" state, after a therapeutic or sometimes supratherapeutic dose of levodopa [16].

A secondary purpose of such a levodopa challenge is to identify patients with a suboptimal response to levodopa, which may represent patients with atypical parkinsonian disorders, previously considered as PD, for whom DBS may lead to unsustained benefits at best or even accelerated decline at worst [19]. A thorough preoperative neurocognitive and behavioral assessment is performed in order to exclude patients with overt or emerging dementia, or with underlying psychiatric conditions that could be exacerbated by, or lessen the response to, surgery. Depression should be optimally treated prior to considering surgery. The presence or absence of depression could influence the choice of target, as some data suggest that STN stimulation may worsen depression, whereas GPi stimulation may alleviate it [20]. Psychosis is not an absolute contraindication to DBS but is frequently a harbinger of an emerging dementia; therefore extreme caution is needed. Mild cognitive impairment in one area, such as executive functioning, is common in PD and is not necessarily an exclusionary factor. However, involvement of multiple domains, particularly localizable to posterior cortical functioning, suggests an atypical parkinsonism or comorbid Alzheimer's dementia. In either case, DBS can be associated with deterioration of cognitive function and the development of frank dementia. Finally, it is important to manage patient expectations by educating prospective surgical candidates on what DBS can and cannot accomplish, and on the potential risks. This includes ensuring that the goal for DBS (e.g. dyskinesias or reduction in "off" time) corresponds to what the patient finds troublesome and is worthy of assuming the surgical risks. Postoperative questionnaires have demonstrated a high degree of satisfaction, with 89% of patients believing that they made the right decision to undergo DBS, 78% making the same decision again and 72% recommending DBS to another patient in a similar situation [21].

In terms of the timing of STN-DBS, by the time medically intractable fluctuations and dyskinesias occur, patients often find themselves with impaired quality of life, and with social and professional disability [22]. For this reason, DBS is increasingly being considered earlier in the disease process, in an attempt to prevent disability from accruing. The EARLYSTIM trial demonstrated superiority of STN-DBS over medical therapy in patients with early motor complications [23], with quality-of-life measurements improving in parallel with motor improvements. However, several pitfalls in the design of this study, including a 7-year disease duration (which is not easily defined as "early" by most definitions) and the "lessebo" effect shown by those allocated to the best medical therapy arm (who had presumably become study subjects with the expectation of receiving surgery rather than oral medications) cast doubt on the generalizability of their conclusions [24]. Indeed, a recent study applying more stringent criteria for "early" DBS demonstrated no differences in motor function between the surgical and best medical therapy arms [25]. While there remains cautious reluctance in offering an invasive therapy to patients still adequately managed by oral therapies, the prevention of accumulating disability and the resultant improvement in quality of life are attractive possibilities that warrant further study. Currently, however, disease progression following STN-DBS appears to continue at the same rate as in those who are medically treated [26, 27]. The long-term effects of STN-DBS stimulation remain beneficial, and the improvements found from stimulation can persist for over a decade [10, 13], although nonmotor and axial motor features, which are less responsive to STN-DBS, dominate the clinical picture in advanced stages, detracting from its overall benefit [28, 29].

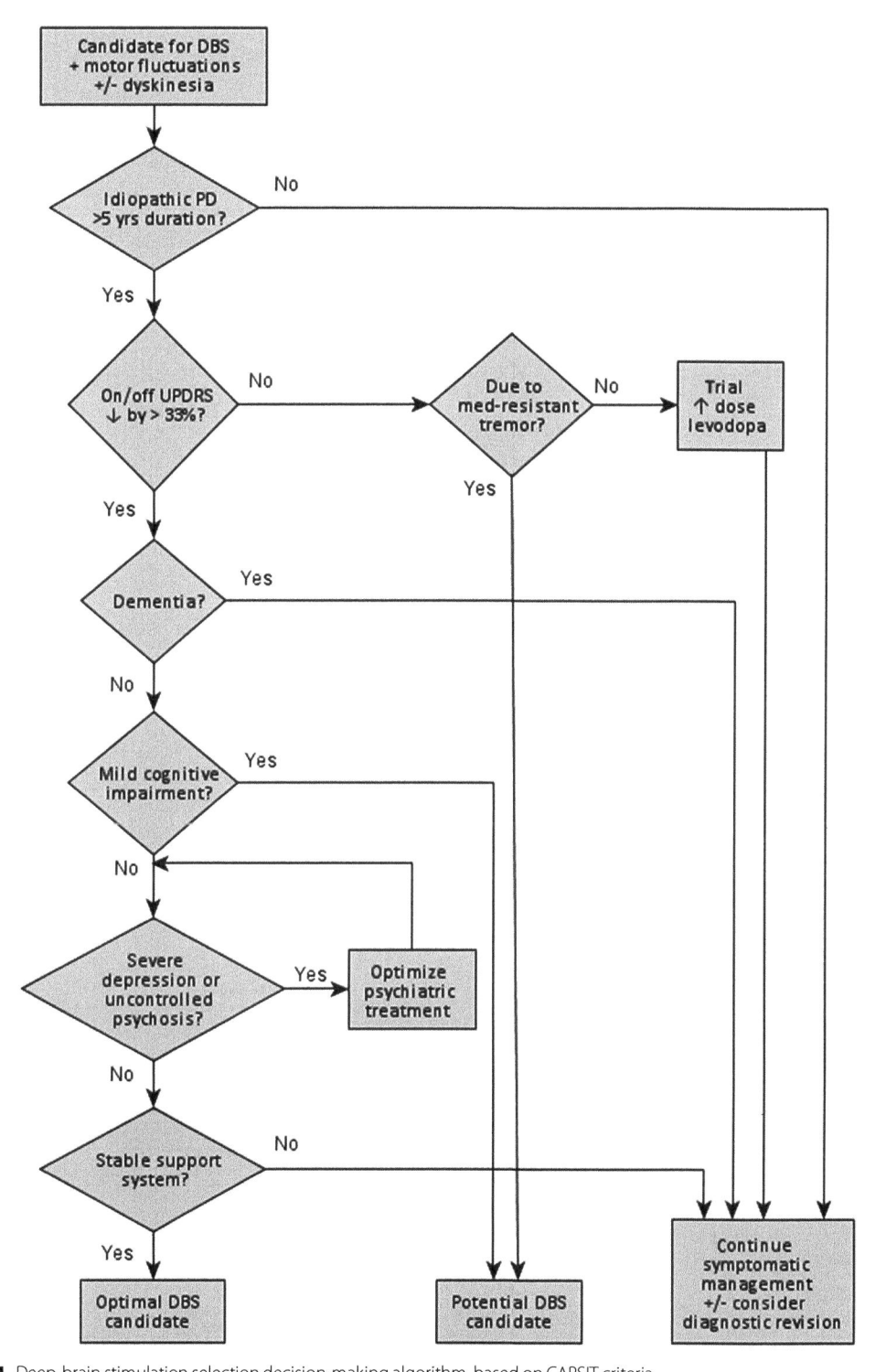

Figure 19.1 Deep-brain stimulation selection decision-making algorithm, based on CAPSIT criteria.
Reproduced with permission from Duker AP, Espay AJ. Surgical Treatment of Parkinson Disease: Past, Present, and Future. *Neurol Clin* 2013; 31: 799–808 [18].

The procedure

The neurosurgical procedure of selection and implantation of the DBS electrodes has been well described elsewhere [30, 31]. Electrodes are typically implanted under local anesthesia, although some centers may use general anesthesia. Prior to the procedure, the neurosurgeon plans the surgery with targeting based on MRI localization of visual landmarks and brain atlases using brain-mapping software. Targeting is also compared with expected three-dimensional coordinates, established by a frame placed around the patient's skull or alternatively with other markers if a frameless system is used. Once the coordinates and trajectory have been mapped, a burr hole is made for each respective electrode.

The microelectrode is channeled down the mapped trajectory and the STN target is confirmed via microelectrode recording, typically performed by an electrophysiologist or trained movement disorder specialist (Figure 19.2). After the target is confirmed, the microelectrode is removed and replaced with a stimulating macroelectrode. The stimulating macroelectrode is tested during surgery to determine optimal benefits and identify side effects and the threshold for their effect (Table 19.1). The final position of the macroelectrode is that at which the greatest efficacy on rigidity and motor symptoms is obtained with the lowest stimulation intensity and highest threshold for side effect. Quadripolar electrode models are frequently used, and bilateral placement in a single operative session is typically performed. Although unilateral stimulation may

Table 19.1 Possible intraoperative subthalamic nucleus stimulation-induced side effects

Stimulation-induced side effect	Localization of electrical stimulation
Paresthesias	Medial lemniscus (posterior)
Photopsia	Medial lemniscus (posterior)
Eyelid opening apraxia	Oculomotor basal ganglia loop
Gaze deviation	Oculomotor basal ganglia loop
Diplopia	Fascicles of CNIII or supranuclear oculomotor system
Ataxia or vertigo	Red nucleus (medial)
Face or arm muscle contraction	Internal capsule
Dysphagia	Corticobulbar fibers
Dysarthria	Corticobulbar fibers
Sweating or flushing	Hypothalamus (anterior)
Dyskinesias	Indicative of proper subthalamic nucleus placement

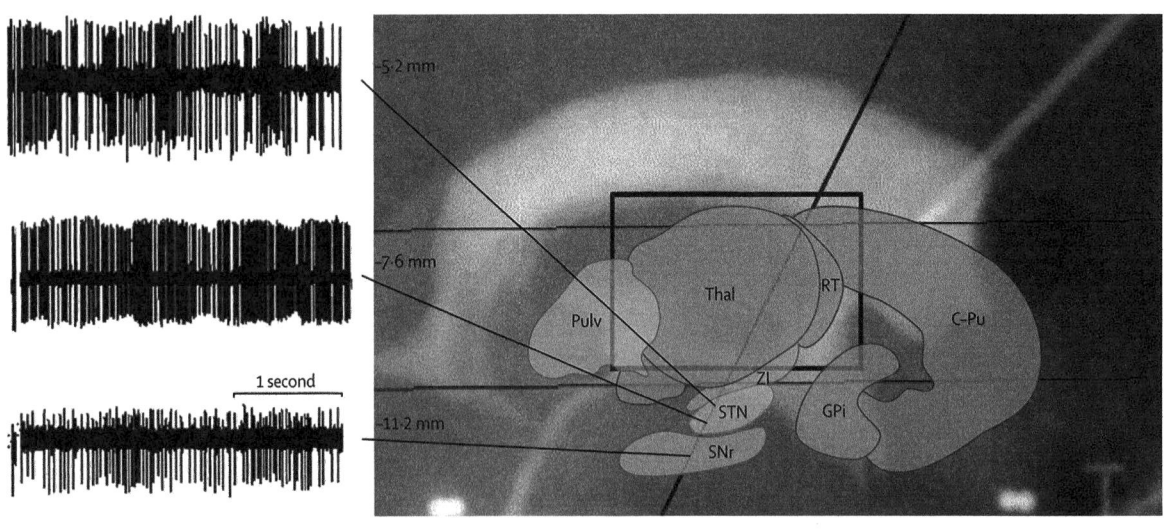

Figure 19.2 Stereotactic localization of the subthalamic nucleus using firing patterns from microelectrode recordings. The microelectrode trajectory (black oblique line) encounters the thalamus and then the zona incerta, followed by a rich, irregular burst of neural activity in the kinesthetic neurons of the subthalamic nucleus (STN; 5.2 and 7.6 mm below the commissural line in this patient), and high-amplitude, regular and unresponsive neural activity in the substantia nigra pars reticulata (SNr; 11.2 mm below the commissural line). C-Pu, caudate and putamen (striatum); GPi, internal globus pallidus; Pulv, pulvinar; RT, reticularis thalami; Thal, thalamus; ZI, zona incerta. (A black and white version of this figure will appear in some formats. For the color version, please refer to the plate section.)
Reproduced with permission from Benabid AL *et al.* Deep brain stimulation of the subthalamic nucleus for the treatment of Parkinson's disease. *The Lancet Neurology.* 2009;8[1]: 67–81 [32].

benefit a subset of patients [33], its benefit is typically limited to contralateral symptoms and may not provide maximal improvement in walking [34].

After successful determination of the position, the macroelectrode is secured, the surgical site is closed and typically within a week or two the implantable pulse generator is surgically placed. Following surgery, patients may experience a "lesion effect" whereby symptoms are transiently improved due to the placement of the electrode alone. This effect generally disappears after several days to weeks.

Outcomes/proof of efficacy

Randomized controlled trials comparing STN-DBS with best medical therapy (levodopa) have consistently demonstrated that neurostimulation produces a greater improvement from baseline in the UPDRS and 39-Item Parkinson's disease Quality of Life Questionnaire (PDQ-39) [10, 35]. A trial by Deuschl et al. [10] demonstrated PDQ-39 improvements of 24–38% compared with medication management alone when examining the subscales for mobility, activities of daily living (ADLs), emotional well-being, stigma and bodily discomfort (Table 19.2).

One of the greatest effects from STN-DBS (unlike pallidal stimulation) is the ability to reduce dopaminergic medication postoperatively, with an average drug dosage reduction of 40–65% [11, 13, 38, 39]. "Off"-period impairment is also reduced; patients assessed on neurostimulation alone have demonstrated over a 40% improvement in their UPDRS score, as well as improvements in ADLs, as evidenced by improvements on the Schwab and England Scale [10]. Overall, the average change in ADL scores estimated by Kleiner-Fishman et al. [35] in a meta-analysis of outcomes was nearly a 50% improvement from baseline, although largely affecting motor aspects of function. Disease progression following STN-DBS appears to continue at the same rate as for those who are medically treated [26]. The long-term effect of STN-DBS stimulation remains beneficial, and the improvements found from stimulation do persist over several years [10, 13].

Dyskinesias are perhaps the source of disability exhibiting the greatest magnitude of improvement after STN-DBS [11, 12], with a 54% reduction in the neurostimulation group found by Deuschl et al. [10] compared with no changes in the medication group. These patients demonstrated a longer duration of "on" time without dyskinesias, gaining on average 4.4 h "on" and 4.2 fewer "off" hours [10]. Rigidity and tremor improved by 70% with STN stimulation, and bradykinesia was reduced by over 50% [13]. Speech and other axial symptoms such as postural reflexes and gait tend not to improve as much as appendicular motor symptoms with STN-DBS [11, 13]. Dysarthria may even be aggravated if stimulation affects the corticobulbar fibers [40]. Cognitive outcomes following STN-DBS remain relatively similar compared with best medical management, although verbal fluency scores are consistently decreased, whereas working memory and processing speed typically are stable [41].

The optimal anatomical location within the STN is still debated. Stimulation of the dorsolateral sensorimotor portion of the STN is more effective for improvement in motor symptoms, but attempts to separate out discrete localizations responsible for tremor, bradykinesia, rigidity and other symptoms have been fraught with inconsistent results. Ultimately, individual patient differences in response to stimulation are the driving force tailoring DBS programming.

Mechanism of action

The technique of STN-DBS requires high-frequency stimulation (greater than 130 Hz) to be effective [42]. Lower frequencies (60–80 Hz) have been utilized in some patients to treat freezing of gait [43], although results have been inconsistent. Low-frequency DBS below 20 Hz typically worsens bradykinesia [42, 44]. High-frequency stimulation of the STN is thought to exert its effects through changes in the pattern of neuronal firing [45], rather than simply changes in the firing rate, as was thought previously. Microelectrode recording in the STN during DBS reveals local field potentials with specific frequencies, which are the product of the synchronicity of neuronal oscillations. In PD, frequencies between 11 and 30 Hz (the "beta band") have been found to be associated with worsened motor function [46]. These same oscillatory frequencies are attenuated by voluntary movement, dopaminergic medication and DBS [47], and are replaced by low-frequency oscillations (1–7 Hz) whose significance remains unknown; however, they are hypothesized to reflect the effect of electrical polarization around the stimulating electrode that may be normalizing STN hyperactivity [48–50].

Complications and side effects

Compared with medical management, DBS surgery produces a higher frequency of serious adverse events, 13% compared with 4% in the 2006 study by Deuschl

Section III: Surgical Management of Parkinson's Disease

Table 19.2 Clinical trials comparing deep-brain stimulation with best medical therapy
The data below depict changes from baseline of each surgical group versus medical therapy

Study	Surgical site	Mean age (years)	Duration of disease	Mean decrease in "off" time	Mean increase in "on" time	UPDRS-III change (STN vs medical)	Dyskinesia scale or change	PDQ-39 summary index mean change[a]	Duration of follow-up
Deuschl et al., 2006 [10]	STN	60.5 (±7.4 SD; maximum age 75)	Unknown; mean stage 4	4.2 vs 0 h	4.4 vs −0.5 h	41 vs 1% improvement	Scale: 6.7 vs 0, a 54 vs 0% improvement	−9.5 (−13.1 to −5.9) vs +0.2 (2.4−2.9)	6 months
Weaver et al., 2009 [36]	STN or GPi	62.4 (range 37−83)	12.4 years (± 5.8 SD)	2.4 h vs 0 h	4.6 vs 0 h	71 vs 32% improvement	Unknown	−7.7 (−9.7 to −5.6) vs 0.4 (−1.0 to 1.8)	6 months
Williams et al., 2010 [37]	STN or Gpi	59 (range 37−79)	11.5 years (2.0−32.2)	Unknown	Unknown	17 vs −4% improvement	Unknown	−5.0 (± 14.1 SD) vs −0.3 (± 11.1 SD)	12 months
Schuepbach et al., 2013 [23]	STN	52.9 (±6.6 SD). Maximum age 60.	7.3 years (± 3.1 SD; minimum 4-year duration)	17.5 vs 1.2 h	3.2 vs −1.3 h	26 vs −11% improvement	2.1 vs 0.2 h improvement in dyskinesias	−7.8 (± 1.2 SD) vs +0.2 (± 1.1 SD), a 26% improvement vs 1% worsening	24 months

[a] PDQ-39 range is 0−100; higher scores = worse reported quality of life; a negative change represents an improvement.

Table 19.3 Common possible complications of subthalamic nucleus deep-brain stimulation

Complication	Relative risk (%)
Fatal intracranial hemorrhage	3.9
Surgical or device infection	3.6
Device dysfunction	3
Migration of leads	1.5
Seizures	1.5
Ischemic stroke	1

Adapted from [35].

et al. [10]. Serious adverse events include seizures in up to 3% of patients, ischemic stroke in nearly 1% of patients, fatal intracranial hemorrhage occurring in about 2–4% of patients and surgical-site infections occurring in up to 8% (Table 19.3) [20, 35, 37, 51]. Device failure is possible as well, with possible complications including lead breaks, dermal erosion, seromas, excessive battery consumption and pulse generator failure [52]. Patient discomfort can be seen, with tightness of the extension lead, scars and subdermal bumps along the duration of the lead [32]. Stimulation-related complications generally result from the unintentional spread of current into neighboring structures surrounding the STN, which can occur in up to 30% of patients [35]. These effects fortunately are often transient, reversible and adjustable with modification of the stimulation parameters (Figure 19.3). Another possible complication of STN-DBS surgery is weight gain, with reports varying from 8.4% [35] to an incidence approaching 100% in some small studies [53]. The cause of this is likely multifactorial and may be influenced by a decrease in dyskinesias or decreased serum cortisol [54], or potentially related to electrode location, with greater risk associated with closer proximity to more medial regions within the STN [55].

The incidence of certain complications can be prevented or reduced by adhering to strict patient selection criteria, as outlined above. Neuropsychological evaluation is performed to avoid surgery in patients who have significant cognitive impairment or uncontrolled depression. Perioperative confusion and psychosis can be risk factors for further cognitive decline [56]. While uncommon, some patients undergoing STN-DBS have attempted or completed suicide [10, 57]. Rates of attempt have been seen at nearly 0.90% and rate of completion at 0.45% [58]. The reason for such behavior is unclear, although it may be associated with a decrease in the dopaminergic tone, associated with reductions in levodopa and dopamine agonist dosage made possible after surgery, which could contribute to the magnification of postsurgical behavioral disturbances, including depression. Neurosurgery may impact the patients' perception of themselves and their body, experiencing apathy, a sense of loss of vitality, and strangeness [59]. Furthermore, "in spite of the excellent motor outcome, it is clear that the operation can result in poor adjustment of the patient to his or her personal, family, and

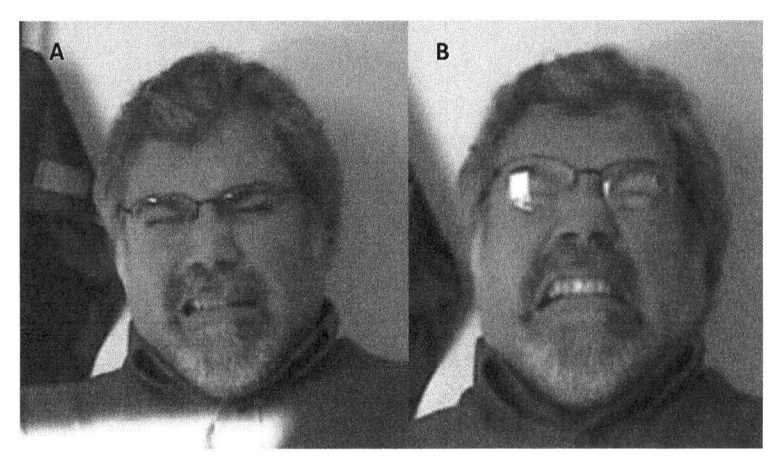

Figure 19.3 A man with facial dystonia as a stimulation-induced side effect from subthalamic nucleus deep-brain stimulation. Note that the contraction of facial muscles at rest (A) is magnified when attempting to speak (B), a typical expression of focal dystonias. Dystonia substantially improved with lowered stimulation amplitude.

socio-professional life" [59]. For this reason, a strong social support network is important to help care for the patient following surgery. For patients requiring a substantial decrease in levodopa dose, monitoring of behavioral "at-risk" changes is warranted. Other complications of STN-DBS exist, including dysexecutive syndrome [41] and psychiatric symptoms [60]. Certain complications have been associated with the location of stimulation within the STN area. Patients who have received stimulation being slightly too ventral, closer to the limbic system, have experienced postsurgical hypomania, typically transient or alleviated with a change in DBS programming [61, 62]. Generally, patients who experience cognitive decline postsurgically have been found to have electrode placements with deeper and more posterior/ventral contacts [56].

Future uses of subthalamic nucleus deep-brain stimulation

The future of STN-DBS may include a wider opportunity for patients to be considered eligible and more patient-specific programming. Animal data had provided optimism that STN-DBS could be neuroprotective [63, 64], although supportive data in humans have been so far elusive. Based on prior studies demonstrating that those with "early" motor complications receiving STN-DBS with best medical therapy versus medical therapy alone had an improved quality of life in the DBS group [23], future research endeavors will examine the extent to which early STN-DBS may have disease-modifying properties. The intermediate-frequency range between 60 and 80 Hz is being evaluated for possible improvements in freezing and gait [43]. With research into specific frequency-related treatments comes the potential for clinical trials into adaptive technology, such as an adaptive or "closed-loop" DBS [65], which has been demonstrated in primate models to be more effective than the standard open-loop treatment [66]. The ability to shape electrical fields to focus stimulation in desired structures and minimize side effects is being developed with the use of segmented electrodes [67, 68]. With the greater complexity of programming DBS electrodes that have an increased number of contacts or segmented contacts, it is likely that software will assist the neurologist with steering the DBS current in the intended direction and translating this into the appropriate parameters.

Alternative targets and conclusion

There are multiple other targets being considered for electrode placement, some of which will be covered elsewhere in this book. The STN has consistently remained an effective location for placement due to the consistency of its benefit on motor symptoms, the reduction in fluctuations and the ability to decrease dopaminergic medication. Ventral intermediate thalamic stimulation is effective at tremor reduction in PD but does not adequately address bradykinesia and other motor symptoms, which become prominent with disease progression [69, 70]. The technique of GPi-DBS may be more effective at reducing dyskinesias [71], although randomized and blinded studies comparing STN with GPi stimulation have shown similar motor benefits [20, 72]. Thus, GPi stimulation may be less likely to cause cognitive complications [20], but the differential effect may be slight. Some small, open-label studies have targeted both the STN and the PPN for symptoms typically refractory to STN-DBS treatment, with some improvement to axial symptoms and a reduction in falls [71, 73]. Despite these alternatives, STN-DBS remains a difficult standard to surpass, given the large motor improvement it produces through reduced "off" time and improved dyskinesias. Current decision making on targeting remains largely based on the patient and the surgeon's preference and experience. New technologies and research stand to help refine and improve this procedure with more nuanced targeting and adaptive technology.

Acknowledgements

DAS has received personal compensation as a consultant for Merz Pharmaceuticals. AJE is supported by the K23 career development award (NIMH, 1K23MH092735) and has received grant support from CleveMed/Great Lakes Neurotechnologies, and the Michael J Fox Foundation; personal compensation as a consultant/scientific advisory board member for Abbvie, Chelsea Therapeutics, TEVA, Impax, Merz, Pfizer, Acadia, Cynapsus, Solstice Neurosciences, Eli Lilly, Lundbeck, and USWorldMeds; royalties from Lippincott Williams & Wilkins and Cambridge University Press; and honoraria from UCB, TEVA, the American Academy of Neurology, and the Movement Disorders Society. He serves as Associate Editor of *Movement Disorders, Frontiers in Movement Disorders* and *Journal of Clinical Movement Disorders*, and is on the editorial boards of *Parkinsonism and Related*

Disorders and the *European Neurological Journal*. APD has received personal compensation as a consultant for USWorldMeds.

References

1. Hullay J, Velok J, Gombi R, Boczan G. Subthalamotomy in Parkinson's disease. *Confin Neurol* 1970; 32: 345–8.
2. Bechtereva NP, Bondartchuk AN, Smirnov VM, Meliutcheva LA, Shandurina AN. Method of electrostimulation of the deep brain structures in treatment of some chronic diseases. *Confin Neurol* 1975; 37: 136–40.
3. Benabid AL, Pollak P, Louveau A, Henry S, de Rougemont J. Combined (thalamotomy and stimulation) stereotactic surgery of the VIM thalamic nucleus for bilateral Parkinson disease. *Appl Neurophysiol* 1987; 50: 344–6.
4. Albin RL, Young AB, Penney JB. The functional anatomy of basal ganglia disorders. *Trends Neurosci* 1989; 12: 366–75.
5. Benazzouz A, Gross C, Feger J, Boraud T, Bioulac B. Reversal of rigidity and improvement in motor performance by subthalamic high-frequency stimulation in MPTP-treated monkeys. *Eur J Neurosci* 1993; 5: 382–9.
6. Limousin P, Pollak P, Benazzouz A, et al. Effect of parkinsonian signs and symptoms of bilateral subthalamic nucleus stimulation. *Lancet* 1995; 345: 91–5.
7. Schrag A, Jahanshahi M, Quinn N. What contributes to quality of life in patients with Parkinson's disease? *J Neurol Neurosurg Psychiatry* 2000; 69: 308–12.
8. Olanow CW, Obeso JA, Stocchi F. Continuous dopamine-receptor treatment of Parkinson's disease: scientific rationale and clinical implications. *Lancet Neurol* 2006; 5: 677–87.
9. Goetz CG, Poewe W, Rascol O, Sampaio C. Evidence-based medical review update: pharmacological and surgical treatments of Parkinson's disease: 2001 to 2004. *Mov Disord* 2005; 20: 523–39.
10. Deuschl G, Schade-Brittinger C, Krack P, et al. A randomized trial of deep-brain stimulation for Parkinson's disease. *N Engl J Med* 2006; 355: 896–908.
11. Limousin P, Krack P, Pollak P, et al. Electrical stimulation of the subthalamic nucleus in advanced Parkinson's disease. *N Engl J Med* 1998; 339: 1105–11.
12. Deep-Brain Stimulation for Parkinson's Disease Study Group. Deep-brain stimulation of the subthalamic nucleus or the pars interna of the globus pallidus in Parkinson's disease. *N Engl J Med* 2001; 345: 956–63.
13. Krack P, Batir A, Van Blercom N, et al. Five-year follow-up of bilateral stimulation of the subthalamic nucleus in advanced Parkinson's disease. *N Engl J Med* 2003; 349: 1925–34.
14. Lang AE. Surgery for Parkinson disease: a critical evaluation of the state of the art. *Arch Neurol* 2000; 57: 1118–25.
15. Langston JW, Widner H, Goetz CG, et al. Core assessment program for intracerebral transplantations (CAPIT). *Mov Disord* 1992; 7: 2–13.
16. Defer GL, Widner H, Marie RM, Remy P, Levivier M. Core assessment program for surgical interventional therapies in Parkinson's disease (CAPSIT-PD). *Mov Disord* 1999; 14: 572–84.
17. Lang AE, Widner H. Deep brain stimulation for Parkinson's disease: patient selection and evaluation. *Mov Disord* 2002; 17 (Suppl. 3): S94–101.
18. Duker AP, Espay AJ. Surgical treatment of Parkinson disease: past, present, and future. *Neurol Clin* 2013; 31: 799–808.
19. Shih LC, Tarsy D. Deep brain stimulation for the treatment of atypical parkinsonism. *Mov Disord* 2007; 22: 2149–55.
20. Follett KA, Weaver FM, Stern M, et al. Pallidal versus subthalamic deep-brain stimulation for Parkinson's disease. *N Engl J Med* 2010; 362: 2077–91.
21. Hasegawa H, Samuel M, Douiri A, Ashkan K. Patients' expectations in subthalamic nucleus deep brain stimulation surgery for Parkinson disease. *World Neurosurg* 2014; 82: 1295–9.
22. Marinus J, Visser M, Martinez-Martin P, van Hilten JJ, Stiggelbout AM. A short psychosocial questionnaire for patients with Parkinson's disease: the SCOPA-PS. *J Clin Epidemiol* 2003; 56: 61–7.
23. Schuepbach WM, Rau J, Knudsen K, et al. Neurostimulation for Parkinson's disease with early motor complications. *N Engl J Med* 2013; 368: 610–22.
24. Mestre TA, Espay AJ, Marras C, et al. Subthalamic nucleus-deep brain stimulation for early motor complications in Parkinson's disease – the EARLYSTIM trial: early is not always better. *Mov Disord* 2014; 29: 1751–6.
25. Charles D, Konrad PE, Neimat JS, et al. Subthalamic nucleus deep brain stimulation in early stage Parkinson's disease. *Parkinsonism Relat Disord* 2014; 20: 731–7.
26. Hilker R, Portman AT, Voges J, et al. Disease progression continues in patients with advanced Parkinson's disease and effective subthalamic nucleus stimulation. *J Neurol Neurosurg Psychiatry* 2005; 76: 1217–21.
27. Lilleeng B, Bronnick K, Toft M, Dietrichs E, Larsen JP. Progression and survival in Parkinson's disease with subthalamic nucleus stimulation. *Acta Neurol Scand* 2014; 130: 292–8.
28. Fasano A, Romito LM, Daniele A, et al. Motor and cognitive outcome in patients with Parkinson's disease 8 years after subthalamic implants. *Brain* 2010; 133: 2664–76.

29. Castrioto A, Lozano AM, Poon YY, *et al.* Ten-year outcome of subthalamic stimulation in Parkinson disease: a blinded evaluation. *Arch Neurol* 2011; **68**: 1550–6.
30. Bejjani BP, Dormont D, Pidoux B, *et al.* Bilateral subthalamic stimulation for Parkinson's disease by using three-dimensional stereotactic magnetic resonance imaging and electrophysiological guidance. *J Neurosurg* 2000; **92**: 615–25.
31. Machado A, Rezai AR, Kopell BH, *et al.* Deep brain stimulation for Parkinson's disease: surgical technique and perioperative management. *Mov Disord* 2006; **21** (Suppl. 14): S247–58.
32. Benabid AL, Chabardès S, Mitrofanis J, Pollak P. Deep brain stimulation of the subthalamic nucleus for the treatment of Parkinson's disease. *Lancet Neurology* 2009; **8**: 67–81.
33. Taba HA, Wu SS, Foote KD, *et al.* A closer look at unilateral versus bilateral deep brain stimulation: results of the National Institutes of Health COMPARE cohort. *J Neurosurg* 2010; **113**: 1224–9.
34. Bastian AJ, Kelly VE, Revilla FJ, Perlmutter JS, Mink JW. Different effects of unilateral versus bilateral subthalamic nucleus stimulation on walking and reaching in Parkinson's disease. *Mov Disord* 2003; **18**: 1000–7.
35. Kleiner-Fisman G, Herzog J, Fisman DN, *et al.* Subthalamic nucleus deep brain stimulation: summary and meta-analysis of outcomes. *Mov Disord* 2006; **21** (Suppl. 14): S290–304.
36. Weaver FM, Follett K, Stern M, *et al.* Bilateral deep brain stimulation vs best medical therapy for patients with advanced Parkinson disease: a randomized controlled trial. *JAMA* 2009; **301**: 63–73.
37. Williams A, Gill S, Varma T, *et al.* Deep brain stimulation plus best medical therapy versus best medical therapy alone for advanced Parkinson's disease (PD SURG trial): a randomised, open-label trial. *Lancet Neurol* 2010; **9**: 581–91.
38. Moro E, Scerrati M, Romito LM, *et al.* Chronic subthalamic nucleus stimulation reduces medication requirements in Parkinson's disease. *Neurology* 1999; **53**: 85–90.
39. Kumar R, Lozano AM, Kim YJ, *et al.* Double-blind evaluation of subthalamic nucleus deep brain stimulation in advanced Parkinson's disease. *Neurology* 1998; **51**: 850–5.
40. Pinto S, Gentil M, Krack P, *et al.* Changes induced by levodopa and subthalamic nucleus stimulation on parkinsonian speech. *Mov Disord* 2005; **20**: 1507–15.
41. Parsons TD, Rogers SA, Braaten AJ, Woods SP, Tröster AI. Cognitive sequelae of subthalamic nucleus deep brain stimulation in Parkinson's disease: a meta-analysis. *Lancet Neurol* 2006; **5**: 578–88.
42. Moro E, Esselink RJ, Xie J, *et al.* The impact on Parkinson's disease of electrical parameter settings in STN stimulation. *Neurology* 2002; **59**: 706–13.
43. Moreau C, Defebvre L, Destée A, *et al.* STN-DBS frequency effects on freezing of gait in advanced Parkinson disease. *Neurology* 2008; **71**: 80–4.
44. Eusebio A, Chen CC, Lu CS, *et al.* Effects of low-frequency stimulation of the subthalamic nucleus on movement in Parkinson's disease. *Exp Neurol* 2008; **209**: 125–30.
45. Meissner W, Leblois A, Hansel D, *et al.* Subthalamic high frequency stimulation resets subthalamic firing and reduces abnormal oscillations. *Brain* 2005; **128**: 2372–82.
46. Brown P. Oscillatory nature of human basal ganglia activity: relationship to the pathophysiology of Parkinson's disease. *Mov Disord* 2003; **18**: 357–63.
47. Bronte-Stewart H, Barberini C, Koop MM, Hill *et al.* The STN beta-band profile in Parkinson's disease is stationary and shows prolonged attenuation after deep brain stimulation. *Exp Neurol* 2009; **215**: 20–8.
48. Rossi L, Marceglia S, Foffani G, *et al.* Subthalamic local field potential oscillations during ongoing deep brain stimulation in Parkinson's disease. *Brain Res Bull* 2008; **76**: 512–21.
49. Priori A, Ardolino G, Marceglia S, *et al.* Low-frequency subthalamic oscillations increase after deep brain stimulation in Parkinson's disease. *Brain Res Bull* 2006; **71**: 149–54.
50. Giannicola G, Rosa M, Servello D, *et al.* Subthalamic local field potentials after seven-year deep brain stimulation in Parkinson's disease. *Exp Neurol* 2012; **237**: 312–7.
51. Odekerken VJ, van Laar T, Staal MJ, *et al.* Subthalamic nucleus versus globus pallidus bilateral deep brain stimulation for advanced Parkinson's disease (NSTAPS study): a randomised controlled trial. *Lancet Neurol* 2013; **12**: 37–44.
52. Guridi J, Rodriguez-Oroz MC, Alegre M, Obeso JA. Hardware complications in deep brain stimulation: electrode impedance and loss of clinical benefit. *Parkinsonism Relat Disord* 2012; **18**: 765–9.
53. Barichella M, Marczewska AM, Mariani C, *et al.* Body weight gain rate in patients with Parkinson's disease and deep brain stimulation. *Mov Disord* 2003; **18**: 1337–40.
54. Ruzicka E, Novakova L, Jech R, *et al.* Decrease in blood cortisol corresponds to weight gain following deep brain stimulation of the subthalamic nucleus in Parkinson's disease. *Stereotact Funct Neurosurg* 2012; **90**: 410–11.
55. Ruzicka F, Jech R, Novakova L, *et al.* Chronic stress-like syndrome as a consequence of medial site subthalamic stimulation in Parkinson's disease. *Psychoneuroendocrinology* 2015; **52**: 302–10.
56. Welter ML, Schüpbach M, Czernecki V, *et al.* Optimal target localization for subthalamic stimulation in

patients with Parkinson disease. *Neurology* 2014; **82**: 1352–61.

57. Doshi PK, Chhaya N, Bhatt MH. Depression leading to attempted suicide after bilateral subthalamic nucleus stimulation for Parkinson's disease. *Mov Disord* 2002; **17**: 1084–5.

58. Voon V, Krack P, Lang AE, *et al.* A multicentre study on suicide outcomes following subthalamic stimulation for Parkinson's disease. *Brain* 2008; **131**: 2720–8.

59. Schüpbach M, Gargiulo M, Welter ML, *et al.* Neurosurgery in Parkinson disease: a distressed mind in a repaired body? *Neurology* 2006; **66**: 1811–16.

60. Voon V, Kubu C, Krack P, Houeto JL, Tröster AI. Deep brain stimulation: neuropsychological and neuropsychiatric issues. *Mov Disord* 2006; **21** (Suppl. 14): S305–27.

61. Ulla M, Thobois S, Llorca PM, *et al.* Contact dependent reproducible hypomania induced by deep brain stimulation in Parkinson's disease: clinical, anatomical and functional imaging study. *J Neurol Neurosurg Psychiatry* 2011; **82**: 607–14.

62. Mallet L, Schüpbach M, N'Diaye K, *et al.* Stimulation of subterritories of the subthalamic nucleus reveals its role in the integration of the emotional and motor aspects of behavior. *Proc Natl Acad Sci U S A* 2007; **104**: 10661–6.

63. Spieles-Engemann AL, Behbehani MM, Collier TJ, *et al.* Stimulation of the rat subthalamic nucleus is neuroprotective following significant nigral dopamine neuron loss. *Neurobiol Dis* 2010; **39**: 105–15.

64. Wallace BA, Ashkan K, Heise CE, *et al.* Survival of midbrain dopaminergic cells after lesion or deep brain stimulation of the subthalamic nucleus in MPTP-treated monkeys. *Brain* 2007; **130**: 2129–45.

65. Marceglia S, Rossi L, Foffani G, *et al.* Basal ganglia local field potentials: applications in the development of new deep brain stimulation devices for movement disorders. *Expert Rev Med Devices* 2007; **4**: 605–14.

66. Rosin B, Slovik M, Mitelman R, *et al.* Closed-loop deep brain stimulation is superior in ameliorating parkinsonism. *Neuron* 2011; **72**: 370–84.

67. Martens HC, Toader E, Decre MM, *et al.* Spatial steering of deep brain stimulation volumes using a novel lead design. *Clin Neurophysiol* 2011; **122**: 558–66.

68. Chaturvedi A, Foutz TJ, McIntyre CC. Current steering to activate targeted neural pathways during deep brain stimulation of the subthalamic region. *Brain Stimul* 2012; **5**: 369–77.

69. Benabid AL, Pollak P, Gao D, *et al.* Chronic electrical stimulation of the ventralis intermedius nucleus of the thalamus as a treatment of movement disorders. *J Neurosurg* 1996; **84**: 203–14.

70. Rehncrona S, Johnels B, Widner H, *et al.* Long-term efficacy of thalamic deep brain stimulation for tremor: double-blind assessments. *Mov Disord* 2003; **18**: 163–70.

71. Stefani A, Lozano AM, Peppe A, *et al.* Bilateral deep brain stimulation of the pedunculopontine and subthalamic nuclei in severe Parkinson's disease. *Brain* 2007; **130**: 1596–607.

72. Okun MS, Fernandez HH, Wu SS, *et al.* Cognition and mood in Parkinson's disease in subthalamic nucleus versus globus pallidus interna deep brain stimulation: the COMPARE trial. *Ann Neurol* 2009; **65**: 586–95.

73. Moro E, Hamani C, Poon YY, *et al.* Unilateral pedunculopontine stimulation improves falls in Parkinson's disease. *Brain* 2010; **133**: 215–24.

Chapter 20

Deep-brain stimulation of the thalamic ventral intermediate nucleus in the management of Parkinson's disease

Diana Apetauerova, Jay L. Shils and Peter K. Dempsey

Introduction

Deep-brain stimulation (DBS) of the thalalmic ventral intermediate nucleus (VIM) was introduced by Benabid et al. [1] as a new surgical procedure for the treatment of tremor-dominant Parkinson's disease (PD). Prior to this procedure, thalamotomy had been used for decades as the primary weapon against resting and essential tremors [2–4, 5] but had much less success with the rigidity and bradykinesia aspects of PD. Thalamotomy involves the creation of a destructive lesion in the thalamus with a chance of permanent adverse side effects, especially when bilateral lesions are created [6]. The long-term complication rates of thalamotomy are estimated to affect between 9 and 23% of patients and are similar with both PD and essential tremor [3, 7, 8]. Bilateral thalamotomy carries an even higher risk of complications [9], including impaired speech and cognitive function [10], and is no longer recommended [11].

Historically, prior to placing the lesion in the thalamus, an electrical signal was passed through the lead to "simulate" the effects of the lesion (i.e. a reversible lesion). Additionally, this electrical stimulus would affect tremor intensity; when located in the most appropriate place for the lesion, there would be a reduction in the tremor intensity [12]. Benabid et al. [1, 13] were the first to observe that reduction of tremor was consistently associated with high-frequency stimulation, while low-frequency (lower than 100 Hz) stimulation would be ineffective or possibly increase tremor amplitude.

The advantage of VIM-DBS over thalamotomy is its reversibility and adjustability. It offers the same clinical effect as thalamotomy but without the need to make a destructive lesion. Deep-brain stimulation in the VIM consists of applying high-frequency stimulation using an implanted electrode connected to a subcutaneously placed neuropacemaker, which has the same effect as a thalamic lesion. Chronic stimulation of the VIM is considered a valid and safe method of alleviating tremor; since August 1997, unilateral thalamic DBS (Activa Tremor Control Therapy; Medtronic, Inc., Minneapolis, MN, USA) for refractory essential and parkinsonian tremors has been approved in the USA.

Neuroanatomy

The most common nomenclature for naming the nuclei of the thalamus is attributed to Jones [14]; however, for DBS and lesioning procedures, the nomenclature of Hassler [15] is more commonly used (for a helpful cross-reference between each of the nomenclatures, see Table 1 in Krack et al. [8]). The VIM nucleus is anterior to the ventral oralis posterior nucleus (the cerebellar receiving area) and posterior to the ventralis caudalis (VC) nucleus (the sensory receiving nucleus). The electrode is typically placed more anterior than a lesion would be to ensure that stimulation does not extend posteriorly to the VC, evoking intolerable paresthesias. Lenz et al. [16] demonstrated that the most common location for tremogenic cells in the VIM is approximately 2 mm anterior to the VIM/VC border. Somatotopic representation of body segments within the VIM nucleus is as follows, moving medially to laterally: face, hand and arm, torso and lower limbs. Once the area is mapped out, it is critically important to test the implanted lead with intraoperative stimulation through a temporarily connected external pulse generator (Figure 20.1). This method allows the confirmation of successful tremor suppression with high-frequency stimulation, and the thresholds for stimulation-induced side effects can be measured.

Parkinson's Disease: Current and Future Therapeutics and Clinical Trials, ed. Gálvez-Jiménez et al. Published by Cambridge University Press. © Cambridge University Press 2016.

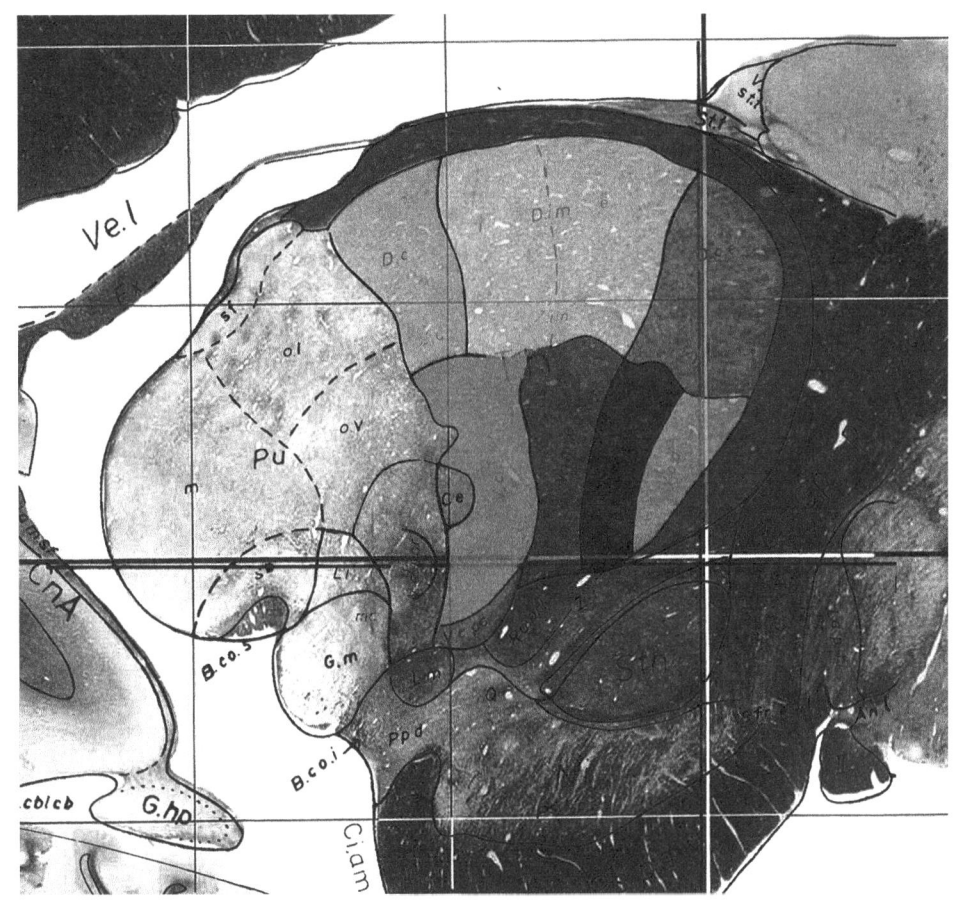

Figure 20.1 A sagittal slice through the thalamus taken 14.5 mm from the midline. The ventral intermediate nucleus, shown in red, is the target for tremor therapy in deep-brain stimulation (DBS). The initial target for the DBS lead is 14.5 mm from the midline and is then fine-tuned using intraoperative neurophysiological mapping techniques. (A black and white version of this figure will appear in some formats. For the color version, please refer to the plate section.)
From [17].

Neurophysiology of the ventral intermediate nucleus

The VIM in general has tonic cells with a frequency range of 20–50 Hz. Many of the cells in the lower two-thirds of the nucleus respond to joint movements. Important to the placement of the DBS lead are cells that have a bursting pattern that are highly correlated to the tremor activity [18].

The close temporal relationship between tremors and bursts of thalamic neuronal activity has led to the suggestion that these thalamic tremor cells could act as tremorigenic pacemakers. Intraoperative electrical stimulation in areas of the thalamus that are populated by tremor-synchronous cells momentarily arrests tremor, an observation that is important in the selection of the most effective target for tremor control [19]. It is thought that VIM stimulation desynchronizes neuronal overactivity within the VIM and leads to "functional ablation" [20, 21]. The VIM, as part of the nucleus ventralis lateralis (VL), seems to be the last relay of a complex of neuronal loops that finally projects to the motor and premotor cortex [22]. Moreover, the complete ventral thalamic nuclei are considered to act not only as relays but also as convergence points for pallidal and cerebellar afferent pathways [23].

The ventral intermediate nucleus procedure

The VIM-DBS procedure is divided into the following stages: stereotactic imaging, thalamic mapping, electrode implantation, implantation of the pulse generator and programming. Physiological mapping is carried out to identify the tremogenic region of the VIM and the location of the VC nucleus (somatosensory relay nucleus) that lies immediately posterior to the VIM. Stimulation of this nucleus produces paresthesias in the corresponding part of the body. Historically, prior to microelectrode recording, the VC nucleus was targeted, and once the area that responded to brushing of the thumb was located, the electrode was moved anteriorly. The VIM nucleus of the thalamus is located anterior to the VC and has characteristic features of VIM neurons, which include response of neurons to kinesthetic inputs and the spontaneous tremor-synchronous activity. Sites within the VIM in which tremor is arrested with stimulation are potential surgical targets.

Results of ventral intermediate nucleus surgery

The results of VIM-DBS show that this procedure is highly beneficial for tremor control in patients with PD but ineffective for the other disabling features of PD, including bradykinesia, rigidity, gait and postural disturbances. Unilateral or bilateral stimulation of the VIM is therefore considered only for tremor-dominant PD with a long duration of disease and in the absence of pronounced rigidity or bradykinesia. It has largely been replaced by subthalamic nucleus (STN) and globus pallidus interna (GPi) stimulation [24].

There have been several studies showing lack of efficacy of the thalamic target on the other symptoms of PD, namely rigidity, bradykinesia and dyskinesias [1, 11, 13, 20, 25–32].

As seen in Table 20.1, symptom control with DBS tends to be stable over time, although as many as 20% of patients with VIM stimulation experience reduced efficacy over time, and between 22 and 57% may develop rebound tremor upon discontinuation of stimulation [40], which is in contradiction to lesioning procedures [38].

The effectiveness of VIM-DBS for tremor has been established; however, the long-term studies pay little attention to progression of other signs of parkinsonism. All of the studies included a relatively small number of patients with PD. Benabid et al. [20] studied 26 patients with PD and six patients with essential tremor; seven of these patients had already undergone thalamotomy contralateral to the stimulated side, and 11 others had bilateral VIM stimulation at the same time. In patients with PD, rigidity was moderately improved but akinesia was not. Levodopa (L-DOPA) treatment had to be continued in all but two patients, but doses were reduced by more than 30% in ten patients.

Blond et al. [27] studied ten patients with parkinsonian tremor. Three of the ten parkinsonian patients had previously undergone contralateral thalamotomy. The follow-up period ranged from 6 to 26 months (mean 19.4 months). The intensity that effectively suppressed tremor was low (1–1.5 V) during the first 2 months but was increased in seven patients to maintain tremor alleviation. During the follow-up period, tremor reappeared transiently in three patients. Akinesia and rigidity were not changed by stimulation. Dyskinesias affecting limbs disappeared in all cases. Dystonic dyskinesias disappeared in two out of three patients after surgery. Neuropsychological evaluation failed to reveal memory, speech or praxis skill disorders.

Benabid et al. [26] followed 80 patients with PD for up to 8 years. Tremor was essentially the only symptom that was substantially influenced by VIM stimulation. Rigidity was slightly affected but was most likely due to a reduction in cogwheeling when the tremor was suppressed. There was almost no change in bradykinesia or any other symptom of PD.

Benabid et al. [41] followed 91 patients with PD, with a follow-up period of up to 17 months; 11 patients had contralateral thalamotomy and 43 patients had bilateral implants. Tremor was the only parkinsonian symptom that was greatly influenced by VIM stimulation. Parkinsonian resting tremor had the best benefit after surgery. Similarly, rigidity was only slightly affected, most likely due to a reduction in cogwheeling when the tremor was suppressed. There was no change in bradykinesia or in other parkinsonian symptoms. The effect on tremor was scored independently by the neurologist on a 5-point scale. At 3 months after the procedure, 86% of patients had a global score of 3 + 4 (permanent suppression of tremor or only slight recurrence on rare occasions) in the upper limbs and lower limbs. Resting tremor was better controlled than action tremor, distal-limb tremor was better controlled than proximal or axial tremor, and upper-limb tremor was better controlled than lower-limb tremor. In all patients, the effect was strictly coincident with stimulation, and there was no significant delay at the onset or after the effect at the cessation of stimulation. Thirty-nine of 80 patients (48.7%) had their levodopa dosage decreased by 20% at their 3-month follow-up. Because of disease progression, there were only 12 patients

Table 20.1 Long-term (greater than 12 months) efficacy studies of deep-brain stimulation for Parkinson's disease

Reference	n	Description of last follow-up group	n at last follow-up (% retained)	Site	Results of long-term assessment
Albanese et al. (1999) [33]	27	Not stated after 12 months (M = 10 months)	25 (93)	VIM	Tremor remained stable during follow-up period; rebound tremor in 22%; stimulation parameters stabilized after first 3 months
Benabid et al. (1996) [26]	91	At least 6 months (maximum 7 years)	80 (88)	VIM	Stable stimulation efficacy in 96% of operative sides; rebound tremor in 42%; stable stimulation parameters after first few months
Blond et al. (1992) [27]	10	Range of 6–26 months, (M = 19 months)	10 (100)	VIM	Long-term tremor control maintained; rebound tremor in 57% (not separated by diagnosis); voltage increased over time
Hariz et al. (2008) [34]	22	More than 12 months (M = 21 months)	17 (77)	VIM	Those with "good" effect decreased from 90 to 70% from week 1 to last follow-up; rebound tremor in 32%; stimulation parameters after 6 months
Krauss et al. (2001) [35]	45	Not stated (M = 12 months)	NR	VIM	Marked or excellent tremor control in 87% (only results of last follow-up reported)
Kumar et al. (1999) [36]	11	Every 6 months after the first year (M = 16 months)	NR	VIM	Long-term tremor control maintained; stimulation parameters stabilized after 3 months; rebound tremor in 27%
Lyons et al. (2001) [37]	12	Yearly after 12 months (M = 40 months)	9 (75)	VIM	Stable tremor control; however, UPDRS motor score not significantly different than baseline at long-term follow-up; no change in stimulation parameters
Tasker (1998) [38]	16	Range of 3–36 months (M = 15 months)	16 (100)	VIM	Long-term control of tremor and other PD symptoms; voltage increased over time in 32% of cases
Rehncrona et al. (2003) [39]	20	Range of 2 and 6–7 years	16 at 2 years and 12 at 6–7 years	VIM	Efficient tremor suppression at 6–7 years after surgery; stimulation parameters stable over time
Putzke et al. (2003) [40]	19	12 months to 3 years			Significant tremor improvement in follow-up period; stimulation parameters little or no change over time

NR, not reported by disease group; VIM, ventral intermediate nucleus; DBS, deep-brain stimulation; UPDRS, Unified Parkinson's Disease Rating Scale; ADL, activities of daily living; M, mean.

(15%) at the last follow-up. Rigidity and pain, as well as levodopa-induced dyskinesias, were partly reduced. Akinesia was not modified. The effect of VIM stimulation remained stable in 96%.

Hariz et al. [42] followed 22 patients with PD for up to 21 months (range 3–52 months). Seventeen patients were followed for more than 1 year. Seventeen patients had stimulation of the left thalamus. Five patients (23%) had previous contralateral thalamotomy, nine patients (41%) had a contralateral pallidotomy and three patients (14%) had a pallidotomy ipsilateral to the DBS side. All patients needed incremental increases in their stimulation parameters during the first 6–12 months after surgery. Ninety percent of patients with PD initially had good tremor control after surgery. At 1 year, 70% of patients with PD still exhibited good tremor control. Beyond 1 year, stimulation parameters and the effect on tremor seemed to stabilize. There was also an overall improvement of the Unified Parkinson's Disease Rating Scale (UPDRS) scores at 1 year, with the greatest improvement on the tremor items of the contralateral limb. Mean UPDRS-III motor scores improved from 37.2 preoperatively to 26.6 postoperatively while the stimulation was on ($P < 0.01$). However, the contralateral tremor scores showed a tendency to increase after the stimulation was switched off, compared with the preoperative values ($P = 0.007$).

Kumar et al. [36] followed seven patients; four had a bilateral procedure and three had a unilateral procedure. The mean follow-up time was 16.2 ± 7.0 months. The Schwab and England score and the total UDPRS score showed significant improvement at 1 week postoperatively ($P < 0.01$). However, long-term follow-up at 16.2 ± 7.0 months failed to show any significant change in these scores. Contralateral arm and leg resting tremor and ipsilateral resting leg tremor were found to be significantly decreased 1 week postoperatively ($P < 0.04$) and at follow-up ($P < 0.02$). Ipsilateral arm tremor did not show any statistically significant change. No significant improvement was seen in rigidity, bradykinesia, gait, speech or postural stability at immediate or long-term follow-up. Dopamine dosage was decreased by about 20% over early follow-up, but there was a tendency for this dose to increase with later follow-up. There was no significant difference in medication usage at long-term follow-up.

Lyons et al. [37] followed 12 patients with PD. Nine patients had follow-up evaluation for longer than 24 months; three patients were lost to follow-up. The last postsurgical evaluation occurred on average at 40 months after surgery. Motor UPDRS scores did not change significantly from baseline to long-term follow-up (40.7 at baseline to 35.6 at long-term follow-up; P value not significant). However, tremor scores for the targeted side were significantly improved when stimulation was on at long-term follow-up, compared with baseline (7.2 at baseline to 0.9 at long-term follow-up; $P = 0.007$). There were no significant changes in any stimulation parameters from follow-up at 3 months to the last follow-up at 40 months.

Krauss et al. [35] prospectively assessed 45 patients with PD with a mean follow-up of 11.9 months (range 3–24 months). Symptomatic improvement of tremor was rated as excellent in 51% of the patients. There was no description of other symptoms of PD.

Pollak et al. [43] followed 81 patients. Use of VIM surgery alleviated contralateral tremor in approximately 85% of these patients. "Off"-period dystonia related to chronic levodopa treatment was not alleviated, and VIM stimulation was ineffective on akinesia.

Kumar et al. [44] followed eight patients with a mean follow-up of 49 months (range 44–62 months). Contralateral arm tremor mean scores were improved with stimulation compared with baseline by 82% at 1 year ($n = 8$, $P < 0.05$) and by 86% at the final follow-up ($n = 7$). Total body tremor scores improved by 62% with stimulation at 1 year ($n = 8$, $P < 0.05$) and by 44% at the final follow-up ($n = 4$). Patients showed varied long-term responses. Three patients had excellent relief of disabling tremor. Two patients had some improvement in tremor with stimulation; however, tremor was no longer the major source of disability since levodopa-induced dyskinesias, motor fluctuations and bradykinesia had become most problematic, despite stimulation-off tremor ratings, which were worse than baseline in one patient. Three patients did not use stimulation as their tremor progressively declined.

Rehncrona et al. [49] studied 20 patients, with follow-up at 2 years and 6–7 years after DBS. The UPDRS evaluations were done in a double-blinded manner. Stimulation significantly ($P < 0.025$) suppressed tremor in both the upper and lower extremities at 2 years as well as at 6–7 years after surgery. Tremor suppression was also statistically significant compared with baseline (before operation) for both follow-up periods. In the majority of patients, resting tremor in the upper extremity improved two grades or more and in the lower extremity at least by one grade. In some patients, stimulation completely suppressed tremor. One of these patients had microthalamotomy effect at operation and only mild tremor (grade 1) without stimulation at the first follow-up. At the 6–7 year follow-up, this patient had no tremor, irrespective of whether the stimulator was activated or not. Stimulation also significantly ($P < 0.025$) suppressed kinetic tremor in PD patients. Use of DBS (stimulation on compared with off) improved the total motor score at 6–7 years, not only by suppressing tremor but also by decreasing akinesia ($P < 0.025$) in the side contralateral to the implanted electrode. Speech and postural stability deteriorated at the last visit and were not improved by stimulation. The mean daily intake of levodopa in the entire group increased at the last visit.

Putzke et al. [40] followed 23 patients for up to 3 years. Stimulation was associated with significant improvement in both subjective and objective measures of performance of activities of daily living, midline tremor, and contralateral upper- and lower-extremity tremor, including parkinsonian resting and action tremors, over the follow-up period. Ipsilateral tremor showed little or no effect of stimulation after the first 3 months. Use of antiparkinsonian medications and stimulation parameters showed little or no change over the course of follow-up.

Tarsy et al. [24] followed 17 patients for up to 4.5–7.3 years (mean 5.5 years). There was significant improvement in resting and postural/action tremor in the target upper extremity at both the 12-month and last visit with the DBS on compared with the DBS off. Tremor severity was not significantly increased at the last visit compared with the 12-month visit, with the DBS either on or off. However, there was no significant improvement in rigidity at either 12 months or the last visit, and rigidity was not significantly increased at the last visit compared with the 12-month visit with the DBS either on or off. Thalamic DBS produced significant improvement in upper-extremity akinesia in the target extremity (contralateral extremity) at the 12-month visit but not at the last visit. Three of four measures of upper-extremity akinesia were improved at the last visit compared with the 12-month visit with the DBS off but not with the DBS on. Leg agility was improved at the last visit compared with the 12-month visit only with the DBS on. The total UPDRS motor scores were significantly improved with the DBS on compared with the DBS off at 12 months and at the last visit, which was attributable to improved tremor and akinesia scores with the DBS on. There was no improvement in speech, facial expression, postural stability and gait disturbance at either the 12-month or the last visit.

Finally, Hariz *et al.* [34] described 38 patients with PD, with up to 6 years of follow-up. Tremor was still effectively controlled by DBS, and appendicular rigidity and akinesia remained stable compared with baseline. Axial scores (speech, gait and postural instability), however, worsened, and the initial improvement in activities of daily living scores at the 1-year follow-up had disappeared at 6 years, despite sustained improvement of tremor. Remarkably, neither daily doses of dopaminergic medication nor fluctuations and dyskinesias had changed at 6 years compared with baseline in this patient group.

Stimulation parameters

Stimulation parameters showed little or no change over time [37, 39, 40]. Voltage and pulse width showed an increase in stimulus frequency and only a slight increase in pulse width. Impedance increased over time.

The voltage intensity that effectively suppressed tremor was low (1–1.5 V) during the first 2 months but was increased over time [27]. Similar results were seen by Benabid *et al.* [41] when voltage increased from an average initial value of 1 ± 0.5 to approximately 4 ± 0.5 V, reaching a plateau after approximately 2 months, with a mean value of 3.06 V. Hariz *et al.* [34] found lower stimulation amplitudes of 1.9 V at 3 months and 2.14 V at 12 months. Pulse width was 73.7 μs at 1 year. Koller *et al.* [11] found slightly higher amplitudes and pulse widths (3.03 V at 12 months and 117.5 μs at 12 months). Kumar *et al.* [36] found the mean stimulus intensity was 1.86 ± 00.83 V at 7 days post-operatively and increased to 2.9 ± 01.0 V at 120 days postoperatively. The impedance also increased from a mean of 738 Ω postoperatively to 1032 Ω by day 120. This increase in impedance was thought to be responsible for the increase in voltage needed to control the tremors. Lyons *et al.* [37] found that amplitude did not change significantly from the third postoperative month to follow-up at more than 12 months (from 3.2 to 3.6 V). Pulse width changed from 76.7 μs at 3 months to 80.0 μs at more than 12 months. There was no significant change in rate from 3 months to long-term follow-up (from 155.0 to 158.3 Hz). Benabid *et al.* [26] found that amplitude reached a plateau after approximately 2 months, with a mean value of 3.06 V. They also found increased impedances from a mean of 794 Ω on postoperative day 14 to 1057 Ω at day 106. They also suggested that an increase in impedance could account for the increase in threshold voltage intensity. Limousin *et al.* [29], in their multicenter study, found that voltage was slightly but significantly increased over 1 year, and changes in pulse width and frequency were small. Monopolar stimulation was used in most of the patients in this study. Bipolar stimulation was used when tremor reduction was obtained, with fewer adverse effects than monopolar stimulation.

Rebound effect

Rebound phenomenon was noticed in patients whose stimulation was cycled in order to prolong the battery life of the pulse generator. Discontinuation of stimulation tended to produce a tremor of greater amplitude. This might also be explained by habituation (decreased biological response of the neuronal network).

Adverse effects

The same side effects that are encountered with thalamotomy are also seen with unilateral or bilateral VIM-DBS, but they can be modulated, to a great extent, with adjustments of the stimulation parameters. Bilateral procedures tend to have higher rates of side effects, especially dysarthria. The most commonly reported stimulation-related adverse events are paresthesias (10–20%) [25, 11], dysarthria (10%) [25, 30], ataxia (5%) [20], limb weakness (5%) [11] and dystonia (5%) [11, 13], although they are frequently viewed as mild and tolerable and amenable to reprogramming in many cases.

Complications related to hardware are inherent to this type of surgery and have been reported to occur in 4% to as high as 20–25% of patients [20, 37, 45]. Infection occurs in 2–3% of patients, while the hemorrhage rate is less than 1% [31, 46]. Cognitive side effects are very poorly studied in this group and appear to be associated with low cognitive morbidity [47]. The most common adverse events seen in various studies are summarized in the Table 20.2.

Table 20.2 Most common adverse events with ventral intermediate nucleus deep-brain stimulation

Reference	Number of patients	Side effects related to stimulation (n)	Side effects related to hardware (n)	Side effects related to procedure (n)	Neuropsychological disturbance
Benabid et al. [20]	26 PD, six ET	Paresthesias (3), dystonia (2), cerebellar ataxia (2), disequilibrium (2), dysarthria (5)		No hemorrhage or infection reported	Not reported
Blond et al. [27]	10 PD, four ET	Tonic posture of the fingers (1), persistent paresthesias (1)			No memory, speech, praxis skill disorder
Pollak et al. [48]	47 PD, 11 ET	Limb or hemifacial paresthesias (6), limb dystonia (6), disequilibrium (5), dysarthria (10)		I.c. microhematomas (3), removal of the lead due to healing problem (1)	Not reported
Benabid et al. [26]	80 PD, 20 ET	Dysarthria (18), disequilibrium (10), contralateral (4), paresthesia (1)		Asymptomatic microhematoma (3), symptomatic hematoma (2), skin infections (5), required removal with replacement (3)	Slight decrease in performance fluency, especially verbal performance with left VIM
Koller et al. [11]	24 PD, 29 ET	Generalized motor seizure (1), paresthesias (19), disequilibrium (3), gait disorder (1), dystonia (1), dysarthria (1)	Lead dislodgement during surgery (1)	I.c. hemorrhage (1), subdural hemorrhage (1)	
Pollak et al. [49]	80 PD	Dysarthria (15), disequilibrium (10), limb dystonia (10), numbness (6)	Extension lead break (3)	I.c. hemorrhage (8; 2 asymptomatic), infection (2), skin necrosis (1)	
Kumar et al. [38]	7 PD, four ET	Transient dystonia (2), transient nightmares (1), seizures (2)		Transient facial droop (1), transient confusion (1)	
Limousin et al. [29]	74 PD, 37 ET	Dysarthria (7), disequilibrium (3), dystonia (1)		Extracerebral hemorrhage without sequel (2), intracranial hemorrhage (1)	
Benabid et al. [41]	91 PD, 23 ET	Contralateral paresthesias (12), limb dystonia (12), disequilibrium (10), dysarthria (bilateral stimulation) (10)		Scalp infection (3), granuloma along connector extension track (2), transient fluid collection in the subclavian pocket of the stimulator (1), i.c. microhematoma with long-term thalamotomy effect (3), asymptomatic i.c. hematoma (3), transient confusion (5)	No spontaneous psychological disturbance noted; 29 patients with formal neuropsychological testing did not detect any impairment
Schuurman et al. [50]	45 PD, 13 ET	Dysarthria (2)		Infection (1), hematoma near IPG (1)	
Krauss et al. [37]	45 PD, 42 ET	Dystonia (3), diplopia (2), paresthesias (6), gait disturbance (22), dysarthria (16)	Wire breakage (1)	Cortical venous infarction (1), intraventricular hemorrhage (1), transient mental status changes (2)	
Rehncrona et al. [40]	20 PD, 19 ET	Paresthesias (1)	Lead fracture (1)		

(continued)

Table 20.2 (cont.)

Reference	Number of patients	Side effects related to stimulation (n)	Side effects related to hardware (n)	Side effects related to procedure (n)	Neuropsychological disturbance
Pahwa et al. [51]	19 PD, 26 ET	Pain (38), paresthesias (13), dysarthria (88)	Device replacement (25), surgical revisions other than IPG replacement (12)		
Hariz et al. [36]	66 PD	Dystonia (2), dysarthria (2), disequilibrium (3), hallucination (1), "nonclassified" adverse events (gait disorder, paresthesias, paresis, dyskinesias, proximal limb ataxia, migraine, neck pain) (11)	Replacement of the IPG due to battery expiration (17), repositioning of the stimulator (1), DBS lead reposition (1), infections (3), skin erosion without infection (1)		Dementia (1)

n, Number of patients, i.c., intracerebral; DBS, deep-brain stimulation; IPG, implantable pulse generator.

Benign tremulous parkinsonism

It is well accepted that VIM-DBS surgery has been replaced by STN-DBS or GPi-DBS in idiopathic PD, yet there is one group of patients – those with benign tremulous parkinsonism – who responds very well to VIM stimulation. Benign tremulous parkinsonism is characterized by prominent resting and action tremor, mild parkinsonism with limited disability or progression apart from tremor, and a less-robust response to levodopa therapy. This disorder has an uncertain pathophysiological relationship to idiopathic PD. Savica et al. [52] performed a retrospective study in 15 patients, with eight patients undergoing unilateral VIM-BDS and four patients undergoing bilateral VIM-DBS. They found excellent tremor outcomes in these patients; however, larger studies are needed.

Conclusion

In summary, VIM-DBS in patients with parkinsonian tremor has been shown to be safe and effective overall. The use of VIM-DBS is highly beneficial for tremor control. Thalamic DBS is safer than thalamotomy and can be carried out bilaterally in either one or two stages, although bilateral VIM-DBS is associated with a greater risk of adverse effects. Patients whose functional disability is due to tremor rather than other motor signs of PD have been considered suitable candidates for this procedure. However, reduced tremor may not improve the functional disabilities in patients with PD. Disability is more closely related to bradykinesia, which is not significantly improved after thalamic DBS. In addition, other cardinal features of PD such as rigidity, postural stability, gait, speech, facial expression and bradykinesia are not improved by thalamic DBS. This type of surgery does not prevent progression of other PD motor signs. This procedure might be a reasonable option only for patients with long-standing, nonprogressive, tremor-predominant PD, especially in elderly or cognitively impaired patients.

Acknowledgements

The authors thank Nicholas Ventura for editing assistance.

References

1. Benabid AL, Pollak P, Louveau A, Henry S, de Rougemont J. Combined (thalamotomy and stimulation) stereotactic surgery of the VIM nucleus for bilateral Parkinson disease. *Appl Neurophysiol* 1987; **50**: 344–6.
2. Derome PJ, Jedynak CP, Visot A, Delalande O. Traitement des mouvements anormaux par lesions thalamiques. *Rev Neurol* 1986; **142**: 391–7.
3. Fox MW, Ahlskog JE, Kelly PJ. Stereotactic ventrolateralis thalamotomy for medically refractory tremor in post-levodopa era Parkinson's disease patients. *J Neurosurg* 1991; **75**: 723–30.

4. Goldman MS, Ahlskog JE, Kelly PJ. The symptomatic and functional outcome of stereotactic thalamotomy for medically intractable essential tremor. *J Neurosurg* 1992; **76**: 924–8.

5. Narabayashi H. Stereotaxis Vim thalamotomy for treatment of tremor. *Eur Neurol* 1989; **29**: 29–32.

6. Tasker RR, Siqueira J, Hawrylyshyn P, Organ LW. What happened to VIM thalamotomy for Parkinson's disease? *Appl Neurophysiol*. 1983; **46**: 68–83.

7. Jankovic J, Cardoso F, Grossman RG, Hamilton WJ. Outcome after stereotactic thalamotomy for parkinsonian, essential, and other types of tremor. *Neurosurgery* 1995; **37**: 680–6.

8. Krack P, Dostrovsky J, Ilinsky I, et al. Surgery of the motor thalamus: problems with the present nomenclatures. *Movement Disord* 2002; **17**: S2–8.

9. Matsumoto K, Asano T, Baba T, Miyamuto T, Ohmouto T. Long-term follow up results of bilateral thalamotomy for parkinsonism. *Appl Neurophysiol* 1976; **39**: 257–60.

10. Selby G. Stereotaxic surgery for the relief of Parkinson's disease: Part 2. An analysis of the results of a series of 303 patients (413 operations). *J Neurol Sci* 1967; **5**: 343–75.

11. Koller W, Pahwa R, Busenbark K, et al. High-frequency unilateral thalamic stimulation in the treatment of essential and parkinsonian tremor. *Ann Neurol* 1997; **42**: 292–9.

12. Ohye C, Nakamura R, Fukamachi A, Narabayashi H. Recording and stimulation of the ventralis intermedius nucleus of the human thalamus. *Appl Neurophysiol* 1975; **37**: 258.

13. Benabid AL, Pollak P, Seigneuret D, et al. Chronic VIM thalamic stimulation in Parkinson's disease, essential tremor and extra-pyramidal dyskinesias. *Acta Neurochir Suppl (Wein)* 1993; **58**: 39–44.

14. Jones EG, Steriade M, McCormick D. *The Thalamus*. New York: Plenum Press; 1985.

15. Hassler R. Anatomy of the thalamus. In: Schaltenbrand G, Baily P, eds. *Introduction to Stereotaxis with an Atlas of the Human Brain*. Stuttgart: Thieme, 1959; 230–90.

16. Lenz FA, Normans SL, Kwan HC, et al. Statistical prediction of the optimal site for thalamotomy in Parkinsonian tremor. *Mov Disord* 1995; **10**: 318–28.

17. Shils JL, Tagliati M, Alterman RL. Neurophysiological monitoring during neurosurgery for movement disorders. In: Deletis V, Shils JL, eds. *Neurophysiology in Neurosurgery: a Modern Approach*. New York: Academic Press; 2002; 405–48.

18. Hua SE, Lenz FA, Zirh TA, Reich SG, Dougherty PM. Thalamic neuronal activity correlated with essential tremor. *J Neuol Neurosurg Psychiatry*. 1998; **64**: 273–6.

19. Tasker RR, Organ LW, Hawrylyshyn P. *The Thalamus and Midbrain of Man: a Physiological Atlas Using Electrical Stimulation*. Springfield: Charles C. Thomas; 1982.

20. Benabid AL, Pollak P, Hoffmann D, et al. Long- term suppression of tremor by chronic stimualation of the ventral intermediate thalamic nucleus. *Lancet* 1991; **337**: 403–6.

21. Blond S, Siefried J. Thalamic stimulation for the treatment of tremor and other movement disorders. *Acta Neurochir Suppl* 1991; **52**: 109–11.

22. DeLong M. Primate model of movements disorder of basal ganglia origin. *Trends Neursci* 1990; **13**: 281–5.

23. Alexander GE, Crutcher MD, De Long MR. Basal ganglia-thalamocortical circuits: parallel substrates for motor, oculomotor, prefrontal and limbic functions. *Prog Brain Res* 1991; **85**: 119–46.

24. Tarsy D, Scollins L, Corapi K, et al. Progression of Parkinson's disease following thalamic deep brain stimulation for tremor. *Stereotact Funct Neurosurg* 2005; **83**: 222–7.

25. Alesch F, Pinter MM, Helscher RJ, et al. Stimulation of the ventralis intermediate thalamic nucleus in tremor dominated Parkinson's disease and essential tremor. *Acta Neurochir (Wien)* 1995; **136**: 75–81.

26. Benabid AL, Pollak P, Gao D, et al. Chronic electrical stimulation of the ventralis intermedius nucleus of the thalamus as a treatment of movement disorders. *J Neurosurg* 1996; **84**: 203–14.

27. Blond S, Caparros-Lefebvre D, Parker F, et al. Control of tremor and involuntary movement disorders by chronic stereotactic stimulation of the ventral intermediate thalamic nucleus. *J Neurosurg* 1992; **77**: 62–8.

28. Hariz GM, Bergenheim AT, Hariz MI, Lindberg M. Assessment of ability/disability in patients treated with chronic thalamic stimulation for tremor. *Mov Disord* 1998; **13**: 78–83.

29. Limousin P, Speelman JD, Gielen F, Janssens M. Multicentre European study of thalamic stimulation in parkinsonian and essential tremor. *J Neurol Neurosurg Psychiatry* 1999; **66**: 289–96.

30. Ondo W, Jankovic J, Schwartz K, Almaguer M, Simpson RK. Unilateral thalamic deep brain stimulation for refractory essential tremor and Parkinson's disease tremor. *Neurology* 1998; **51**: 1063–9.

31. Siegfried J, Blond S. *The Neurosurgical Treatment of Parkinson's Disease and Other Movement Disorders*. Baltimore: Williams and Wilkins; 1997.

32. Speelman JD, Schuurman PR, de Bie RMA, Bosch DA. Thalamic surgery and tremor. *Mov Disord* 1998; **113**: 103–6.

33. Albanese A, Nordera GP, Caraceni T, Moro E. Long-term ventralis intermedius thalamic stimulation for parkinsonian tremor. Italian Registry for Neuromodulation in Movement Disorders. *Adv Neurol* 1999; **80**: 631–4.

34. Hariz MI, Krack P, Alesch F, et al. Multicentre European study of thalamic stimulation for parkinsonian tremor: a 6 year follow-up. *J Neurol Neurosurg Psychiatry* 2008; **79**: 694–9.
35. Krauss JK, Simpson RK, Ondo WG, et al. Concepts and methods in chronic thalamic stimulation for treatment of tremor: technique and application. *Neurosurgery* 2001; **48**: 535–41.
36. Kumar K, Kelly M, Toth C. Deep brain stimulation of the ventral intermediate nucleus of the thalamus for control of tremors in Parkinson's disease and essential tremor. *Stereotact Funct Neurosurg* 1999; **72**: 47–61.
37. Lyons KE, Koller WC, Wilkinson SB, Pahwa R. Long term safety and efficacy of unilateral deep brain stimulation of the thalamus for parkinsonian tremor. *J Neurol Neurosurg Psychiatry* 2001; **71**: 682–4.
38. Tasker, RR. Deep brain stimulation preferable to thalamotomy for tremor suppression. *Surgical Neurol* 1998; **49**: 145–53.
39. Rehncrona S, Johnels B, Widner H, et al. Long-term efficacy of thalamic deep brain stimulation for tremor:double-blind assessments. *Mov Disord* 2003; **18**: 163–70.
40. Putzke JD, Wharen RE, Wszolek ZK, et al. Thalamic deep brain stimulation for tremor-predominant Parkinson's disease. *Parkinsonism Relat Disord* 2003; **10**: 81–8.
41. Benabid AL, Benazzouz A, Gao D, et al. Chronic electrical stimulation of the ventralis intermedius nucleus of the thalamus and of other nuclei as a treatment for Parkinson's disease. *Tech Neurosurg* 1999; **5**: 5–30.
42. Hariz MI, Shamsgovara P, Johansson F, Hariz GM, Fodstad H. Tolerance and tremor rebound following long-term chronic thalamic stimulation for parkinsonian and essential tremor. *Stereot Funct Neurosurg*. 1999; **72**: 208–18.
43. Pollak P, Fraix V, Krack P, et al. Treatment results: Parkinson's disease. *Mov Disord* 2002; **17**: S75–83.
44. Kumar R, Lozano A, Sime E, Lang A. Long-term follow-up of thalamic deep brain stimulation for essential and parkinsonian tremor. *Neurology* 2003; **61**: 1601–4.
45. Joint C, Nardi D, Parkin S, Gregory R, Aziz T. Hardware-related problems of deep brain stimulation. *Mov Disord* 2002; **17**: S175–80.
46. Binder DK, Rau G, Starr PA. Hemorrhagic complications of microelectrode-guided deep brain stimulation. *Stereotact Funct Neurosurg* 2003; **80**: 28–31.
47. Woods SP, Fields JA, Lyons KE, et al. Neuropsychological and quality of life changes following unilateral thalamic deep brain stimulation in Parkinson's disease: a one -year follow-up. *Acta Neurochir (Wein)*. 2001; **143**: 1273–7.
48. Pollak P, Benabid AL, Gervason CL, et al. Long-term effects of chronic stimulation of the ventral intermediate thalamic nucleus in different types of tremor. *Adv Neurol* 1993; **60**: 408–13.
49. Pollak P, Benabid AL, Limousin P, Benazzouz A. Chronic intracerebral stimulation in Parkinson's disease. *Adv Neurol* 1997; **74**: 213–20.
50. Schuurman PR, Bosch DA, Bossuyt PMM, et al. A comparison of continuous thalamic stimulation and thalamotomy for suppression of severe tremor. *N Engl J Med.* 2000; **342**: 461–8.
51. Pahwa R, Lyons KE, Wilkinson SB, et al. Long-term evaluation of deep brain stimulation of the thalamus. *J Neurosurg* 2006; **104**: 506–12.
52. Savica R, Matsumoto JY, Josephs KA, et al. Deep brain stimulation in benign tremulous parkinsonism. *Arch Neurol* 2011; **68**: 1033–6.

Chapter 21

Emerging targets and other stimulation-related procedures in the management of Parkinson's disease

Tiago A. Mestre and Elena Moro

Introduction

Since the first report from Benabid et al. [1] about the stimulation of the ventral intermediate nucleus (VIM) of the thalamus as a successful treatment for tremor, deep-brain stimulation (DBS) has revolutionized the management of movement disorders, especially Parkinson's disease (PD).

Along the years, the therapeutic value of DBS of other brain targets in PD has been firmly established, such as the subthalamic nucleus (STN) and the globus pallidus internus (GPi) [2]. Between the two nuclei, the STN has become the most widely used target for DBS in PD. The significant improvement in motor complications and quality of life in PD patients brought about by STN-DBS has prompted research on new brain targets that could become an option for patients who are not candidates for STN-DBS or GPi-DBS. Indeed, STN-DBS and GPi-DBS are effective treatments for levodopa (L-DOPA)-responsive signs and symptoms but not for manifestations of PD that are nonresponsive to dopaminergic treatment such as axial signs and cognitive decline, the main determinants of disability and quality of life in advanced stages of PD.

In this chapter, we will present the most recent targets investigated for DBS for the treatment of motor and/or nonmotor symptoms in PD. For each target, we will provide the fundamental anatomical and physiopathological data that support its consideration for the management of PD, and will describe the advances made in clinical studies to assess its therapeutic value. In addition, we will review the advances made in noninvasive brain stimulation and introduce novel stimulation paradigms for DBS.

The pedunculopontine nucleus

The pedunculopontine nucleus (PPN) is a structure bounded laterally by the medial lemniscus and medially by the superior cerebellar peduncle and its decussation [3]. Superiorly, it reaches the retrorubral field dorsally and the substantia nigra (SN) anteriorly. The most dorsal aspect of the PPN contacts the pontine reticular formation, and the cuneiform and subcuneiform nuclei from a dorsal–ventral axis [3]. The most inferior portion of the PPN is adjacent to the locus coeruleus [3]. The PPN is divided into two parts based on cell density: the pars dissipata, composed of cholinergic, glutamatergic and other neuronal subtypes; and the pars compacta, containing mainly cholinergic neurons [3]. The PPN is, together with the cuneiform and the subcuneiform nucleus, the major component of the mesencephalic locomotor region [4], in which stimulation has been able to elicit controlled locomotion in decerebrated animals [3]. The PPN is richly connected with several structures, receiving inputs from the cortex, the limbic system, the basal ganglia, the spinal cord and the brainstem, especially the ascending activating reticular system. The efferent pathways ascend toward the thalamus and the basal ganglia (mainly the STN and the SN), and descend toward the cerebellum and the spinal cord [3]. With such a rich and wide network of connections, the PPN has been proposed as a relay station for the modulation of gait and posture [3]. Most of the studies conducted to determine the connectivity of the PPN were done in rat and primate models, although an overlap has been founded in the few rare human studies [5]. In PD patients, there is a reduction of neurons (average 40%) within the pars compacta [6], which strengthens the rational for an involvement of the PPN in the pathophysiology of PD and for exploring its therapeutic potential by directly modulating PPN activity with DBS.

The first reports of bilateral PPN stimulation in PD patients had promising results [7, 8]. Since then, several studies with variable methodological quality have assessed the effects of PPN-DBS in PD but with inconsistent results [9–14] (Table 21.1). The only two randomized, double-blinded studies available did not show any significant improvement in the objective ratings using the Unified Parkinson's Disease Rating Scale (UPDRS)-III 1 year after surgery. Both studies reported significant improvements in secondary outcomes when measured in the off-medication condition: the item "falls" of the UPDRS-II [11] and freezing of gait using a walking protocol that included environmental triggers [10]. The improvements associated with PPN stimulation were still present after an average postoperative follow-up of 4 years in one of these studies [11] (T. A. Mestre and E. Moro, unpublished data). Overall, these clinical studies suggest that low-frequency stimulation (below 70 Hz) is more effective, although different ranges of frequencies have been used [15]. Possible stimulation-related side effects

Table 21.1 Literature about pedunculopontine nucleus (PPN) stimulation in Parkinson's disease patients; case reports have been excluded

Study	Sample size (n)	Target	Study design	Study duration (months)	Stimulation details	Results
Stefani et al. [9]	6	Bilateral PPN + STN	Assessments pre-op, 2–3 months (off med), 6 months (on med); physician rater blinded to condition	6	Bipolar contacts, 25 Hz, 60 μs, 1.5–2.0 V	*PPN only*: improvement in total UPDRS-III (33–44%) and items 27–30 (off- and on-medication). Decline of PPN-DBS efficacy overtime
Moro et al. [11]	6	Unilateral PPN	Double-blinded assessments pre-op, 3, 12 months	12	Mono/bipolar contacts, 66.7 Hz, 70 μs, 2.0 V (mean values)	Improvement in falls (item 13, UPDRS-II) off and on med, at 3 and 12 months. No significant improvement in UPDRS-III and items 27–30
Ferraye et al. [10]	6	Bilateral PPN + STN	Unblinded assessments pre-op, 12 months *plus* double-blinded crossover between months 4 and 6	12	Bipolar contacts (5/6 patients), 15–25 Hz, 1.2–3.8 V, 60–90 μs	*PPN only*: improvement of freezing (item 14, UPDRS-II). Freezing episodes significantly improved ($P = 0.046$) only off med. No improvement in the double-blinded assessment
Thevastan et al. [13]	5	Bilateral PPN	Unblinded assessments pre-op, 6 and 24 months	24	Monopolar contacts, 35 Hz, 60 μs, 3.5 V (mean values)	UPDRS-III (total, items 27–30) – no significant improvement. Gait and Falls Questionnaire – sustained improvement until 24 months
Khan et al. [12, 14]	7	Bilateral PPN + cZi	Unblinded assessments pre-op, 12 months	10–13 ($n=7$)	Bi-/tripolar contacts, 60 Hz, 60 μs, 2.6 V (mean values)	*PPN only*: improvement in UPDRS-III (total, items 27–30, tremor, bradykinesia) both off and on med. PDQ-39 – n/a. Longer f/u at 12–60 months ($n=5$) – no significant improvement in UPDRS-III (total, items 27–30)

STN, subthalamic nucleus; cZi, caudal zona incerta; med, PD medications; op, operative; n/a, not applicable; f/u, follow-up; stim, stimulation; UPDRS, Unified Parkinson Disease Rating Scale.

included contralateral paresthesias due to current diffusion to the medial lemniscus, oscillopsia [16] likely due to current diffusion to fibers from the uncinate fasciculus of the cerebellum and the superior cerebellar peduncle [17], and myoclonus due to stimulation of the thalamic projections [10, 16]. Despite the small and inconsistent therapeutic effects so far observed, PPN stimulation has not been dismissed as a target for axial levodopa-resistant signs and symptoms in PD patients. Indeed, there are several issues that may have interfered with the different outcomes and require clarification. One fundamental aspect is that the optimal site for stimulation of the PPN region and surrounding areas has not been fully established. There is an ongoing discussion about the best site being in the actual PPN or in adjacent areas such as the subcuneiform nucleus [10]. In one study, a more posterior location of the electrodes was associated with greater improvement, which was interpreted as a possible involvement of the cuneiform and subcuneiform nuclei [10]. However, this remains far from consensual, with other authors indicating other nuclei such as the peripeduncular nucleus [18] and the existence of inconsistent clinical/anatomical correlations (T. A. Mestre and E. Moro, unpublished data). Moreover, targeting the PPN raises important technical issues. The electrode location seems to vary greatly among the studies [4, 10, 11, 18–22]. Such findings can be justified by the absence of a specific identifying neurophysiological activity and of any acute clinical benefit with a localizing value, after electrode placement and stimulation. A novel alternative MRI-based targeting has been proposed as a more accurate method compared with traditional atlas-based methodologies [23].

Although there is some evidence suggesting that bilateral PPN stimulation might be more effective than unilateral stimulation [14], this remains to be fully established. In addition, the sample size of these studies has been small, and the potential poor sensitivity of the clinical rating scales used to measure gait-related outcomes such as freezing of gait deserves further appraisal, as the UPDRS-III does not incorporate environmental triggers for freezing of gait in its administration [10, 11].

The PPN has also been studied as part of multitarget DBS strategies. Combination of PPN and caudal zona incerta (cZi) stimulation was associated with a cumulative effect compared with the isolated stimulation of each target for the motor UPDRS axial subscore in the on-medication condition [12, 14]. A corresponding cumulative effect was observed in the regional cerebral blood flow using $^{15}O H_2 O$ positron emission tomography (PET) [24]. Bilateral combined STN and PPN stimulation has been suggested to provide a potential synergistic effect, as measured by gait kinematics [25] during the off-medication condition. More importantly, bilateral combined STN and PPN stimulation had a cumulative effect for improvement in the UPDRS-III and its axial item scores 3 months after surgery, in both the off-medication and on-medication conditions, as well as for measures of activities of daily living [9]. Nevertheless, the antiparkinsonian effects related to PPN stimulation waned in a period of 6 months, while the effects related to STN stimulation were more sustained during the same period of time [9]. This observation has been interpreted as tolerance to DBS, and an intermittent stimulation with an overnight arrest of PPN stimulation was adopted in another study [10], although it was never compared with continuous PPN stimulation.

Modulation of sleep and alertness was observed in PD patients with PPN-DBS operated on for levodopa-resistant gait and balance impairment. Unilateral PPN-DBS increased the duration of rapid eye movement (REM) sleep using a wide range of frequencies (5–70 Hz) in stimulation [26], whereas the N1 stage sleep was induced with higher-frequency (80 Hz) PPN stimulation [27]. More importantly, low-frequency (20–30 Hz) PPN stimulation was associated with increased alertness [27]. The increase alertness could partially explain the improvement of freezing of gait and falls observed in PD patients with PPN stimulation. Another interesting finding related to PPN stimulation has been the potential improvement in cognition documented together with a corresponding activation of bilateral prefrontal and frontal cortical areas in ^{18}F-fluorodeoxyglucose PET [28]. These nonmotor effects of PPN stimulation warrant further exploration for the treatment of sleep disorders and cognitive impairment, although the benefits would have to be clinically significant to outweigh the surgical risk.

The posterior subthalamic area

The posterior subthalamic area (PSA) is delimited anteriorly by the posterior border of the STN, posteriorly by the medial lemniscus, inferiorly by the dorsal SN, superiorly by the ventral thalamic nuclei, laterally by the posterior limb of the internal capsule, posteromedially by the red nucleus and posterolaterally by the ventrocaudal nucleus [29, 30]. The PSA is formed by the nucleus of the zona incerta (Zi) and the white fiber tracts of the prelemniscal radiations [31].

The Zi, or the "region of which nothing certain can be said," as described by Forel in 1877, is a small diencephalic nucleus that covers the STN and lies between the bundles of the pallidothalamic tract [31]. The Zi is considered a connecting node for basal ganglia and thalamocortical and cerebellar thalamocortical circuits [30]. The pallidothalamic tract has its origin in the GPi and is composed of the ansa lenticularis and the fasciculus lenticularis (or Forel H2 field in classical nomenclature), which have different trajectories and progressively merge to form the Forel H1+H2 field and, finally, the fasciculus thalamicus before entering the ventral thalamus [29]. The prelemniscal radiations lie posterior to the STN and are composed of the mesencephalic reticular formation projections to the thalamus and the ascending cerebellothalamic tract. The cerebellothalamic tract, or brachium conjuntivum, connects the dentate, interposed and fastigial cerebellar nuclei with the thalamus (ventral division of the ventral lateral posterior nucleus) passing through the superior cerebellar pedunculus and its decussation, and the red nucleus anteriorly [29]. It is important to recognize that the Zi and the prelemniscal radiations are difficult to distinguish on MRI [30], even on a 3-tesla device [32].

The exploration of the therapeutic potential of the Zi in PD patients is not novel. In the 1960s, there were multiple clinical studies on the effect of subthalamotomy for different types of tremor, including PD tremor and essential tremor but also dystonia and other movement disorders [30, 33]. Most of the subthalamotomies corresponded to lesions in the PSA [30, 33] and the studies reported a consistent effect for tremor as well as for rigidity in PD [30, 34]. Indirect evidence of the potential therapeutic benefit of stimulating the Zi was provided by studies of clinical/anatomical correlation after STN-DBS, suggesting that the Zi was directly involved in the therapeutic effects observed with stimulation [35–37], together with dorsal–lateral STN and Forel fields, although this interpretation is not consensual [38]. In addition, evidence suggests a specific effect in the reduction of dyskinesias and of the levodopa-equivalent daily dose [39]. In the past decade, five studies have assessed in a systematic fashion the effect of PSA stimulation on tremor, rigidity and bradykinesia in a total of 51 PD patients [40–44] (Table 21.2). Although these studies report consistent positive efficacy results for PD cardinal signs, these should be interpreted with caution, due to their small sample size and the poor methodological quality: the studies were nonrandomized, open label and most of them were noncontrolled. Stimulation of the PSA has been considered a safe procedure. Worsening of depression, pyramidal effects, dysarthria and dizziness were rarely reported as chronic stimulation-induced effects, although, at times, with a suboptimal control of tremor [43, 44]. Irritability, psychomotor agitation, severe progressive insomnia [45] and persistent apathy [46] have also been reported in isolated case reports. In a case series of 19 PD patients with a mean long-term follow-up of 4 years, PSA stimulation (both cZi and prelemniscal radiations) was associated with an incidence of depression and speech impairment comparable with the known incidence in STN-DBS, although the patient group in these case series already had mild speech impairment and/or behavioral disease (depression and apathy) preoperatively [47]. Potential deleterious effects in speech were assessed for stimulation of the Zi in a direct comparison with STN-DBS: a slight worsening in voice intensity [48] and articulation rate [49] was associated with Zi stimulation, but there was no difference in the control of onset/offset of phonation [50] and no change in pitch variability, while STN-DBS improved the latter [51]. Swallowing functioning was not affected [52]. In addition, current spread to neighboring cerebellothalamic tract and pallidothalamic fibers has to be considered with the potential risk of dysarthria and postural instability [53, 54] and blocking of levodopa effects [55–57], respectively.

The substantia nigra pars reticulata

The substantia nigra pars reticulata (SNr) is the main output nucleus of the basal ganglia, along with the GPi. The SNr projects ascending fibers to the thalamus with its inhibitory efferents to cortical areas [59] and to the mesopontine tegmental area [60]. In animals, modulation of SNr activity modifies both locomotion and control of posture [60]. The effect of bilateral SNr-DBS on different parameters of gait was compared with STN stimulation in seven PD patients initially treated with STN-DBS but later found to have the most ventral contact of the electrodes located within the SNr [60]. In a head-to-head comparison for the same patient and lead, SNr stimulation alone improved only axial signs (reduction of 44%), measured by an axial score composed of the sum of items 27–30 of the UPDRS-III (rising from chair, posture, postural stability and gait). Stimulation of the STN improved axial and distal parkinsonian signs by 74 and by 77%, respectively, the latter defined as the sum of nonaxial items of the UPDRS-III. The effect of

Table 21.2 Literature about posterior subthalamic area stimulation in Parkinson's disease patients

Study	Patients (n)	Target	Study design	Study duration (months)	Stimulation details	Tremor	Rigidity	Bradykinesia
Velasco et al. [40]	10	Uniteral Raprl	Unblinded assessments pre-op, 3, 6, 9 and 12 months	12	Bipolar contacts, 130 Hz, 232 μs, 2.8 V (mean values)	Pre-op vs 12 months ↓ on vs off stim (off med) ↓	→ =	=
Kitagawa et al. [41]	8	Unilateral Zi/Raprl	Unblinded assessments pre-op, 6, 12, 18 and 24 months, on vs off stim (off med)	24	Monopolar contacts, 132.5 Hz, 86.3 μs, 2.3 V (mean values)	↓ (78.3%)	↓ (92.7%)	↓ (65.7%)
Plaha et al. [58]	14	Unilateral (n = 13)/ bilateral (n = 1) cZi	Unblinded assessments pre-op, 6 months, on vs off stim (off med) (cZi vs STN vs dorsomedial to STN)	6 (median value)	Mono/bipolar contacts, 150 Hz, 82 μs, 2.7 V (mean values)	↓ (93%)	↓ (76%)[a]	↓ (65%)
Carrilo-Ruiz et al. [43]	5	Bilateral Raprl	Unblinded assessments pre-op, 3, 6, 9 and 12 months, pre-op vs post-op	12 (n = 4)	Bipolar contacts, 130 Hz, 90–330 μs, 2.5–4.0 V	↓ (90%)	↓ (94%)	↓ (75%)
Blomstedt et al. [44]	14	Unilateral (13)/ staged bilateral (1) cZi	Unblinded assessments pre-op, 12 months, on vs off stim (off med)	18 (mean value)	Mono (n = 12)/ bipolar contacts, 160, 66 μs, 2.6 V (mean values)	↓ (82.2%)	↓ (34.3%)	↓ (26.7%)

Raprl, prelemniscal radiation; cZi, caudal zona incerta; STN, subthalamic nucleus; med, PD medications; op, operative; stim, stimulation. Statistically significant results are presented for comparison.

[a] Significantly different from STN or dorsomedial to the STN.

SNr stimulation on the biomechanics of gait was also assessed [60] and was associated with a significant improvement of braking capacity but no change in step length or peak velocity for both natural and fast gait conditions. Stimulation of the STN improved the three gait parameters. The changes in the three gait parameters correlated with the "axial" score. More recently, a double-blind, randomized, crossover study compared STN stimulation alone with interleaving stimulation of the STN and SNr in 12 PD patients [61]. This novel advanced programming modality allows the alternate stimulation of different contacts of the same lead with different amplitudes and pulse widths, at a common frequency, which was 125 Hz for this study. The contacts of electrodes were located in the STN area and in the caudal STN–SNr border zone. After 3 weeks of continuous stimulation, either combined STN–SNr interleaving stimulation or isolated STN stimulation did not improve the compounded score of axial items combining corresponding items of the UPDRS-II and -III [61]. The Freezing of Gait Assessment Course suggested a greater improvement of freezing of gait with combined STN–SNr interleaving stimulation than with isolated STN stimulation [61]. Four patients prematurely discontinued isolated STN stimulation due to gait impairment [61]. Combined STN–SNr interleaving stimulation was safe and well tolerated [61]. Two patients developed dyskinesias that remitted with the adjustment of stimulation. To further test the apparent effect of combined STN and SNr interleaving stimulation on freezing of gait, a larger phase 3 study is warranted.

The centromedian–parafascicular complex

The centromedian–parafascicular complex (CM-Pf), or central complex, is part of the caudal intralaminar nuclei of the thalamus [62]. The CM-Pf is composed of several subdivisions with highly organized efferent projections into sensorimotor, limbic and associative parallel circuits of the basal ganglia [62]. The CM-Pf receives afferents from the SNr, PPN and GPi, but has reduced synaptic interactions with dopaminergic axonal projections [62]. The CM-Pf has marked neuronal loss (40–55%) in PD [62], further strengthening the rational to explore its therapeutic potential in PD. Lesions to the CM-Pf with therapeutic goals in parkinsonian patients were first reported in the 1960s [63]. The effects of CM-Pf stimulation were reported initially in anecdotal cases of patients with chronic pain syndrome submitted to thalamic DBS, in whom an improvement of concomitant hyperkinesias as varied as tremor, stump dyskinesia or athetosis was observed [64, 65]. The combined approach of CM-Pf stimulation with standard targets for DBS in PD (bilateral STN or GPi) has been formally reported in eight PD patients [66–68]: CM-Pf stimulation alone was associated with a significant reduction in UPDRS-III scores, although GPi stimulation alone provided a greater improvement than CM-Pf stimulation alone. Combined CM-Pf and GPi stimulation had a significant synergistic effect [66]. In addition, CM-Pf stimulation caused a significant improvement in freezing of gait, while GPi stimulation did not [66]. These results were maintained for 3 years post-surgery [68]. Combined stimulation of the CM-Pf and bilateral STN was assessed in two PD patients [67]. After 6 months of continuous stimulation, the blinded assessed UPDRS-III score improved more with bilateral STN stimulation alone than with CM-Pf stimulation alone, while resting tremor improved more with CM-Pf stimulation alone. In these studies, a high-frequency (185 Hz) stimulation was used [66]. An anecdotal report of improvement of limb tremor in two PD patients after CM-Pf stimulation alone has since been published [47]. Limiting stimulation-induced side effects can be persistent paresthesias, facial muscle contraction or dystonia [66]. In a single case report, CM-Pf stimulation was tried in combination with the contralateral ventralis oralis posterior nucleus of the thalamus and the cZi for refractory PD tremor [47]. Good tremor control was reported but at the expense of severe speech impairment that only improved with switching-off of stimulation in either side [47]. The potential reduction in treatment-induced dyskinesias in PD was suggested in a group of patients submitted to VIM-DBS, in which a more posterior and deeper position of the electrodes, corresponding to the CM-Pf complex, was associated with an improvement of tremor and better control of peak-dose dyskinesias than the accurately located VIM stimulation [69]. In contrast, studies using a combined approach of CM-Pf and GPi stimulation did not report a significant antidyskinesia effect with CM-Pf stimulation alone [66]. Further studies are necessary to support these preliminary observations.

The nucleus basalis of Meynert

The nucleus basalis of Meynert (NBM) is an important cholinergic nucleus located in the basal forebrain and extends from the olfactory tubercle anteriorly to the level of the uncus of the hippocampus posteriorly [70]. The NBM is divided into six sectors with ascending projections to the neocortex, mainly with connections with the medial temporal structures, amygdala, and frontoparietal and temporoparietal cortices. There is a considerable overlap between individual subsectors for some innervated neocortical areas, which potentially makes these areas more protected from the effects of neuronal loss within specific sectors of the NBM [70]. Although dementia represents a brain neurodegenerative process and DBS has not been shown to be neuroprotective for currently used targets, it is postulated that stimulation of these pathways might enhance cholinergic activity in the innervated cortical regions and improve cognitive function, including memory and attention [70]. The case of a single patient with PD and PD dementia (PDD) has been reported after chronic combined stimulation of the NBM and STN. The laterodorsal portion of the intermediate part (Ch4 intermedius sector) was targeted, which corresponds to the largest section of the NBM [71], in the expectation of achieving a more widespread neocortical projection of the stimulation effects. Low-frequency stimulation (20 Hz) was used in order to induce an excitatory effect [72]. At 24 weeks after implantation, NBM stimulation alone was associated with cognitive improvement compared with the preoperative assessment, STN stimulation alone and sham NBM stimulation [72]. Performance in the Auditory–Verbal Learning and Memory Test and the Trail Making and Clock Drawing tests improved, but there was no change for delayed recognition and recall [72]. Ideomotor and ideational apraxia improved up to 18 months after the onset of NBM stimulation [73]. Phase 1 and 2 trials are ongoing to assess the effect of NBM stimulation in PDD and dementia with Lewy bodies (ClinicalTrials.gov identifiers: NCT01701544 and NCT01340001). Other targets, such as the fornix, which have been assessed in Alzheimer's disease, could potentially be assessed for PDD in the future [74, 75].

Motor cortex stimulation

Motor cortex stimulation (MCS) has been proposed as an alternative surgical procedure in PD patients with motor fluctuations and dyskinesias with a contraindication for either STN-DBS or GPi-DBS. Motor cortical activity has been shown to be dysfunctional in PD patients: the primary motor cortex (M1) has reduced intra-cortical inhibition [76] and an increased metabolism with disease progression [77]. Motor cortex stimulation in PD was first introduced by Canavero in 2000 [78], after a seminal observation by Woolsey *et al.* [79]. Since then, a few human studies were conducted targeting of the M1 area (Table 21.3). Most of these studies adopted an epidural placement of the electrodes, with the exception of one study that used a subdural implantation, with the rational of achieving a more precise placement of the electrodes and a more direct stimulation, without the interposition of cerebrospinal fluid [80]. Most of these studies were case series, with the exception of one study [80]. The results have been mixed, ranging from the observation of no therapeutic effect to a long-lasting improvement of parkinsonian disability measured by the UPDRS-III or its item scores of rigidity and axial signs. When reported, the improvement could be observed on both sides of the body, even for unilateral MCS. A reduction in treatment-induced dyskinesias has also been reported. Most of the clinical studies were small in sample size, as well as nonrandomized and open label. In addition, MCS lacked a standardized approach regarding stimulation parameters, duration of stimulation, laterality of electrodes and localization techniques. Overall, MCS appears to be a safe procedure, without changes in cognition or behavior [80]. Nevertheless, the risk for seizures and surgical complications such as venous brain infarction has to be considered [82]. Other potentially valuable cortical targets such as the supplementary motor area (SMA) and the dorsolateral prefrontal cortex (DLPFC) have not been explored.

Epidural spinal cord stimulation

Currently, epidural spinal cord stimulation (eSCS) is used for chronic pain syndromes such as failed back surgery syndrome and complex regional pain syndrome [89]. Based on animal models, eSCS has been proposed to have a putative therapeutic in PD, mediated through the activation of the dorsal columns with the putative effect of disrupting aberrant low-frequency synchronous corticostriatal oscillations by ascending pathways reaching thalamic nuclei and/or the PPN [90]. There have been a total of 20 PD patients operated on using eSCS reported in the literature [91–96], with preliminary results that are mixed in terms of rigidity, bradykinesia, tremor, gait and postural stability and, anecdotally, bladder incontinence. There are many confounding factors to be considered: the role of the concomitant relief of pain, as in most of these cases the primary indication for eSCS was a concomitant chronic pain syndrome, the different

Table 21.3 Literature about motor cortex stimulation in Parkinson's disease patients

Study	Patients (n)	Target	Study design	Study duration (months)	Stimulation details	Efficacy results
Bentivoglio et al. (2012) [80]; Giuda et al. (2012) [81]	11	Unilateral M1	Unblinded assessments, pre-op, 1, 3, 6 and 12 months, pre-op vs on stim (off and on med)	12 (n = 9)	Epidural bipolar contacts, 80 Hz, 125 μs, 3.7 V (mean values)	↓ UPDRS-III (13.2% at 12 months), significant reduction in rigidity and axial symptoms. On med – no significant change
Moro et al. (2011) [82]	5	Unilateral M1	Unblinded assessments, pre-op, 12 months. Double-blinded (3 months), randomized on vs off stim (off and on med)	12	Subdural mono/bipolar contacts, 108 Hz, 76 μs, 3.3 V (mean values)	UPDRS-III – nonsignificant changes ($P > 0.05$), 3 and 12 months
Arle et al. (2008) [83]	4	Bilateral M1 (n = 3)	Unblinded assessments, pre-op, 1, 3, 6 and 12 months, pre-op vs on stim, off med and on stim vs on med and on stim	12 (n = 2)	Epidural mono/bipolar contacts, 100–130 Hz, 210–240 μs, 3.2–3.5 V	UPDRS-III – nonsignificant changes at 1, 3, 6 and 12 months ($P > 0.05$)
Cilia et al. (2007) [84]	5	Left M1	Rater-blinded assessment, pre-op, 6 months. Pre-op vs on stim, and off vs on stim (off and on med)	6	Epidural mono/multiple bipolar contacts, 40–60 Hz, 180–210 μs, 3–4 V	UPDRS-II and -III and Item 39, medication dosage and dyskinesias – no significant mean changes
Cioni et al. (2007) [85]	7	Unilateral M1 (n3); bilateral M1 (n = 4)	Unblinded assessments, pre-op, 1, 3, 6 and 12 months. Pre-op vs on stim, (off and on med)	12	Epidural bipolar contacts; 80 Hz, 120 μs, 3–4 V	UPDRS-III (off-med) – mean improvement of 30% at 3 months, 22% at 12 months (no statistical testing)
Pagni et al. (2008) [86]	41	Unilateral M1	Unblinded assessments, pre-op, 1, 3, 6 and 12, up to 36 months, on stim (on vs off med)	3–36	25–80 Hz, 90–180 μs, 2.5–6 V	↓ UPDRS-III (19.1% at 36 months); ↓ axial item score, UPDRS-III (only at 24 months). On med – no consistent significant change. Reduction in UPDRS-IV scores (up to 24 months), no change in LEDD
Gutiérrez et al. (2009) [87]	6	Unilateral M1	Unblinded assessments, pre-op, 1, 3, 6 and 12 months, off stim vs off med and on stim vs on med and on stim	12	Epidural bipolar contacts; 21.7 Hz, 421 μs, 3.6 V	UPDRS-III – no apparent change (only individual patient description)
DeRose et al. (2012) [88]	10	Unilateral M1	Unblinded assessments, pre-op, 1, 3, 6, 12, 18, 24 and 36 months. pre-op vs on stim (off vs on med)	36	Epidural bipolar contacts; 20–40 Hz, 120–240 μs, 2.5–4.0 V	↓ UPDRS-III – sustained (13% at 36 months), greater improvement on axial signs (28% at 36 months). On med – no significant change. Reduction in LEDD (at 36 months), treatment-induced dyskinesias (18 months)

M1, primary motor cortex; LEDD, levodopa-equivalent daily dose; med, PD medications; op, operative; stim, stimulation; UPDRS, Unified Parkinson's Disease Rating Scale.

locations of the eSCS either at a high cervical level or mid-to-low thoracic levels, the orientation of the electrode poles, the latency between onset of stimulation and documentation of the therapeutic effect, and use of a wide range of frequencies from 40 to 300 Hz. Potential stimulation-related limiting side effects are paresthesias and startle reaction [92]. Clinical studies are being planned to assess, in a more systematic fashion, the validity and significance of eSCS as a new target in the surgical management of PD patients.

Noninvasive brain stimulation

Historically, electroconvulsive therapy was the first attempt at using noninvasive brain stimulation for the treatment of motor symptoms of PD [97]. Presently, repetitive transcranial magnetic stimulation (rTMS) is the form of noninvasive brain stimulation that has been more extensively evaluated for various therapeutic goals, including the improvement of parkinsonian disability, as well as specific parkinsonian features such as gait, bradykinesia, tremor and other motor symptoms such as diphasic dyskinesia, off-time dystonia and phonation, and nonmotor features such as depression, cognition and sleep. Different stimulation areas have been explored, including the M1, SMA, DLPFC and cerebellum. Recent meta-analyses of the effect of rTMS in parkinsonian disability [98, 99] concluded that high-frequency (>1 Hz) rTMS slightly improves bradykinesia, an effect that can last up to 2 months. Low-frequency (1 Hz) rTMS is suggested to have a small and transient antidyskinesia effect [98–101]. From a mechanistic perspective, high-frequency rTMS seems to increase cortical excitability, while low-frequency rTMS decreases cortical excitability, but further standardization of the stimulation paradigm for rTMS is required. A larger, multicenter, randomized controlled study is warranted, further supported by the importance of the placebo effect in rTMS [102]. A future clinical use of rTMS for parkinsonian disability or depression must outweigh the cost of the equipment and the need for multiple rTMS sessions that may condition patient adherence in regular clinical practice [103].

Another paradigm of noninvasive brain stimulation is transcranial direct current stimulation (tDCS). In tDCS, a low-amplitude direct current is applied via scalp electrodes [104]. In the single randomized, double-blinded, sham-controlled study conducted with tDCS, the authors reported a long-lasting (3 months) effect on bradykinesia, although only when measured by timed tests and not by the UDPRS-III [104].

Novel stimulation paradigms and devices

Recent advances in DBS technology have provided novel stimulation paradigms, with the ultimate goal of tailoring the stimulation to the individual patient and to specific symptoms of PD. A closed-loop device is an example of a new paradigm of stimulation, in which current parameters are modulated on a continuous basis, according to changing neural activity [105], as cardiac pacemakers currently can function. The closed-loop stimulation is conceptually appealing for its adaptability and potential advantage of lengthening the battery life due to better energy use. Nevertheless, it can be challenging to find a suitable neurophysiological signal that can serve as a source signal for its correlation with PD motor symptoms and signs. The wireless instantaneous neurochemical concentration sensor (WINCS) has been suggested as a potential electrochemical feedback strategy for a closed-loop DBS system. The WINCS is able to perform an almost real-time detection (in the range of milliseconds) of changes in the neurotransmitters dopamine, adenosine and serotonin by means of fast-scan cyclic voltammetry and amperometry [106]. Another approach is to use neurophysiological recordings as the source signal. In the 1-methyl-4-phenyl-1,2,3,6-tetrahydropyridine (MPTP) non-human primate model, neural activity in the GPi and M1 was used as source signals and electrodes located in the GPi were used for stimulation. Closed-loop stimulation of the GPi was associated with a greater improvement of primate akinesia compared with the "classical" GPi continuous stimulation [105]. More recently, a pilot study assessed the safety and efficiency of brain–computer interfaces as a neurophysiological feedback for a closed-loop DBS system in PD patients [107]. In this closed-loop DBS system, local field potentials recorded from electrodes implanted in the STN were used as the source signal. The authors reported a greater motor improvement compared with continuous DBS and a reduction in energy requirements [107], fulfilling the goal of lengthening the lifespan of the internal pulse generators in DBS without compromising clinical benefit. These results will encourage new studies to confirm the safety, feasibility and efficacy of the closed-loop stimulation paradigm. An intuitive indication for a closed-loop DBS system is the treatment of paroxystic phenomenon in PD, such as freezing of gait.

The constant voltage model, as opposed to the constant current model, is another stimulation paradigm for DBS devices. The constant voltage stimulator delivers electric current, independent of changes in impedance. Recently, an open-label, randomized controlled trial [108] reported a significant clinical benefit in the reduction of "off" time without dyskinesias that warrants a head-to-head comparison with the "classical" constant paradigm of stimulation. Another technological aspect in DBS technology is innovation in lead design with the use of multiple independent current sources that can potentially provide the ability to "steer" the volume of activated tissue to increase the therapeutic window of DBS, by avoiding side effects secondary to current spread and to specifically target the adequate structures [109].

Concluding remarks

In last two decades, DBS therapy has greatly improved the quality of life of patients with PD. This history-making success has also created new expectations of managing additional symptoms in PD using the same paradigm, especially in patients excluded from the currently accepted indications for DBS. Up to now, multiple targets have been explored with DBS but with variable results and these remain to be fully and comprehensively assessed. Larger and better-designed clinical studies with randomization, allocation concealment and blinded assessments are warranted, as well as improved targeting techniques and new devices that can provide a more accurate implantation of electrodes and improve stimulation paradigms. The latter two points are paramount in defining the real therapeutic effect associated with stimulation of a specific brain area or nucleus, and in avoiding erroneous conclusions. Technological advances in stimulation paradigms could be the next revolution in DBS.

References

1. Benabid AL, Pollak P, Hommel M, *et al.* [Treatment of Parkinson tremor by chronic stimulation of the ventral intermediate nucleus of the thalamus]. *Rev Neurol (Paris)* 1989; **145**: 320–3.
2. Odekerken VJ, van Laar T, Staal MJ, *et al.* Subthalamic nucleus versus globus pallidus bilateral deep brain stimulation for advanced Parkinson's disease (NSTAPS study): a randomised controlled trial. *Lancet Neurology* 2013; **12**: 37–44.
3. Pahapill PA, Lozano AM. The pedunculopontine nucleus and Parkinson's disease. *Brain* 2000; **123**: 1767–83.
4. Alam M, Schwabe K, Krauss JK. The pedunculopontine nucleus area: critical evaluation of interspecies differences relevant for its use as a target for deep brain stimulation. *Brain* 2011; **134**: 11–23.
5. Aravamuthan BR, Muthusamy KA, Stein JF, Aziz TZ, Johansen-Berg H. Topography of cortical and subcortical connections of the human pedunculopontine and subthalamic nuclei. *Neuroimage* 2007; **37**: 694–705.
6. Zweig RM, Jankel WR, Hedreen JC, Mayeux R, Price DL. The pedunculopontine nucleus In Parkinson's disease. *Ann Neurol* 1989; **26**: 41–6.
7. Mazzone P, Lozano A, Stanzione P, *et al.* Implantation of human pedunculopontine nucleus: a safe and clinically relevant target in Parkinson's disease. *Neuroreport* 2005; **16**: 1877–81.
8. Plaha P, Gill SS. Bilateral deep brain stimulation of the pedunculopontine nucleus for Parkinson's disease. *Neuroreport* 2005; **16**: 1883–7.
9. Stefani A, Lozano AM, Peppe A, *et al.* Bilateral deep brain stimulation of the pedunculopontine and subthalamic nuclei in severe Parkinson's disease. *Brain* 2007; **130**: 1596–607.
10. Ferraye MU, Debû B, Fraix V, *et al.* Effects of pedunculopontine nucleus area stimulation on gait disorders in Parkinson's disease. *Brain* 2010; **133**: 205–14.
11. Moro E, Hamani C, Poon YY, Al-Khairallah T, *et al.* Unilateral pedunculopontine stimulation improves falls in Parkinson's disease. *Brain* 2010; **133**: 215–24.
12. Khan S, Mooney L, Plaha P, *et al.* Outcomes from stimulation of the caudal zona incerta and pedunculopontine nucleus in patients with Parkinson's disease. *Brit J Neurosurg* 2011; **25**: 273–80.
13. Thevathasan W, Coyne TJ, Hyam JA, *et al.* Pedunculopontine nucleus stimulation improves gait freezing in Parkinson disease. *Neurosurgery* 2011; **69**: 1248–53; discussion 1254.
14. Khan S, Javed S, Mooney L, *et al.* Clinical outcomes from bilateral versus unilateral stimulation of the pedunculopontine nucleus with and without concomitant caudal zona incerta region stimulation in Parkinson's disease. *Brit J Neurosurg* 2012; **26**: 722–5.
15. Ferraye MU, Debû B, Fraix V, *et al.* Subthalamic nucleus versus pedunculopontine nucleus stimulation in Parkinson disease: synergy or antagonism? *J Neural Transm* 2011; **118**: 1469–75.
16. Ferraye MU, Gerardin P, Debû B, *et al.* Pedunculopontine nucleus stimulation induces monocular oscillopsia. *J Neurol Neurosurg Psychiatry* 2009; **80**: 228–31.
17. Jenkinson N, Brittain JS, Hicks SL, Kennard C, Aziz TZ. On the origin of oscillopsia during pedunculopontine stimulation. *Stereotact Funct Neurosurg* 2012; **90**: 124–9.

18. Zrinzo L, Zrinzo LV, Hariz M. The peripeduncular nucleus: a novel target for deep brain stimulation? *Neuroreport* 2007; **18**: 1301–2.
19. Mazzone P, Insola A, Lozano A, et al. Peripeduncular and pedunculopontine nuclei: a dispute on a clinically relevant target. *Neuroreport* 2007; **18**: 1407–8.
20. Yelnik J. PPN or PPD, what is the target for deep brain stimulation in Parkinson's disease? *Brain* 2007; **130**: e79; author reply e80.
21. Zrinzo L, Hariz M. The peripeduncular nucleus: a novel target for deep brain stimulation? *Neuroreport* 2007; **18**: 1631–2; author reply 1632–3.
22. Zrinzo L, Zrinzo LV, Hariz M. The pedunculopontine and peripeduncular nuclei: a tale of two structures. *Brain* 2007; **130**: e73; author reply e74.
23. Zrinzo L, Zrinzo LV, Massey LA, et al. Targeting of the pedunculopontine nucleus by an MRI-guided approach: a cadaver study. *J Neural Transm* 2011; **118**: 1487–95.
24. Khan S, Gill SS, Mooney L, et al. Combined pedunculopontine-subthalamic stimulation in Parkinson disease. *Neurology* 2012; **78**: 1090–5.
25. Peppe A, Pierantozzi M, Chiavalon C, et al. Deep brain stimulation of the pedunculopontine tegmentum and subthalamic nucleus: effects on gait in Parkinson's disease. *Gait Posture* 2010; **32**: 512–18.
26. Lim AS, Moro E, Lozano AM, et al. Selective enhancement of rapid eye movement sleep by deep brain stimulation of the human pons. *Ann Neurol* 2009; **66**: 110–14.
27. Arnulf I, Ferraye M, Fraix V, et al. Sleep induced by stimulation in the human pedunculopontine nucleus area. *Ann Neurol* 2010; **67**: 546–9.
28. Stefani A, Pierantozzi M, Ceravolo R, et al. Deep brain stimulation of pedunculopontine tegmental nucleus (PPTg) promotes cognitive and metabolic changes: a target-specific effect or response to a low-frequency pattern of stimulation? *Clin EEG Neurosci* 2010; **41**: 82–6.
29. Gallay MN, Jeanmonod D, Liu J, Morel A. Human pallidothalamic and cerebellothalamic tracts: anatomical basis for functional stereotactic neurosurgery. *Brain Struct Funct* 2008; **212**: 443–63.
30. Blomstedt P, Sandvik U, Fytagoridis A, Tisch S. The posterior subthalamic area in the treatment of movement disorders: past, present, and future. *Neurosurgery* 2009; **64**: 1029–38.
31. Morel A. *Stereotactic Atlas of the Human Thalamus and Basal Ganglia*. London: CRC Press, 2007.
32. Kerl HU, Gerigk L, Huck S, et al. Visualisation of the zona incerta for deep brain stimulation at 3.0 tesla. *Clin Neuroradiol* 2012; **22**: 55–68.
33. Andy OJ, Jurko MF, Sias FR. Subthalamotomy in treatment of parkinsonian tremor. *J Neurosurg* 1963; **20**: 860–70.
34. Mundinger F. Stereotaxic interventions on the zona incerta area for treatment of extrapyramidal motor disturbances and their results. *Confin Neurol* 1965; **26**: 222–30.
35. Saint-Cyr JA, Hoque T, Pereira LC, et al. Localization of clinically effective stimulating electrodes in the human subthalamic nucleus on magnetic resonance imaging. *J Neurosurg* 2002; **97**: 1152–66.
36. Voges J, Volkmann J, Allert N, et al. Bilateral high-frequency stimulation in the subthalamic nucleus for the treatment of Parkinson disease: correlation of therapeutic effect with anatomical electrode position. *J Neurosurg* 2002; **96**: 269–79.
37. Caire F, Ranoux D, Guehl D, Burbaud P, Cuny E. A systematic review of studies on anatomical position of electrode contacts used for chronic subthalamic stimulation in Parkinson's disease. *Acta Neurochir (Wien)* 2013; **155**: 1647–54; discussion 1654.
38. Herzog J, Fietzek U, Hamel W, et al. Most effective stimulation site in subthalamic deep brain stimulation for Parkinson's disease. *Mov Disord* 2004; **19**: 1050–4.
39. Herzog J, Pinsker M, Wasner M, et al. Stimulation of subthalamic fiber tracts reduces dyskinesias in STN-DBS. *Mov Disord* 2007; **22**: 679–84.
40. Velasco F, Jimenez F, Perez ML, et al. Electrical stimulation of the prelemniscal radiation in the treatment of Parkinson's disease: An old target revised with new techniques. *Neurosurgery* 2001; **49**: 293–306.
41. Kitagawa M, Murata J, Uesugi H, et al. Two-year follow-up of chronic stimulation of the posterior subthalamic white matter for tremor-dominant Parkinson's disease. *Neurosurgery* 2005; **56**: 281–7; discussion 281–9.
42. Plaha P, Ben-Shlomo Y, Patel NK, Gill SS. Stimulation of the caudal zona incerta is superior to stimulation of the subthalamic nucleus in improving contralateral parkinsonism. *Brain* 2006; **129**: 1732–47.
43. Carrillo-Ruiz JD, Velasco F, Jimenez F, et al. Bilateral electrical stimulation of prelemniscal radiations in the treatment of advanced Parkinson's disease. *Neurosurgery* 2008; **62**: 347–57.
44. Blomstedt P, Fytagoridis A, Astrom M, et al. Unilateral caudal zona incerta deep brain stimulation for Parkinsonian tremor. *Parkinsonism Relat Disord* 2012; **18**: 1062–6.
45. Merello M, Cavanagh S, Perez-Lloret S, et al. Irritability, psychomotor agitation and progressive insomnia induced by bilateral stimulation of the area surrounding the dorsal subthalamic nucleus (zona incerta) in Parkinson's disease patients. *J Neurol* 2009; **256**: 2091–3.
46. Czernecki V, Schüpbach M, Yaici S, et al. Apathy following subthalamic stimulation in Parkinson disease: a dopamine responsive symptom. *Mov Disord* 2008; **23**: 964–9.

47. Franzini A, Cordella R, Messina G, et al. Deep brain stimulation for movement disorders. Considerations on 276 consecutive patients. *J Neural Transm* 2011; **118**: 1497–510.

48. Lundgren S, Saeys T, Karlsson F, et al. Deep brain stimulation of caudal zona incerta and subthalamic nucleus in patients with Parkinson's disease: effects on voice intensity. *Parkinsons Dis* 2011; **2011**: 658956.

49. Karlsson F, Unger E, Wahlgren S, et al. Deep brain stimulation of caudal zona incerta and subthalamic nucleus in patients with Parkinson's disease: effects on diadochokinetic rate. *Parkinsons Dis* 2011; **2011**: 605607.

50. Karlsson F, Blomstedt P, Olofsson K, et al. Control of phonatory onset and offset in Parkinson patients following deep brain stimulation of the subthalamic nucleus and caudal zona incerta. *Parkinsonism Relat Disord* 2012; **18**: 824–7.

51. Karlsson F, van Doorn J. Effects of deep brain stimulation of caudal zona incerta and subthalamic nucleus on pitch level in speech of patients with Parkinson's disease. *Mov Disord* 2012; **27**: S161.

52. Sundstedt S, Olofsson K, van Doorn J, et al. Swallowing function in Parkinson's patients following Zona Incerta deep brain stimulation. *Acta Neurol Scand* 2012; **126**: 350–6.

53. Tripoliti E, Zrinzo L, Martinez-Torres I, et al. Effects of subthalamic stimulation on speech of consecutive patients with Parkinson disease. *Neurology* 2011; **76**: 80–6.

54. Fytagoridis A, Astrom M, Wardell K, Blomstedt P. Stimulation-induced side effects in the posterior subthalamic area: distribution, characteristics and visualization. *Clin Neurol Neurosurg* 2013; **115**: 65–71.

55. Bejjani B, Damier P, Arnulf I, et al. Pallidal stimulation for Parkinson's disease. Two targets? *Neurology* 1997; **49**: 1564–9.

56. Krack P, Pollak P, Limousin P, et al. Opposite motor effects of pallidal stimulation in Parkinson's disease. *Ann Neurol* 1998; **43**: 180–92.

57. Tommasi G, Lopiano L, Zibetti M, et al. Freezing and hypokinesia of gait induced by stimulation of the subthalamic region. *J Neurol Sci* 2007; **258**: 99–103.

58. Plaha P, Bunnage M, Gill S. Bilateral deep brain stimulation of the caudal zona Incerta for Parkinson's disease: A one-year clinical, cognitive, and quality-of-life outcome study. *J Neurosurg* 2006; **104**: A640–1.

59. Alexander GE, DeLong MR, Strick PL. Parallel organization of functionally segregated circuits linking basal ganglia and cortex. *Annu Rev Neurosci* 1986; **9**: 357–81.

60. Chastan N, Westby GW, Yelnik J, et al. Effects of nigral stimulation on locomotion and postural stability in patients with Parkinson's disease. *Brain* 2009; **132**: 172–84.

61. Weiss D, Wachter T, Meisner C, et al. Combined STN/SNr-DBS for the treatment of refractory gait disturbances in Parkinson's disease: study protocol for a randomized controlled trial. *Trials* 2011; **12**: 222.

62. Benarroch EE. The midline and intralaminar thalamic nuclei: anatomic and functional specificity and implications in neurologic disease. *Neurology* 2008; **71**: 944–9.

63. Adams JE, Rutkin BB. Lesions of the centrum medianum in the treatment of movement disorders. *Confin Neurol* 1965; **26**: 231–45.

64. Andy OJ. Parafascicular-center median nuclei stimulation for intractable pain and dyskinesia (painful-dyskinesia). *Appl Neurophysiol* 1980; **43**: 133–44.

65. Krauss JK, Pohle T, Weigel R, Burgunder JM. Deep brain stimulation of the centre median-parafascicular complex in patients with movement disorders. *J Neurol Neurosurg Psychiatry* 2002; **72**: 546–8.

66. Mazzone P, Stocchi F, Galati S, et al. Bilateral implantation of centromedian-parafascicularis complex and GPi: a new combination of unconventional targets for deep brain stimulation in severe Parkinson disease. *Neuromodulation* 2006; **9**: 221–8.

67. Peppe A, Gasbarra A, Stefani A, et al. Deep brain stimulation of CM/PF of thalamus could be the new elective target for tremor in advanced Parkinson's Disease? *Parkinsonism Relat Disord* 2008; **14**: 501–4.

68. Stefani A, Peppe A, Pierantozzi M, et al. Multi-target strategy for Parkinsonian patients: The role of deep brain stimulation in the centromedian-parafascicularis complex. *Brain Res Bull* 2009; **78**: 113–18.

69. Caparros-Lefebvre D, Blond S, Feltin MP, Pollak P, Benabid AL. Improvement of levodopa induced dyskinesias by thalamic deep brain stimulation is related to slight variation in electrode placement: possible involvement of the centre median and parafascicularis complex. *J Neurol Neurosurg Psychiatry* 1999; **67**: 308–14.

70. Gratwicke J, Kahan J, Zrinzo L, et al. The nucleus basalis of Meynert: a new target for deep brain stimulation in dementia? *Neurosci Biobehav Rev* 2013; **37**: 2676–88.

71. Mesulam MM and Geula C 1988 Nucleus basalis (Ch4) and cortical cholinergic innervation in the human brain: observations based on the distribution of acetylcholinesterase and choline acetyltransferase. *J Comp Neurol* **275**: 216–40.

72. Freund HJ, Kuhn J, Lenartz D, et al. Cognitive functions in a patient with Parkinson-dementia syndrome undergoing deep brain stimulation *Arch Neurol* 2009; **66**: 781–5.

73. Barnikol TT, Pawelczyk NB, Barnikol UB, et al. Changes in apraxia after deep brain stimulation of the nucleus basalis Meynert in a patient with Parkinson dementia syndrome. *Mov Disord* 2010; **25**: 1519–20.

74. Laxton AW, Tang-Wai DF, McAndrews MP, et al. A phase I trial of deep brain stimulation of memory

circuits in Alzheimer's disease. *Ann Neurol* 2010; **68**: 521–34.

75. Hardenacke K, Shubina E, Buhrle CP, et al. Deep brain stimulation as a tool for improving cognitive functioning in Alzheimer's dementia: a systematic review. *Front Psychiatry* 2013; **4**: 159.

76. Lefaucheur JP. Treatment of Parkinson's disease by cortical stimulation. *Expert Rev Neurother* 2009; **9**: 1755–71.

77. Huang C, Tang C, Feigin A, et al. Changes in network activity with the progression of Parkinson's disease. *Brain* 2007; **130**: 1834–46.

78. Canavero S, Paolotti R. Extradural motor cortex stimulation for advanced Parkinson's disease: case report. *Mov Disord* 2000; **15**: 169–71.

79. Woolsey CN, Erickson TC, Gilson WE. localization in somatic sensory and motor areas of human cerebral-cortex as determined by direct recording of evoked potentials and electrical stimulation. *J Neurosurg* 1979; **51**: 476–506.

80. Bentivoglio AR, Fasano A, Piano C, et al. Unilateral extradural motor cortex stimulation is safe and improves Parkinson disease at 1 year. *Neurosurgery* 2012; **71**: 815–25.

81. Di Giuda D, Calcagni ML, Totaro M, et al. Chronic motor cortex stimulation in patients with advanced Parkinson's disease and effects on striatal dopaminergic transmission as assessed by 123I-FP-CIT SPECT: a preliminary report. *Nucl Med Commun* 2012; **33**: 933–40.

82. Moro E, Schwalb JM, Piboolnurak P, et al. Unilateral subdural motor cortex stimulation improves essential tremor but not Parkinson's disease. *Brain* 2011; **134**: 2096–105.

83. Arle JE, Apetauerova D, Zani J, et al. Motor cortex stimulation in patients with Parkinson disease: 12-month follow-up in 4 patients. *J Neurosurg* 2008; **109**: 133–9.

84. Cilia R, Landi A, Vergani F, et al. Extradural motor cortex stimulation in Parkinson's disease. *Mov Disord* 2007; **22**: 111–14.

85. Cioni B. Motor cortex stimulation for Parkinson's disease. *Acta Neurochir Suppl* 2007; **97**: 233–8.

86. Pagni CA, Albanese A, Bentivoglio A, et al. Results by motor cortex stimulation in treatment of focal dystonia, Parkinson's disease and post-ictal spasticity. The experience of the Italian Study Group of the Italian Neurosurgical Society. *Acta Neurochir Suppl* 2008; **101**: 13–21.

87. Gutiérrez JC, Seijo FJ, Alvarez Vega MA, et al. Therapeutic extradural cortical stimulation for Parkinson's disease: report of six cases and review of the literature. *Clin Neurol Neurosurg* 2009; **111**: 703–7.

88. De Rose M, Guzzi G, Bosco D, et al. Motor cortex stimulation in Parkinson's disease. *Neurol Res Int* 2012; **2012**: 502096.

89. Simpson EL, Duenas A, Holmes MW, Papaioannou D, Chilcott J. Spinal cord stimulation for chronic pain of neuropathic or ischaemic origin: systematic review and economic evaluation. *Health Technol Assess* 2009; **13**: iii, ix–x, 1–154.

90. Fuentes R, Petersson P, Siesser WB, Caron MG, Nicolelis MA. Spinal cord stimulation restores locomotion in animal models of Parkinson's disease. *Science* 2009; **323**: 1578–82.

91. Nicolelis MA, Fuentes R, Petersson P. Spinal cord stimulation failed to relieve akinesia or restore locomotion in Parkinson disease. *Neurology* 2010; **75**: 1484; author reply 1484–5.

92. Thevathasan W, Mazzone P, Jha A, et al. Spinal cord stimulation failed to relieve akinesia or restore locomotion in Parkinson disease. *Neurology* 2010; **74**: 1325–7.

93. Agari T, Date I. Spinal cord stimulation for the treatment of abnormal posture and gait disorder in patients with Parkinson's disease. *Neurologia Med Chir (Tokyo)* 2012; **52**: 470–4.

94. Fenelon G, Goujon C, Gurruchaga JM, et al. Spinal cord stimulation for chronic pain improved motor function in a patient with Parkinson's disease. *Parkinsonism Relat Disord* 2012; **18**: 213–4.

95. Hassan S, Amer S, Alwaki A, Elborno A. A patient with Parkinson's disease benefits from spinal cord stimulation. *J Clin Neurosci* 2013; **20**: 1155–6.

96. Landi A, Trezza A, Pirillo D, et al. Spinal cord stimulation for the treatment of sensory symptoms in advanced Parkinson's disease. *Neuromodulation* 2013; **16**: 276–9.

97. Andersen K, Balldin J, Gottfries CG, et al. A double-blind evaluation of electroconvulsive therapy in Parkinson's disease with "on–off" phenomena. *Acta Neurol Scand* 1987; **76**: 191–9.

98. Fregni F, Simon DK, Wu A, Pascual-Leone A. Non-invasive brain stimulation for Parkinson's disease: a systematic review and meta-analysis of the literature. *J Neurol Neurosurg Psychiatry* 2005; **76**: 1614–23.

99. Elahi B, Chen R. Effect of transcranial magnetic stimulation on Parkinson motor function – systematic review of controlled clinical trials. *Mov Disord* 2009; **24**: 357–63.

100. Brusa L, Versace V, Koch G, et al. Low frequency rTMS of the SMA transiently ameliorates peak-dose LID in Parkinson's disease. *Clin Neurophysiol* 2006; **117**: 1917–21.

101. Filipović SR, Rothwell JC, van de Warrenburg BP, Bhatia K. Repetitive transcranial magnetic stimulation for levodopa-induced dyskinesias in Parkinson's disease. *Mov Disord* 2009; **24**: 246–53.

102. Strafella AP, Ko JH, Monchi O. Therapeutic application of transcranial magnetic stimulation in Parkinson's disease: the contribution of expectation. *Neuroimage* 2006; **31**: 1666–72.

103. Chen R. Repetitive transcranial magnetic stimulation as treatment for depression in Parkinson's disease. *Mov Disord* 2010; **25**: 2272–3.
104. Benninger DH, Lomarev M, Lopez G, *et al.* Transcranial direct current stimulation for the treatment of Parkinson's disease. *J Neurol Neurosurg Psychiatry* 2010; **81**: 1105–11.
105. Rosin B, Slovik M, Mitelman R, *et al.* Closed-loop deep brain stimulation is superior in ameliorating parkinsonism. *Neuron* 2011; **72**: 370–84.
106. Van Gompel JJ, Chang SY, Goerss SJ, *et al.* Development of intraoperative electrochemical detection: wireless instantaneous neurochemical concentration sensor for deep brain stimulation feedback. *Neurosurg Focus* 2010; **29**: E6.
107. Little S, Pogosyan A, Neal S, *et al.* Adaptive deep brain stimulation in advanced Parkinson disease. *Ann Neurol* 2013; **74**: 449–57.
108. Okun MS, Gallo BV, Mandybur G, *et al.* Subthalamic deep brain stimulation with a constant-current device in Parkinson's disease: an open-label randomised controlled trial. *Lancet Neurol* 2012; **11**: 140–9.
109. Chaturvedi A, Foutz TJ, McIntyre CC. Current steering to activate targeted neural pathways during deep brain stimulation of the subthalamic region. *Brain Stimul* 2012; **5**: 369–77.

Section IV Clinical Trials in Parkinson's Disease: Lessons, Controversies and Challenges

Chapter 22 Rating scales and clinical outcome measures in the evaluation of patients with Parkinson's disease

Pablo Martinez-Martin and Carmen Rodríguez-Blázquez

Introduction

In recent years, the use of rating scales for Parkinson's disease (PD) has been expanding in clinical practice and research, allowing clinicians and researchers to assess PD manifestations, the course of the disease and the response to treatment. However, the situation has been characterized by great variability in the content and quality of available scales, making comparisons between studies using different tools somewhat difficult.

As a whole, rating scales can be classified as: (i) rater based, used mainly by clinicians for assessment of motor and nonmotor manifestations, complications and treatment effects; and (ii) self-administered instruments commonly known as "patient-reported outcomes" (PROs) [1]. The use of PROs reflects a trend toward a more active role of patients in their treatment and highlights that interventions should be evaluated by using outcomes that are meaningful to patients. Patient-reported outcomes represent the patient's report of a health condition and its treatment [1], and include a variety of subjective aspects of the disease (symptoms, functioning, quality of life, perceived change, satisfaction with treatment). They are essential for understanding the impact of the disease, evaluating treatment efficacy and interpreting the significance of clinical outcomes, and for evidence-based decision making.

Rating scales are very useful when they are developed following rigorous methodological standards and procedures that guarantee the appropriateness and quality of the data they provide. Development and validation of rating scales are based on two main approaches: the Classical Test Theory (CTT) and the Latent Trait Theories (LTT), which includes the Item Response Theory (IRT) and the Rasch measurement theory.

The development and validation of a rating scale is a complex task, involving several steps: (i) definition and operationalization of the concept to be measured, the target population and the purpose (evaluative, discriminative, predictive); (ii) components of the scale (items, subscales, response options); (iii) style and format; (iv) evaluation of a preliminary version (pilot testing); and finally (v) implementation of the first validation study. The main properties to be tested during the validation process are acceptability, reliability, validity, precision and responsiveness [2, 3]. Interpretability of scale scores is not a measurement property but is an important aspect of the scale usefulness. The definition and standard criteria for assessment of these attributes are described in Table 22.1. Acceptability, reliability, validity and responsiveness are especially relevant when rating scales are used as endpoints in clinical trials. The indexes related to the magnitude and meaningfulness of the change (responsiveness and interpretability) are of utmost importance in the context of intervention outcomes. Responsiveness or sensitivity to change is defined as "the ability of an instrument to detect true change" [2], and it is related to the presence of floor and ceiling effects, the reliability and the precision of the instrument. Several methods for assessing responsiveness exist but the most used are the effect size (ES) and the standardized response mean (SRM), both of them with standardized values for interpretation of change [4]. Interpretability is the extent to which a qualitative meaning can be assigned to quantitative scores. For health measures, it is represented by the minimally important change (MIC)

Parkinson's Disease: Current and Future Therapeutics and Clinical Trials, ed. Gálvez-Jiménez et al. Published by Cambridge University Press. © Cambridge University Press 2016.

Table 22.1 Main psychometric attributes of rating scales

Attribute and definition	Standard criteria (examples)
Feasibility: the extent to which the measure can be used in the intended context	Missing data < 5–10%
Acceptability: how acceptable is the scale for the target population?	Observed vs theoretical range coincident Mean vs median coincident Floor and ceiling effects < 15% Skewness −1 to +1
Reliability: degree to which a scale is free of random error	
Internal consistency: the extent to which the items measure the same construct	Cronbach's $\alpha > 0.70$ (group) Inter-item correlation: $r > 0.20$ and $r < 0.75$ Item-total correlation: $r = 0.20–0.40$ Item homogeneity coefficient > 0.30
Reproducibility: stability of scores over time or across different raters	Inter-observer and test-retest reliability: κ (nominal/ordinal data) > 0.60 or > 0.70 Intraclass correlation coefficient (continuous data) > 0.70
Validity: the extent to which an instrument measures the construct it is intended to measure	
Content validity: the degree to which the content of an instrument covers the main aspects of the construct to be measured	Expert opinion Lynn's Content Validity Index
Construct validity (hypothesis testing): the extent to which the scale's scores are consistent with hypothesis regarding the construct	Convergent validity: $r > 0.60$ Divergent validity: $r < 0.30$ Internal validity: $r = 0.30–0.70$ Known-groups validity: significant difference between groups
Criterion validity: the degree of relationship of a scale with a "gold standard"	$R > 0.60$

or difference (MID), which can be ascertained by two groups of techniques: anchor-based and distribution-based approaches. The first operationalizes the change by assigning the subjects to groups (stable, worse or better) using an anchor (a clinical or patient-based measure of change). The distribution-based approaches use statistical tests to determine the ability of the scale to detect a clinically important change. There is no agreement about which approach is more suitable to calculate MIC or MID, so the use of several methods (triangulation) has been proposed to offer a range of figures that is likely to contain the real value [5].

Rating scales for Parkinson's disease
Clinician-based rating scales

In PD, clinicians need strategies and measures capable not only of detecting symptoms but also of identifying the progression of disability and the effects of treatment. For years, the main rating scales for assessing PD were rater based, focused on directly observable signs, such as the core PD manifestations (tremor, bradykinesia and rigidity), and functional ability, and most of them lacked full validation studies. At present, that situation has been deeply modified with the development of comprehensive rater-based scales and PROs for a wide array of motor and nonmotor manifestations, with formal validation studies.

The most frequently studied clinical outcomes include severity of motor manifestations, magnitude of disability, and long-term motor and nonmotor complications (e.g. fluctuations, dyskinesias, hallucinations), although nonmotor aspects of PD are currently receiving rapidly increasing attention. Some of the frequently used and tested rating scales in clinical practice and research are the Hoehn and Yahr staging (HY) for global disability appraisal; the Clinical Impression of Severity Index – Parkinson's Disease (CISI-PD), for global severity appraisal; the Unified Parkinson's Disease Rating Scale (UPDRS) and its clinimetrically enhanced form, the Movement Disorders Society-sponsored version of the UPDRS (MDS-UPDRS), for multidomain severity and disability evaluations; the Scales for Outcomes in Parkinson's Disease (SCOPA) Motor, and the Schwab and England Scale (SES) to assess motor impairment and disability, respectively; the Abnormal Involuntary Movement Scale (AIMS), Rush Dyskinesia Rating Scale (RDRS) and Unified Dyskinesia Rating Scale (UDysRS), for evaluating motor complications and dyskinesias; and the Non-Motor Symptoms Scale (NMSS), SCOPA Cognition (SCOPA-Cog), and SCOPA Psychiatric Complications (SCOPA-PC), for assessing nonmotor symptoms.

Global severity and disability scales

The HY staging is the universally accepted system to classify and characterize the stages of disability of the disease [6]. It consists of a single item addressing the functional and clinical status of the patient on a five-point scale, based on the clinical judgment of the health professional. Although widely used, its properties have barely been assessed [7]. It captures PD progression and change due to treatment, and there is evidence that a change from one stage to another is clinically relevant. Its simplicity and ease of use have made it a common measure in clinical trials, mainly for selection of patients into relatively homogeneous disability groups [7].

The CISI-PD is a global severity/disability index formed by four items – motor signs, disability, cognitive status and motor complications – scored from 0 (not at all) to 6 (very severe or very disabled). The components of the CISI-PD explained 92% of the Clinical Global Impression of Severity variability [8]. It is able to discriminate between PD severity levels, and shows good psychometric properties [9]. As an approach to the minimal detectable change or MID, the standard error of measurement (SEM) resulted in a range between 3.8 and 5.4 [9]. However, there is still a lack of studies on the responsiveness and interpretability of the CISI-PD.

Multidomain scales

The UPDRS assesses motor impairment and complications, through 42 items grouped in four subscales: I, Mentation, Behavior and Mood (four items); II, Activities of Daily Living (ADLs) (13 items); III, Motor (14 items, 27 scores); and IV, Complications of Therapy (11 items) [10]. It also includes a modified HY and the SES. The UPDRS properties have been tested in several studies, applied in most studies on interventions with medication, surgery and other therapies, and it is the primary outcome measure for establishing the effectiveness of PD therapies for the European and US regulatory agencies [11]. The responsiveness of the UPDRS is well established, and its scores are considered for clinical decision making regarding therapy. In consequence, some responsiveness indexes of the UPDRS have been calculated, such as the minimally detectable change (MDC), which was 13 for total score [12]; the minimal clinically relevant incremental difference (MCRID), which was established in a range from 4 to 10 points for UPDRS motor section [13]; and the minimal clinically important change (MCIC) of the total score, which was –3.5 [14].

The MDS-UPDRS was designed to retain the UPDRS strengths and overcome some of its weaknesses [11, 15]. The MDS-UPDRS maintains the UPDRS sections, but they have been renamed: Part I: Non-Motor Experiences of Daily Living, with six rater-based items and seven for self-assessment; Part II: Motor Experiences of Daily Living, with 13 patient-rated items; Part III: Motor Examination, 18 items (33 scores); and Part IV: Motor Complications, with six items. Validation and translation programs have been carefully designed to ensure the instrument's psychometric quality and its applicability across the spectrum of PD and in different cultural settings [16, 17]. The MDS-UPDRS has been replacing the UPDRS as reference scale for clinical trials and practice. It has been shown to be responsive to changes over time and to treatment, including surgery [18, 19], and minimal clinically relevant difference (MCRD) and minimal clinically important difference (MCID) have been calculated for Part III [20, 21]. However, to date no new treatment has been approved using the MDS-UPDRS as the primary outcome measure, and more research is needed to test its responsiveness. Some formulas have been elaborated to transform the scores from the UPDRS [22, 23] and SPES/SCOPA (SCOPA-Motor) [24] to corresponding MDS-UPDRS scores and vice versa.

Motor impairment and disability scales

The SCOPA-Motor assesses motor signs (10 items), impairments in activities of daily living (seven items) and motor complications (four items) [25]. Items are scored in a 4-point scale ranging from 0 (normal) to 3 (severe). The scale is short, easily administered, reliable and valid for PD patients at all stages of disease [25, 26]. The motor section scores can be converted to MDS-UPDRS scores and vice versa [24]. The SCOPA-Motor showed better precision than UPDRS, with SEMs ranging from 0.40 (dyskinesias) to 2.46 (motor examination) [26], but there have been no studies on the scale's responsiveness and interpretability.

The SES has been the reference scale for assessing PD-related disability as it was included in the UPDRS, although it was not designed specifically for this disease [10]. It consists of a one-item scale, scored from 100% (completely independent) to 0% (vegetative functions, bedridden) [27]. Although it has several shortcomings such as the lack of standardization in its administration, its psychometric properties are satisfactory as a whole. The SES has proved to be sensitive to changes [28, 29].

Motor complications and dyskinesia scales

The AIMS is an extensively used scale for screening and rating the severity of dyskinetic complications in PD, although it was originally developed for psychiatric patients [30]. The AIMS counts with ten items scoring the presence and severity of abnormal movements in several parts of the body from 0 (absent) to 4 (severe). The scale includes specific instructions for the rater, its psychometric properties are adequate and it fulfills the criteria for a recommended scale by the MDS [31]. The AIMS has been widely used to assess the effects of interventions, although there is no firm evidence about its ability to detect changes in dyskinesias across the different stages of PD and it is not superior to other dyskinesia scales in responsiveness [31, 32].

The RDRS is a PD specifically designed scale that assesses the interference due to dyskinesias in three standardized motor tasks: walking, drinking from a cup and dressing [33]. It meets the criteria for a recommended scale by the MDS, as it has been applied extensively in PD patients in clinical trials and practice and has undergone some clinimetric testing [31]. However, its ability to detect response to treatment is limited [34].

The UDysRS is the most recent scale specifically designed to assess dyskinesias in PD patients, but it has been already used in numerous clinical trials and counts with excellent clinimetric properties and a teaching program and detailed instructions for standardized administration [35]. It has two primary sections: Historical, with Part 1 (On-Dyskinesia) and Part 2 (Off-Dystonia), whose items are answered by interview and self-report; and Objective, with Part 3 (Impairment) and Part 4 (Disability), answered by the clinician based on observation of the patient performing four tasks. Among the existing dyskinesia scales, the UDysRS is superior for detecting treatment effects and sets a clear standard for comparison for new dyskinesia agents, with an effect size of around 0.14, although more research is needed to confirm its properties [32]. It has been classified as "recommended" by the MDS [36].

Nonmotor symptoms scales

The NMSS is the first instrument developed to assess a wide range of nonmotor symptoms (NMSs) in PD [37]. It is composed of nine domains and 30 items: cardiovascular (two items); sleep/fatigue (four items); mood/apathy (six items); perceptual problems/hallucinations (three items); attention/memory (three items); gastrointestinal tract (three items); urinary (three items); sexual function (two items); and miscellaneous (four items). The score for each item is the result of the multiplication of severity (from 0 to 3) and frequency scores (from 1 to 4), with higher scores meaning more severity and frequency (burden) of NMSs. The NMSS psychometric properties are satisfactory, and it has been translated into and validated in several languages and used in several clinical trials [38]. Regarding responsiveness, the SEM has been deemed acceptable (13.91 for total score and 1.71–4.73 for domains), with effect size values confirming its ability to detect changes [38–40].

The SCOPA-Cog is a ten-item scale for assessing cognitive deficits in PD through tasks related to visual and verbal memory, delayed recall, executive and visuospatial functions, and attention [41]. The maximum score, indicative of good cognitive status, is 43. Its psychometric properties have been tested using both CTT and IRT approaches [42, 43] and it has been translated into several languages. The SEM and smallest real difference for SCOPA-Cog have been estimated, and its sensitivity to change has been tested in a cognitive training program, but information on the SCOPA-Cog responsiveness is still limited [42, 44].

The SCOPA-PC is a scale aimed at assessing psychotic and compulsive disorders in PD, developed from the modified Parkinson Psychosis Rating Scale (mPPRS) [45, 46]. It is composed of seven items, answered in a scale from 0 (absent) to 3 (severe), with a total score of 21 indicative of greater psychiatric complications. The SCOPA-PC has adequate psychometric properties, but its responsiveness needs additional testing.

Patient-reported outcome measures

In recent years, there have been significant efforts toward the development, validation and use of PRO measures in PD. As explained above, PROs measure a wide array of areas: symptoms, functional status, psychological well-being, quality of life, satisfaction with care, and others. Some of them (quality of life, psychological well-being and some NMSs such as sleeping disorders and pain) have been recognized as the most relevant for PD patients and therefore must be taken into account in clinical research and practice. The PRO measures used in PD can be classified into two main groups: generic and specific scales. For years, generic instruments have been used in PD, sometimes without a formal validation in this population. Only in the last decade have researchers assessed the validity of these measures or developed specific PROs for PD evaluation. The most-used PD-specific PRO measures, which are the scope of this section, are addressed to assess perceived motor manifestations, disability, NMSs and health-related quality of life (HRQoL) measures.

Motor manifestations and disability scales

Several scales can be considered in this section: the Motor Aspects of Experiences of Daily Living (M-EDL) section of the MDS-UPDRS, the Wearing-Off Questionnaires (WOQ), the Freezing of Gait Questionnaire (FOGQ), and the Parkinson Disease Dyskinesia Scale (PDYS-26).

The M-EDL section of the MDS-UPDRS is composed of 13 items, each ranging from 0 (normal) to 4 (severe), and assesses difficulties related to speech, saliva and drooling, chewing and swallowing, eating tasks, dressing, hygiene, handwriting, hobbies and other activities, turning in bed, tremor, getting out of bed, car seat or deep chair, walking and balance, and freezing of gait [16]. The M-EDL section is a valid, reliable and useful self-reported measure for PD-related disability, with better sensitivity than other disability instruments [47]. Its longitudinal metric properties have been tested, with good sensitivity to change that surpasses the responsiveness of the UPDRS-II [19].

The WOQ is a screening tool to identify patients with wearing off with several versions composed of 32 (WOQ-32), 19 (WOQ-19, Patient Card Questionnaire or Quick Questionnaire), ten (Q10) and nine (WOQ-9) items [48–52]. The WOQ-32 is a suggested screening tool for wearing off, while the WOQ-19 and WOQ-9 are recommended by the MDS [53]. These two latter questionnaires have been used in several studies as screening instruments, and the WOQ-9 was sensitive to dopaminergic treatment, but the information about their responsiveness is still scarce.

The FOGQ is a scale composed of six items, scored from 0 (normal) to 4 (inability to walk), for assessing the difficulties in walking, freezing-related circumstances and duration of blocks while walking [54]. There have been several validation studies and translation into several languages, and a revised version is available [55]. Both versions have been used as outcome measures in trials, but their sensitivity to change needs more research.

The PDYS-26 is a scale aimed at quantifying the impact of dyskinesias on daily living activities, designed following the Rasch analysis methodology and tested using both IRT and CTT approaches [56]. Items are scored from 0 (not at all) to 4 (activity impossible). Its clinimetric properties are excellent, the scale is easy to use, with clear and concise instructions to patients, and it deserves the status of a recommended scale by the MDS [36]. However, PDYS-26 responsiveness is not satisfactory [34].

NMS scales

The development and use of NMS scales have undergone considerable growth as a result of the increased awareness of the NMS consequences in PD patients. Nonmotor symptoms include neuropsychiatric and cognitive, sleep-related, autonomic, gastrointestinal, fatigue, sexual and sensory disturbances, contributing to disability and impacting on a patient's social role, daily activities and HRQoL. In the last decade, several initiatives such as those carried out by the SCOPA Group, Non-Motor Symptoms Group and MDS-UPDRS Task Force have developed specific NMS measures for application in clinical practice and research.

Comprehensive questionnaires

The NMS Questionnaire (NMSQuest) is the first comprehensive, screening tool of NMSs in PD [57]. It is composed of 30 items, grouped into ten domains, with yes/no score options. The NMSQuest is useful for highlighting symptoms needing attention in clinical practice and for epidemiological studies [58], but its usefulness as an evaluative instrument has not been tested.

The Non-Motor Aspects of Experiences of Daily Living (nM-EDL) section of the MDS-UPDRS contains six rater-based items (cognitive impairment, hallucinations, anxiety, depression, apathy and dopamine dysregulation syndrome) and seven self-assessed items (sleep problems, daytime sleepiness, pain, urinary problems, constipation, light-headedness and fatigue) [16]. The nM-EDL is highly correlated with the NMSS [59] and is able to detect improvements in NMSs following deep-brain stimulation, particularly those that are self-assessed (constipation, light-headedness and fatigue), and changes over time [19, 60].

Neuropsychiatric symptom scales

The MDS Task Force has published reviews about the scales for neuropsychiatric disorders, including depression, anxiety, anhedonia, apathy and psychotic manifestations, used in studies on PD populations (available at http://www.movementdisorders.org/MDS/Resources/Publications-Reviews/Task-Force-Papers.htm).

Two other PD-specific instruments have appeared recently: the Questionnaire for Impulsive–Compulsive Disorders in Parkinson's Disease – Rating Scale (QUIP-RS) [61] and the Scale for Evaluation of Neuropsychiatric Disorders in Parkinson's Disease (SEND-PD) [62].

The QUIP has been available since 2012 [63], but as a screening instrument, it is not applicable for evaluative purposes. The QUIP-RS is aimed at assessing the severity of impulse control behaviors (compulsive gambling, buying, eating and sexual behavior) and related disorders (medication use, punding and hobbyism) for purposes of diagnosis and monitoring over time [61]. It consists of four core questions about thoughts, urges/desires, and difficulty controlling and engaging in behaviors for each of the seven ICDs, with responses scored in a Likert-type scale from 0 (never) to 4 (very often). It is a promising scale, due to its good psychometric properties, and it has been incorporated into ongoing clinical trials of symptomatic therapies. There is still limited information about its sensitivity to change.

The SEND-PD is an interview-based scale for assessment of neuropsychiatric symptoms that consists of 12 items, each one scoring for severity from 0 (no) to 4 (very severe) [62]. Items are grouped into three subscales: psychotic symptoms, mood/apathy, and impulse control disorders (ICDs). The SEND-PD showed good psychometric properties and potential responsiveness, with a precision (SEM) ranging from 0.71 (ICD subscales) to 1.43 (mood/apathy). Additional analyses are needed to confirm these results and confirm the validation data of the scale.

Sleep disorder scales

Two main PD-specific rating scales for sleep disorders are available: the Parkinson's Disease Sleep Scale (PDSS) [64] and SCOPA-Sleep [65].

The PDSS contains 14 items measuring nocturnal sleep problems and one item addressed to excessive daytime sleepiness. Each item is rated on a visual analog scale from 0 (severe or always present) to 10 (never or not present). A revised version has recently been published, the PDSS-2, focused only on nocturnal sleep problems and with items scored on a Likert-type scale from 0 (never) to 4 (very frequent) [66]. The PDSS has good clinimetric properties and meets the criteria for a recommended scale for screening of sleep disorders [67]. It is also a precise and responsive scale. Regarding the responsiveness of the PDSS-2, there are contradictory results [68, 69].

The SCOPA-Sleep is composed by two parts: nocturnal sleep (NS), with five items, and daytime sleepiness (DS), with six items. Both parts are scored on a scale from 0 (not at all) to 3 (very much) [65]. The SCOPA-Sleep has been validated in several cultural settings with good results and has been listed as recommended by the MDS [67]. The SEM was calculated for both subscales, resulting in 1.4 for the NS and 1.5 for the DS subscale, and it seems to be responsive to treatment, although there is no further information about its responsiveness [70, 71].

Gastrointestinal and autonomic scales

Only two specific scales exist for gastrointestinal dysautonomic symptoms in PD: the Sialorrhea Clinical Scale for PD (SCS-PD) [72] and the Swallowing Disturbance Questionnaire (SDQ) [73]. However, neither meets the criteria for a recommended scale by the MDS and there is no information about their responsiveness [74].

The only specific scale for global assessment of dysautonomia in PD is the SCOPA-Autonomic (SCOPA-AUT) [75]. It is composed of 25 items assessing six dimensions: gastrointestinal, urinary, cardiovascular, thermoregulatory, pupillomotor and sexual dysfunction. Items are scored from 0 (never) to 3 (often), with a maximum possible score of 69. There are several validation studies of the SCOPA-AUT, including CTT and Rasch analysis approaches [76, 77], and the MDS has designed it as a recommended scale, although with some limitations [74]. The SEM has been determined and there is differential item functioning by sex in item 2 (sialorrhea) and by age in item 13 (nocturia) [76, 77]. The scale has been used in several clinical studies in parkinsonian patients but has not been tested for responsiveness.

Fatigue

The Parkinson Fatigue Scale (PFS-16) is the first PD-specific measure of fatigue [78], although other generic instruments, such as the Fatigue Severity Scale (FSS) and the Multidimensional Fatigue Inventory (MFI), have been validated in PD patients with good results [79]. The PFS-16 contains 16 items focused on physical fatigue and its impact on daily living activities. The MDS has classified it as a recommended instrument for fatigue screening and severity ratings [79]. The PFS-16 has demonstrated satisfactory responsiveness related to the effects of treatment [80].

HRQoL scales

The use of HRQoL measures, which rate the subjective perception of the impact of the disease and the treatment, is growing incessantly in clinical trials. Some generic HRQoL scales have been successfully tested and used in PD and therefore they are recommended by the MDS [112]: the Nottingham Health Profile (NHP), the EQ-5D, the 36-Item Short-Form Health Survey (SF-36) and the Sickness Impact Profile (SIP).

However, PD-specific instruments are more adequate and sensitive for the assessment of treatment effects. Several have been developed and validated in recent years and the following five are recommended by the MDS Task Force: Parkinson's Disease Questionnaire, 39- and eight-item versions (PDQ-39 and PDQ-8), Parkinson's Disease Quality of Life Questionnaire (PDQL), Parkinson's Impact Scale (PIMS) and SCOPA-Psychosocial Questionnaire (SCOPA-PS) [81].

The SIP contains 136 items grouped into 12 categories and two dimensions (physical and psychosocial) [82]. The SIP covers areas of interest for PD patients and has good psychometric properties in this population. Responsiveness for PD treatment has been reported, although there is no information about its MID.

The NHP is a scale that contains 38 items addressed to measure emotional reactions, energy, pain, physical mobility, sleep and social isolation [83]. It has population normative values and is sensitive to changes due to PD treatment.

The EQ-5D is a short and useful scale widely used in clinical and economic evaluation and for comparing different health conditions and populations [84]. It provides a descriptive profile and a single index value for health status and is responsive to medical and surgical interventions in PD.

The SF-36 is a scale comprising 36 items grouped into eight domains: physical function, physical role functioning, bodily pain, general health, vitality, social role functioning, emotional role functioning and mental health [85]. Although it has good psychometric properties in PD, when used to measure change due to treatment it was less sensitive than specific instruments.

The PDQ-39 is the most-used HRQoL instrument in PD clinical trials, in research and in practice [81, 86, 87]. It is formed by 39 items grouped into eight domains: mobility, activities of daily living, emotional well-being, stigma, social support, cognitions, communication and bodily discomfort. Items are scored from 0 (never) to 4 (always) and a transformed total score ranging from 0 to 100 and a summary index can be obtained. The PDQ-39 has shown satisfactory metric properties and is sensitive to changes due to medical or surgical interventions [88, 89]. The ES, the MID and other interpretability parameters have been also calculated, varying across dimensions and between studies [90, 91].

The PDQ-8 is a shorter version of the PDQ-39, with one item from each of the PDQ-39 domains [92]. It has been widely used and tested in different PD settings, with good psychometric properties. It is sensitive to changes in health status and has several responsiveness indexes that can be calculated.

The PDQL has 37 items classified into four domains: parkinsonian symptoms, systemic symptoms, social function and emotional function [93]. Items are scored on a Likert-type scale from 1 (all the time) to 5 (never), and a summary index can be extracted from the sum of items. Data about its psychometric properties and responsiveness are satisfactory, revealing that PDQL scores showed significant changes following treatment [29, 88].

The PIMS contains ten items addressed to rate physical, psychological and social aspects of the disease and sexuality [94]. Although it has good psychometric properties and is moderately sensitive to changes, the scale has scarcely been used beyond its original developers.

The SCOPA-PS is a questionnaire developed to quantify the psychosocial impact of the disease, and is composed of 11 items [95]. It has good psychometric properties and has been tested in different cultural settings. The SCOPA-PS is sensitive to changes, and several responsiveness parameters have been calculated [96].

Conclusions

In recent years, there have been important efforts toward the development of PD-specific outcome measures, the guidelines that must follow their development, and the procedures for inclusion and interpretation of these measures in clinical trials. Rating scales provide data with an inferential component from the rater or patient, as subjectivity influences the score assignment. Nonetheless, valid scales provide information that is indispensable for, among other applications, epidemiological studies, management of patients in daily practice, outcomes analysis in research and decision making in health policy.

Parkinson's disease is a complex disease, with a multitude of motor and nonmotor symptoms and complications that impact on patients' functioning and psychosocial aspects. Another feature of PD is its variability, both intra- and inter-subject. The patient condition evolves over time, not only increasing the severity of their disability but also modifying the symptoms that are present at different points in time. On the other hand, some subtypes are widely recognized and patients belonging to one of these subtypes have manifestations, complications and a disease course over time that differs from the other groups.

This chapter has focused on valid, commonly used and pragmatic scales (Table 22.2), with emphasis on their

Table 22.2 Comprehensive assessments in Parkinson's disease

Global severity/disability and multidomain

Hoehn and Yahr staging (HY) [7]

Clinical Impression of Severity Index – Parkinson's Disease (CISI-PD) [8]

Unified Parkinson's Disease Rating Scale (UPDRS) [10]

Movement Disorders sponsored version of the UPDRS (MDS-UPDRS) [15]

Scales for Outcomes in PD-Motor (SPES-SCOPA, SCOPA-Motor) [25]

Nonmotor symptoms

Non-Motor Symptoms Scale (NMSS) [37]

Non-Motor Symptoms Questionnaire (NMSQuest) [57]

Parkinson's Disease Sleep Scale [64]

Parkinson's Disease Sleep Scale – version 2 [66]

Scales for Outcomes in PD-Sleep (SCOPA-Sleep) [65]

Scales for Outcomes in PD-Autonomic (SCOPA-Autonomic) [75]

Scale for Evaluation of Neuropsychiatric Disorders in PD (SEND-PD) [62]

Health-related quality of life

Parkinson's Disease Questionnaire – 39 items (PDQ-39) [86, 87]

Parkinson's Disease Questionnaire – eight items (PDQ-8) [92]

Parkinson's Disease Quality of Life Questionnaire (PDQL) [93]

Parkinson's Impact Scale (PIMS) [94]

SCOPA-Psychosocial questionnaire (SCOPA-PS) [95]

most relevant characteristics and, specifically, their ability for estimating changes as effects of interventions or passage of time. Additional information can be obtained from the reviews carried out by the MDS Task Force – Committee on Rating Scales Development (available at http://www.movementdisorders.org/MDS/About/Committees--Other-Groups/MDS-Committees/Committee-on-Rating-Scales-Development.htm).

References

1. Acquadro C, Berzon R, Dubois D, et al. Incorporating the patient's perspective into drug development and communication: an ad hoc task force report of the Patient-Reported Outcomes (PRO) Harmonization Group meeting at the Food and Drug Administration, February 16, 2001. *Value Health* 2003; **6**: 522–31.

2. Scientific Advisory Committee of the Medical Outcomes Trust. Assessing health status and quality-of-life instruments: attributes and review criteria. *Qual Life Res* 2002; **11**: 193–205.

3. Mokkink LB, Terwee CB, Patrick DL, et al. The COSMIN checklist for assessing the methodological quality of studies on measurement properties of health status measurement instruments: an international Delphi study. *Qual Life Res* 2010; **19**: 539–49.

4. Terwee CB, Dekker FW, Wiersinga WM, Prummel MF, Bossuyt PMM. On assessing responsiveness of health-related quality of life instruments: guidelines for instrument evaluation. *Qual Life Res* 2003; **12**: 349–62.

5. Wyrwich KW, Metz SM, Kroenke K, et al. Triangulating patient and clinician perspectives on clinically important differences in health-related quality of life among patients with heart disease. *Health Serv Res* 2007; **42**: 2257–74.

6. Hoehn MM, Yahr MD. Parkinsonism: onset, progression and mortality. *Neurology* 1967; **17**: 427–42.

7. Goetz CG, Poewe W, Rascol O, et al. Movement Disorder Society Task Force report on the Hoehn and Yahr staging scale: status and recommendations. *Mov Disord* 2004; **19**: 1020–8.

8. Martínez-Martín P, Forjaz MJ, Cubo E, Frades B, de Pedro Cuesta J. Global versus factor-related impression of severity in Parkinson's disease: a new clinimetric index (CISI-PD). *Mov Disord* 2006; **21**: 208–14.

9. Martínez Martín P, Rodríguez-Blázquez C, Forjaz MJ, de Pedro J. The Clinical Impression of Severity Index for Parkinson's Disease: international validation study. *Mov Disord* 2009; **24**: 211–17.

10. Fahn S, Elton R, UPDRS Program Members. Unified Parkinson's Disease Rating Scale. In: Fahn S, Marsden C, Goldstein M, Calne D, eds. *Recent Developments in Parkinson's Disease*. Florham Park, NJ: Macmillan Healthcare Information; 1987; 153–63.

11. Movement Disorder Society Task Force on Rating Scales for Parkinson's Disease. The Unified Parkinson's Disease Rating Scale (UPDRS): status and recommendations. *Mov Disord* 2003; **18**: 738–50.

12. Steffen T, Seney M. Test-retest reliability and minimal detectable change on balance and ambulation tests, the 36-item Short-Form Health Survey, and the unified Parkinson disease rating scale in people with parkinsonism. *Phys Ther* 2008; **88**: 733–46.

13. Oertel WH, Wolters E, Sampaio C, et al. Pergolide versus levodopa monotherapy in early Parkinson's disease patients: the PELMOPET study. *Mov Disord* 2006; **21**: 343–53.

14. Hauser RA, Auinger P, Parkinson Study Group. Determination of minimal clinically important change in early and advanced Parkinson's disease. *Mov Disord* 2011; **26**: 813–8.

15. Goetz CG, Fahn S, Martinez-Martin P, et al. Movement Disorder Society-sponsored revision of the Unified Parkinson's Disease Rating Scale (MDS-UPDRS): process, format, and clinimetric testing plan. *Mov Disord* 2007; **22**: 41–7.

16. Goetz CG, Tilley BC, Shaftman SR, *et al.* Movement Disorder Society-sponsored revision of the Unified Parkinson's Disease Rating Scale (MDS-UPDRS): scale presentation and clinimetric testing results. *Mov Disord* 2008; **23**: 2129–70.

17. Goetz CG, Stebbins GT, LaPelle N, Huang J, Tilley BC. MDS-UPDRS non-English translation program. *Mov Disord* 2012; **27** (Suppl. 1): S96.

18. Poewe W, Hauser R, Lang AE. Rasagiline 1 mg/day provides benefits in the progression of nonmotor symptoms in patients with early Parkinson's disease: Assessment with the revised MDS-UPDRS. *Mov Disord* 2009; **24** (Suppl. 1): S272.

19. Lang AE, Eberly S, Goetz CG, *et al.* Movement Disorder Society Unified Parkinson Disease Rating Scale experiences in daily living: longitudinal changes and correlation with other assessments. *Mov Disord* 2013; **28**: 1980–6.

20. Goetz CG, Stebbins GT, Simkus V. Severity ranges on the MDS-UPDRS motor examination: comparison to CGI-severity scores. *Mov Disord* 2009; **24** (Suppl. 1): S434.

21. Stebbins GT, Goetz CG, Simkus V. Minimal clinically important change and the MDS-UPDRS motor examination. *Mov Disord* 2009; **24** (Suppl. 1): S436.

22. Merello M, Gerschcovich ER, Ballesteros D, Cerquetti D. Correlation between the Movement Disorders Society Unified Parkinson's Disease Rating Scale (MDS-UPDRS) and the Unified Parkinson's Disease Rating Scale (UPDRS) during l-dopa acute challenge. *Parkinsonism Relat Disord* 2011; **17**: 705–7.

23. Goetz CG, Stebbins GT, Tilley BC. Calibration of Unified Parkinson's Disease Rating Scale scores to Movement Disorder Society – Unified Parkinson's Disease rating scale scores. *Mov Disord* 2012; **27**: 1239–42.

24. Verbaan D, van Rooden SM, Benit CP, *et al.* SPES/SCOPA and MDS-UPDRS: formulas for converting scores of two motor scales in Parkinson's disease. *Parkinsonism Relat Disord* 2011; **17**: 632–4.

25. Marinus J, Visser M, Stiggelbout AM, *et al.* A short scale for the assessment of motor impairments and disabilities in Parkinson's disease: the SPES/SCOPA. *J Neurol Neurosurg Psychiatry* 2004; **75**: 388–95.

26. Martínez-Martín P, Benito-León J, Burguera JA, *et al.* The SCOPA-Motor Scale for assessment of Parkinson's disease is a consistent and valid measure. *J Clin Epidemiol* 2005; **58**: 674–9.

27. Schwab R, England A. *Third Symposium for Parkinson's Disease*. Edinburgh, UK: Livingstone; 1969; 152–7.

28. Martinez-Martin P, Prieto L, Forjaz MJ. Longitudinal metric properties of disability rating scales for Parkinson's disease. *Value Health* 2006; **9**: 386–93.

29. Schrag A, Spottke A, Quinn NP, Dodel R. Comparative responsiveness of Parkinson's disease scales to change over time. *Mov Disord* 2009; **24**: 813–18.

30. Guy W. Abnormal involuntary movement scale. In: *ECDEU Assessment Manual for Psychopharmacology*. Washington, DC: US Government Printing Office; 1976; 534–7.

31. Colosimo C, Martínez-Martín P, Fabbrini G, *et al.* Task force report on scales to assess dyskinesia in Parkinson's disease: critique and recommendations. *Mov Disord* 2010; **25**: 1131–42.

32. Goetz CG, Stebbins GT, Chung KA, *et al.* Which dyskinesia scale best detects treatment response? *Mov Disord* 2013; **28**: 341–6.

33. Goetz CG, Stebbins GT, Shale HM, *et al.* Utility of an objective dyskinesia rating scale for Parkinson's disease: inter- and intrarater reliability assessment. *Mov Disord* 1994; **9**: 390–4.

34. Goetz CG, Stebbins GT, Chung KA, *et al.* Which dyskinesia scale best detects treatment response? *Mov Disord* 2013; **28**: 341–6.

35. Goetz CG, Nutt JG, Stebbins GT. The Unified Dyskinesia Rating Scale: presentation and clinimetric profile. *Mov Disord* 2008; **23**: 2398–403.

36. Colosimo C. Dyskinesia rating scales in Parkinson's disease. In: Sampaio C, Goetz CG, Schrag A, eds. *Rating Scales in Parkinson's Disease*. New York: Oxford University Press; 2012; 84–98.

37. Chaudhuri KR, Martinez-Martin P, Brown RG, *et al.* The metric properties of a novel non-motor symptoms scale for Parkinson's disease: results from an international pilot study. *Mov Disord* 2007; **22**: 1901–11.

38. Martinez-Martin P, Rodriguez-Blazquez C, Abe K, *et al.* International study on the psychometric attributes of the non-motor symptoms scale in Parkinson disease. *Neurology* 2009; **73**: 1584–91.

39. Reddy P, Martinez-Martin P, Rizos A, *et al.* Intrajejunal levodopa versus conventional therapy in Parkinson disease: motor and nonmotor effects. *Clin Neuropharmacol* 2012; **35**: 205–7.

40. Chaudhuri KR, Martinez-Martin P, Antonini A, *et al.* Rotigotine and specific non-motor symptoms of Parkinson's disease: post hoc analysis of RECOVER. *Parkinsonism Relat Disord* 2013; **19**: 660–5.

41. Marinus J, Visser M, Verwey NA, *et al.* Assessment of cognition in Parkinson's disease. *Neurology* 2003; **61**: 1222–8.

42. Carod-Artal FJ, Martínez-Martín P, Kummer W, Ribeiro LdaS. Psychometric attributes of the SCOPA-COG Brazilian version. *Mov Disord* 2008; **23**: 81–7.

43. Forjaz MJ, Frades-Payo B, Rodriguez-Blazquez C, Ayala A, Martinez-Martin P. Should the SCOPA-COG be modified? A Rasch analysis perspective. *Eur J Neurol* 2010; **17**: 202–7.

44. Reuter I, Mehnert S, Sammer G, Oechsner M, Engelhardt M. Efficacy of a multimodal cognitive

rehabilitation including psychomotor and endurance training in Parkinson's disease. *J Aging Res* 2012; **2012**: 235765.

45. Visser M, Verbaan D, van Rooden SM, *et al.* Assessment of psychiatric complications in Parkinson's disease: the SCOPA-PC. *Mov Disord* 2007; **22**: 2221–8.

46. Friedberg G, Zoldan J, Weizman A, Melamed E. Parkinson Psychosis Rating Scale: a practical instrument for grading psychosis in Parkinson's disease. *Clin Neuropharmacol* 1998; **21**: 280–4.

47. Rodriguez-Blazquez C, Rojo-Abuin JM, Alvarez-Sanchez M, *et al.* The MDS-UPDRS Part II (motor experiences of daily living) resulted useful for assessment of disability in Parkinson's disease. *Parkinsonism Relat Disord* 2013; **19**: 889–93.

48. Stacy M, Bowron A, Guttman M, *et al.* Identification of motor and nonmotor wearing-off in Parkinson's disease: Comparison of a patient questionnaire versus a clinician assessment. *Mov Disord* 2005; **20**: 726–33.

49. Stacy M, Hauser R. Development of a Patient Questionnaire to facilitate recognition of motor and non-motor wearing-off in Parkinson's disease. *J Neural Transm* 2007; **114**: 211–17.

50. Stacy MA, Murphy JM, Greeley DR, *et al.* The sensitivity and specificity of the 9-item Wearing-off Questionnaire. *Parkinsonism Relat Disord* 2008; **14**: 205–12.

51. Martinez-Martin P, Tolosa E, Hernandez B, Badia X, ValidQUICK Study Group. Validation of the "QUICK" questionnaire – a tool for diagnosis of "wearing-off" in patients with Parkinson's disease. *Mov Disord* 2008; **23**: 830–6.

52. Martinez-Martin P, Hernandez B. The Q10 questionnaire for detection of wearing-off phenomena in Parkinson's disease. *Parkinsonism Relat Disord* 2012; **18**: 382–5.

53. Antonini A, Martinez-Martin P, Chaudhuri RK, *et al.* Wearing-off scales in Parkinson's disease: Critique and recommendations. *Mov Disord* 2011; **26**: 2169–75.

54. Giladi N, Shabtai H, Simon ES, *et al.* Construction of freezing of gait questionnaire for patients with Parkinsonism. *Parkinsonism Relat Disord* 2000; **6**: 165–70.

55. Nieuwboer A, Rochester L, Herman T, *et al.* Reliability of the new freezing of gait questionnaire: agreement between patients with Parkinson's disease and their carers. *Gait Posture.* 2009; **30**: 459–63.

56. Katzenschlager R, Schrag A, Evans A, *et al.* Quantifying the impact of dyskinesias in PD: the PDYS-26: a patient-based outcome measure. *Neurology* 2007; **69**: 555–63.

57. Chaudhuri KR, Martinez-Martin P, Schapira AHV, *et al.* International multicenter pilot study of the first comprehensive self-completed nonmotor symptoms questionnaire for Parkinson's disease: the NMSQuest study. *Mov Disord* 2006; **21**: 916–23.

58. Martinez-Martin P, Schapira AHV, Stocchi F, *et al.* Prevalence of nonmotor symptoms in Parkinson's disease in an international setting; study using nonmotor symptoms questionnaire in 545 patients. *Mov Disord* 2007; **22**: 1623–9.

59. Martinez-Martin P, Chaudhuri KR, Rojo-Abuin JM, *et al.* Assessing the non-motor symptoms of Parkinson's disease: MDS-UPDRS and NMS Scale. *Eur J Neurol* 2013; **22**: 37–43.

60. Chou KL, Taylor JL, Patil PG. The MDS-UPDRS tracks motor and non-motor improvement due to subthalamic nucleus deep brain stimulation in Parkinson disease. *Parkinsonism Relat Disord* 2013; **19**: 966–9.

61. Weintraub D, Mamikonyan E, Papay K, *et al.* Questionnaire for Impulsive-Compulsive Disorders in Parkinson's Disease – Rating Scale. *Mov Disord* 2012; **27**: 242–7.

62. Martinez-Martin P, Frades-Payo B, Agüera-Ortiz L, Ayuga-Martinez A. A short scale for evaluation of neuropsychiatric disorders in Parkinson's disease: first psychometric approach. *J Neurol* 2012; **259**: 2299–308.

63. Weintraub D, Stewart S, Shea JA, *et al.* Validation of the Questionnaire for Impulsive-Compulsive Behaviors in Parkinson's Disease (QUIP). *Mov Disord* 2009; **24**: 1461–7.

64. Chaudhuri KR, Pal S, DiMarco A, *et al.* The Parkinson's disease sleep scale: a new instrument for assessing sleep and nocturnal disability in Parkinson's disease. *J Neurol Neurosurg Psychiatry* 2002; **73**: 629–35.

65. Marinus J, Visser M, van Hilten JJ, Lammers GJ, Stiggelbout AM. Assessment of sleep and sleepiness in Parkinson disease. *Sleep.* 2003; **26**: 1049–54.

66. Trenkwalder C, Kohnen R, Högl B, *et al.* Parkinson's disease sleep scale – validation of the revised version PDSS-2. *Mov Disord* 2011; **26**: 644–52.

67. Högl B, Arnulf I, Comella C, *et al.* Scales to assess sleep impairment in Parkinson's disease: critique and recommendations. *Mov Disord* 2010; **25**: 2704–16.

68. Zibetti M, Rizzone M, Merola A, *et al.* Sleep improvement with levodopa/carbidopa intestinal gel infusion in Parkinson disease. *Acta Neurol Scand* 2013; **127**: e28–32.

69. Takanashi M, Shimo Y, Hatano T, Oyama G, Hattori N. Efficacy and safety of a once-daily extended-release formulation of pramipexole switched from an immediate-release formulation in patients with advanced Parkinson's disease: results from an open-label study. *Drug Res.* 2013; **63**: 639–43.

70. Martinez-Martin P, Visser M, Rodriguez-Blazquez C, *et al.* SCOPA-sleep and PDSS: two scales for assessment of sleep disorder in Parkinson's disease. *Mov Disord* 2008; **23**: 1681–8.

71. Chahine LM, Daley J, Horn S, *et al.* Association between dopaminergic medications and nocturnal

71. sleep in early-stage Parkinson's disease. *Parkinsonism Relat Disord* 2013; **19**: 859–63.

72. Perez Lloret S, Pirán Arce G, Rossi M, et al. Validation of a new scale for the evaluation of sialorrhea in patients with Parkinson's disease. *Mov Disord* 2007; **22**: 107–11.

73. Manor Y, Giladi N, Cohen A, Fliss DM, Cohen JT. Validation of a swallowing disturbance questionnaire for detecting dysphagia in patients with Parkinson's disease. *Mov Disord* 2007; **22**: 1917–21.

74. Evatt ML, Chaudhuri KR, Chou KL, et al. Dysautonomia rating scales in Parkinson's disease: sialorrhea, dysphagia, and constipation – critique and recommendations by movement disorders task force on rating scales for Parkinson's disease. *Mov Disord* 2009; **24**: 635–46.

75. Visser M, Marinus J, Stiggelbout AM, van Hilten JJ. Assessment of autonomic dysfunction in Parkinson's disease: the SCOPA-AUT. *Mov Disord* 2004; **19**: 1306–12.

76. Rodriguez-Blazquez C, Forjaz MJ, Frades-Payo B, de Pedro-Cuesta J, Martinez-Martin P. Independent validation of the scales for outcomes in Parkinson's disease-autonomic (SCOPA-AUT). *Eur J Neurol* 2010; **17**: 194–201.

77. Forjaz MJ, Ayala A, Rodriguez-Blazquez C, Frades-Payo B, Martinez-Martin P. Assessing autonomic symptoms of Parkinson's disease with the SCOPA-AUT: a new perspective from Rasch analysis. *Eur J Neurol* 2010; **17**: 273–9.

78. Brown RG, Dittner A, Findley L, Wessely SC. The Parkinson fatigue scale. *Parkinsonism Relat Disord* 2005; **11**: 49–55.

79. Friedman JH, Alves G, Hagell P, et al. Fatigue rating scales critique and recommendations by the Movement Disorders Society task force on rating scales for Parkinson's disease. *Mov Disord* 2010; **25**: 805–22.

80. Rascol O, Fitzer-Attas CJ, Hauser R, et al. A double-blind, delayed-start trial of rasagiline in Parkinson's disease (the ADAGIO study): prespecified and post-hoc analyses of the need for additional therapies, changes in UPDRS scores, and non-motor outcomes. *Lancet Neurol* 2011; **10**: 415–23.

81. Martinez-Martin P, Jeukens-Visser M, Lyons KE, et al. Health-related quality-of-life scales in Parkinson's disease: critique and recommendations. *Mov Disord* 2011; **26**: 2371–80.

82. Bergner M, Bobbitt RA, Carter WB, Gilson BS. The Sickness Impact Profile: development and final revision of a health status measure. *Med Care* 1981; **19**: 787–805.

83. Hunt SM, McEwen J, McKenna SP. Measuring health status: a new tool for clinicians and epidemiologists. *J R Coll Gen Pract* 1985; **35**: 185–8.

84. EuroQol Group. EuroQol – a new facility for the measurement of health-related quality of life. *Health Policy* 1990; **16**: 199–208.

85. Ware JE Jr, Sherbourne CD. The MOS 36-item Short-Form Health Survey (SF-36). I. Conceptual framework and item selection. *Med Care* 1992; **30**: 473–83.

86. Peto V, Jenkinson C, Fitzpatrick R, Greenhall R. The development and validation of a short measure of functioning and well being for individuals with Parkinson's disease. *Qual Life Res*. 1995; **4**: 241–8.

87. Jenkinson C, Fitzpatrick R, Peto V, Greenhall R, Hyman N. The Parkinson's Disease Questionnaire (PDQ-39): development and validation of a Parkinson's disease summary index score. *Age Ageing* 1997; **26**: 353–7.

88. Martinez-Martin P, Deuschl G. Effect of medical and surgical interventions on health-related quality of life in Parkinson's disease. *Mov Disord* 2007; **22**: 757–65.

89. Martinez-Martin P, Kurtis MM. Health-related quality of life as an outcome variable in Parkinson's disease. *Ther Adv Neurol Disord* 2012; **5**: 105–17.

90. Peto V, Jenkinson C, Fitzpatrick R. Determining minimally important differences for the PDQ-39 Parkinson's Disease Questionnaire. *Age Ageing* 2001; **30**: 299–302.

91. Fitzpatrick R, Norquist JM, Jenkinson C. Distribution-based criteria for change in health-related quality of life in Parkinson's disease. *J Clin Epidemiol* 2004; **57**: 40–4.

92. Jenkinson C, Fitzpatrick R, Peto V, Greenhall R, Hyman N. The PDQ-8: development and validation of a short-form Parkinson's Disease Questionnaire. *Psychol Health* 1997; **12**: 805–14.

93. De Boer AG, Wijker W, Speelman JD, de Haes JC. Quality of life in patients with Parkinson's disease: development of a questionnaire. *J Neurol Neurosurg Psychiatry* 1996; **61**: 70–4.

94. Calne S, Schulzer M, Mak E, et al. Validating a quality of life rating scale for idiopathic parkinsonism: Parkinson's Impact Scale (PIMS). *Parkinsonism Relat Disord* 1996; **2**: 55–61.

95. Marinus J, Visser M, Martínez-Martín P, van Hilten JJ, Stiggelbout AM. A short psychosocial questionnaire for patients with Parkinson's disease: the SCOPA-PS. *J Clin Epidemiol* 2003; **56**: 61–7.

96. Martínez-Martin P, Carod-Artal FJ, da Silveira Ribeiro L, et al. Longitudinal psychometric attributes, responsiveness, and importance of change: an approach using the SCOPA-Psychosocial questionnaire. *Mov Disord* 2008; **23**: 1516–23.

Chapter 23

Functional imaging markers as outcome measures in clinical trials for Parkinson's disease

Ryan R. Walsh

Introduction

There is currently no validated functional imaging marker (FIM) that is universally accepted for use as an outcome measure for clinical trials in Parkinson's disease (PD). This is reflected in a summary statement from a key review of the field by leading investigators: "...no imaging technique should be considered [a surrogate endpoint] in PD" [1]. This chapter will examine the reasons why this is the case by exploring what "functional imaging" means in PD, considering what an FIM in PD could include, identifying challenges in the use of FIMs in PD, and reviewing how this informs the development of FIMs useful as outcome measures in PD clinical trials.

Functional imaging in Parkinson's disease

The first step in discussing FIMs in PD must consider what "functional imaging" means. Functional imaging can be broadly defined as the ability to detect any change in the brain over time, with the corollary that such change reflects or correlates with underlying PD brain function/dysfunction. Current brain imaging techniques in PD permit dynamic investigation of a variety of physical measures ranging from micro- to macrostructural changes and from within-synapse to whole-brain-network changes. Furthermore, this range of dynamic measures may correlate with disease progression, symptom response, both or another pathophysiological or compensatory process in PD. All of these concepts are important in considering FIMs as outcome measures in PD, and a brief review of current PD functional imaging techniques (broadly defined) will serve as a platform for considering what functional imaging means in PD.

Imaging dopamine system integrity

Perhaps the most explored functional imaging area in PD is that addressing dopamine neurotransmission integrity. This reflects the importance of dopaminergic dysfunction underlying PD symptoms, symptom response to dopaminergic therapies and the classic nigrostriatal pathological features identified in PD [2]. These imaging techniques provide the ability to assess pre-, intra- and postsynaptic dopaminergic transmission [3, 4]. Presynaptic dopaminergic imaging relies primarily on positron emission tomography (PET)- and single-photon-emission computed tomography (SPECT)-based modalities: levodopa (L-DOPA) that has been radiolabeled (^{18}F-DOPA) is taken up and processed presynaptically; radiolabeled dihydrotetrabenazine binds vesicular monoamine transporter type 2 (VMAT2), important for presynaptic vesicle processing; and radiolabeled cocaine-like agents (tropanes) bind to the dopamine transporter, which is located presynaptically and is important in clearance of dopamine from the synaptic cleft [5]. Presynaptic radiotracers have been shown to have reduced uptake in the posterior more than the anterior striatum, correlate with nigrostriatal pathological features and correlate with bradykinesia (but not tremor) in PD [6]. Despite these clinical and pathological correlates with PD, changes in presynaptic cellular mechanisms (pathological or compensatory) may impact measured outcomes and there are inconsistent findings regarding clinical and pathological progression relative to radiotracer-based imaging [7]. Furthermore, subjects

Parkinson's Disease: Current and Future Therapeutics and Clinical Trials, ed. Gálvez-Jiménez et al. Published by Cambridge University Press. © Cambridge University Press 2016.

with clinical parkinsonism but without evidence of dopaminergic deficiency (known as SWEDDs [scans without evidence of dopamine deficits]) as measured by such imaging techniques represent another challenge in correlating dopaminergic imaging output with clinical syndrome [8].

Intra- and postsynaptic dopaminergic imaging techniques also rely primarily on PET and SPECT [9], including the ability to secondarily detect changes in synaptic cleft dopamine levels as indicated by alterations in D2-receptor availability for radiolabeled agents with low binding affinity (e.g. ^{11}C-raclopride). Changes in synaptic dopamine as measured by these techniques have been correlated with clinical and pathological features in PD, but this is complicated by the difficulty in accounting for the impact of receptor internalization and endogenous dopamine processing and by observations that certain clinical features do not correlate with these imaging measures [10]. Changes in postsynaptic dopamine-receptor levels have also been evaluated in PD, including the employment of several radiolabeled agents capable of binding D1, D2 and D3 receptors both within and outside the striatum. The interpretation of these data faces challenges similar to those mentioned for intrasynaptic imaging.

Structural imaging

Structural imaging in PD is dominated by MRI, which has permitted investigation of brain functional pathology from micro- to macroscales [11]. Changes in brain microstructure in PD as identified by MRI include abnormalities in substantia nigra morphology identified with high-field magnetic imaging [12], as well as changes in white and gray matter integrity identified by diffusion-tensor imaging. Whole-brain and brain subregion changes have been identified in PD with MRI volumetric studies, and changes in local brain chemistry in PD can be identified with magnetic resonance spectroscopy. Most structural imaging studies in PD to date have focused on correlating imaging findings with diagnosis or symptoms with varying results, with particular attention paid to discrimination of PD versus atypical parkinsonisms (e.g. multiple-system atrophy). Prospective structural imaging studies utilizing MRI in PD are lacking, as are consistent results from large, well-characterized cohorts in cross-sectional studies [13]. Nevertheless, the potential utility of structural MRI in PD was evident in a study incorporating multiple structural measures simultaneously, which reported high accuracy in distinguishing PD from controls when combining three different measurements [14].

Brain-network imaging

There has been a rapid recent expansion in reports of brain-network investigations in PD. The majority of these studies have employed PET-based evaluation of blood flow (H$_2$^{15}O-PET) and glucose metabolism (FDG-PET) to investigate brain activity and putative functional connectivity between brain regions, while the potential utility of functional MRI (fMRI) has been explored more recently. Analyses of spatial covariance patterns of PET-derived cerebral metabolism or blood flow measures have reported diagnostic capacity, correlation with symptom manifestation and response to therapy in PD as well [15]. In addition, some PET-based investigations have employed fully automated analytic paradigms, which avoid a priori assumptions regarding connectivity, investigate whole-brain-network function and address potential confounds associated with data acquisition and analysis in PD. Functional MRI-based investigations have also employed network analyses, with particular focus on "activation" patterns and resting-state putative functional connectivity across cortical and subcortical brain regions [11, 16]. These studies have typically used smaller numbers of participants and have yielded less consistent results between studies to date compared with PET-based studies [17, 18], and such techniques must currently be viewed as more speculative.

Other imaging methodologies of interest

Transcranial ultrasound is an inexpensive and accessible imaging technique that has demonstrated increased echogenicity of the substantia nigra in PD, but this finding has also been noted in other parkinsonisms as well as in nonparkinsonian conditions; it appears to be a static measure and has an unclear relationship to PD pathology, symptomatology and disease progression [19]. Imaging of neuroinflammation utilizes a radiolabeled ligand that binds to peripheral benzodiazepine receptors expressed in active microglia, and this technique has been used to demonstrate putative inflammation in the PD brain [20]. There are limited reports using this technique in PD, however, and its relationship to underlying PD pathology, symptomatology and progression is currently unclear. Imaging of neurotransmission beyond dopamine has also been reported in PD [4], with a consistently demonstrated relationship between cognitive impairment in PD and PET-based imaging of reductions in acetylcholine receptor-binding and acetylcholinesterase activity in particular [21]. Imaging the core pathologies of PD (e.g. α-synuclein aggregation) has proved challenging, but recent advances in this area provide reason for optimism for future development of such markers [22].

Multimodal imaging

Given the wide range of potential targets for functional imaging in PD, in combination with the broad pathology, pathophysiology, symptomatology and patterns of PD presentation and progression, a multimodal approach could be important in developing PD FIMs [23]. Recent reports demonstrate the evolving feasibility of multimodal imaging, including the MRI study mentioned above utilizing multiple MRI-based structural measures simultaneously. The capacity to image neurotransmitter, synaptic, structural and network dynamics contemporaneously in PD using a system that combines the molecular sensitivity, spatial and temporal capabilities of PET and MRI is also tantalizing [24], but currently this area is experimental.

Functional imaging markers in Parkinson's disease

The variety of functional imaging possibilities evident in the brief overview above encourages exploration of their different meanings regarding the development of functional imaging *markers* as clinical trials outcome measures. For example, structural/molecular imaging may be needed as a measure of anatomic disease progression and functional pathology, connectivity measures may be desired as indices of brain-network function, and intrasynaptic imaging may be indicated as a marker of dopaminergic transmission depending on the hypothesized mechanisms of action of an experimental therapeutic in a PD clinical trial. Furthermore, the emerging recognition that PD is a pathologically, symptomatically and neurophysiologically diverse syndrome impacts the meaning and utility of an FIM in PD [25]. What a PD FIM useful in clinical trials could or should entail, FIM usage in PD clinical trials to date and challenges in the use of PD FIMs are thus important concepts to consider.

Consideration of functional imaging marker criteria in Parkinson's disease

Criteria have previously been proposed regarding PD FIM usage to measure disease progression [26] and as a surrogate for a clinical endpoint [1]. In tracking PD progression, suggested FIM criteria included the ability to measure a process that changes with anatomic and symptomatic disease progression, objectivity, reproducibility, specificity, safety and availability. Considering FIM use as a surrogate endpoint for a clinical outcome, suggested biomarker criteria include the ability to measure disease processes, enabling of diagnosis/prognosis, evaluating therapeutic efficacy and mechanism, guiding therapeutic choice, and being tightly correlated with its associated clinical endpoint.

No single currently available functional imaging measure meets all of these criteria. Furthermore, it can be argued that no one FIM *could* meet all the criteria: given the varied pathological, neurophysiological and clinical PD sequelae, it is difficult to conceive of a single imaging measure that could capture all of these signals with equal validity at all stages of disease. In addition, a given PD FIM may have more relevance for one particular disease subtype (e.g. tremor-predominant PD), pathological hallmark, symptom, treatment response or disease complication than for another. Indeed, the same FIM that may tightly correlate with early disease pathology and symptomatology could lack utility as PD progresses, yet could still meet the criteria mentioned above at a given disease stage. Such challenges for an FIM in PD are exemplified by the use of dopaminergic imaging in PD clinical trials to date, and this will be expanded on to further consider the meaning of an FIM in PD.

Discordance between clinical and functional imaging marker outcomes in Parkinson's disease clinical trials

Several clinical trials in PD have attempted to use radiotracer imaging of dopamine system integrity as a biomarker of disease progression correlated with clinical outcome, yet these trials have demonstrated some discordance in this regard [27]. The CALM-PD (Comparison of the Agonist Pramipexole versus Levodopa on Motor complications of Parkinson's Disease) trial investigated the effect of pramipexole versus levodopa both clinically and with regard to impact on dopamine transporter (DaT) binding as a presumed measure of dopamine neuron degeneration [28]. The primary outcome was a reduction in loss of DaT binding in the pramipexole cohort, which was discordant with greater clinical improvement in the levodopa group. Similarly, REAL-PET examined the impact of ropinirole versus levodopa clinically and with regard to impact on an ^{18}F-DOPA uptake measure of dopamine terminal function, again as a presumed marker of neurodegeneration [29]. The primary outcome was a reduction in decreased ^{18}F-DOPA uptake in the ropinirole cohort, also discordant with observed greater clinical improvement in the levodopa group. Subsequent analyses of data from these clinical trials have suggested that the imaging findings could be explained by differential impact on DaT binding and ^{18}F-DOPA uptake by levodopa versus pramipexole or ropinirole, respectively, rather than by the reduction in neurodegeneration [7]. Furthermore, similar discordance between clinical improvement and the rate of decrease in DaT binding was noted in ELLDOPA (Early versus Later Levodopa in Parkinson Disease) study, which was designed to investigate the impact of levodopa (including dose) on rate of disease progression in PD [30].

In summary, clinical trials utilizing imaging of dopamine system integrity as presumed outcome measures related to neurodegeneration have yielded results that are not fully reconciled with observed clinical responses to medication. This discordance between imaging and clinical outcomes has been interpreted as a possible result of the direct impact medications have on the dopaminergic system, which in turn impacts the imaging measures themselves and confounds their interpretation. This highlights a fundamental problem in developing FIMs as outcome measures in PD trials: can the direct impact of an experimental therapeutic on an imaging measure be fully known to enable the correct interpretation of an FIM as an outcome metric? If not, how tight does the correlation between an FIM and a clinical outcome then need to be and can this be quantified in a manner useful for data analysis in clinical trials? These and other challenges facing FIMs in PD will become important to explore.

Challenges in the use of functional imaging markers as outcome measures in Parkinson's disease clinical trials

It is illustrative to consider FIM challenges in the context of three key outcome areas in PD clinical trials: progression of neurodegeneration, symptom response and/or progression, and brain function. Each of these PD outcome areas is in urgent need of novel therapeutics, and each manifests its own challenges in FIM utility.

In clinical trials where progression of neurodegeneration is hypothesized to be reduced by an experimental therapeutic, it would be helpful to include *direct* measures of neuronal loss and/or proteinopathy burden (e.g. synuclein aggregation) to confirm or refute a theorized effect on functional pathology in PD. This could avoid potential confounds related to indirect measurement of neurodegeneration (e.g. dopaminergic imaging), and could also provide insights into the anatomical distribution of therapeutic impact beyond the nigrostriatal system. Structural imaging, particularly MRI-based and proteinopathy-ligand-based imaging, has the potential to provide cross-sectional and longitudinal insight into the functional pathological processes associated with PD clinical presentation and progression, respectively. Although presently such imaging methods remain to be validated as FIMs in PD, their clinical and clinical trial utility in Alzheimer's disease provides a potential roadmap for development in PD [31]. This becomes complicated in PD, however, given the molecular and temporal heterogeneity of functional pathology over the course of the disease and the unclear relationship between anatomical pathology and symptom presence [32]. In addition, the ability for clinical parkinsonism to be present without significant synuclein pathology highlights the challenges that can impact proteinopathy imaging in PD [33]. Furthermore, basic technical considerations for structural (and other) imaging modalities are not trivial in PD and include the impact of patient movement (e.g. tremor, dyskinesias), tolerability of prolonged imaging protocols in rigid/dystonic patients, difficulty in protocol cooperation with cognitively impaired patients and limited access to specialized nuclear imaging currently required for proteinopathy imaging.

Symptom response and progression in PD are also complicated in considering FIM utility as they include not only cardinal PD motor symptoms but also complications related to antiparkinsonian medication (e.g. dyskinesias), development of new nonmotor as well as motor symptoms with progression of disease, and variable rates of symptom and dopaminergic as well as nondopaminergic pathology progression [3, 34]. Indeed, several of these issues could impact a PD clinical trial participant simultaneously, further clouding an imaging outcome's interpretation relative to clinical effect. Although strides have been made with dopaminergic imaging as well as PET-based spatial covariance analyses in particular in addressing these problems, there remain significant and currently unresolved issues in understanding a functional imaging measure's relevance for and relationship to a symptomatic therapeutic outcome.

The impact of a clinical trial agent on brain function is a third area of particular interest and complication in PD, because it relates to clinical outcome. Intracellular function, synaptic function, neuronal function and neural network function can all be (and likely are) impacted by a given neurological therapeutic in PD either directly or indirectly, yet measurement of such functions *in vivo* remains challenging, as does understanding such measurements relative to disease progression and symptomatology. For example, the ability to measure dopaminergic transmission secondarily via dopamine tracer-based imaging is of potential utility, but this is complicated by previously discussed difficulties in interpreting the measured output in the presence of an experimental therapeutic. Direct neuronal output can be assessed, but currently this is largely limited to intraoperative techniques performed during deep-brain stimulation surgery, which limits their utility and skews and restricts the cohort investigated. Whole-brain-distributed networks can be evaluated via PET-based imaging as mentioned above, and this presents arguably the most mature imaging method to date for evaluation of distributed brain-network function in PD. Indeed, such PET-based networks can tightly correlate with specific symptoms in PD including tremor and cognitive impairment [15]. Furthermore, some of these PET networks modulate with dopaminergic or deep-brain stimulation therapy providing an index of brain function relative to treatment. The relationship of such networks to neurodegeneration, proteinopathic distribution and burden, and other structural pathology remains unclear, however, and the statistical and analytic techniques required to interpret these network data are not trivial and may prove difficult to standardize and generalize more broadly.

Lastly, understanding the required sample size and power for a presumptive outcome marker to guide PD clinical trial design represents another important challenge in FIM utility. For example, one can imagine that an FIM for symptom response may require a different cohort size from a neurodegenerative FIM and may also require a different time frame of investigation, yet both could be required in the same PD study in order to test the hypothesized impact of an experimental therapeutic. In addition, the same FIM may vary in power and sample size requirements depending on the duration, severity or phenotype of PD, and the PD population investigated may thus impact the study design as well. Although FIMs inherently hold promise to reduce the duration of trials and the required sample sizes, they must first be well characterized to permit appropriate clinical trial design and prespecification of statistical analyses. The understanding of many currently available functional imaging methods falls short of this goal presently. Furthermore, the substantial impact of placebo effect in PD [35], including on dopaminergic transmission [36], makes even more urgent the need to develop objective, rater-independent and well-characterized FIMs that eliminate the impact of this important confound in powering and analyzing PD clinical trials.

Considerations for development of functional imaging markers as Parkinson's disease outcome measures

Despite the challenges associated with the development of FIMs in PD, there is legitimate reason to be hopeful for their continued (and perhaps more rapid) development and ultimate realization as outcome measures for clinical trials. The breadth and depth of available techniques continues to grow, which is important to permit investigation of the complex and varied functional pathology and pathophysiology of PD. The correlation of imaging output with PD neurodegeneration, proteinopathy burden, symptom progression and response to therapeutic intervention has made substantial strides in the last decade. Improvement in the imaging techniques themselves continues apace, as does attention to technique validation in different PD populations. Improved protocol standardization, increased availability of sophisticated imaging technology and analytic software, and enhanced technical ability to account for challenges inherent in imaging PD patients all reflect significant advances in imaging required for utility of FIMs in clinical trials. These necessary steps toward FIM development are inherently complicated in a heterogeneous and slowly progressive disease such as PD, and such challenges continue to impact the evolution of PD imaging. Nevertheless, PD functional imaging is poised to offer further insights into clinical trials, including as outcome measures.

The panoply of emerging imaging techniques also serves as its own issue to be addressed, however: with the ability to image so many aspects of the brain, what is the most efficient path to mature, validated PD FIMs? This question is important in PD, given both the urgent need to develop novel therapeutics (particularly disease-modifying ones) and the equally urgent need to shorten trial duration, reduce cohort size and improve clarity of outcome interpretation in clinical trials. As alluded to previously, perhaps the most promising route forward in addressing these needs involves particular attention paid to multimodal imaging. As experimental therapeutics with real potential for disease modification develop, and as questions continue to surround the impact of currently available therapeutics on disease progression versus symptoms, it can be argued that multimodal imaging represents an important potential tool to simultaneously improve our understanding of PD pathophysiology and fully capture the response to therapeutic intervention.

As exemplified in the Parkinson Progression Marker Initiative and Alzheimer's Disease Neuroimaging Initiative [23, 37], sampling multiple imaging markers (along with nonimaging markers) is possible to pursue in a standardized prospective manner. Further carefully designed longitudinal observational trials incorporating well-characterized cohorts along with multiple simultaneous nigrostriatal and whole-brain imaging methods could be important in hastening the development of FIMs in PD. It is intriguing to consider the combined application of dopaminergic, proteinopathy ligand, metabolic, blood flow, structural and brain-network imaging to contemporaneously capture important temporal, spatial, structural and network level dynamics in PD. Such rich multimodal imaging is becoming feasible, and could represent an important step to carefully yet broadly and efficiently correlate functional imaging with PD clinical symptomatology. This, in turn, could hasten the development of standardized and widely accepted and utilized criteria for quantification and qualification of imaging data in PD. Although significant challenges persist in developing FIMs as clinical trial outcomes, there has been important work done to date in technique development and characterization toward this goal. The evolution of dopaminergic and PET imaging in particular highlights how far the field has already come, and provides insight into its potential for further development. It is an exciting time for FIM development in PD, and a time that holds real promise to deliver FIMs useful as outcome measures in clinical trials for PD.

References

1. Ravina B, Eidelberg D, Ahlskog JE, *et al.* The role of radiotracer imaging in Parkinson disease. *Neurology* 2005; **64**: 208–15.
2. Bernheimer H, Birkmayer W, Hornykiewicz O, Jellinger K, Seitelberger F. Brain dopamine and the syndromes of Parkinson and Huntington. Clinical, morphological and neurochemical correlations. *J Neurol Sci* 1973; **20**: 415–55.
3. Stoessl AJ, Martin WW, McKeown MJ, Sossi V. Advances in imaging in Parkinson's disease. *Lancet Neurol* 2011; **10**: 987–1001.
4. Brooks DJ, Pavese N. Imaging biomarkers in Parkinson's disease. *Prog Neurobiol* 2011; **95**: 614–28.
5. Brooks DJ. The role of structural and functional imaging in parkinsonian states with a description of PET technology. *Semin Neurol* 2008; **28**: 435–45.
6. Vingerhoets, FJ, Schulzer M, Calne DB, Snow BJ. Which clinical sign of Parkinson's disease best reflects the nigrostriatal lesion? *Ann Neurol*, 1997; **41**: 58–64.
7. de la Fuente-Fernandez R, Schulzer M, Mak E, Sossi V. Trials of neuroprotective therapies for Parkinson's disease: problems and limitations. *Parkinsonism Relat Disord* 2010; **16**: 365–9.
8. Scherfler C, Schwarz J, Antonini A, *et al.* Role of DAT-SPECT in the diagnostic work up of parkinsonism. *Mov Disord* 2007; **22**: 1229–38.
9. Laruelle M. Imaging synaptic neurotransmission with in vivo binding competition techniques: a critical review. *J Cereb Blood Flow Metab* 2000; **20**: 423–51.
10. Pavese N, Evans AH, Tai YF, *et al.* Clinical correlates of levodopa-induced dopamine release in Parkinson disease: a PET study. *Neurology* 2006; **67**: 1612–17.
11. Baglieri A, Marino MA, Morabito R, *et al.* Differences between conventional and nonconventional MRI techniques in Parkinson's disease. *Funct Neurol* 2013; **28**: 73–82.
12. Cho ZH, Oh SH, Kim JM, *et al.* Direct visualization of Parkinson's disease by in vivo human brain imaging using 7.0T magnetic resonance imaging. *Mov Disord* 2011; **26**: 713–18.
13. Mahlknecht P, Hotter A, Hussl A, *et al.* Significance of MRI in diagnosis and differential diagnosis of Parkinson's disease. *Neurodegener Dis* 2010; **7**: 300–18.
14. Peran P, Cherubini A, Assogna F, *et al.* Magnetic resonance imaging markers of Parkinson's disease nigrostriatal signature. *Brain* 2010; **133**: 3423–33.
15. Tang CC, Eidelberg D. Abnormal metabolic brain networks in Parkinson's disease from blackboard to bedside. *Prog Brain Res* 2010; **184**: 161–76.
16. Niethammer M, Feigin A, Eidelberg D. Functional neuroimaging in Parkinson's disease. *Cold Spring Harb Perspect Med* 2012; **2**: a009274.
17. Stoessl AJ. Neuroimaging in Parkinson's disease. *Neurotherapeutics* 2011; **8**: 72–81.
18. Nandhagopal R, McKeown MJ, Stoessl AJ. Functional imaging in Parkinson disease. *Neurology* 2008; **70**: 1478–88.

19. Berg D. Hyperechogenicity of the substantia nigra: pitfalls in assessment and specificity for Parkinson's disease. *J Neural Transm* 2011; **118**: 453–61.
20. Ouchi Y, Yagi S, Yokokura M, Sakamoto M. Neuroinflammation in the living brain of Parkinson's disease. *Parkinsonism Relat Disord* 2009; **15** (Suppl. 3): S200–4.
21. Yarnall A, Rochester L, Burn DJ. The interplay of cholinergic function, attention, and falls in Parkinson's disease. *Mov Disord* 2011; **26**: 2496–503.
22. Vernon AC, Ballard C, Modo M. Neuroimaging for Lewy body disease: is the in vivo molecular imaging of α-synuclein neuropathology required and feasible? *Brain Res Rev* 2010; **65**: 28–55.
23. Parkinson Progression Marker Initiative. The Parkinson Progression Marker Initiative (PPMI). *Prog Neurobiol* 2011; **95**: 629–35.
24. Catana C, Drzezga A, Heiss WD, Rosen BR. PET/MRI for neurologic applications. *J Nucl Med* 2012; **53**: 1916–25.
25. Stern MB, Lang A, Poewe W. Toward a redefinition of Parkinson's disease. *Mov Disord* 2012; **27**: 54–60.
26. Brooks DJ, Frey KA, Marek KL, *et al.* Assessment of neuroimaging techniques as biomarkers of the progression of Parkinson's disease. *Exp Neurol* 2003; **184** (Suppl. 1): S68–79.
27. Agarwal PA, Stoessl AJ. Biomarkers for trials of neuroprotection in Parkinson's disease. *Mov Disord* 2013; **28**: 71–85.
28. Parkinson Study Group. Dopamine transporter brain imaging to assess the effects of pramipexole vs levodopa on Parkinson disease progression. *JAMA* 2002; **287**: 1653–61.
29. Whone AL, Watts RL, Stoessl AJ, *et al.* Slower progression of Parkinson's disease with ropinirole versus levodopa: the REAL-PET study. *Ann Neurol* 2003; **54**: 93–101.
30. Fahn S, Parkinson Study Group. Does levodopa slow or hasten the rate of progression of Parkinson's disease? *J Neurol* 2005; **252** (Suppl. 4): IV37–42.
31. Jack CR Jr, Holtzman DM. Biomarker modeling of Alzheimer's disease. *Neuron* 2013; **80**: 1347–58.
32. Lim SY, Fox SH, Lang AE. Overview of the extranigral aspects of Parkinson disease. *Arch Neurol* 2009; **66**: 167–72.
33. Doherty KM, Silveira-Moriyama L, Parkkinen L, *et al.* Parkin disease: a clinicopathologic entity? *JAMA Neurol* 2013; **70**: 571–9.
34. Alves G, Wentzel-Larsen T, Aarsland D, Larsen JP. Progression of motor impairment and disability in Parkinson disease: a population-based study. *Neurology* 2005; **65**: 1436–41.
35. Benedetti F, Carlino E, Pollo A. How placebos change the patient's brain. *Neuropsychopharmacology* 2011; **36**: 339–54.
36. Lidstone SC, Schulzer M, Dinelle K, *et al.* Effects of expectation on placebo-induced dopamine release in Parkinson disease. *Arch Gen Psychiatry* 2010; **67**: 857–65.
37. Weiner MW, Veitch DP, Aisen PS, *et al.* The Alzheimer's Disease Neuroimaging Initiative: a review of papers published since its inception. *Alzheimers Dement* 2012; **8** (Suppl.): S1–68.

Chapter 24

Cerebrospinal fluid and blood biomarkers as outcome measures in clinical trials for Parkinson's disease

Thomas F. Tropea and Claire Henchcliffe

Introduction

There is an urgent need to develop improved treatments for Parkinson's disease (PD), and frustration has mounted over recent years due to difficulties translating promising preclinical and early-phase clinical data into approved therapies. This has in turn prompted examination of the likely roadblocks, including limitations in clinical trial outcome measures.

Measurement of response to intervention in the short term or in changes in PD over time currently relies on observation of signs and/or patients' perceptions of symptoms. These are typically recorded using clinical rating scales that incorporate information provided by the patient and/or caregiver, and by the investigator. A number of valuable validated rating scales exist that address motor and nonmotor symptoms, as well as quality-of-life measures (as detailed in Chapter 22, this volume). In terms of determining the impact of PD on a person's function and well-being, such scales are critically important. However, this approach has many disadvantages. First, sensitivity may be limited and large phase 3 clinical trials that are costly and time-consuming are required to demonstrate efficacy. Secondly, clinical rating scales do not distinguish short-term symptomatic benefits from neuroprotective effects, again resulting in the need for large trials over extended time periods. Thirdly, clinical findings do not determine whether a given treatment engages its predicted target – this is important information in terms of go/no go decisions during early phases of drug development, and also in understanding negative trial results. Fourthly, clinical measures do not determine whether there are changes in function that might be predicted to have long-term advantages or disadvantages, for example whether antibodies develop to a given treatment. In 2001, a Biomarkers Working Definition Working Group was convened by the National Institutes of Health and defined a biomarker as a "characteristic that is objectively measured and evaluated as an indicator of normal biological processes, pathogenic processes, or pharmacologic responses to a therapeutic intervention" [1].

The hope is that development of validated biomarkers will provide sensitive and reliable measures of treatment effects to rationally inform go/no go decisions, to improve the pace of bringing new drugs to the clinic, and to decrease the cost of drug development. One specific need is a biomarker incorporated as a primary outcome measure in clinical trials designed to track progression of PD and test an intervention's potential for neuroprotection, a so-called "surrogate marker." This requires evidence that changes in the biomarker reflect, and therefore may substitute for, a clinically meaningful measure such as patient function or survival. Although this has not yet been achieved in PD research, there are many examples of the usefulness of surrogate markers in other areas of clinical research (for example, human immunodeficiency virus PCR tests) and therefore their role has been discussed extensively by regulatory bodies.

Although biomarker development in PD has traditionally been strongly focused on neuroimaging, recent breakthroughs in the neuroscience and molecular genetics of PD are helping to shape thinking about potential serum and cerebrospinal fluid (CSF) biomarkers. In this chapter, we describe previous efforts to incorporate biomarkers into PD clinical trials, examine serum- and CSF-based biomarkers studied in PD, and, although still in its infancy, discuss initial studies that have already been undertaken and potential future directions.

Biomarkers in Parkinson's disease clinical trials: lessons from neuroimaging

So far, PD biomarker incorporation into clinical trials has focused almost exclusively on neuroimaging techniques, making use of single-photon-emission computed tomography (SPECT) and positron emission tomography (PET). Three studies comparing neuroimaging versus clinical outcome measures have been encouraging in demonstrating the feasibility of biomarker use in PD clinical trials but have also highlighted difficulties in the interpretation of results. First, in the CALM-PD (Comparison of the Agonist Pramipexole versus Levodopa on Motor complications of Parkinson's Disease) phase 3 clinical trial of pramipexole versus levodopa (L-DOPA) in early PD, the primary outcome was the development of motor complications. However, a subgroup of participants underwent SPECT imaging to detect the dopamine transporter (DAT) with [^{123}I]β-CIT(2β-carbomethoxy-3β-[4-iodophenyl]tropane)[2]. Those assigned to pramipexole (plus supplemental levodopa) had less decline in striatal [^{123}I]β-CIT uptake versus those assigned to levodopa (16% decline vs 25.5% decline at 46 months, $P = 0.01$). Secondly, the REAL-PET (Requip as Early Therapy versus L-DOPA – PET) study measured the reduction in ^{18}F-DOPA uptake in the putamen using PET [3]. Once again, there was less decline in those assigned to ropinirole (plus supplemental levodopa) versus levodopa (13 vs 20%; $P = 0.022$, at 2 years). Thirdly, the ELLDOPA (Early versus Later Levodopa in Parkinson Disease) study comparing levodopa versus placebo in early PD included a substudy of [^{123}I]β-CIT SPECT imaging in 116 subjects [4]. Decline in ligand uptake was between −4 and −7.2% in the three groups receiving levodopa versus −1.4% in the placebo group. If changes in ligand uptake indeed reflected dopaminergic neuron survival, this has far-reaching implications and would suggest possible levodopa toxicity or neuroprotection by dopamine agonists. However, imaging changes did not reflect clinically meaningful differences between groups as measured by clinical rating scale scores, a condition required of a surrogate marker. The studies raised the fundamental question of how directly ligand uptake was related to the underlying disease process, and whether target availability for binding (rather than the number of healthy dopaminergic cells and/or terminals present) was influenced by the treatment administered. This prompted much discussion, temporarily halted efforts to incorporate biomarkers into clinical trials, and served to emphasize that a sound fundamental understanding of potential fluid-based biomarkers will be needed if they are to serve as surrogate markers.

The use of neuroimaging in surgical interventions has been less controversial, albeit with more limited interpretation. For example, ^{18}F-DOPA-PET has been successful in determining the maintenance of fetal mesencephalic tissue grafts in PD [5,6]. Fluorodeoxyglucose (^{18}F-FDG)-PET examinations also demonstrated the ability to reflect change in 12 individuals with PD who had undergone "gene therapy," unilateral subthalamic nucleus infusion of the glutamic acid decarboxylase gene expressed in an adeno-associated virus vector [7]. In these cases, an abnormal baseline elevation in a previously defined motor-related network activity declined after surgery but not that of a cognitive-related pattern. As the fields of gene therapy and cell-based therapies move ahead, these findings therefore strongly support the use of neuroimaging biomarkers in exploratory trials, and, by analogy, it seems likely that blood and CSF biomarkers might be designed to augment information in such trials.

Cerebrospinal fluid and blood biomarkers in Parkinson's disease: the developing landscape

Despite the lead time of neuroimaging over fluid-based biomarkers in PD, a "next generation" of biomarkers is now the subject of intensive investigation. Fluid-derived biomarkers have the potential for greater accessibility, faster development of novel assays and therefore the ability to reflect a wider range of fundamental disease processes. While CSF is theoretically preferable since it is more proximal to the major sites of neurodegeneration, obtaining plasma, serum and other blood components is simpler and less invasive. Ideally, any fluid-based biomarker would be reliable and sensitive to change, simple to use, noninvasive or minimally invasive, and have good tolerability and acceptability.

The advent of increasingly sophisticated technology has opened the door to future use of fluid-based biomarkers in PD clinical trials. Improved understanding of the molecular and genetic underpinnings of PD have identified "key players" as biomarker candidates in pathways as diverse as aberrant protein aggregation, oxidative stress, mitochondrial dysfunction, inflammation, transcriptional dysregulation, destruction of pigmented cells releasing neuromelanin and disruption of dopamine metabolism. Development of increasingly sensitive measurements of proteins, polynucleotides and small molecules, as well as their modifications, has expanded the breadth of potential targets that may be measured. Finally, more sophisticated bioinformatics technology has allowed identification of combinatorial markers, and has facilitated the use of untargeted "omics" approaches.

With the rapid development of new technologies, it is imperative that there are adequate resources for discovery and validation in the PD research arena. Various initiatives are now testing how a collaborative approach for comparison and combination of markers may be beneficial. The Parkinson's Progression Markers Initiative (PPMI; National Institutes of Health clinical trials registry [ClinicalTrials.gov]: NCT01141023) is an international longitudinal observational study, now following 400 subjects with early PD who are drug naive, collecting clinical data, DAT imaging, and serum and CSF samples [8]. Control subjects are also included in the study, facilitating comparison. The BioFIND study (Fox Investigation for New Discovery of Biomarkers in Parkinson's disease) is an ongoing initiative intended to provide a platform for discovery and validation of biomarkers in a well-characterized moderate to advanced PD cohort. Clinical data, as well as blood, DNA, RNA and CSF samples from 120 individuals with PD and 120 control subjects will be made available for discovery and validation studies, which may then be extended to longitudinal and/or more heterogeneous PD cohorts [9]. Although not intended for this purpose, the value of such biosample repositories is nicely illustrated by published studies of CSF, plasma and urine samples from the DATATOP (Deprenyl and Tocopherol Antioxidant Treatment On Parkinson's disease) study [10], several of which are included in the following sections.

This field is in very early development. It must be emphasized that as yet there is no accepted fluid-based biomarker for PD. However, a core set of criteria are proposed in Table 24.1, in part based on previous proposals [11, 12], to help evaluate the work so far. Like drug development, discovery and validation of biomarkers will take several steps from discovery to testing in cross-sectional cohorts and then larger prospective studies (Figure 24.1). To validate a surrogate marker, it

Table 24.1 Ideal Parkinson's disease (PD) biomarker characteristics for a candidate neuroprotection clinical trial endpoint

Marker is linked to fundamental PD pathology

Changes predictably with a change in disease status

Unaffected by short-term symptomatic treatment

Sensitive enough to reflect small changes

Captures all change with minimal or no loss of data

Confirmed by at least two peer-reviewed published independent studies

Based on [11, 12].

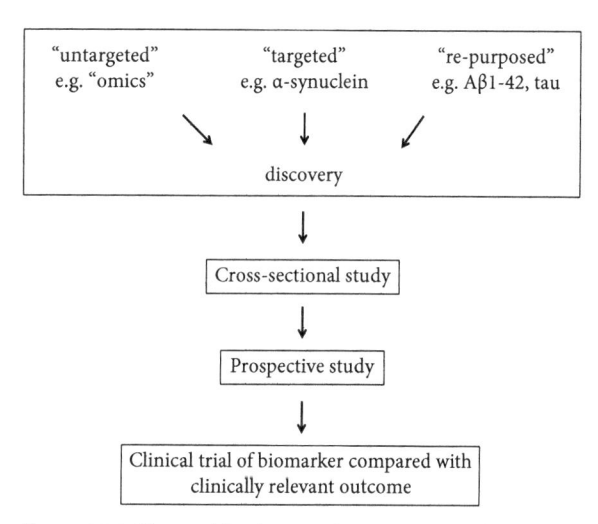

Figure 24.1 Phases of development for a surrogate marker of progression in Parkinson's disease (PD). Biomarker discovery leads to identification of species that are most often first studied in cross-sectional cohorts to provide information on disease association and also disease characteristics. This needs to be followed by characterization of biomarker performance in longitudinal cohorts. To validate a surrogate marker of PD progression, the biomarker will finally need to be tested in longitudinal clinical trials in which it is compared with a meaningful clinical outcome to determine that it will potentially substitute for that outcome in future clinical trials.

will need to be compared in a clinical trial with a relevant clinical endpoint. The following section, while not an exhaustive list, seeks to describe work on potential biomarkers that are candidates for future development (Table 24.2). Most of the data so far is concerned with association with PD diagnosis. While all such markers will not be useful as clinical trial outcome measures, this does provide a first step. Where more relevant data for measuring disease progression or response to treatment has been captured, it is mostly in cross-sectional studies that identify changes in biomarker status associated with disease stage or severity. The much-needed

Table 24.2 Potential CSF and blood biomarkers for PD: hypothetical uses as clinical trial outcome measures

Biomarker	CSF	Blood	Potential outcome measure
Dopamine-based marker			
HVA	Increased xanthine/HVA ratio in PD		Progression Dopamine metabolism, e.g. for gene therapy or cell transplant
PD genetic marker			
α-Synuclein	Decreased in PD	Variable	Nonmotor i.e. link to cognitive decline Target engagement for anti-α-synuclein immunotherapy
AD-associated markers			
t-tau; $A\beta_{1-42}$/t-tau; p-tau/$A\beta_{1-42}$	t-tau decrease associated with motor disability and progression p-tau/$A\beta_{1-42}$ and $A\beta_{1-42}$/t-tau associates with motor progression		Motor progression Target engagement for immunotherapy, e.g. anti-Aβ antibodies
$A\beta_{1-42}$; t-tau; $A\beta_{1-42}$/t-tau	$A\beta_{1-42}$ and t-tau decrease associated with cognitive decline $A\beta_{1-42}$/t-tau associates with cognition		Nonmotor Target engagement for immunotherapy, e.g. anti-Aβ antibodies
Oxidative stress markers			
Glutathione		Increased oxidized form in PD	Central and peripheral target engagement of interventions predicted to alter levels, e.g. N-acetyl cysteine
Coenzyme Q10	Decreased oxidized/total CoQ10 in PD	Decreased redox ratio in PD	Target engagement by antioxidants
Malondialdehyde		Increased in PD	Target engagement by antioxidants
F2-isoprostanes and cholesterol oxidation products		Increased in PD	Target engagement by antioxidants
8-OHdG	Increased in PD	Increased in PD	Target engagement by antioxidants
Urate	Decreased in PD and decrease associated with faster progression	Decreased in PD and decrease associated with faster progression	Measure of ability of inosine to increase urate as possible neuroprotectant progression
Immune system markers			
IL-10, RANTES		Increased in PD	Physiological effects of anti-inflammatory intervention
TNF-α	Increased in PD (not all studies)	Increased in PD	Physiological effects of anti-inflammatory intervention
CRP, IL-6, TNFα, IFN-10, MCP-1 and macrophage inflammatory protein 1-β	Associated with depression, anxiety, fatigue and cognition		Nonmotor-related physiological effects of anti-inflammatory intervention
TNF receptor R1 and R2		Increased in PD	Physiological effects of anti-inflammatory intervention
"Omics" approaches			
Detection of RNA transcripts by transcriptomics		Specific PD-associated transcripts	Future measures of progression and target engagement
Detection of proteins by proteomics	Specific PD-associated proteins (single and combinations)	Specific PD-associated proteins (single and combinations)	Future measures of progression and target engagement

8OHdG, 8-hydroxy-2 deoxyguanosine; $A\beta_{1-42}$, β-amyloid 42 aa isoform; CoQ10, coenzyme Q10; CRP, C-reactive protein; CSF, cerebrospinal fluid; HVA, homovanillic acid; IL-6, interleukin 6; IL-10, interleukin 10; MCP-1, monocyte chemotactic protein 1; PD, Parkinson's disease; p-tau, phosphorylated tau; RANTES, regulated on activation, normal T-cell-expressed and -secreted chemokine; t-tau, total tau; TNF-α, tumor necrosis factor-α.

longitudinal studies now have a foundation upon which to begin but have not yet been completed or undertaken.

Targeted markers

Dopamine-based markers

Although measuring dopamine directly in fluids has not proved useful as a PD biomarker, studies of CSF have identified altered levels of related compounds. Particular attention has been paid to CSF homovanillic acid (HVA) levels, as HVA is the breakdown product of central dopamine (Figure 24.2). The ratio of HVA:xanthine is significantly different between the CSF of patients with PD and that of controls, and changed with time in one longitudinal study, suggesting its potential as a progression marker [13, 14]. In contrast, other potential dopamine-related markers are lacking longitudinal data that would provide information on changes with disease status. These include platelet monoamine oxidase B activity, responsible for dopamine breakdown, which has been found to be increased in the plasma of patients with PD [15]; reduced dopamine content, tyrosine hydroxylase immunoreactivity, and expression and density of dopamine receptors in peripheral blood lymphocytes [16]; and dopamine D2 and D3 receptor transcripts [17].

Disease-related protein biomarkers

Advances in our understanding of PD etiopathogenesis have now identified a number of proteins that are key in cellular pathways perturbed in the disease. The first gene determined to lead to PD, α-synuclein (*SNCA*), allowed identification of a protein in which oxidative damaged and misfolding is now thought to be the major molecular factor underlying PD pathogenesis in the majority of cases. Multiple other genes have now been identified in which mutations either lead to or increase the risk of PD. Their transcripts and protein products are now under intensive investigation as potential biomarkers.

α-Synuclein

α-Synuclein is a major component of Lewy bodies and Lewy neurites, which represent the pathological hallmarks of PD. Although the focus has been on Lewy bodies present in surviving dopaminergic neurons of the substantia nigra, these structures are widespread within the central nervous system (CNS), and in peripheral autonomic nerves [18, 19], in salivary glands [20] and within skin tissue [21]. At least some such changes may occur in the "premotor" phase of PD, making α-synuclein a future candidate for monitoring prior to diagnosis on the basis of motor symptoms ("phenoconversion"). Although primarily intracellular, α-synuclein is detectable in plasma [22–24] and CSF [25].

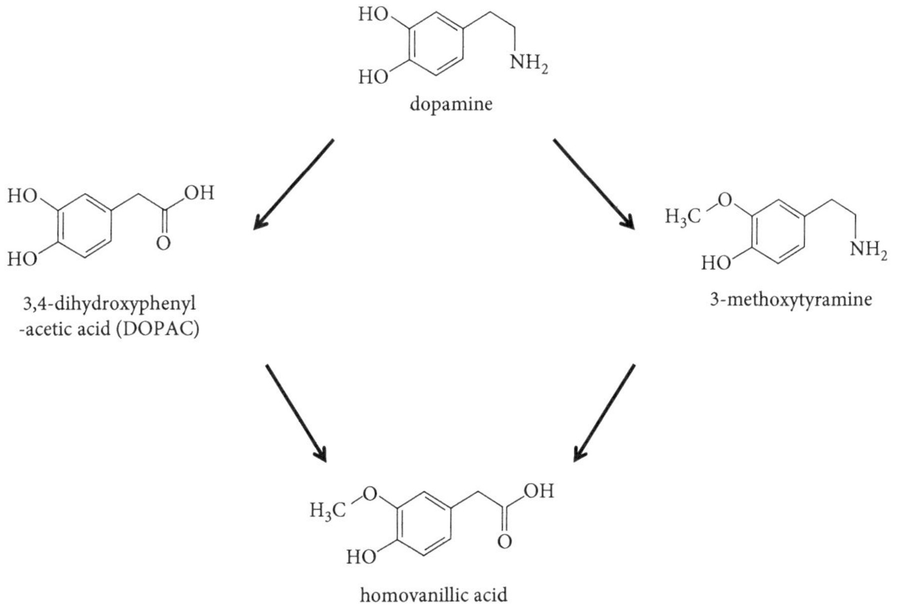

Figure 24.2 Dopamine metabolism and the relationship of homovanillic acid, a potential Parkinson's disease biomarker, to dopamine.

Unfortunately, measuring α-synuclein in blood samples may be more difficult than anticipated, due to different forms that may be measured, as well as technical confounders. α-Synuclein total level [26], oligomeric form [22] and phosphorylated α-synuclein [24] have all been found to be elevated in blood in PD, but there are differences among studies. Others have found a trend for decreased α-synuclein [27] and Li et al. [28] found a greater decrement in α-synuclein in early-onset PD versus late-onset PD when measured by western blotting. Over 95% of α-synuclein in blood samples is thought to be located in red blood cells, with 1% or less in plasma, and therefore even a small variation in hemolysis would have a large confounding effect on results.

Measuring α-synuclein in CSF has been more robust. Decreased α-synuclein levels in CSF of individuals with PD versus controls have now been documented in a number of independent studies [25, 29–36]. Although the majority of these studies involved more advanced PD patients, similar results have been found in early PD compared with control subjects [35, 36], demonstrating that such a difference is not due to unanticipated medication treatment effects. How specific this finding will be to PD is uncertain. In one study, a lower level of α-synuclein was measured in CSF from Alzheimer's disease (AD) versus controls, leading the investigators to postulate that it is a marker of loss of synapses in general [29], as opposed to a PD-specific process. A more recent study found decreased CSF α-synuclein not only in PD but also in dementia with Lewy bodies (DLB) and multiple-system atrophy (MSA) [34]. It will likely be important to examine different species of α-synuclein to obtain the full picture and appreciate its potential usefulness as a biomarker. Another important issue to consider is whether a combination of protein measurements, incorporating α-synuclein, might constitute a superior biomarker. In one study, a panel of seven proteins comprising α-synuclein, DJ-1, total tau, phosphorylated tau, fractalkine, Flt3 ligand, and β-amyloid 42 aa isoform differed in CSF samples from PD when compared with normal controls, AD and MSA [37].

Whether α-synuclein will ultimately turn out to be helpful in tracking PD progression remains to be seen. However, in the PPMI study [8], decreased α-synuclein was associated with increased motor severity in PD [35]. Moreover, a recent study has suggested that lower α-synuclein levels may be associated with a longitudinal cognitive decline, based on post-hoc analysis of CSF α-synuclein levels in samples stored from the DATATOP study of selegiline and α-tocopherol in PD [38].

Immunotherapy targeting α-synuclein has recently been investigated as a potential PD treatment. Active immunization with recombinant human α-synuclein reduces α-synuclein accumulation in neuronal cell bodies and synapses in a mouse model of PD, and was also demonstrated to reduce neurodegeneration in that model [39]. A vaccine, PD01A (AFFITOPE®; AFFiRiS), is now in an extension study following a phase 1 clinical trial. Passive immunization with an anti-α-synuclein monoclonal antibody has also been shown to reduce motor deficits and reduce α-synuclein expression on synapses and axons in an animal model [40]. It is thought that these effects occur through inhibiting the early stages of α-synuclein aggregation, thus preventing the development of oligomeric deposits [41]. Given these promising preclinical results and current translational initiatives, it is tempting to speculate that biomarkers centered on α-synuclein may be helpful in monitoring the response to intervention, and particularly in demonstrating target engagement, as has been described for AD markers [42–45].

DJ-1

Mutations in the *DJ-1* gene are a rare cause of autosomal-recessive forms of PD. It is detected in blood and CSF. Similarly to α-synuclein, only a small fraction of DJ-1 is present in plasma compared with blood cells and platelets, making variable hemolysis or residual platelets in sample preparation a potential confounder [27]. No significant difference between PD versus control plasma levels of DJ-1 was detected by Maita et al. [46]. However, another study demonstrated a significantly higher concentration of plasma DJ-1 in PD compared with control subjects, and plasma levels of DJ-1 correlated with PD disease severity [47]. A recent large study of DJ-1 in CSF found decreased DJ-1 levels associated with PD, with 90% sensitivity and 70% specificity for the diagnosis of PD [30]. This study also measured α-synuclein and found that α-synuclein and DJ-1 levels in CSF were correlated. However, there are some differences in findings between groups, and a previous study actually suggested that DJ-1 levels were increased in CSF in PD, particularly in early stages [48]. Moreover, DJ-1 may not be a marker of disease severity [27, 37]. The picture is likely to be more complicated, since DJ-1 exists in multiple isoforms. Lin et al. [49] found that of seven isoforms detected in blood, those with posttranslational 4-hydroxy-2-nonenal modifications were altered in late PD. Additionally, a form of DJ-1 oxidized at cysteine-106 is elevated in red blood cells in PD versus control blood samples [50]. To fully explore whether and how DJ-1 might act as a biomarker of PD and progression, more careful consideration of its various isoforms including posttranslational modifications is needed.

β-Amyloid and tau

β-Amyloid (Aβ) and tau proteins have been under intensive scrutiny in AD. Specifically, the 42 aa isoform of β-amyloid ($A\beta_{1-42}$) and total (t-tau) and hyperphosphorylated tau (p-tau) concentrations in the CSF have recently been included in diagnostic criteria, and may be of use not only in the diagnosis of AD with dementia but also in predicting AD [51]. Parkinson's disease ventricular CSF from post-mortem cases [52] showed that the p-tau-181:$A\beta_{1-42}$ ratio and ApoA-1 levels were significantly associated with PD versus controls, demonstrating that AD markers may also be of use in PD. Reduced CSF $A\beta_{1-42}$ levels have been suggested to be an independent predictor of cognitive decline in PD patients [53]. A combination of proteins examined by Shi et al. [37] found that the ratio of fractalkine:$A\beta_{1-42}$ in CSF samples not only correlated with disease severity in a cross-sectional cohort of PD but also with disease progression in longitudinal samples. A recent study of CSF samples from the PPMI cohort described lower $A\beta_{1-42}$ and p-tau associated with the diagnosis of PD, and also decreased t-tau levels associated with increased motor severity [35]. Differences between tremor-predominant and postural instability and gait disorder (PIGD) subtypes of PD suggested a potential association with prognosis: lower $A\beta_{1-42}$ and p-tau were both associated with PIGD and not with the tremor-predominant phenotype of PD. Both PD severity and cognitive impairment/dementia in another study associated with the CSF complement 3:$A\beta_{1-42}$ ratio and factor H:$A\beta_{1-42}$ ratio [54], again supporting the usefulness of $A\beta_{1-42}$. In 22 nondemented individuals with PD, CSF levels of $A\beta_{1-42}$, t-tau and $A\beta_{1-42}$:total tau correlated with various scores of cognition, including Logical Memory (delayed), Category Fluency, Digit Symbol, and Trails B minus A [55]. Recently, analysis of the DATATOP CSF samples from 403 participants measured t-tau, p-tau and $A\beta_{1-42}$. In early PD, $A\beta_{1-42}$ levels were found to have a weak negative correlation with total Unified Parkinson's Disease Rating Scale (UPDRS) scores, and baseline p-tau:t-tau and p-tau:$A\beta_{1-42}$ ratios were found to have a negative correlation with the rate of UPDRS change. While medications (selegiline and/or tocopherol) did not appear to alter biomarkers appreciably, a weak but significant positive correlation between the rate of change in t-tau level or t-tau:$A\beta_{1-42}$ ratio and the change in UPDRS score was observed.

Antibodies targeting Aβ in AD are now under intensive study. If successful, repurposing such treatments from AD to PD will need to be considered. In this situation, prior experience with CSF protein biomarkers in AD will be invaluable, including help in anticipating potential pitfalls. In a phase 2 clinical trial of the anti-Aβ monoclonal antibody bapineuzumab in mild to moderate AD, reduced CSF t-tau and p-tau concentrations were associated with the study intervention, possibly reflecting an effect on the disease process [42]. Unfortunately, a phase 3 clinical trial detected no clinical benefit [43]. Solanezumab, an anti-Aβ antibody, was also recently tested in phase 2 and phase 3 randomized, double-blind, placebo-controlled trials in mild to moderate AD [44, 45]. The CSF unbound $A\beta_{1-42}$ increased while the CSF unbound $A\beta_{1-40}$ decreased in both phase 2 and phase 3 trials, suggesting a change in equilibrium in Aβ in the central compartment. The investigators interpreted the increase in CSF unbound $A\beta_{1-42}$ as indicating a shift in "equilibrium" as the plaque was modified, yet phase 3 trials failed to meet their clinical primary endpoints, with no demonstration of significant cognitive improvement or functional improvement [45]. This echoes the situation in the CALM-PD, REAL-PET and ELLDOPA trials in PD described in above, in which biomarker changes did not reflect clinical outcomes. It remains to be determined whether the changes measured are truly irrelevant to clinical outcome, or whether the discordance arose from clinical aspects of the trial design. The CSF biomarker results in these AD studies nonetheless supported a central effect. With the possibility that intervention was made too late in the disease process, testing of solanezumab in an earlier "at-risk" population is now being pursued.

Markers of oxidative stress

Increased levels of oxidative stress contribute to PD pathogenesis, and not only are mitochondria the major source of cellular free radicals but defects in their biogenesis are now well documented in PD [56, 57]. Oxidative stress markers, including markers of redox status and oxidative damage, have therefore been of great interest in studies of various blood components and CSF in PD.

There are many potential species that have demonstrated initial promise. Glutathione is a potent antioxidant, and an increase in its oxidized form was reported in plasma in PD versus control subjects [58]. Similarly for coenzyme Q10 (CoQ10), another potent antioxidant, two studies found its redox ratio in blood samples to be decreased in PD versus controls [59, 60], and in CSF the oxidized:total CoQ10 ratio was increased in PD [61]. Malondialdehyde is a product formed as reactive oxygen species degrade polyunsaturated lipids, and two studies have found significantly increased plasma levels of malondialdehyde associated with PD [58, 62]. Other markers of oxidative damage to lipids may be similarly elevated. In a study of PD compared with healthy controls, plasma F2-isoprostanes (a fatty acid peroxidation product) and cholesterol oxidation products were elevated in PD [63]. Oxidative damage to DNA has been recognized in plasma and CSF in PD, and notably 8-hydroxy-2 deoxyguanosine (8-OHdG), formed by direct oxidative damage to nucleosides, is elevated in plasma and urine in PD [64, 65].

None of these markers has yet been linked to PD progression, and therefore they are not helpful at this point in tracking the effect of potential neuroprotectants on disease progression. However, in clinical trials, they have the potential to determine the effects of an intervention on redox status in blood or CSF. This is important in understanding why (or sometimes more importantly, why not) a given drug may be effective. There are now a number of potential therapeutic agents acting on the interrelated pathways of mitochondrial dysfunction and oxidative stress [66], making this an ideal area to incorporate biomarkers for target engagement into clinical trials. With the recent lack of benefit in a large phase 3 clinical trial of high-dose CoQ10, inclusion of such markers might have proved informative. A recent study, however, suggested that findings may be more complex than anticipated. In an open-label, dose-escalation clinical trial testing CoQ10 up to 2400 mg daily in 16 individuals with early PD, plasma F2 isoprostanes and serum phospholipase A2 were reduced at CoQ10 doses of 400–1200 mg daily (as expected) but were actually increased at a dose of 2400 mg daily [67]. This serves to illustrate the potential complexities in translating preclinical promise into a clinically useful intervention.

Urate and other purine pathway compounds

Urate is a potent antioxidant, a metal chelator capable of binding iron, and in several rodent models of PD is neuroprotective [68–70]. In humans, it is the end product of the metabolic pathway for purines, and is subject to dietary influences. Independent studies have now detected decreased urate concentration in serum (for example [71]) and in CSF [72] in strong association with PD in men (although less so in women). Moreover, higher serum and CSF urate concentrations in post-hoc analyses of two large clinical trials have been associated with slower PD progression [72, 73]. Urate is therefore a high priority for interventional testing as a potential neuroprotectant in PD. Urate itself is rapidly degraded by intestinal bacteria after oral ingestion. However, its precursor, inosine (Figure 24.3), may be orally administered and has been shown to elevate serum urate. Recently, a phase 2 clinical trial of inosine was undertaken in individuals with de novo PD. Primary endpoints were safety and tolerability but also included a primary endpoint of ability to elevate serum and CSF urate concentration, i.e. as a means of testing "target engagement." In this study, serum urate levels were elevated in the mild and moderate inosine dose treatment arms by 2 weeks, and were back to baseline at 1 month after cessation of the study drug. A single measurement of CSF urate levels found elevations in the mild (40%) and moderate (50%) inosine dose treatment arms in 44/75 participants from whom CSF was collected [74]. These findings therefore provide encouraging data upon which to proceed with larger-scale testing in which manipulated urate changes can be examined for correlation with clinical outcomes.

In addition to urate, altered purine metabolism (Figure 24.3) has been demonstrated in PD. Hypoxanthine concentration, and hypoxanthine:xanthine as well as xanthosine:xanthine ratios were found to be reduced in PD versus controls [75]. In a study of 217 unmedicated PD subjects compared with 26 control subjects, the mean xanthine:homovanillic acid ratio was significantly higher in PD subjects, and this ratio was further elevated at the 24-month repeat testing, raising the possibility that the degree of abnormality of the xanthine:homovanillic acid ratio might reflect disease progression [14]. Further longitudinal studies are now warranted, as this seems to be a promising pathway in studying PD progression.

Markers of inflammation

Inflammatory pathways are now thought to play a significant role in PD pathogenesis. Microglial activation has been well documented in autopsy specimens in PD. Moreover, neuroimaging using the peripheral

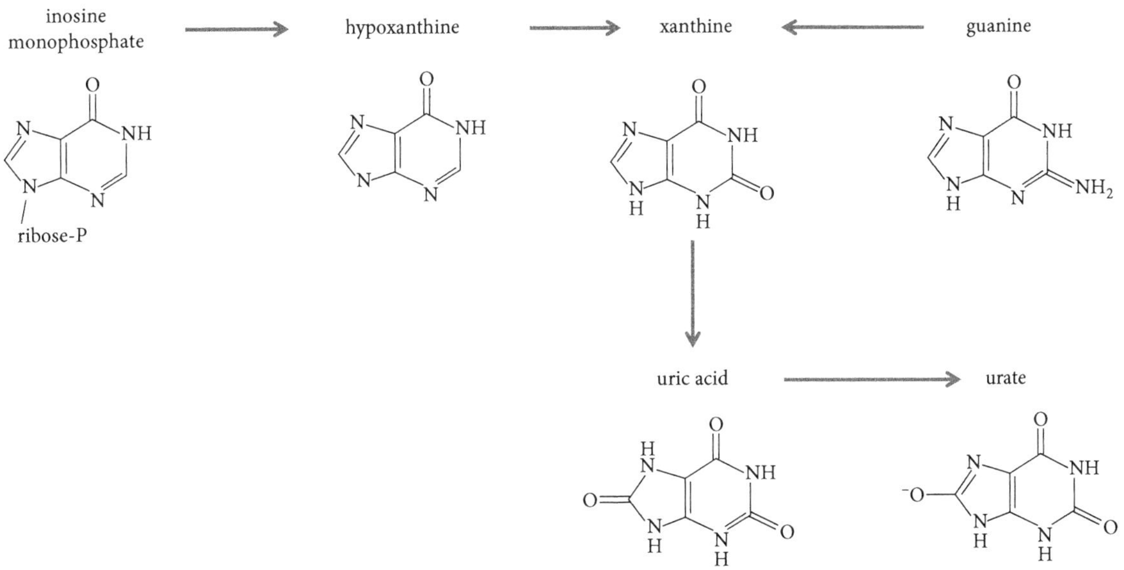

Figure 24.3 Metabolic pathway depicting the synthesis of urate from its precursor, inosine. Inosine has been tested in a phase 2 clinical trial with primary outcome measures of safety, tolerability and ability to elevate urate levels.

benzodiazepine receptor ligand PK11195 supports ongoing microglial activation during a patient's lifetime [57]. Although studying inflammatory markers has not yet revealed candidates for use in delineating the progression of motor PD, it is possible that such markers will be useful in demonstrating target engagement and pathway effects for future anti-inflammatory intervention. Several studies have now described disrupted inflammatory pathways in blood and CSF, although many of these findings remain to be replicated.

Interleukin (IL)-10 and the chemokine RANTES (Regulated on Activation, Normal T-cell Expressed and Secreted) have been found at increased levels in serum in PD compared with controls [76]. Decreased mannan-binding lectin levels and elevated tumor necrosis factor (TNF)-α levels have been detected in association with PD [77]. In addition to this finding in plasma, an increase in TNF-α has been reported in CSF in patients with PD versus controls [78]. One interesting possibility is that nonmotor symptoms may be associated with a pro-inflammatory state [79]. In one study, not only PD severity but also cognitive impairment and dementia were associated with the CSF complement 3:Aβ_{1-42} ratio and factor H:Aβ_{1-42} ratio [54]. Increased plasma levels of the soluble TNF receptors TNFR1 and TNFR2 were associated in one study with worse scores on psychometric testing [80]. In a study of CSF from 87 PD patients and 33 controls, measures of inflammatory markers including C-reactive protein, IL-6, TNF-α, interferon γ-induced protein-10, monocyte chemotactic protein-1 and macrophage inflammatory protein 1-β did not differ between groups, but instead inflammatory markers were significantly associated with worse measures of depression, anxiety, fatigue and cognition within the PD group [81]. These independent findings therefore suggest a potential area of focus upon cognitive dysfunction in PD that warrants further study.

Perturbations in cellular components of the immune system have been documented. A higher population of circulating CD4-bright$^+$/CD8-dull$^+$ lymphocytes (usually seen in the thymus) has been demonstrated in PD compared with control subjects [82]. Decreased numbers of CD4$^+$CD45RA$^+$ (naive) T cells and increased numbers of CD4$^+$CD45RO$^+$ (memory) T cells and TCRγδ$^+$ cells have also been observed [83], and this same study found increased HLA-DR expression on CSF monocytes. Whether these will provide benefit as PD biomarkers remains to be seen.

Abnormal antibody expression has also been detected in PD. Increased levels of anti-melanin antibodies detected by ELISA were observed in one study in serum from individuals with PD versus age-matched controls, and levels were inversely correlated with PD duration [84]. Of particular interest, however, are two examples of studies in which antibody measures were incorporated into clinical trials [85]. The CSF was examined for antineuronal antibodies in clinical trial participants who had undergone adrenal medulla cell transplantation as a potential treatment for PD, and transplantation was found to affect the presence of these antibodies. The measurement of anti-glutamic acid decarboxylase (GAD) antibodies also serves to illustrate a potential use of biomarkers in clinical trials – that of detecting potentially undesirable outcomes. When the first human phase 1 study of GAD gene therapy was performed in PD, a potential concern was that a "host" immune response might be mounted. Serum samples from participants with PD in this open-label trial were therefore tested for the presence of neutralizing antibodies. No induction of such antibodies was observed over the 1-year clinical trial period [86]. Although these are two isolated examples, it should stimulate more thoughtful inclusion of antibody measures in future clinical trials that involve the introduction of a "foreign" biological material. Recently, the existence of anti-α-synuclein antibodies has also been associated with PD [87, 88].

Untargeted approaches: the "omics"

In contrast to the targeted markers discussed above, the "omics" approach makes use of emerging technologies and bioinformatics for unbiased and systematic evaluation of patterns of variations in RNAs (transcriptomics), proteins (proteomics) or small molecules (metabolomics), and has been highly promising as a means to develop disease biomarkers in neurodegenerative diseases including PD [89]. Sophisticated statistical methods allow large amounts of data to be organized for data mining and informatics, making these techniques potentially extremely powerful. In general, "omics" offers the possibility for identification of one or more species (protein, peptide, RNA or small molecule) or a composite "fingerprint" that could potentially reflect disease progression and/or response to a specific treatment. Although early in application to PD, those studies that have successfully identified potential PD biomarkers are outlined below. Most of the findings described still require independent validation, are cross-sectional and are focused on markers that differ between PD and healthy or disease controls. Longitudinal changes and changes in response to treatment remain to be investigated in the majority of cases. At the present time, "omics" studies remain highly technically challenging.

Transcriptomics

The transcriptome comprises all mRNAs present in a given sample and therefore reflects both transcription from DNA and post-transcriptional regulation. Transcript patterns are determined using high-throughput microarray techniques, and multiple studies have demonstrated disruption of gene expression in PD brain tissue [90–92], providing hope that such changes may be reflected in the CSF and/or blood. There are now multiple studies that support this possibility. Grunblatt *et al.* [91] selected 12 candidate transcripts upon differential expression in brain tissue, and used quantitative reverse transcription PCR to demonstrate that the combination of transcripts (encoding proteasome subunit-α type 2, laminin β-2, aldehyde dehydrogenase 1 family-member A1 and histone cluster-1 H3e) in blood achieved a sensitivity and specificity of over 80% for association with PD. A case–control study of 66 subjects similarly defined a combination of eight transcripts whose levels were associated with risk of PD, and these results were then validated in a smaller set of independent samples [94]. Many transcripts identified in such studies fit into known pathways: for example, in a study of 22 mRNAs found to differ between PD and controls, the co-chaperone ST13 stands out as a stabilizer of heat-shock protein 70, known to modify α-synuclein misfolding and toxicity, among numerous other roles. Differences are evident in early PD: for example, transcriptomic analysis of blood samples identified altered levels in p19 S-phase kinase-associated protein 1A, huntingtin-interacting protein-2, aldehyde dehydrogenase family 1 subfamily A1, 19S proteasomal protein PSMC4 and heat-shock 70 kDa protein 8 [95]. A panel of these transcripts had high sensitivity and specificity in identifying PD cases, was validated in advanced PD and was unaffected by medication status. Regarding the utility of defining a response to treatment, although the above study found no difference according to PD medication, other studies have found a number of effects of antidepressant and antipsychotic medications on transcripts with potential effects in PD [96]. Lithium and bupropion, for example, downregulate brain-derived neurotrophic factor (*BDNF*) transcripts, and amitriptyline upregulates the dopamine-receptor D2 (*DRD2*) and *DRD3* genes. These provide a proof of principle that changes in the transcriptome might be sensitive and informative to treatment interventions. Perhaps defining transcriptome responses to potential neuroprotectants might be informative in future studies as a measure of target pathway engagement.

Proteomics

Proteomic analysis involves separation of the protein or peptide constellation of a given biosample, followed by their identification by mass spectrometry-based techniques and advanced bioinformatics to determine species or combinations of species that may be associated with a specific state. The first proteomics study in PD used two-dimensional gel electrophoresis in substantia nigra pars compacta extracts to identify a set of nine proteins that were differentially expressed in PD compared with healthy controls [97], and further analysis increased this number to 221 [98]. The study is encouraging in identifying proteins likely to be involved in PD pathogenesis, such as glutathione S-transferase and other genes involved in glutathione metabolism, and suggests that these are worthy of more targeted studies. In a separate study by Abdi et al. [99], over 1500 CSF proteins were analyzed using isobaric tagging for relative and absolute protein quantification (iTRAQ), followed by mass spectrometry in samples from individuals with PD (clinical diagnosis), DLB (autopsy confirmed), AD (autopsy confirmed) and controls. Seventy-two of these manifested altered expression in PD. Matrix-assisted laser desorption/ionization time-of-flight mass spectrometry (MALDI-TOF MS) has also been used to identify a set of proteins that are differentially expressed between PD and controls [1, 100, 101]. Furthermore, recent analysis of proteins captured by magnetic bead-based weak cation exchange followed by MALDI-TOF MS identified a combination of five biomarkers discriminating PD and healthy controls with high sensitivity (85%) and specificity (70%) in a blinded analysis [102]. Other approaches, including two-dimensional gel electrophoresis and MS, are also highly encouraging that differentiation of PD is possible on the basis of such proteomic fingerprints [103, 104].

These potential markers have yet to be examined in longitudinal cohorts, and how they respond to PD treatment is unknown. However, a recent proteomic analysis of CSF obtained from a small number of subjects before and after deep-brain stimulation therapy for PD involved two-dimensional differential gel electrophoresis, in combination with MALDI-TOF and tandem TOF MS, or electrospray ionization MS. The investigators determined that two proteins, extracellular superoxide dismutase (SOD) and tetranectin, were significantly elevated in samples taken after DBS [105]. In one patient, a further CSF sample was analyzed with the stimulator present but turned off, and it was found that extracellular SOD and tetranectin had now declined. The authors suggested that changes were therefore due to stimulation. This is a highly preliminary observation but nonetheless suggests that proteomic analysis will be sensitive enough to detect at least some treatment-related changes.

Metabolomics

Metabolomic analysis focuses on the array of low-molecular-weight species in a given sample, usually CSF or plasma. Metabolomic profiling using plasma samples has now been used to successfully distinguish subjects with PD versus healthy controls using high-performance liquid chromatography with electrochemical coulometric array detection to quantitatively assess approximately 2000 small analytes [64]. In a small number of samples (PD nonmedicated: $n = 15$; control: $n = 25$) metabolomics analysis was able to completely distinguish the two groups ($P < 0.01$). Using this same platform, it was demonstrated that individuals with idiopathic PD and leucine-rich repeat kinase 2 (LRRK2)-associated PD could also be distinguished from each other and from control subjects on the basis of their metabolomics profile [75]. As discussed above, when examining levels of individual analytes, urate was found to be lower in idiopathic and LRRK2 PD than in control samples [64, 75]. A smaller, nonstatistically significant decrease was measured in LRRK2 nonmanifesting carriers [75], leaving the question as to whether this would be a helpful premotor-phase tool unanswered. Other specific purine metabolites (hypoxanthine, HVA:xanthine ratio, xanthosine:xanthine ratio) have been demonstrated to be significantly reduced in a small number of unmedicated PD patients versus controls [75]. Although most of these metabolomics analyses did not involve a longitudinal component, in one study, as noted earlier, metabolomic analysis was instrumental in detecting HVA:xanthine ratio abnormalities in PD that changed with disease progression over a 2-year period [13, 14].

Conclusions and future directions

Development of validated PD biomarkers to track disease progression or measure responses to therapeutic interventions is increasingly recognized as a critical need in identifying and developing new treatments. It is concerning that encouraging preclinical data regarding neuroprotection has not yet translated to disease modification in clinical trials. Biomarker development will take several steps, from discovery, to small- to medium-scale studies in cross-sectional cohorts, through to large-scale prospective studies in which ideally the biomarker performance will be compared with relevant clinical endpoints. The examples mentioned above have not yet reached the final stages of validation, and since many candidates will likely fail at one of these steps of development, a healthy pipeline is needed. However, although we are not yet at the point of having identified surrogate markers for clinical trials, there are a number of candidate markers that are ready for incorporation into larger trials.

At the present time, we seem to be closer to having diagnostic biomarkers rather than progression biomarkers. This reflects work in largely cross-sectional analyses of patients, usually compared with healthy controls or disease controls. A focus on longitudinal studies will be now be needed to examine performance over time. However, the search for a marker of progression should not be limited to those that are useful in diagnosis. Abnormalities in certain protein levels, such as tau or α-synuclein, may not be specific for PD but might provide valuable information on progression. Furthermore, it is important to appreciate that a single marker will likely not suffice. A marker of motor progression may well be different from a marker of progressive cognitive decline. Matching the right biomarker to the required task of measuring a clinical trial outcome will be critical, and in the immediate future it seems logical to include candidate biomarkers in clinical trials where appropriate as exploratory measures. It may be advisable to develop a battery of validated biomarkers that would be standardized for use in diverse clinical trials, thus allowing comparison across studies, similar to the concept of the NIH Toolbox, which incorporates "standard" clinical measures for assessment of neurological and behavioral function [106]. A biomarker "kit" for defining changes in various aspects of PD, including motor and nonmotor features, could be envisioned.

The use of surrogate markers has been established in other fields from a regulatory perspective, for example antihypertensive drugs, or agents that lower cholesterol. A recent FDA draft guideline (http://www.fda.gov/downloads/Drugs/GuidanceCom-pliance RegulatoryInformation/Guidances/UCM338287.pdf) has kick-started discussion of biomarkers in AD drug development [107]. Furthermore, a recent report from the EU/US/CTAD Task Force included recommendations on obtaining evidence of target engagement as well as downstream effects on biomarkers prior to beginning large phase III studies [108]. If this is to progress in the field of PD research, there remain some critical needs. A major issue remains variability between laboratory measures. For example, in AD a study of measures from 84 laboratories indicated too much variability to determine cut-off values [109]. Efforts have therefore been initiated to harmonize and standardize laboratory protocols and sample collection. For example, the Alzheimer's Association created the Global Biomarkers Standardization Consortium (GBSC) in 2010, bringing together representatives from academia, industry and the regulatory community [110]. The Human Plasma Proteome Project (HPPP; http://www.hupo.org/initiatives/plasma-proteome-project) is addressing the need for standard operating procedures in this area. There will also be issues of sensitivity to change, floor and ceiling effects, and precise definition of the appropriate situation to apply a given biomarker, for example disease stage, or which feature of the disease is of interest.

If such markers can be successfully identified, this will revolutionize drug development in PD, exploratory testing as part of a go/no go decision process, and phase 3 clinical trials for neuroprotection. Biomarkers that measure undesirable effects, such as antibody production in response to particular therapies, will also be useful in contributing to our understanding of the full complement of a treatment effect, possibly prompting enhancements of that therapy. Ultimately, biomarkers are desirable for application in premotor PD, as part of the strategy to develop and implement neuroprotective/preventative interventions in at-risk populations. In the future, it is predicted that the incorporation of appropriate biomarkers may not only enhance the number of treatments available but may well open the door to theragnosis in PD, with more informed and precise treatment improving patient outcomes.

References

1. Biomarkers Definitions Working Group. Biomarkers and surrogate endpoints: preferred definitions and conceptual framework. *Clin Pharmacol Ther* 2001; **69**: 89–95.
2. Parkinson Study Group. Dopamine transporter brain imaging to assess the effects of pramipexole vs

levodopa on Parkinson disease progression. *JAMA* 2002; **287**: 1653–61.

3. Whone AL, Watts RL, Stoessl AJ, *et al.* Slower progression of Parkinson's disease with ropinirole versus levodopa: the REAL-PET study. *Ann Neurol* 2003; **54**: 93–101.

4. Fahn S, Oakes D, Shoulson I, *et al.* Levodopa and the progression of Parkinson's disease. *N Engl J Med* 2004; **351**: 2498–508.

5. Freed CR, Greene PE, Breeze RE, *et al.* Transplantation of embryonic dopamine neurons for severe Parkinson's disease. *N Engl J Med* 2001; **344**: 710–19.

6. Olanow CW, Goetz CG, Kordower JH, *et al.* A double-blind controlled trial of bilateral fetal nigral transplantation in Parkinson's disease. *Ann Neurol* 2003; **54**: 403–14.

7. Feigin A, Kaplitt MG, Tang C, *et al.* Modulation of metabolic brain networks after subthalamic gene therapy for Parkinson's disease. *Proc Natl Acad Sci U S A* 2007; **104**: 19559–64.

8. Parkinson Progression Marker Initiative. The Parkinson Progression Marker Initiative (PPMI). *Prog Neurobiol* 2011; **95**: 629–35.

9. Kang UJ, Alcalay R, Goldman JG, *et al.* The BioFIND study (Fox Investigation for New Discovery of Biomarkers in Parkinson's disease): design and methodology. *Neurology* 2014; **10** (Suppl.): P4.043.

10. Parkinson Study Group. DATATOP: a decade of neuroprotective inquiry. Deprenyl And Tocopherol Antioxidative Therapy Of Parkinsonism. *Ann Neurol* 1998; **44**: S160–6.

11. Gerlach M, Maetzler W, Broich K, *et al.* Biomarker candidates of neurodegeneration in Parkinson's disease for the evaluation of disease-modifying therapeutics. *J Neural Transm* 2012; **119**: 39–52.

12. Michell AW, Lewis SJ, Foltynie T, Barker RA. Biomarkers and Parkinson's disease. *Brain* 2004; **127**: 1693–705.

13. LeWitt P. Recent advances in CSF biomarkers for Parkinson's disease. *Parkinsonism Relat Disord* 2012; **18** (Suppl. 1): S49–51.

14. LeWitt P, Schultz L, Auinger P, *et al.* CSF xanthine, homovanillic acid, and their ratio as biomarkers of Parkinson's disease. *Brain Res* 2011; **1408**: 88–97.

15. Zhou G, Miura Y, Shoji H, Yamada S, Matsuishi T. Platelet monoamine oxidase B and plasma β-phenylethylamine in Parkinson's disease. *J Neurol Neurosurg Psychiatry* 2001; **70**: 229–31.

16. Barbanti P, Fabbrini G, Ricci A, *et al.* Increased expression of dopamine receptors on lymphocytes in Parkinson's disease. *Mov Disord* 1999; **14**: 764–71.

17. Gui YX, Wan Y, Xiao Q, *et al.* Verification of expressions of Kir2 as potential peripheral biomarkers in lymphocytes from patients with Parkinson's disease. *Neurosci Lett* 2011; **505**: 104–8.

18. Iwanaga K, Wakabayashi K, Yoshimoto M, *et al.* Lewy body-type degeneration in cardiac plexus in Parkinson's and incidental Lewy body diseases. *Neurology* 1999; **52**: 1269–71.

19. Minguez-Castellanos A, Chamorro CE, Escamilla-Sevilla F, *et al.* Do α-synuclein aggregates in autonomic plexuses predate Lewy body disorders? A cohort study. *Neurology* 2007; **68**: 2012–18.

20. Beach TG, Adler CH, Dugger BN, *et al.* Submandibular gland biopsy for the diagnosis of Parkinson disease. *J Neuropathol Exp Neurol* 2013; **72**: 130–6.

21. Wang N, Gibbons CH, Lafo J, *et al.* α-Synuclein in cutaneous autonomic nerves. *Neurology* 2013; **81**: 1604–10.

22. El-Agnaf OM, Salem SA, Paleologou KE, *et al.* Detection of oligomeric forms of α-synuclein protein in human plasma as a potential biomarker for Parkinson's disease. *Faseb J* 2006; **20**: 419–25.

23. Tinsley RB, Kotschet K, Modesto D, *et al.* Sensitive and specific detection of α-synuclein in human plasma. *J Neurosci Res* 2010; **88**: 2693–700.

24. Foulds PG, Mitchell JD, Parker A, *et al.* Phosphorylated α-synuclein can be detected in blood plasma and is potentially a useful biomarker for Parkinson's disease. *FASEB J* 2011; **25**: 4127–37.

25. Tokuda T, Salem SA, Allsop D, *et al.* Decreased α-synuclein in cerebrospinal fluid of aged individuals and subjects with Parkinson's disease. *Biochem Biophys Res Commun* 2006; **349**: 162–6.

26. Lee PH, Lee G, Park HJ, *et al.* The plasma α-synuclein levels in patients with Parkinson's disease and multiple system atrophy. *J Neural Transm* 2006; **113**: 1435–9.

27. Shi M, Zabetian CP, Hancock AM, *et al.* Significance and confounders of peripheral DJ-1 and α-synuclein in Parkinson's disease. *Neuroscience Lett* 2010; **480**: 78–82.

28. Li QX, Mok SS, Laughton KM, *et al.* Plasma α-synuclein is decreased in subjects with Parkinson's disease. *Exp Neurol* 2007; **204**: 583–8.

29. Ohrfelt A, Grognet P, Andreasen N, *et al.* Cerebrospinal fluid α-synuclein in neurodegenerative disorders-a marker of synapse loss? *Neurosci Lett* 2009; **450**: 332–5.

30. Hong Z, Shi M, Chung K, *et al.* DJ-1 and α-synuclein in human cerebrospinal fluid as biomarkers of Parkinson's disease. *Brain* 2010; **133**: 713–26.

31. Waragai M, Sekiyama K, Sekigawa A, *et al.* α-Synuclein and DJ-1 as potential biological fluid biomarkers for Parkinson's Disease. *Int J Mol Sci* 2010; **11**: 4257–66.

32. Mollenhauer B, Locascio JJ, Schulz-Schaeffer W, *et al.* α-Synuclein and tau concentrations in cerebrospinal fluid of patients presenting with parkinsonism: a cohort study. *Lancet Neurol* 2011; **10**: 230–40.

33. Wennstrom M, Surova Y, Hall S, et al. Low CSF levels of both α-synuclein and the α-synuclein cleaving enzyme neurosin in patients with synucleinopathy. *PLoS One* 2013; **8**: e53250.

34. Hall S, Ohrfelt A, Constantinescu R, et al. Accuracy of a panel of 5 cerebrospinal fluid biomarkers in the differential diagnosis of patients with dementia and/or parkinsonian disorders. *Arch Neurol* 2012; **69**: 1445–52.

35. Kang JH, Irwin DJ, Chen-Plotkin AS, et al. Association of cerebrospinal fluid beta-amyloid 1–42, T-tau, P-tau181, and α-synuclein levels with clinical features of drug-naive patients with early Parkinson disease. *JAMA Neurol* 2013; **70**: 1277–87.

36. Mollenhauer B, Trautmann E, Taylor P, et al. Total CSF α-synuclein is lower in de novo Parkinson patients than in healthy subjects. *Neurosci Lett* 2013; **532**: 44–8.

37. Shi M, Bradner J, Hancock AM, et al. Cerebrospinal fluid biomarkers for Parkinson disease diagnosis and progression. *Ann Neurol* 2011; **69**: 570–80.

38. Stewart T, Liu C, Ginghina C, et al. Cerebrospinal fluid α-synuclein predicts cognitive decline in Parkinson disease progression in the DATATOP cohort. *Am J Pathol* 2014; **184**: 966–75.

39. Masliah E, Rockenstein E, Adame A, et al. Effects of α-synuclein immunization in a mouse model of Parkinson's disease. *Neuron* 2005; **46**: 857–68.

40. Masliah E, Rockenstein E, Mante M, et al. Passive immunization reduces behavioral and neuropathological deficits in an α-synuclein transgenic model of Lewy body disease. *PLoS One* 2011; **6**: e19338.

41. Nasstrom T, Goncalves S, Sahlin C, et al. Antibodies against α-synuclein reduce oligomerization in living cells. *PLoS One* 2011; **6**: e27230.

42. Blennow K, Zetterberg H, Rinne JO, et al. Effect of immunotherapy with bapineuzumab on cerebrospinal fluid biomarker levels in patients with mild to moderate Alzheimer disease. *Arch Neurol* 2012; **69**: 1002–10.

43. Salloway S, Sperling R, Fox NC, et al. Two phase 3 trials of bapineuzumab in mild-to-moderate Alzheimer's disease. *N Engl J Med* 2014; **370**: 322–33.

44. Farlow M, Arnold SE, van Dyck CH, et al. Safety and biomarker effects of solanezumab in patients with Alzheimer's disease. *Alzheimers Dement* 2012; **8**: 261–71.

45. Doody RS, Thomas RG, Farlow M, et al. Phase 3 trials of solanezumab for mild-to-moderate Alzheimer's disease. *N Engl J Med* 2014; **370**: 311–21.

46. Maita C, Tsuji S, Yabe I, et al. Secretion of DJ-1 into the serum of patients with Parkinson's disease. *Neurosci Lett* 2008; **431**: 86–9.

47. Waragai M, Nakai M, Wei J, et al. Plasma levels of DJ-1 as a possible marker for progression of sporadic Parkinson's disease. *Neurosci Lett* 2007; **425**: 18–22.

48. Waragai M, Wei J, Fujita M, et al. Increased level of DJ-1 in the cerebrospinal fluids of sporadic Parkinson's disease. *Biochem Biophys Res Commun* 2006; **345**: 967–72.

49. Lin X, Cook TJ, Zabetian CP, et al. DJ-1 isoforms in whole blood as potential biomarkers of Parkinson disease. *Sci Rep* 2012; **2**: 954.

50. Saito Y, Hamakubo T, Yoshida Y, et al. Preparation and application of monoclonal antibodies against oxidized DJ-1. Significant elevation of oxidized DJ-1 in erythrocytes of early-stage Parkinson disease patients. *Neurosci Lett* 2009; **465**: 1–5.

51. Rosén C, Hansson O, Blennow K, Zetterberg H. Fluid biomarkers in Alzheimer's disease – current concepts. *Mol Neurodegener* 2013; **8**: 20–31.

52. Maarouf CL, Beach TG, Adler CH, et al. Quantitative appraisal of ventricular cerebrospinal fluid biomarkers in neuropathologically diagnosed Parkinson's disease cases lacking Alzheimer's disease pathology. *Biomark Insights* 2013; **8**: 19–28.

53. Siderowf A, Xie SX, Hurtig H, et al. CSF amyloid β1–42 predicts cognitive decline in Parkinson disease. *Neurology* 2010; **75**: 1055–61.

54. Wang Y, Hancock AM, Bradner J, et al. Complement 3 and factor h in human cerebrospinal fluid in Parkinson's disease, Alzheimer's disease, and multiple-system atrophy. *Am J Pathol* 2011; **178**: 1509–16.

55. Leverenz JB, Watson GS, Shofer J, et al. Cerebrospinal fluid biomarkers and cognitive performance in non-demented patients with Parkinson's disease. *Parkinsonism Relat Disord* 2011; **17**: 61–4.

56. Henchcliffe C, Beal MF. Mitochondrial biology and oxidative stress in Parkinson disease pathogenesis. *Nat Clin Pract Neurol* 2008; **4**: 600–9.

57. Hauser DN, Hastings TG. Mitochondrial dysfunction and oxidative stress in Parkinson's disease and monogenic parkinsonism. *Neurobiol Dis* 2013; **51**: 35–42.

58. Younes-Mhenni S, Frih-Ayed M, Kerkeni A, Bost M, Chazot G. Peripheral blood markers of oxidative stress in Parkinson's disease. *Eur Neurol* 2007; **58**: 78–83.

59. Götz ME, Gerstner A, Harth R, et al. Altered redox state of platelet coenzyme Q10 in Parkinson's disease. *J Neural Transm* 2000; **107**: 41–8.

60. Sohmiya M, Tanaka M, Tak NW, et al. Redox status of plasma coenzyme Q10 indicates elevated systemic oxidative stress in Parkinson's disease. *J Neurol Sci* 2004; **223**: 161–6.

61. Isobe C, Abe T, Terayama Y. Levels of reduced and oxidized coenzymeQ-10 and 8-hydroxy-2'-deoxyguanosine in the cerebrospinal fluid of patients with living Parkinson's disease demonstrate that mitochondrial oxidative damage and/or oxidative DNA damage contributes to the neurodegenerative process. *Neurosci Lett* 2010; **469**: 159–63.

62. Ilic TV, Jovanovic M, Jovicic A, Tomovic M. Oxidative stress indicators are elevated in de novo Parkinson's disease patients. *Funct Neurol* 1999; **14**: 141–7.

63. Seet RC, Lee CY, Lim EC, et al. Oxidative damage in Parkinson disease: Measurement using accurate biomarkers. *Free Radic Biol Med* 2010; **48**: 560–6.

64. Bogdanov M, Matson WR, Wang L, et al. Metabolomic profiling to develop blood biomarkers for Parkinson's disease. *Brain* 2008; **131**: 389–96.

65. Gmitterova K, Heinemann U, Gawinecka J, et al. 8-OHdG in cerebrospinal fluid as a marker of oxidative stress in various neurodegenerative diseases. *Neurodegener Dis* 2009; **6**: 263–9.

66. Andreux PA, Houtkooper RH, Auwerx J. Pharmacological approaches to restore mitochondrial function. *Nat Rev Drug Discov* 2013; **12**: 465–83.

67. Seet RC, Lim EC, Tan JJ, et al. Effects of high-dose coenzyme Q10 on biomarkers of oxidative damage and clinical outcomes in Parkinson disease. *Antioxidants & Redox Signaling* 2014; **21**: 211–17.

68. Cipriani S, Desjardins CA, Burdett TC, et al. Urate and its transgenic depletion modulate neuronal vulnerability in a cellular model of Parkinson's disease. *PLoS One* 2012; **7**: e37331.

69. Gong L, Zhang QL, Zhang N, et al. Neuroprotection by urate on 6-OHDA-lesioned rat model of Parkinson's disease: linking to Akt/GSK3β signaling pathway. *J Neurochem* 2012; **123**: 876–85.

70. Chen X, Burdett TC, Desjardins CA, et al. Disrupted and transgenic urate oxidase alter urate and dopaminergic neurodegeneration. *Proc Natl Acad Sci U S A* 2013; **110**: 300–5.

71. Cipriani S, ChenX, Schwarzschild MA. Urate: a novel biomarker of Parkinson's disease risk, diagnosis and prognosis. *Biomark Med* 4: 701–12.

72. Ascherio A, LeWitt PA, Xu K, et al. Urate as a predictor of the rate of clinical decline in Parkinson disease. *Arch Neurol* 2009; **66**: 1460–8.

73. Schwarzschild MA, Schwid SR, Marek K, et al. Serum urate as a predictor of clinical and radiographic progression in Parkinson disease. *Arch Neurol* 2008; **65**: 716–23.

74. The Parkinson Study Group. Inosine to increase serum and cerebrospinal fluid urate in Parkinson disease: a randomized clinical trial. *JAMA Neurol* 2014; **71**: 141–50.

75. Johansen KK, Wang L, Aasly JO, et al. Metabolomic profiling in LRRK2-related Parkinson's disease. *PLoS One* 2009; **4**: e7551.

76. Rentzos M, Nikolaou C, Andreadou E, et al. Circulating interleukin-15 and RANTES chemokine in Parkinson's disease. *Acta Neurol Scand* 2007; **116**: 374–9.

77. Dufek M, Hamanova M, Lokaj J, et al. Serum inflammatory biomarkers in Parkinson's disease. *Parkinsonism Relat Disord* 2009; **15**: 318–20.

78. Mogi M, Harada M, Riederer P, et al. Tumor necrosis factor-α (TNF-α) increases both in the brain and in the cerebrospinal fluid from parkinsonian patients. *Neurosci Lett* 1994; **165**: 208–10.

79. Barnum CJ, Tansey MG. Neuroinflammation and non-motor symptoms: the dark passenger of Parkinson's disease? *Curr Neurol Neurosci Rep* 2012; **12**: 350–8.

80. Rocha NP, Teixeira AL, Scalzo PL, et al. Plasma levels of soluble tumor necrosis factor receptors are associated with cognitive performance in Parkinson's disease. *Mov Disord* 2014; **29**: 527–31.

81. Lindqvist D, Hall S, Surova Y, et al. Cerebrospinal fluid inflammatory markers in Parkinson's disease – associations with depression, fatigue, and cognitive impairment. *Brain Behav Immun* 2013; **33**: 183–9.

82. Hisanaga K, Asagi M, Itoyama Y, Iwasaki Y. Increase in peripheral CD4 bright+ CD8 dull+ T cells in Parkinson disease. *Arch Neurol* 2001; **58**: 1580–3.

83. Fiszer U, Mix E, Fredrikson S, Kostulas V, Link H. Parkinson's disease and immunological abnormalities: increase of HLA-DR expression on monocytes in cerebrospinal fluid and of CD45RO+ T cells in peripheral blood. *Acta Neurol Scand* 1994; **90**: 160–6.

84. Double KL, Rowe DB, Carew-Jones FM, et al. Anti-melanin antibodies are increased in sera in Parkinson's disease. *Exp Neurol* 2009; **217**: 297–301.

85. McRae-Degueurce A, Klawans HL, Penn RD, et al. An antibody in the CSF of Parkinson's disease patients disappears following adrenal medulla transplantation. *Neurosci Lett* 1988; **94**: 192–7.

86. Kaplitt MG, Feigin A, Tang C, et al. Safety and tolerability of gene therapy with an adeno-associated virus (AAV) borne GAD gene for Parkinson's disease: an open label, phase I trial. *Lancet* 2007; **369**: 2097–105.

87. Papachroni KK, Ninkina N, Papapanagiotou A, et al. Autoantibodies to α-synuclein in inherited Parkinson's disease. *J Neurochem* 2007; **101**: 749–56.

88. Yanamandra K, Gruden MA, Casaite V, et al. α-synuclein reactive antibodies as diagnostic biomarkers in blood sera of Parkinson's disease patients. *PLoS One* 2011; **6**: e18513.

89. Caudle WM, Bammler TK, Lin Y, Pan S, Zhang J. Using 'omics' to define pathogenesis and biomarkers of Parkinson's disease. *Expert Rev Neurother* 2010; **10**: 925–42.

90. Grunblatt E, Mandel S, Jacob-Hirsch J, et al. Gene expression profiling of parkinsonian substantia nigra pars compacta; alterations in ubiquitin-proteasome, heat shock protein, iron and oxidative stress regulated proteins, cell adhesion/cellular matrix and vesicle trafficking genes. *J Neural Transm* 2004; **111**: 1543–73.

91. Moran LB, Graeber MB. Towards a pathway definition of Parkinson's disease: a complex disorder with links to

cancer, diabetes and inflammation. *Neurogenetics* 2008; **9**: 1–13.
92. Sutherland GT, Matigian NA, Chalk AM, et al. A cross-study transcriptional analysis of Parkinson's disease. *PLoS One* 2009; **4**: e4955.
93. Grunblatt E, Zehetmayer S, Jacob CP, et al. Pilot study: peripheral biomarkers for diagnosing sporadic Parkinson's disease. *J Neural Transm* 2010; **117**: 1387–93.
94. Scherzer CR, Eklund AC, Morse LJ, et al. Molecular markers of early Parkinson's disease based on gene expression in blood. *Proc Natl Acad Sci U S A* 2007; **104**: 955–60.
95. Molochnikov L, Rabey JM, Dobronevsky E, et al. A molecular signature in blood identifies early Parkinson's disease. *Mol Neurodegener* 2012; **7**: 26.
96. Lauterbach EC. Psychotropic drug effects on gene transcriptomics relevant to Parkinson's disease. *Prog Neuropsychopharmacol Biol Psychiatry* 2012; **38**: 107–15.
97. Basso M, Giraudo S, Corpillo D, et al. Proteome analysis of human substantia nigra in Parkinson's disease. *Proteomics* 2004; **4**: 3943–52.
98. Werner CJ, Heyny-von Haussen R, Mall G, Wolf S. Proteome analysis of human substantia nigra in Parkinson's disease. *Proteome Science* 2008; **6**: 8–22.
99. Abdi F, Quinn JF, Jankovic J, et al. Detection of biomarkers with a multiplex quantitative proteomic platform in cerebrospinal fluid of patients with neurodegenerative disorders. *J Alzheimers Dis* 2006; **9**: 293–348.
100. Jin J, Hulette C, Wang Y, et al. Proteomic identification of a stress protein, mortalin/mthsp70/GRP75: relevance to Parkinson disease. *Mol Cell Proteomics* 2006; **5**: 1193–204.
101. Pan S, Rush J, Peskind ER, et al. Application of targeted quantitative proteomics analysis in human cerebrospinal fluid using a liquid chromatography matrix-assisted laser desorption/ionization time-of-flight tandem mass spectrometer (LC MALDI TOF/TOF) platform. *J Proteome Res* 2008; **7**: 720–30.
102. Li YH, Wang J, Zheng XL, et al. Matrix-assisted laser desorption/ionization time-of-flight mass spectrometry combined with magnetic beads for detecting serum protein biomarkers in parkinson's disease. *Eur Neurol* 2011; **65**: 105–11.
103. Zhao X, Xiao WZ, Pu XP, et al. Proteome analysis of the sera from Chinese Parkinson's disease patients. *Neurosci Lett* 2010; **479**: 175–9.
104. Mila S, Albo AG, Corpillo D, et al. Lymphocyte proteomics of Parkinson's disease patients reveals cytoskeletal protein dysregulation and oxidative stress. *Biomark Med* 2009; **3**: 117–28.
105. Wang ES, Yao HB, Chen YH, et al. Proteomic analysis of the cerebrospinal fluid of Parkinson's disease patients pre- and post-deep brain stimulation. *Cell Physiol Biochem* 2013; **31**: 625–37.
106. Gershon RC, Cella D, Fox NA, et al. Assessment of neurological and behavioural function: the NIH Toolbox. *Lancet Neurolo* 2010; **9**: 138–9.
107. Kozauer N, Katz R. Regulatory innovation and drug development for early-stage Alzheimer's disease. *New Engl J Med* 2013; **368**: 1169–71.
108. Vellas B, Carrillo MC, Sampaio C, et al. Designing drug trials for Alzheimer's disease: what we have learned from the release of the phase III antibody trials: a report from the EU/US/CTAD Task Force. *Alzheimers Dement* 2013; **9**: 438–44.
109. Mattsson N, Andreasson U, Persson S, et al. CSF biomarker variability in the Alzheimer's Association quality control program. *Alzheimers Dement* 2013; **9**: 251–61.
110. Carrillo MC, Blennow K, Soares H, et al. Global standardization measurement of cerebral spinal fluid for Alzheimer's disease: an update from the Alzheimer's Association Global Biomarkers Consortium. *Alzheimers Dement* 2013; **9**: 137–40.

Chapter 25

Lessons learned: neuroprotective trials in Parkinson's disease

Isabelle Beaulieu-Boire and Anthony E. Lang

Introduction

Over the past 50 years, treatment of Parkinson's disease (PD) has greatly evolved. The arrival of levodopa (L-DOPA) as a symptomatic treatment for the dopamine deficiency of PD has markedly changed the course of PD, especially in the early years of the disease. However, as the disease evolves, motor complications such as dyskinesias and wearing off, and nonmotor symptoms including autonomic dysfunction, cognitive and behavioral changes, and sleep issues, among others, develop and eventually become the major source of disability for the patient. Currently, there are no interventions that have been proven to slow the progression of PD. It is acknowledged that neuroprotective treatment is a major unmet need in PD [1]. Multiple preclinical studies have provided considerable hope; however, translation to human clinical trials has generally proven disappointing.

Neuroprotection and disease modification are often considered synonyms; however, they refer to different concepts. Neuroprotection is defined as prevention of cell death and progression of degeneration by modification of the pathophysiological process itself, while disease modification indicates slowing of clinical progression, without regard to the mechanism. Even though this theoretical distinction exists, in clinical practice, any agent that would slow down progression of the disease would be a real breakthrough for patients and physicians dealing with PD.

In this chapter, we will discuss the limitations in investigating neuroprotective agents. We will describe the strengths and weaknesses of measures to document the progression of PD, clinical trial designs and animal models. We will also review the main clinical trials that have been done in this field and the lessons that have been learned, and how the resulting expanding knowledge and experience may be applied to future studies.

Limitations of neuroprotective studies

No candidate for neuroprotection has yet shown unequivocal positive results in clinical studies. There are many limitations to studying neuroprotective agents in PD [2–4]. First, there are no validated methods for quantifying progression of the disease. Usual endpoints in studies include clinical rating scales such as the Unified Parkinson's Disease Rating Scale (UPDRS), or time to a clinical event such as the need for symptomatic treatment. However, these endpoints do not reflect the whole disease process and may be influenced by symptomatic effects of therapeutic agents. Imaging studies have been developed as surrogate markers, but none of these has been shown to accurately predict disease progression.

Design of clinical trials has proven challenging, especially when it comes to differentiating symptomatic effects from true neuroprotection. Any clinical difference at the end of the study period in trials involving parallel groups may be explained by symptomatic or disease-modifying effects, and the distinction cannot be made simply on the basis of these results. Washout designs have been used to minimize this problem; however, the duration of the washout period is limited for ethical reasons, and the time frame for elimination of symptomatic effects is not clearly defined. The delayed-start design has been conceived specifically for neuroprotection studies, and although it probably remains the best way to investigate neuroprotective candidates, some argue that this method has major drawbacks [5].

The choice of which population to study has been questioned. Most studies choose to test neuroprotective candidates in early PD patients, although some argue

Parkinson's Disease: Current and Future Therapeutics and Clinical Trials, ed. Gálvez-Jiménez et al. Published by Cambridge University Press. © Cambridge University Press 2016.

that these patients may already be too far advanced in the disease process to benefit from neuroprotective interventions, as the symptoms of PD are known to appear only after >30–50% of substantia nigra dopaminergic cells are lost [6]. However, including pre-symptomatic cases presents a major challenge since we still do not have reliable predictive biomarkers, and concentrating on very early PD patients carries the risk of selecting patients with an alternative diagnosis (i.e. another degenerative type of parkinsonism), or cases that do not actually have degenerative parkinsonism, as approximately 15% of patients in clinical studies are shown to have negative dopamine imaging (SWEDDs, i.e. scans without evidence of dopamine deficits) [7–9].

Moreover, the lack of a good animal model makes preclinical studies difficult to apply in a PD population. There is currently no animal model that accurately reflects the whole evolution of idiopathic PD, and it has been argued that this is the main reason for the failure of animal studies to translate into human trials. The therapeutic dose range is also difficult to predict, as uncertainty about bioavailability and passage through the blood–brain barrier further complicate application to clinical trials. Thus, the types of biomarkers needed to confirm pathogenic models and assist in defining necessary drug doses include markers of the disease trait itself for accurate diagnosis, and markers of the severity or state of the disease to monitor the disease course and the effects of treatment, as well as markers of target engagement of the therapeutic intervention.

Finally, our incomplete understanding of the pathophysiology of PD almost certainly accounts for the difficulties in finding an effective neuroprotective agent. Indeed, there might be different mechanisms involved at the beginning of the disease compared with during its evolution, and a molecule may be effective early in the evolution but not as the disease progresses. Furthermore, cell death may be due to multiple mechanisms, and a cocktail of neuroprotective agents might be needed to obtain significant benefit.

Methods to evaluate progression of Parkinson's disease

Clinical measures

In the perspective of studying neuroprotective effects in PD, there is a crucial need for validated markers of disease progression. Clinical trials have so far focused mainly on progression of symptoms and signs on a clinical rating scale (UPDRS) or the time to requiring symptomatic treatment. However, as stated above, neither of these measures reflects the whole constellation of clinical features of patients with PD. The UPDRS mainly emphasizes motor features, and although a new clinical scale has been developed by the Movement Disorders Society (MDS-UPDRS) [10], with more focus on nonmotor features, it has not yet been used in neuroprotection trials. Furthermore, there is no consensus on the definition of minimal clinically significant changes on the UPDRS [11], and aspects of this scale have low inter-rater reliability [12]. Furthermore, clinical ratings are subject to the effects of placebo [13] and, obviously, of symptomatic treatment, which complicates the design of neuroprotective trials.

In some studies, the primary outcome measure was time to a clinical event, such as time to needing a symptomatic treatment. This type of outcome is often confounded, because the decision to start symptomatic treatment is dependent on many factors besides progression of symptoms, including baseline disability levels, depression, education, employment status and many others [14–16]. Longer-term measures such as time to cognitive changes or loss of ambulation may be used, but again they are subject to the effects of different variables, including the effects of symptomatic treatment and of other comorbidities.

Biomarkers

An objective, quantifiable method for measuring progression and response to therapeutic interventions is much needed [17–19]. A biomarker that would not be influenced by the treatment, and that would reflect the progression of both clinical features and neuropathology would be ideal. Biomarkers would be useful not only to follow the progression of PD but also to assist with early diagnosis. Having a method to diagnose PD with more certainty in its earliest stages would allow inclusion of individuals in preclinical or prodromal disease stages into trials of neuroprotective therapies, before major cell loss has occurred.

Dopaminergic neuroimaging

[^{18}F]-Fluoro-L-DOPA positron emission tomography (^{18}FD-PET), which reflects dopamine nigrostriatal integrity, has been studied extensively in PD (Table 25.1). It has been shown to correlate with nigral cell counts and striatal dopamine levels in animal models of parkinsonism and in humans [20]. The decreased uptake of ^{18}FD has an anterior–posterior gradient

Table 25.1 Functional neuroimaging biomarkers

Measured function	Type of scan	Findings in PD	Changes in early PD
Presynaptic dopamine nigrostriatal integrity (DOPA decarboxylase function)	^{18}FD-PET	Decreased uptake in the striatum, anterior–posterior gradient, asymmetrical	Compensatory increase (underestimation of changes)
Dopamine transporter levels	[^{131}I]β-CIT SPECT and others	Decreased uptake in the striatum, anterior–posterior gradient, asymmetrical	Compensatory decrease (overestimation of changes)
Vesicular monoamine transporter 2 (VMAT2) levels	[^{11}C]DTBZ	Decreased uptake in the striatum, anterior–posterior gradient, asymmetrical	Less affected by regulatory changes
Glucose metabolism	^{18}FDG-PET	Hypermetabolism in putamen/thalamus/pons with hypometabolism in motor and association cortices (PD-related spatial covariance pattern)	Less affected by regulatory changes

PD, Parkinson's disease; ^{18}FD PET, [^{18}F]-fluoro-L-DOPA positron emission tomography; [^{131}I]β-CIT SPECT, [^{131}I]β-2β-carbomethoxy-3β-(4-iodophenyl)tropane single-photon-emission computed tomography; [^{11}C]DTBZ, 11-C-dihydrotetrabenazine; ^{18}FDG-PET, [^{18}F]-fluorodeoxyglucose positron emission tomography.

in the putamen, which remains present throughout the evolution of the disease [21]. The levels have been shown to correlate with clinical symptoms, mostly with bradykinesia [22]. Changes in ^{18}FD-PET have been reported as early as 6 years before onset of clinical symptoms and may therefore be a marker of early PD. However, in the early phases of the disease, there can be a compensatory increase that may underestimate nigral cell loss initially.

Evaluation of reuptake of dopamine in the synaptic cleft is done by dopamine transporter (DAT) scans, which can be labeled for both PET and single-photon-emission computerized tomography (SPECT). The most frequently used method for DAT imaging in clinical studies has been [^{131}I]β-CIT ([^{131}I]β-2β-carbomethoxy-3β-[4-iodophenyl]tropane) SPECT. The DAT levels correlate with striatal dopamine, and have been shown to decline with increased PD severity [23]. In contrast to ^{18}FD-PET, DAT levels are downregulated early in PD as a compensatory change, and this technique might therefore overestimate nigral cell loss in the early stages.

Vesicular monoamine transporter type 2 (VMAT2), which pumps recycled and newly formed dopamine into vesicles inside the presynaptic neurons, can also be used to measure dopamine function. Such studies are done with [^{11}C]dihydrotetrabenazine (DTBZ), which is nonspecific for dopamine, except in the striatum where dopamine is the main neurotransmitter that binds to [^{11}C]DTBZ. These measures are thought to be less influenced by regulatory changes and might therefore be more useful in the early disease [24].

There are many drawbacks to dopaminergic neuroimaging as a surrogate marker for PD [25]. In multiple studies, there has been a discordance between clinical and neuroimaging endpoints in clinical trials. For instance, both the REAL-PET and CALM-PD studies (see below) [9, 26] demonstrated greater improvement in symptoms with levodopa compared with dopamine agonists, while there was less decline of dopamine indices on imaging with dopamine agonists, as measured by β-CIT SPECT and ^{18}FD-PET, respectively. In the ELLDOPA study [8], which compared levodopa with placebo treatment in early PD, faster declines in β-CIT SPECT were shown in the group treated with levodopa, despite the clear clinical benefit provided by levodopa and additional evidence for less progression of disease than in the placebo group after a washout period (although this may have been too short to eliminate all of the symptomatic effect; see below). Many factors are probably involved in these results, including, most importantly, effects of the therapeutic agents on dopamine imaging. Most studies have demonstrated no change in DAT binding with dopamine agonists; however, results with levodopa treatment have been less consistent [27, 28]. Acute administration of levodopa does not seem to affect radiotracer uptake, but chronic usage of levodopa has induced downregulation of DAT imaging. Moreover, potential effects of compensatory changes in early PD have not been resolved. Furthermore, it is important to remember that dopaminergic imaging does not reflect the whole pathophysiological process of PD, which affects multiple cell groups and neurotransmitter systems.

Glucose metabolism imaging

Methods to measure the rates of glucose metabolism have also been studied in PD [29]. A specific pattern called the PD-related spatial covariance pattern is found in most patients. It is characterized by hypermetabolism of the pallidum, thalamus and pons, associated with decreased metabolism in the motor and association cortices. This pattern is directly correlated with disease severity. The combination of dopaminergic tracers and glucose metabolism imaging might be useful for assessment of early diagnosis and progression of PD.

Structural imaging
Structural imaging is generally normal in patients with PD; however, specific imaging techniques are emerging as sensitive and possibly specific measures of dysfunction in PD. Diffusion-tensor imaging is a relatively new imaging technique that evaluates the integrity of gray-matter and white-matter tracts. Measures of fractional anisotropy are consistently decreased in the substantia nigra of patients with PD [30]. There also seems to be a correlation between this measure and disease progression, as measured by the UPDRS. Findings on 3-tesla MRI and transcranial ultrasound also demonstrate abnormalities in PD, supportive of increased iron content in the substantia nigra compared with controls. Whether this correlates with disease severity and progression of the disease is currently unknown, although most evidence suggests that midbrain hyperechogenicity on transcranial ultrasound is a very early finding that changes little over the course of the disease [31].

Biochemical markers
Biochemical and molecular markers have been investigated to help with early diagnosis of PD and to follow disease progression [17]. So far, none of these biomarkers has been validated. α-Synuclein is known to aggregate in the brains of patients with PD, and levels have been shown to be decreased in the cerebrospinal fluid (CSF) of PD patients; conversely, α-synuclein oligomers are increased in blood and CSF. These markers might be useful for early diagnosis; however, studies to date find considerable overlap between PD patients and controls, and the levels do not seem to correlate with progression of disease. Amyloid-β42 ($A\beta_{1-42}$) and tau protein levels have recently been validated in the diagnosis of preclinical Alzheimer's disease (AD) [32]. In PD, abnormal levels of these markers are found, especially in patients with cognitive changes, who present with decreased $A\beta_{1-42}$ (not as low as in AD) and decreased tau (in contrast to the increased levels in AD). Other markers, such as DJ-1, urate, inflammatory cytokines and epidermal growth factor receptor, and metabolomic markers have been found to be abnormal in PD; however, they are not yet validated for clinical or research use.

Design of clinical trials
One of the major limitations in establishing neuroprotection relates to clinical trial design [33]. Most agents that have shown promise have pro-dopaminergic properties, and dissociating symptomatic from neuroprotective effects has been extremely challenging. In addition to putative direct effects on pathogenesis (e.g. antiapoptotic effects), agents that have a symptomatic effect may also induce disease modification by altering the metabolism and function of dopaminergic neurons, possibly inducing compensatory changes that decrease the progression of symptoms. Distinguishing any of these effects from pure symptomatic benefit is often very difficult. Studies of neuroprotection in PD are further limited because of the availability of highly effective symptomatic treatments, which makes leaving a patient on placebo for a long period ethically unacceptable.

Parallel-group studies
Parallel-group studies (Figure 25.1A–C), although easy to conduct, have the major drawback of being especially subject to symptomatic effects. This type of design may be effective in studying agents that lack symptomatic effects in PD. However, this is not always anticipated (as was the case with the original DATATOP trial, see below) and neuroprotective effects can be both masked by and confused with a pure symptomatic benefit.

Washout period studies
To minimize the symptomatic effects, a washout period design (Figure 25.1D–F) has been proposed and used in some studies. Assuming complete washout of the agent, this theoretically has a significant advantage over parallel-group studies. However, such trials often have limitations in the duration of the washout period, considering the availability of symptomatic treatments and the gradual progression of the disease. Moreover, patients receiving active treatment during the study may not tolerate the washout as well as those who received placebo, and this may lead to differential dropout rates in the two treatment groups. Another related problem is that it is easier to retain patients in an active-treatment arm (due to the symptomatic benefit) than in a placebo arm, and this can also lead

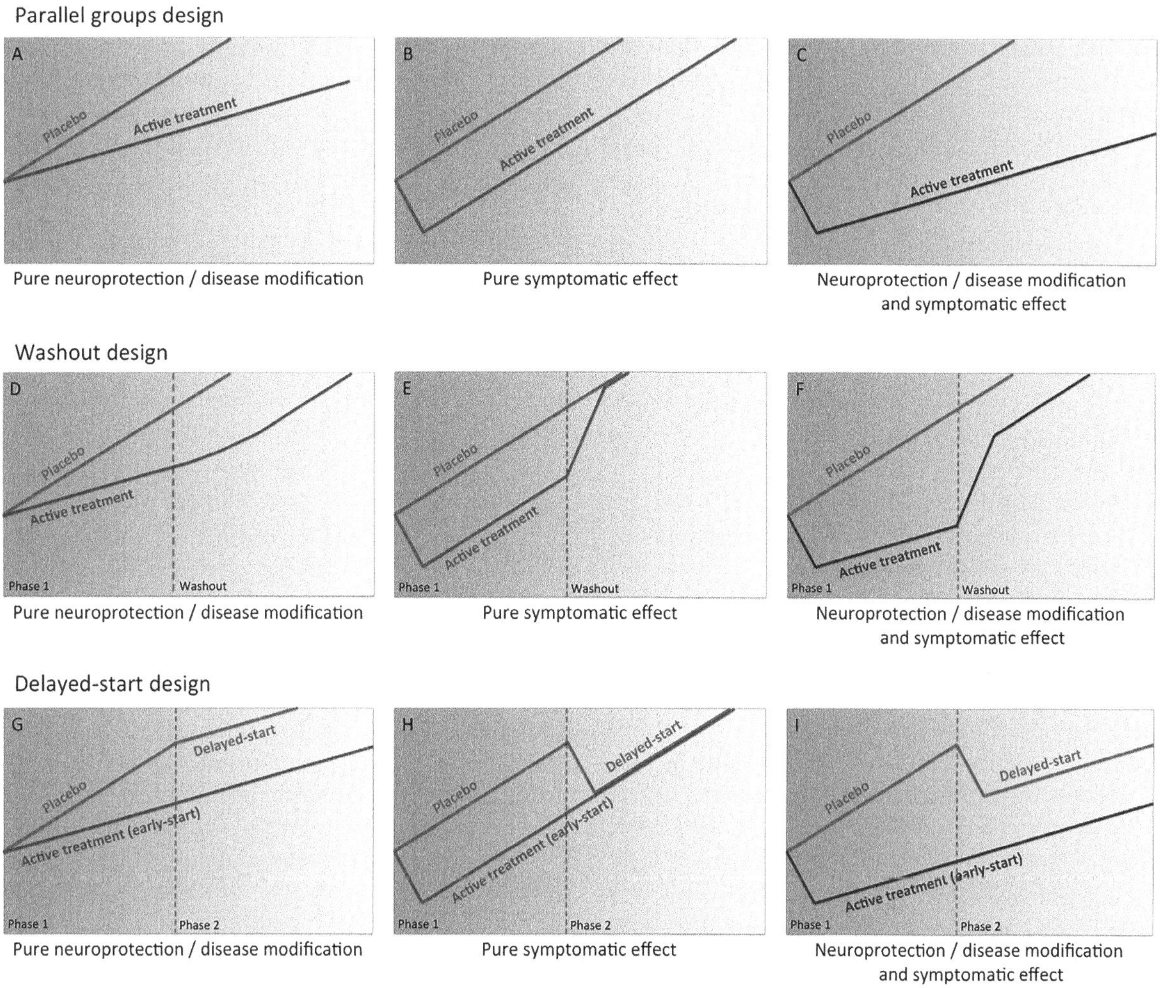

Figure 25.1 Schematic representation of the theoretical effect of neuroprotective, symptomatic, or mixed neuroprotective and symptomatic treatments compared with placebo in different study designs. The x-axis represents time and the y-axis represents the measure of progression, for instance Unified Parkinson's Disease Rating Scale (UPDRS) score. The parallel-group design (A–C), washout design (D–F) and delayed-start design (G–I) are illustrated. The placebo group is depicted as a blue line. The green lines (A, D, G) represent a pure neuroprotective agent, the red lines (B, E, H) represent a pure symptomatic agent, and the purple lines (C, F, I) represent a mixed symptomatic and neuroprotective agent (see text for details). Of note, the curves are artificially simplified; in particular, a beneficial clinical effect of the placebo (i.e. a placebo effect) is not reflected. (A black and white version of this figure will appear in some formats. For the color version, please refer to the plate section.)

to differential dropout during the trial (this is a problem with all studies that have an active versus placebo control period). Furthermore, long-term symptomatic effects persisting after the end of the washout period (as proposed in the ELLDOPA trial, see below) cannot be excluded.

Delayed-start trials

The delayed-start design (Figure 25.1G–I) was conceived with the objective of dissociating neuroprotective effects from confounding symptomatic benefits [5]. This type of study consists of two phases: in phase 1, patients are divided into placebo and active-treatment groups. The primary outcome, usually the UPDRS, is measured at the end of phase 1 to evaluate symptomatic effects, and the slope of progression is also calculated. In phase 2, patients in the placebo group are converted to active treatment, while patients in the early-treatment group maintain the same intervention. Outcomes and slopes are then analyzed the same way as in the initial phase.

The ADAGIO (Attenuation of Disease Progression with Azilect GIven Once daily) trial was the first to formally use the delayed-start design in a neuroprotective trial in PD [34]. In this study, it was determined from the outset that, to establish neuroprotective effects, the intervention had to fulfill all three of its predefined endpoints:

1. A significant difference in the primary outcome at the end of phase 2, favoring the early-treatment group, i.e. an advantage remains in early-treated patients when both groups are receiving the active intervention and the symptomatic effect is presumed to be comparable in both groups.
2. Divergent slopes of progression in phase 1 (slower progression in the early-treatment group than in the placebo group), i.e. the disease-modifying effects are increasing over time.
3. Nonconvergent slopes of progression in phase 2 (parallel slopes or slower progression in the early-treatment group), i.e. the disease-modifying effects are not lost over time.

Although this design seemed promising, many criticisms have emerged [5, 33, 35, 36]. First, the duration of the initial placebo phase is limited ethically by the availability of symptomatic treatments. If the placebo period is too short, an agent that has its maximal effect over a longer period than the duration of phase 1 might be falsely rejected and neuroprotective effects may be missed. Likewise, if the symptomatic effect takes longer to peak than the duration of phase 2, a difference at the end might be misinterpreted as neuroprotection, when in fact the delayed-treatment group has not yet reached maximal benefit. It has also been argued that inclusion criteria in these types of studies might favor slow progressors, as patients are recruited with the expectation that they will not require treatment in the next 6–9 months. This might diminish the power of the study to demonstrate neuroprotection because small changes in endpoints may not be considered statistically significant. A differential placebo response in early-treatment and delayed-treatment groups with an agent that has a symptomatic benefit may also be confused with a neuroprotective effect. Despite these shortcomings, currently this design is probably the best available method to assess neuroprotective effects in PD.

Futility studies

Because of the high number of candidates for neuroprotection, futility studies have been introduced to facilitate selection of agents that have a higher chance of obtaining positive results in phase 3 studies [37]. Futility studies use small groups of patients, which are often compared with a historic control group instead of a placebo group, in order to minimize the sample size. In these studies, the null hypothesis states that the intervention is superior to placebo. If results are positive, the null hypothesis cannot be rejected (the agent does not meet the futility threshold), and the agent can be considered for further studies. To minimize the risk of falsely considering an agent futile (and rejecting a possibly effective neuroprotective agent), the P value is usually set higher, at 0.10 or 0.15. This method minimizes costs and enables the study of more agents with minimal sample sizes. One important challenge in using this approach in PD has been the finding that historical controls may not adequately represent modern patient outcomes and so concurrent placebo groups are deemed necessary (i.e. the sample size advantage to the design no longer applies).

Large simple clinical trials

The progressive nature of PD and the availability of highly effective symptomatic treatments limit the duration of studies in untreated PD. Furthermore, the heterogeneity of clinical manifestations makes the choice of a valid endpoint for neuroprotection difficult. An intervention given over a long time period could make determination of disease modification easier, by permitting symptomatic treatment according to standard practice [33]. Endpoints such as quality of life, necessity of mechanical aids for ambulation, cognitive dysfunction or independence in activities of daily living could reflect disease modification in a more global manner.

Animal models

This topic, which is critical to developing effective neuroprotective treatment in PD, is largely beyond the scope of this chapter. We will only touch briefly on some of the more important issues.

Different types of animal models have been developed; however, none of them has accurately reproduced the complete pathophysiology of PD. The ideal animal model would have a chronic and progressive evolution, and would involve not only dopamine but also multiple other neurotransmitter systems [38]. The variable properties of neurons in different animal species are an issue, and it has been suggested that a neuroprotective agent should be demonstrated to be effective in primate models, which might be closer to human PD.

Age is possibly the most important risk factor for PD, and it should be emphasized that this is largely not considered or accounted for in current animal models.

Toxin-induced models

The most widely used models are toxin-induced models, such the as 1-methyl-4-phenyl-1,2,3,6-tetrahydropyridine (MPTP) mice and nonhuman primates, as well as the 6-hydroxydopamine (6-OHDA) rodent. These models, while useful to evaluate symptomatic treatment and induction of motor complications, are inaccurate in terms of pathophysiology for PD, and neuroprotection studies are therefore difficult to translate into human clinical trials. These models consist of an acute lesion induced by the toxin, followed by a cascade of neurotoxicity and cell death that persists and may progress despite cessation of exposure [39].

The MPTP model was thought to involve primarily the dopaminergic system and therefore to represent only dopaminergic manifestations of PD; however, other monoamines are affected to a lesser extent. The toxin 6-OHDA has less specificity for dopamine neurons, and this model requires pretreatment with selective serotonin reuptake inhibitors, tricyclic antidepressants or monoamine oxidase B (MAO-B) inhibitors to be more similar to PD. Even with these precautions, PD pathophysiology is very complex and cannot be reproduced perfectly in these models. Most notably, we now recognize a critical role for α-synuclein in the pathogenesis of most types of PD, and this is largely lacking in toxin models in current use.

Other criticisms relate to the acute nature of the lesion, which is not believed to be present in idiopathic PD. The introduction of the neuroprotective candidate agent is often made before the lesion is induced; ideally, the agent should be started once the neurodegenerative process is already underway, to more accurately reproduce clinical practice. Furthermore, the cascade of neurotoxic events might be different in toxin-exposed animals compared with idiopathic PD, and the pathological findings are also different, which again raises questions on the reliability of these animal models. One recent model that has been generating considerable interest involves the inoculation of "preformed fibrils" of α-synuclein into the brain of mice [40]. This has been shown to result in cell-to-cell spread (in a prion-like fashion) of α-synuclein pathology similar to that seen in PD [41].

Transgenic models

New animal models are based on genetic forms of PD, most notably (with respect to idiopathic PD) α-synuclein and leucine-rich repeat kinase 2 (LRRK2) [42]. These models might better represent the chronic evolution of PD compared with toxic models. However, they still do not reproduce all of the pathological features of PD, with some showing α-synuclein aggregation but no cell death, and some showing neurodegeneration but no Lewy bodies. Genetic-based models also do not accurately reproduce the presumed contribution from environmental exposures (infections, inflammation, toxins) that may be a determining factor in "sporadic" PD. Vector-based genetic models are currently in development and may be more representative of PD. This method allows the use of older animals, which decreases contributions from adaptive changes, and the chronic evolution is also more similar to PD. In addition, the possibility of injecting the vector unilaterally permits usage of the unaffected side as a control.

Results from major clinical studies

As mentioned above, currently no agent has been unequivocally proven to slow the progression of PD. Multiple studies have been conducted, some with conflicting results, but none with convincing evidence of benefit. Here, we review data from selected major clinical studies, emphasizing the important lessons learned (Table 25.2). A large number of agents have been studied in smaller trials or are currently under evaluation; the reader is referred to a recent review paper in which many more treatments are summarized [43].

Monoamine oxidase B inhibitors

DATATOP

The DATATOP (Deprenyl and Tocopherol Antioxidant Therapy of Parkinson's disease) study [44] was conducted in 800 patients with early PD. This trial involved a 2 × 2 factorial design consisting of four parallel groups: selegiline (10 mg/day) and placebo, tocopherol (2000 IU/day) and placebo, selegiline and tocopherol, or placebo and placebo. The endpoint was the time to progression of disability requiring treatment with levodopa. Selegiline treatment, but not tocopherol, delayed the time to start of levodopa by almost 9 months. Washin and washout effects were observed, consistent with symptomatic benefit from treatment. Symptomatic effects may have

Table 25.2 Results from selected major studies

Study	Agent	Design	Outcome	Results	Lessons learned
DATATOP	Selegiline Tocopherol	Parallel groups	Time to progression of disability requiring treatment with levodopa	Increase in the time to start levodopa by almost 9 months	Symptomatic effect ± neuroprotection
SINDEPAR	Selegiline	Washout study (2 months washout)	UPDRS scores	Difference in UPDRS scores of 5.4 points compared with the placebo group	Neuroprotection vs long-term symptomatic effects
TEMPO	Rasagiline	Parallel groups	UPDRS scores	Improvement in UPDRS for 1 mg (−4.20 points) and 2 mg (−3.56 points)	Symptomatic effects ± neuroprotection
ADAGIO	Rasagiline	Delayed start	Slope of progression in phase 1 UPDRS scores at the end of phase 2 Slope of progression in phase 3	Positive for rasagiline 1 mg (UPDRS: −1.7 points at the end of phase 2) Negative for rasagiline 2 mg/day	Possible neuroprotection with 1 mg/day Post-hoc analysis: positive for 2 mg in quartile with highest UPDRS scores
ELLDOPA	Levodopa/carbidopa	Washout study (2 weeks washout)	UPDRS motor scores [^{123}I]β-CIT SPECT	Dose-response benefit on UPDRS scores Faster decrease in [^{123}I]β-CIT with levodopa	Possible disease modification vs long-term symptomatic effects
REAL-PET	Ropinirole Levodopa/carbidopa	Parallel groups	UPDRS scores [^{18}F]-DOPA PET	UPDRS scores better with levodopa Faster decline in putaminal [^{18}F]-DOPA uptake with levodopa	Possible neuroprotection from ropinirole vs neurotoxicity from levodopa, vs pharmacological interference of levodopa or ropinirole with ^{18}F-DOPA PET imaging
CALM-PD	Pramipexole Levodopa/carbidopa	Parallel groups	[^{123}I]β-CIT SPECT Incidence of motor fluctuations	Faster decline in DAT imaging with levodopa Decreased incidence of motor fluctuations in the pramipexole group	Possible neuroprotection from pramipexole vs neurotoxicity from levodopa, vs pharmacological interference of levodopa or pramipexole with DAT imaging
PROUD	Pramipexole	Delayed start	Slope of progression in phase 1 UPDRS scores at the end of phase 2 Slope of progression in phase 3 [^{123}I]β-CIT SPECT	No difference in UPDRS scores at the end of phase 2 No difference in change of [^{123}I]β-CIT SPECT imaging	Not effective in slowing progression of PD
NET-PD study	Minocycline and creatine	Futility trial	UPDRS scores and subscores	Criteria for futility were not fulfilled by minocycline or creatine (range of effect of creatine seemed better)	Neither intervention could be rejected as futile Placebo group did not evolve similar to the historical control group: need for a calibration group in futility trials
NET-PD LS-1	Creatine	Large simple clinical trial	UPDRS scores	Interim analysis demonstrated futility	No indication to pursue further studies

(continued)

Table 25.2 (cont.)

Study	Agent	Design	Outcome	Results	Lessons learned
PRECEPT	CEP-1347 (antiapoptotic)	Parallel groups	Time to the development of disability requiring dopaminergic therapy UPDRS scores β-CIT SPECT	Interim analysis demonstrated futility Worsening of clinical and neuroimaging parameters with treatment (especially with highest dose), reversal after washout (pharmacological impact on symptoms)	Discrepancy between preclinical studies and the clinical trial questions the applicability of animal models and in vitro studies for neuroprotection Earlier introduction of antiapoptotic treatment may be necessary Worsening of parameters may be a reversible pharmacological effect of intervention
TCH346 study	TCH346 (antiapoptotic)	Parallel groups + washout phase	Time to disability requiring dopaminergic treatment Changes in UPDRS	No symptomatic or neuroprotective effect	THC346 is a propargylamine compound similar to selegiline and rasagiline but has no effects on MAO-B; hence, results from selegiline and rasagiline trials may be related to symptomatic and/or compensatory effects due to inhibition of MAO-B Discordance between animal models and human studies (see above)
AAV2-neurturin	Neurturin (gene delivery via adeno-associated type-2 vector)	Parallel groups (with sham procedure)	Changes in the UPDRS motor score in the practically defined "off" stage	No difference in primary outcome with injection in the putamen or substantia nigra Improvement of 7.6 points on UPDRS at 18 months (in a small subgroup with putaminal injection) Significant improvement in diary "off" score (secondary outcome) with substantia nigra targeting	Histological studies showed that neurturin expression in the substantia nigra was substantially less than expected; hence, neurotrophic therapy probably needs to be applied at a much earlier stage to be effective Marked placebo response in the sham-intervention group
QE3 study	Coenzyme Q10	Parallel groups	UPDRS score	Early termination due to futility in an interim analysis	No evidence of neuroprotection Importance of evaluating positive results of smaller earlier trials with more definitive larger trials
MitoQ	Mitoquinone	Parallel groups	UPDRS score	No improvement in UPDRS scores (trend for worsening)	No evidence of neuroprotection

DATATOP, Deprenyl And Tocopherol Antioxidant Therapy Of Parkinson's disease; SINDEPAR, Sinemet-Deprenyl-Parlodel; TEMPO, TVP-1012 in Early Monotherapy for Parkinson's Disease Outpatients; ADAGIO, Attenuation of Disease Progression with Azilect Given Once-daily; ELLDOPA, Early versus Later Levodopa Therapy in Parkinson Disease; REAL-PET, Requip as Early Therapy versus L-DOPA-PET; CALM-PD, Comparison of the Agonist pramipexole with Levodopa on Motor complications of Parkinson's Disease; PROUD, PRamipexole On Underlying Disease; NET-PD, Neuroprotection Exploratory Trials in Parkinson's Disease; LS1, Long-term Study 1; PRECEPT, Parkinson Research Examination of CEP-1347 Trial; QE3, Effects of Coenzyme Q10 (CoQ) in Parkinson Disease; MAO-B, monoamine oxidase B.

overshadowed possible disease modification, and generally the results have not been interpreted as supporting true neuroprotection.

SINDEPAR

The SINDEPAR (Sinemet-Deprenyl-Parlodel) study [45] compared selegiline versus placebo in patients receiving other treatments for PD. Overall, 101 patients with early untreated PD were included and were divided into four groups after randomization: selegiline and levodopa/carbidopa, placebo and levodopa/carbidopa, selegiline and bromocriptine, or placebo and bromocriptine. The UPDRS scores were analyzed at 14 months, after a washout period of 2 months for the study drug (selegiline) and 7 days for the treatment drug (levodopa/carbidopa or bromocriptine). The effect of selegiline was noted, with a difference in UPDRS scores of 5.4 points compared with the placebo group. The authors concluded that a neuroprotective effect was demonstrated for selegiline, because the washout period was believed to be long enough to exclude a purely symptomatic effect. However, others have suggested that long-term effects of selegiline might explain the difference in motor scores [46].

TEMPO

The TEMPO (TVP-1012 in Early Monotherapy for Parkinson's Disease Outpatients) study [47] examined the effects of rasagiline in early PD. It was designed as a parallel-group, placebo-controlled study. Two doses of rasagiline, 1 and 2 mg/day, were studied. A total of 404 patients with early PD were included. At the end of the study, the UPDRS score was improved with rasagiline compared with placebo, for both 1 mg (−4.20 points) and 2 mg (−3.56 points) groups. An extension study revealed worse scores in patients with deferred treatment (originally receiving placebo), which could be consistent with neuroprotection, although the extension study was not specifically designed for this purpose.

ADAGIO

The ADAGIO (Attenuation of Disease Progression with Azilect Given Once-daily) trial [33] was the first study that used the delayed-start design. Two different doses of rasagiline were studied (1 and 2 mg/day). Early treatment with rasagiline 1 mg resulted in a positive outcome for all three predefined endpoints (as outlined above), with a difference of 1.7 points in the UPDRS score at the end of phase 2. The 2 mg dose group, however, failed to fulfill the predefined criteria. Post-hoc analysis of the 2 mg group data showed that the quartile with the highest UPDRS scores had positive results for all three outcomes. This has been interpreted as possible disease-modifying effects, masked by symptomatic effects. However, other authors have criticized the study and argued that the difference of 1.7 UPDRS points was not clinically significant [36, 48]. The shortcomings of the delayed-start trial design, as described above, have also been cited to claim false-positive results for the 1 mg dose, and the absence of a neuroprotective effect [49, 50].

Levodopa

ELLDOPA

In the past, concern had been raised about the potential toxic effects of levodopa through increased dopamine turnover and resultant increased oxygen reactive species [51, 52]. The ELLDOPA (Earlier versus Later Levodopa Therapy in Parkinson Disease) study [8] was designed to analyze the effects of levodopa on the progression of PD. Patients were randomized to three doses of levodopa/carbidopa (50/12.5 mg three times daily, 100/25 mg three times daily, or 200/50 mg three times daily) or placebo. Assessment of motor scores was done at 42 weeks, after a 2-week washout period from the study drug. A significant dose–response therapeutic benefit was observed, with worsening of UPDRS scores during the washout period, which was more pronounced for the higher dose. After the 2-week washout, the difference in UPDRS scores between active-treatment and placebo groups was sustained, which was interpreted as possible disease modification. However, these results have been contested, because the washout period necessary for complete removal of therapeutic effects might be as long as 1–2 months [53]. An imaging substudy with $[^{123}I]\beta$-CIT SPECT was conducted in a subgroup of 142 patients. When patients with a normal baseline scan were excluded, the decrease in $[^{123}I]\beta$-CIT was faster in levodopa-treated patients (−1.4% with placebo compared with −6.0, −4.0 and −7.2% for the 150, 300 and 600 mg/day levodopa doses, respectively; $P = 0.036$). The discordance between clinical and imaging findings has created problems in interpreting the findings of the ELLDOPA study. Nevertheless, this study reassured patients and physicians about the risk of toxicity induced by levodopa, as a 2-year follow-up did not demonstrate worsening of motor scores.

LEAPS

Whether levodopa does have disease-modifying or neuroprotective effects is being further explored. The LEAPS (Levodopa in Early Parkinson's disease) trial is a delayed-start design study that is currently being conducted in the Netherlands [54]. Patients with early untreated PD are randomized to early and delayed-treatment with levodopa/carbidopa. No other symptomatic treatment will be allowed. The duration of the placebo phase (phase 1) is fixed at 40 weeks, after which all patients will receive active treatment. Results are not available yet.

Dopamine agonists

REAL-PET

Considering the inherent difficulties in neuroprotection clinical trials, some studies have examined neuroimaging as a surrogate marker of the progression of PD. The REAL-PET (Requip as Early Therapy versus L-DOPA-PET) study [9] was a double-blind, double-dummy, parallel-group trial that examined the effects of ropinirole versus levodopa on imaging with ^{18}FD-PET in 162 patients with abnormal scans at baseline (confirming the presence of nigrostriatal degeneration). There was a faster decline in putaminal ^{18}FD uptake with levodopa (20.3% vs 13.4% for ropinirole, $P = 0.022$); however, the UPDRS scores were better with levodopa at 2 years. Different interpretations of these results were suggested, including neuroprotective effects from ropinirole and neurotoxic effects from levodopa, or pharmacological interference of L-DOPA or ropinirole with ^{18}FD-PET imaging.

CALM-PD

The CALM-PD (Comparison of the Agonist pramipexole with Levodopa on Motor complications of Parkinson's Disease) study [25, 55, 56] examined the effects of pramipexole (0.5 mg three times daily) versus levodopa/carbidopa (100/25 mg three times daily) on the development of motor fluctuations. Clinical outcomes showed a decreased incidence of motor fluctuations in the pramipexole group, but levodopa induced more important benefits on UPDRS scores. A subgroup of 82 patients underwent DAT imaging with [^{123}I]β-CIT SPECT. After 23.5 months, the decline in striatal uptake from the baseline scan was 20.0% in the pramipexole group versus 24.8% in patients treated with levodopa/carbidopa ($P=0.15$, not significant). However, this study was not meant to establish neuroprotection.

A major limitation of both the CALM-PD and REAL-PET studies with respect to the interpretation of neuroimaging findings as they inform the neuroprotection question was that neither included a placebo arm.

PROUD

The PROUD (Pramipexole On Underlying Disease) study [57, 58] was conducted to determine whether the dopamine agonist pramipexole has neuroprotective effects. This study used the delayed-start design, with early treatment (pramipexole 1.5 mg/day) versus placebo for the first 9 months (phase 1), followed by active treatment in both groups (phase 2). If symptomatic treatment was needed before the end of phase 1, patients could convert to phase 2 after 6 months. Overall, 535 patients with early idiopathic PD, diagnosed less than 2 years prior to the beginning of the study, were included if they were considered unlikely to need treatment for the next 6–9 months. If another symptomatic treatment was added, such as levodopa, patients were excluded. The predefined clinical endpoints used in the ADAGIO trial were applied (slope of progression in phase 1, UPDRS at the end of phase 2 and slope of progression in phase 2; see above), and a subset of 150 patients was included in an imaging substudy with DAT imaging by [^{123}I]β-CIT SPECT. The UPDRS scores at the end of phase 1 were better in the early-treatment group (difference of –4.8 points in favor of pramipexole, $P < 0.0001$), compatible with the symptomatic benefit in early PD. The slope in phase 1 was less abrupt with pramipexole (0.11 vs 0.22, $P = 0.03$); however, the UPDRS scores at the end of phase 2 failed to show a difference between the two groups. The imaging substudy did not show a difference between pramipexole and placebo groups in the change of DAT uptake at 15 months (–15.1 vs –14.6%, not significant). The authors concluded that pramipexole most probably is not effective in slowing the progression of PD. However, false-negative results might have been seen if there was an overrepresentation of patients with milder disease and slower progression in the trial, or if the active treatment had a longer onset to neuroprotective effects that took more than 6–9 months to become established.

Other agents

NET-PD studies

The National Institute of Neurological Disease and Stroke (NINDS) prioritized different molecules for clinical testing on the basis of preclinical studies.

Minocycline and creatine were selected for the first NET-PD (National Institute of Health Exploratory Trials in PD) futility trial [59]. In total, 200 patients with early untreated PD were assigned to creatine, minocycline or placebo. Neither intervention could be rejected as futile, and the range of effect of creatine seemed better than with minocycline. Recently, a phase 3 study of creatine (NET-PD LS-1 [Long-term Study 1]) in 1741 patients with PD was discontinued prematurely after an interim analysis showed futility [60].

PRECEPT

The antiapoptotic agent CEP-1347 interferes with the c-Jun N-terminal kinase. A large study involving 806 patients with early PD, PRECEPT (Parkinson Research Examination of CEP-1347 Trial), was stopped prematurely after a planned interim analysis at 2 years (average follow-up of 21.4 months) demonstrated futility [61]. No difference was found between treatment groups and placebo in all predetermined clinical outcomes and in a imaging substudy with $[^{123}I]\beta$-CIT SPECT. The prespecified futility analysis permitted earlier termination of a study that had virtually no chance of achieving positive results.

This negative outcome has questioned the applicability of animal models, as discussed above. Questions were also raised about the selection of patients, as antiapoptotic agents may not be useful in patients with clinical manifestations since the neurons may already have sustained irreversible damage. Finally, in contrast to previous trials, there was some clinical and neuroimaging evidence that the active treatment could have worsened the underlying disease. However, follow-up evaluation after a washout period indicated that these effects probably related to reversible pharmacological effects that had not been predicted in preclinical studies.

TCH346 study

TCH346 (*N*-methyl-*N*-propargyl-10-aminomethyl-dibenzo[b,f]-oxepin) is an antiapoptotic drug that was studied in a large, multicenter, randomized controlled trial [62]. Despite the evidence of neuroprotective effects in preclinical models of PD, the study failed to demonstrate benefits in any of the prespecified outcomes (time to disability requiring dopaminergic treatment, changes in UPDRS score, activities of daily living subscores) and no symptomatic effect was found after reviewing the washin and washout assessments.

Again, the discordance between animal and human studies casts doubt on the validity of preclinical models and the timing of introduction of the agent. In addition, the cost associated with such large-scale negative studies justifies futility studies for initial selection of the agents that have a higher chance of being effective in human trials. One potentially important factor to consider in this negative trial result is that TCH346 is a propargylamine similar to selegiline and rasagiline, but, unlike these agents, it lacks effects on MAO-B. Although direct translation of study results is not possible, it could be argued that the suggested neuroprotective effects of selegiline and rasagiline are more likely due to their MAO-B inhibitor properties rather than the glyceraldehyde 3-phosphate dehydrogenase inhibitory and other proposed antiapoptotic effects of the propargylamine moiety.

AAV2-neurturin

In animal and in vitro models of PD, glial-cell-derived neurotrophic factor (GDNF) has a protective effect on dopaminergic cells. However, this finding was not reproduced in human trials where GDNF was infused into the ventricles or the putamen [63, 64]. Gene delivery of neurturin (an analog of GDNF), via an adeno-associated type-2 vector (AAV2), has shown promise in animal models and a small open-label trial. A double-blind, randomized controlled trial in 58 patients with advanced PD and motor complications compared AAV2-neurturin gene transfer in the putamen with sham surgery [65]. Despite some small improvements in secondary endpoints, the study failed to show improvements in the primary outcome (changes in the UPDRS motor score in the practically defined "off" stage) at 12 months. In a subgroup of patients who were followed at 18 months, the patients who had received the intervention had a difference in UPDRS score of 7.6 points on average when compared with the sham surgery group. This encouraged a subsequent sham-controlled trial involving higher doses to the putamen combined with direct substantia nigra targeting [66]. Unfortunately, this study also failed to show a benefit of the active treatment [67]. When histological analysis was performed on two patients who received the gene transfer in earlier trials, the neurturin expression in the substantia nigra was substantially less than expected from animal models, and it has been suggested that the severity of the nigrostriatal degeneration might be responsible for this findings. A further study has shown evidence of profound denervation of the striatum in PD, even after a relatively short disease course [68]. Therefore, one important concern raised by this experience may be that, for neurotrophic therapy to effective, it may need to be applied at a much earlier stage of the disease. However, the risk of serious adverse effects from this invasive intervention will make it challenging to study in early PD patients for ethical reasons.

Coenzyme Q10

Coenzyme Q10 (CoQ10) has received much attention in terms of neuroprotection due to its antioxidant properties and influence on mitochondrial function. Multiple studies have been conducted in PD, most with positive but mild results. A Cochrane review [69] has shown positive results with a 1200 mg/day dose in terms of activities of daily living scores in the UPDRS, and Schwab and England scores. However, a large study in 600 patients with PD using even higher doses, conducted by the Parkinson Study Group, was halted recently due to futility [70] and another trial of the related agent mitoquinone also failed to show evidence of benefit [71].

Conclusion and future directions

Neuroprotection or disease modification is, according to many experts, the single major unmet need in PD. Despite extensive efforts and expense, no treatment has demonstrated unequivocal positive results in clinical trials. Several limitations in animal models and the lack of knowledge of the exact pathophysiology of PD have been highlighted above, and these partially explain the failure of animal studies to successfully translate to human experience. Even more frustrating are the studies that show potential benefit from interventions but are limited by possible confounding symptomatic effects of the treatment.

As our understanding of pathophysiology advances and new targets for neuroprotection are revealed, specific interventions should be applied to target the exact mechanism, instead of using nonspecific treatments that may affect general pathways of cell death or neurodegeneration. Most likely, a combination of different mechanisms at different stages of the disease will be required, and therefore a cocktail of multiple medications targeting different pathways could be necessary.

The timing of the introduction of neuroprotective treatment is also a major issue, as starting a treatment to prevent progression of the disease when significant cell loss has already occurred might be too late to obtain benefit. Better definition of the preclinical stage of PD has to be stressed. This could be done by investigating asymptomatic disease-causing gene mutation carriers (e.g. LRRK2) or individuals who have a strong likelihood of having prodromal PD, with a combination of premotor features such as anosmia, rapid eye movement (REM) sleep behavior disorder and constipation. Imaging and biochemical surrogate biomarkers will be extremely helpful in this regard. Likewise, since PD probably has multiple etiologies, a single agent may not be effective in a general unselected population of PD but may prove valuable in a selected population (e.g. parkin or LRRK2-related PD). Using different candidates in specific populations based on defined pathophysiological mechanisms may be necessary to achieve positive results, and therefore methods to improve selection of patients should be emphasized.

Advancements in our understanding of the pathology of PD have and will continue to enhance the development of biological markers and treatments that may slow or halt the progression of the disease. Clinicians, scientists, patients and regulatory agencies will need to join their efforts to achieve the elusive but critical goals of disease modification and neuroprotection.

References

1. Lang AE. Clinical trials of disease-modifying therapies for neurodegenerative diseases: the challenges and the future. *Nat Med* 2010; **16**: 1223–6.
2. Stocchi F, Olanow CW. Obstacles to the development of a neuroprotective therapy for Parkinson's disease. *Mov Disord* 2013; **28**: 3–7.
3. Olanow CW, Kieburtz K, Schapira AHV. Why have we failed to achieve neuroprotection in Parkinson's disease? *Ann Neurol* 2009; **64** (Suppl. 2): S101–10.
4. Hirsch EC. How to improve neuroprotection in Parkinson's disease? *Parkinsonism Relat Disord* 2007; **13** (Suppl. 3): S332–5.
5. D'Agostino RB. The delayed-start study design. *N Engl J Med* 2009; **361**: 1304–6.
6. Cheng HC, Ulane CM, Burke RE. Clinical progression in Parkinson disease and the neurobiology of axons. *Ann Neurol* 2010; **67**: 715–25.
7. Parkinson Study Group. Pramipexole vs levodopa as initial treatment for Parkinson disease: a randomized controlled trial. *JAMA* 2000; **284**: 1931–8.
8. Fahn S, Oakes D, Shoulson I, *et al.* Levodopa and the progression of Parkinson's disease. *N Engl J Med* 2004; **351**: 2498–508.
9. Whone AL, Watts RL, Stoessl AJ, *et al.* Slower progression of Parkinson's disease with ropinirole versus levodopa: the REAL-PET study. *Ann Neurol* 2003; **54**: 93–101.

10. Goetz CG, Tilley BC, Shaftman SR, et al. Movement Disorder Society-sponsored revision of the Unified Parkinson's Disease Rating Scale (MDS-UPDRS): scale presentation and clinimetric testing results. *Mov Disord* 2008; **23**: 2129–70.

11. Hauser RA, Auinger P, Parkinson Study Group. Determination of minimal clinically important change in early and advanced Parkinson's disease. *Mov Disord* 2011; **26**: 813–8.

12. Richards M, Marder K, Cote L, Mayeux R. Interrater reliability of the Unified Parkinson's Disease Rating Scale motor examination. *Mov Disord* 1994; **9**: 89–91.

13. Goetz CG, Leurgans S, Raman R, Parkinson Study Group. Placebo-associated improvements in motor function: Comparison of subjective and objective sections of the UPDRS in early Parkinson's disease. *Mov Disord* 2002; **17**: 283–8.

14. Parashos SA, Swearingen CJ, Biglan KM, et al. Determinants of the timing of symptomatic treatment in early Parkinson disease: The National Institutes of Health Exploratory Trials in Parkinson Disease (NET-PD) Experience. *Arch Neurol* 2009; **66**: 1099–104.

15. Ravina B, Camicioli R, Como PG, et al. The impact of depressive symptoms in early Parkinson disease. *Neurology* 2007; **69**: 342–7.

16. Marras C, McDermott MP, Marek K, et al. Predictors of time to requiring dopaminergic treatment in 2 Parkinson's disease cohorts. *Mov Disord* 2011; **26**: 608–13.

17. Agarwal PA, Stoessl AJ. Biomarkers for trials of neuroprotection in Parkinson's disease. *Mov Disord* 2012; **28**: 71–85.

18. Pavese N, Kiferle L, Piccini P. Neuroprotection and imaging studies in Parkinson's disease. *Parkinsonism Relat Disord* 2009; **15** (Suppl. 4): S33–7.

19. Ravina B, Eidelberg D, Ahlskog JE, et al. The role of radiotracer imaging in Parkinson disease. *Neurology* 2005; **64**: 208–15.

20. Snow BJ, Tooyama I, McGeer EG, et al. Human positron emission tomographic [18F]fluorodopa studies correlate with dopamine cell counts and levels. *Ann Neurol* 1993; **34**: 324–30.

21. Nandhagopal R, Kuramoto L, Schulzer M, et al. Longitudinal progression of sporadic Parkinson's disease: a multi-tracer positron emission tomography study. *Brain*.2009; **132**: 2970–9.

22. Vingerhoets FJ, Schulzer M, Calne DB, Snow BJ. Which clinical sign of Parkinson's disease best reflects the nigrostriatal lesion? *Ann Neurol* 1997; **41**: 58–64.

23. Pirker W. Correlation of dopamine transporter imaging with parkinsonian motor handicap: how close is it? *Mov Disord* 2003; **18**: S43–51.

24. Martin WRW, Wieler M, Stoessl AJ, Schulzer M. Dihydrotetrabenazine positron emission tomography imaging in early, untreated Parkinson's disease. *Ann Neurol* 2008; **63**: 388–94.

25. Morrish PK. How valid is dopamine transporter imaging as a surrogate marker in research trials in Parkinson's disease? *Mov Disord* 2003; **18** (Suppl. 7): S63–70.

26. Parkinson Study Group. A randomized controlled trial comparing pramipexole with levodopa in early Parkinson's disease: design and methods of the CALM-PD Study. *Clin Neuropharmacol* 2000; **23**: 34–44.

27. Winogrodzka A, Booij J, Wolters EC. Disease-related and drug-induced changes in dopamine transporter expression might undermine the reliability of imaging studies of disease progression in Parkinson's disease. *Parkinsonism Relat Disord* 2005; **11**: 475–84.

28. Eckert T, Eidelberg D. Neuroimaging and therapeutics in movement disorders. *NeuroRx* 2005; **2**: 361–71.

29. Eckert T, Tang C, Eidelberg D. Assessment of the progression of Parkinson's disease: a metabolic network approach. *Lancet Neurol* 2007; **6**: 926–32.

30. Vaillancourt DE, Spraker MB, Prodoehl J, et al. High-resolution diffusion tensor imaging in the substantia nigra of de novo Parkinson disease. *Neurology* 2009; **72**: 1378–84.

31. Berg D. Transcranial ultrasound as a risk marker for Parkinson's disease. *Mov Disord* 2009; **24** (Suppl. 2): S677–83.

32. Sperling RA, Aisen PS, Beckett LA, et al. Toward defining the preclinical stages of Alzheimer's disease: recommendations from the National Institute on Aging-Alzheimer's Association workgroups on diagnostic guidelines for Alzheimer's disease. *Alzheimers Dement* 2011; **7**: 280–92.

33. Lang AE, Melamed E, Poewe W, Rascol O. Trial designs used to study neuroprotective therapy in Parkinson's disease. *Mov Disord* 2012; **28**: 86–95.

34. Olanow CW, Rascol O, Hauser R, et al. A double-blind, delayed-start trial of rasagiline in Parkinson's disease. *N Engl J Med* 2009; **361**: 1268–78.

35. Clarke CE. Are delayed-start design trials to show neuroprotection in Parkinson's disease fundamentally flawed? *Mov Disord* 2008; **23**: 784–9.

36. Ahlskog JE, Uitti RJ. Rasagiline, Parkinson neuroprotection, and delayed-start trials: still no satisfaction? *Neurology* 2010; **74**: 1143–8.

37. Schwid SR, Cutter GR. Futility studies: spending a little to save a lot. *Neurology* 2006; **66**: 626–7.

38. Bezard E, Yue Z, Kirik D, Spillantini MG. Animal models of Parkinson's disease: Limits and relevance to neuroprotection studies. *Mov Disord* 2012; **28**: 61–70.

39. Schober A. Classic toxin-induced animal models of Parkinson's disease: 6-OHDA and MPTP. *Cell Tissue Res* 2004; **J318**: 215–24.

40. Luk KC, Kehm V, Carroll J, et al. Pathological α-synuclein transmission initiates Parkinson-like neurodegeneration in nontransgenic mice. *Science* 2012; **338**: 949–53.
41. Olanow CW, Brundin P. Parkinson's disease and alpha synuclein: is Parkinson's disease a prion-like disorder? *Mov Disord* 2013; **28**: 31–40.
42. Lim KL, Ng CH. Genetic models of Parkinson disease. *Biochim Biophys Acta* 2009; **1792**: 604–15.
43. AlDakheel A, Kalia LV, Lang AE. Pathogenesis-targeted, disease-modifying therapies in Parkinson disease. *Neurotherapeutics* 2013; **11**: 6–23.
44. Parkinson Study Group. Effect of deprenyl on the progression of disability in early Parkinson's disease. *N Engl J Med* 1989; **321**: 1364–71.
45. Olanow CW, Hauser RA, Gauger L, et al. The effect of deprenyl and levodopa on the progression of Parkinson's disease. *Ann Neurol* 1995; **38**: 771–7.
46. Negrotti A, Bizzarri G, Calzetti S. Long-term persistence of symptomatic effect of selegiline in Parkinson's disease. A two-months placebo-controlled withdrawal study. *J Neural Transm* 2001; **108**: 215–19.
47. Parkinson Study Group. A controlled trial of rasagiline in early Parkinson disease: the TEMPO Study. *Arch Neurol* 2002; **59**: 1937–43.
48. Clarke CE, Patel S, Ives N, et al. Should treatment for Parkinson's disease start immediately on diagnosis or delayed until functional disability develops? *Mov Disord* 2011; **26**: 1187–93.
49. de la Fuente-Fernández R, Schulzer M, Mak E, Sossi V. Parkinsonism and related disorders. *Parkinsonism Relat Disord* 2010; **16**: 365–9.
50. Schwarzschild MA. Rasagiline in Parkinson's disease. *N Engl J Med* 2010; **362**: 658; author reply 658–9.
51. Fahn S. Is levodopa toxic? *Neurology* 1996; **47** (Suppl. 3): S184–95.
52. Jenner PG, Brin MF. Levodopa neurotoxicity: experimental studies versus clinical relevance. *Neurology* 1998; **50** (Suppl. 6): S39–48.
53. Hauser RA, Holford NHG. Quantitative description of loss of clinical benefit following withdrawal of levodopa-carbidopa and bromocriptine in early Parkinson's disease. *Mov Disord* 2002; **17**: 961–8.
54. LEAP Study Protocol. Levodopa in early Parkinson's disease: the LEAP study. Availabe at: http://leapamc.nl/wp-content/uploads/2011-12-22-Onderzoeksprotocol.pdf.
55. Parkinson Study Group. Dopamine transporter brain imaging to assess the effects of pramipexole vs levodopa on Parkinson disease progression. *JAMA* 2002; **287**: 1653–61.
56. Parkinson Study Group, CALM Cohort Investigators. Long-term effect of initiating pramipexole vs levodopa in early Parkinson disease. *Arch Neurol* 2009; **66**: 563–70.
57. Schapira AHV, Albrecht S, Barone P, et al. Rationale for delayed-start study of pramipexole in Parkinson's disease: the PROUD study. *Mov Disord* 2010; **25**: 1627–32.
58. Schapira AHV, McDermott MP, Barone P, et al. Pramipexole in patients with early Parkinson's disease (PROUD): a randomised delayed-start trial. *Lancet Neurol* 2013; **12**: 747–55.
59. NINDS NET-PD Investigators. A randomized, double-blind, futility clinical trial of creatine and minocycline in early Parkinson disease. *Neurology* 2006; **66**: 664–71.
60. NET-PD. Study News. Statement on the Termination of NET-PD LS-1 Study. Available at: http://parkinsontrial.ninds.nih.gov/netpd-LS1-study-termination.htm.
61. Parkinson Study Group PRECEPT Investigators. Mixed lineage kinase inhibitor CEP-1347 fails to delay disability in early Parkinson disease. *Neurology* 2007; **69**: 1480–90.
62. Olanow CW, Schapira AHV, LeWitt PA, et al. TCH346 as a neuroprotective drug in Parkinson's disease: a double-blind, randomised, controlled trial. *Lancet Neurol* 2006; **5**: 1013–20.
63. Nutt JG, Burchiel KJ, Comella CL, et al. Randomized, double-blind trial of glial cell line-derived neurotrophic factor (GDNF) in PD. *Neurology* 2003; **60**: 69–73.
64. Lang AE, Gill S, Patel NK, et al. Randomized controlled trial of intraputamenal glial cell line-derived neurotrophic factor infusion in Parkinson disease. *Ann Neurol* 2006; **59**: 459–66.
65. Marks WJ, Bartus RT, Siffert J, et al. Gene delivery of AAV2-neurturin for Parkinson's disease: a double-blind, randomised, controlled trial. *Lancet Neurol* 2010; **9**: 1164–72.
66. Bartus RT, Baumann TL, Siffert J, et al. Safety/feasibility of targeting the substantia nigra with AAV2-neurturin in Parkinson patients. *Neurology* 2013; **80**: 1698–701.
67. PR Newswire. Ceregene reports data from Parkinson's disease phase 2b study. Available at: http://www.prnewswire.com/news-releases/ceregene-reports-data-from-parkinsons-disease-phase-2b-study-203803541.html.
68. Kordower JH, Olanow CW, Dodiya HB, et al. Disease duration and the integrity of the nigrostriatal system in Parkinson's disease. *Brain* 2013; **136**: 2419–31.
69. Liu J, Wang L, Zhan SY, Xia Y. Coenzyme Q10 for Parkinson's disease. *Cochrane Database Syst Rev* 2011; (12): CD008150.
70. National Institute of Neurological Disorders and Stroke. Statement on Termination of QE3 Study. Available at: http://www.ninds.nih.gov/disorders/clinical_trials/CoQ10-Trial-Update.htm.
71. Snow BJ, Rolfe FL, Lockhart MM, et al. A double-blind, placebo-controlled study to assess the mitochondria-targeted antioxidant MitoQ as a disease-modifying therapy in Parkinson's disease. *Mov Disord* 2010; **25**: 1670–4.

Chapter 26

Lessons learned: symptomatic trials in early Parkinson's disease

Ramon Lugo-Sanchez and Néstor Gálvez-Jiménez

Introduction

This chapter will try to explain the concept of "early" Parkinson's disease (PD) and the limitations of the current definition, and will illustrate a few examples of studies that have attempted to give a better understanding of this concept. It is imperative to be able to discern between early and late PD and also to be able to accurately differentiate early PD from a different form of parkinsonism. Currently, the definition that most clinical trials use to classify early PD is using the time of onset of symptoms (less than 3 years) and also a value of 3 or less on the Hoehn and Yahr scale (Table 26.1).

The first limitation of these criteria of "early" PD to be addressed will be the issue of severity in symptoms and onset of symptoms. It is widely believed that patients first start to notice the symptoms of PD when they have already lost so many dompaminergic neurons that they are no longer able to compensate for the deficits. Some scholars refer to a value of more than 70% of dopaminergic neurons lost before onset of symptoms. By this time, the patient must have been suffering from the pathogenesis of PD for several years. Few attempts have been made to describe a prodromal syndrome before the onset of any cardinal PD symptoms. A few of the prodromal symptoms described are anosmia, depression, constipation and rapid eye movement (REM) sleep behavioral disorder among others. The main problem is the lack of specificity of these symptoms with PD. It is not unusual for a patient not to notice anosmia and therefore not to bring it up in a routine medical examination, so the physician would need to be screening patients who are believed to be at risk of developing PD to pick this up. The PROGENI (Parkinson's Research: The Organized Genetics Initiative) study is currently evaluating the prevalence of anosmia in symptomatic and asymptomatic subjects. For depression and constipation, although a relationship with PD has been well documented, these symptoms as a prodrome are not specific enough and there can be plenty of confounding factors. Another approach is to identify an imaging method or blood test that would be sensitive and specific enough to find asymptomatic patients. However, these studies must also be cost-effective. Currently, there is no such test. Another argument for trying to determine asymptomatic patients is the issue of neuroprotection. As mentioned above, if the patients that are recruited for early PD trials are those with one or more cardinal symptoms, then they may already be beyond the point of neuroprotection.

There is yet another issue with the current definition of early PD. In early symptomatic patients, it is very difficult to differentiate among the different parkinsonian syndromes. Certainly, there are clinical criteria and neurological signs that may indicate a more specific diagnosis, but it is only over time, as more

Table 26.1 Modified Hoehn and Yahr scale

Stage	Symtoms
1	Unilateral involvement
1.5	Unilateral and axial involvement
2	Bilateral involvement without impairment of balance
2.5	Mild bilateral disease with recovery on pull test
3	Mild to moderate bilateral disease with some postural instability but physically independent
4	Severe disability but still able to walk or stand unassisted
5	Wheelchair bound or bedridden unless aided

Parkinson's Disease: Current and Future Therapeutics and Clinical Trials, ed. Gálvez-Jiménez *et al*. Published by Cambridge University Press. © Cambridge University Press 2016.

symptoms develop, that there is more certainty about the diagnosis. Some of the trials use the UK Parkinson's Disease Society Brain Bank criteria (Table 26.2). However we have to consider that some of the criteria overlap with other parkinsonian symptoms, especially at the beginning of the disease.

Table 26.2 UK Parkinson's Disease Society Brain Bank criteria

Step 1. Diagnosis of parkinsonian syndrome

Bradykinesia

At least one of the following:
- Muscular rigidity
- 4–6 Hz resting tremor
- Postural instability not caused by primary visual, vestibular, cerebellar or proprioceptive dysfunction

Step 2. Exclusion criteria for Parkinson's disease

History of repeated strokes with stepwise progression of parkinsonian features

History of repeated head injury

History of definite encephalitis

Oculogyric crises

Neuroleptic treatment at onset of symptoms

More than one affected relative

Sustained remission

Strictly unilateral features after 3 years

Supranuclear gaze palsy

Cerebellar signs

Early severe autonomic involvement

Early severe dementia with disturbances of memory, language and praxis

Babinski sign

Presence of cerebral tumor or communication hydrocephalus on imaging study

Negative response to large doses of levodopa (L-DOPA) in absence of malabsorption

MPTP exposure

Step 3. Supportive prospective positive criteria for Parkinson's disease

Three or more required for diagnosis of definite Parkinson's disease in combination with step 1:
- Unilateral onset
- Rest tremor present
- Progressive disorder
- Persistent asymmetry affecting side of onset most
- Excellent response (70–100%) to levodopa
- Severe levodopa-induced chorea
- Levodopa response for 5 years or more
- Clinical course of 10 years or more

In this chapter, we will review some of the approaches that clinical trials have developed to assess different issues in identifying and also in enrolling early PD patients in their different clinical trials.

Early detection with blood tests and imaging studies

Magnetic resonance imaging

There have been several attempts to use this paraclinical test to find and define patients with asymptomatic or very early PD. One study measured the amount of brain atrophy and white-matter hyperintensities compared with healthy individuals [1]. In this study, there was no correlation in the size or number of white-matter changes between early PD patients and healthy controls. In addition, there was no significant difference in the amount of brain atrophy between the early PD patients and normal controls.

Nuclear imaging

There have been several attempts to use nuclear medicine as a reliable method to document or confirm a dopamine-deficient state. Currently, a dopamine transporter scan (DaTscan™) is approved for this use. It is able to differentiate PD with essential tremors, PD versus drug-induced parkinsonism, and psychogenic tremor. However, one of the limitations of this imaging modality is the lack of discrimination between PD and atypical parkinsonian syndrome (APS). In 2009, pre- and postsynaptic dopamine was studied in early parkinsonism using single-photon-emission computed tomography (SPECT) with a combination of [^{123}I] ioflupane (I-FP-CIT), which is a presynaptic ligand for dopamine transporter protein, and [^{123}I]-iolopride (I-IBZM), which is a postsynaptic ligand with affinity to the D2 and D3 receptors located at high concentration in the striatum [2]. When compared with healthy controls, both groups had significantly lower baseline I-FP-CIT ratios. However, there was no significant difference between PD patients and APS patients. The presynaptic phase of the study did not correlate with the disease duration, age of onset or Mini Mental Status Examination (MMSE) scores. When evaluating postsynaptic ratios alone with I-IBZM, there was no significant difference between any of the groups. However, the authors found that by combining the presynaptic and postsynaptic analysis, an accuracy of 85% in excluding APS was found.

One study tried to use a combine striatal binding and cerebral influx analysis of dynamic [^{11}C]raclopride positron emission tomography (PET) in an attempt to improve early differentiation between multiple-system atrophy (MSA) and PD [3]. They divided the study population in three groups: healthy controls, PD patients and MSA patients. When comparing the subjects with healthy controls, the investigators found that the PD patients had slightly lower [^{11}C]raclopride binding in the caudate and slightly higher binding in the posterior putamen. The MSA group showed lower binding in the caudate and in the putamen when compared with healthy controls. When comparing the MSA patients with the PD patients, the MSA patients showed decreased binding in the posterior portions of the putamen bilaterally. On statistical parametric mapping analysis, the PD patients had increased [^{11}C]raclopride binding in the median and left insular cortex, temporofrontal areas, striatum and thalamus when compared with healthy controls. On the other hand, the MSA patients, when compared with the control group, showed decreased cerebellar influx. When comparing the PD group with the MSA group, the MSA group showed decreased striatal, ventral mesencephalic, pontine and cerebellar influx. The investigators concluded that using discriminant analysis combining [^{11}C]raclopride striatal gradient analysis and regional [^{11}C]raclopride influx could distinguish MSA and PD patients with accuracy, and that it showed better performance than the more conventional [^{11}C]raclopride conventional PET analysis.

Vitamin D

Vitamin D deficiency has been reported to be more common in patients with PD. A study was design to evaluate whether this vitamin deficiency is due to lack of mobility and exposure to the sun, or whether it is an integral part of the pathophysiology of PD [4]. the study used a blood bank from the placebo arm of the DATATOP (Deprenyl and Tocopherol Antioxidative Therapy of Parkinsonism) trial and tested the blood samples for vitamin D levels at baseline and at the endpoint. The authors found a higher prevalence of vitamin D deficiency at baseline compared with other studies. However, when testing the endpoint blood samples, they found that the vitamin D levels were higher than the baseline values. They concluded that vitamin insufficiency or deficiency may have been present before the clinical manifestation of PD and therefore may play a role in the pathogenesis of PD.

Somatostatin

Some PD patients suffer from slow gastric emptying and also have significant nausea. This is more prominent with patients who have fluctuations of symptoms. It is thought that either medications or pathology affecting the vagal afferents may be the reason for this phenomenon. One study aimed to clarify whether or not digestive hormone secretions in untreated early PD patients are regulated by central command, and if digestive hormone dynamics in early PD patients with and without nausea or vomiting change after treatment of PD [5]. The authors measured plasma levels of digestive hormones (somatostatin and gastrin) at baseline and 3 weeks after PD medications had been applied. They found that the somatostatin levels at baseline were significantly increased in PD patients compared with the healthy controls, especially in those patients suffering from nausea and vomiting. The increases in somatostatin blood levels were similar in all the treatment groups. Levels of gastrin, serotonin, epinephrine, norepinephrine, dopamine and arginine vasopressin were not significantly different between all the groups at baseline or at the end point. The authors concluded that the increase in somatostatin secretions in PD is centrally mediated via vagal afferent fibers.

Deep-brain stimulation

Deep-brain stimulation (DBS) is an approved treatment for PD patients who have motor fluctuations. It has been shown to improve patients' quality of life. However, recently there have been reports of DBS surgery in early PD patients [6–9]. In one of these studies, it was found that early PD patients were more adept than the more advance population at cooperating during surgery and at articulating stimulation effects. This is believed to be because of better tolerability of the "off" period and decreased disability [6]. In an illustrative case report, it was found that there was an improvement in the Unified Parkinson's Disease Rating Scale (UPDRS) scores over time [7]. The patient showed a 9-point improvement per year; typically, the total UPDRS score worsens by 8–14 points per year in early-stage PD. In addition, focusing only on motor symptoms using the UPDRS-III, it has been shown previously that the usual decline is 1.9–6.7 points per year, while the patient in this study showed only a 2-point decline per year in the "off" state and improved scores in the "on" state. The authors stated that this observation may be an indication that DBS surgery early in the disease may have a disease-modifying effect. However, they also suggested that this reulst may have been due to optimized treatment. In quality-of-life measures, this patient also improvement in the quality-of-life scales. In summary, over a 2-year period, this patient showed improvement in the motor scores of the UPDRS-III and also in quality-of-life measures. In DBS patients, language is known to be affected, with decreased fluency. These are usually advanced PD patients. In early PD patients, a study reported the impact of DBS with regard to language [8]. The authors compared the performance of healthy controls and early PD patients treated with either DBS/medication or medication alone. Patients were assessed on and off treatment, with controls following a parallel testing schedule. The DBS patients showed improved naming of manipulated but not nonmanipulated objects compared both with controls and with patients on medication only. However, the DBS patients performed poorly at grammar but not in lexicon compared with the other two groups. The authors suggested that DBS surgery impacts language in early PD but that this may be specific to grammatical process and not to lexical processes.

Lastly, there was a randomized, double-blinded trial of transcranial electrostimulation in early PD patients [10]. The authors studied the effect of non-invasive transcranial stimulation on the motor and psychological symptoms in early PD. The subjects were treated with 10 days of placebo versus active treatment and were then followed for 14 weeks and assessed using the UPDRS-I and -III. In week 2, the active treatment resulted in a reduction – although nonsignificant – in the UPDRS scores when compared with placebo. Similarly, the anxiety, depression and sleepiness score differences were not significant.

Medications and neuroprotection
Dopamine agonists
A common clinical practice is to start young PD patients on levodopa (L-DOPA)-sparing agents such as dopamine agonists (DAs). In the USA, only three DAs have been approved for widespread use: pramipexole, ropinirole and rotigotine. For pramipexole and ropinirole, there are both short-acting and extended-release (ER) formulations, while rotigotine is available patch form. The rationale of using these medications early is to limit the exposure to levodopa and hopefully delay the complications of motor fluctuations and dyskinesias that occur in most PD patients after extended exposure to levodopa. However, despite these problems, levodopa still remains the most effective therapeutic agent for the treatment of PD.

Pramipexole
This medication can be given in an immediate-release (IR) formulation that is taken three times daily and have been proven to help with PD symptoms. Pramipexole has been associated with several side effects including somnolence, hallucinations and impulse control issues. It can be used as monotherapy in patients with early PD and, as stated above, it helps to decrease levodopa exposure, thus preventing the onset of dyskinesias. In patients already on levodopa, this medication can be used as an adjunct and has been proven to decrease "off" time and improve the motor symptoms of PD. However, this formulation has fluctuating stimulation of the dopamine receptor, requiring frequent dosing. It is believed that in healthy individuals there is constant baseline dopaminergic stimulation and therefore a more physiological formulation was sought. A randomized, multicenter, double-blinded study to evaluate pramipexole ER was carried out in early PD patients [11]. In this study, the subjects were divided into three groups. One group received pramipexole ER, another pramipexole IR and a third group received placebo. These patients were then evaluated using the UPDRS-II and -III. A significant improvement in the score was found in the patients receiving either of the formulations of pramipexole compared with placebo, but there was no significant difference between the two treatment arms. Pramipexole ER was well tolerated but had more side effects when compared with placebo. The most common side effects were somnolence, impulse control disorders, nausea, fatigue and constipation. However, there was no significant difference between the IR and ER formulations with regard to side effects. Patients preferred the once a day dosing as opposed to three times daily [12]. The tolerability and effectiveness of pramipexole ER and pramipexole IR versus placebo were also tested by Poewe *et al.* [13], with similar results. One question remained unanswered by these studies: as many patients were already using the IR formulation, was it safe to switch overnight from the IR to to ER formulation? In 2010, a clinical trial with early PD patients attempted to answer this [14]. The authors defined successful switching as no worsening >15% of baseline in the UPDRS-II plus -III scores when

compared with the IR formulation. They found that although pramipexole ER was not equivalent to IR, the difference was marginal. Furthermore, they concluded that overnight switching may be a feasible clinical practice in most patients.

The Parkinson Study Group CALM Investigators evaluated the long-term effect in patients started on pramipexole compared with patients started on levodopa in early PD [15]. In this study, dopaminergic motor fluctuations were more common in the initial levodopa group than in the pramipexole group. However, somnolence scored by the Epworth Sleepiness Scale was more significant in the initial pramipexole group than in the initial levodopa group. Motor symptoms assessed by the UPDRS-III showed no significant difference between the groups. Another study compared a low-dose twice-daily pramipexole IR with placebo in a randomized, placebo-controlled trial [16]. In this study, the subjects were divided into groups receiving dosages of 0.5 mg twice daily, 0.75 mg twice daily, 0.5 mg three times daily, or placebo. The UPDRS scores were used for comparison from baseline. A significant improvement was found in the UPDRS scores of the treatment groups compared with placebo. However, side effects were more common in the treatment groups. When comparing each of the treatment groups, there was no significant difference in efficacy or side effects.

Ropinirole

Ropinirole is another DA that is commonly used in early PD patients. It also comes in two formulations: IR and ER (also known as XL). A prolonged open-label study of once-daily ropinirole was carried out in early PD patients [17], which found that there was tolerability and that the efficacy of treating early PD symptoms was maintained during the prolonged study period. Since more uniform dopaminergic stimulation may be beneficial, one study used ropinirole XL to assess the onset of dyskinesias in patients requiring adjunct ropinirole XL versus additional levodopa [18]. The authors took patients who were taking levodopa but were not controlled and randomized them between taking the same levodopa dose and adding ropinirole XL versus increasing the levodopa dose. They found a significant difference in the onset of dyskinesias between the group that took ropinirole XL versus the group that took additional levodopa. They also demonstrated no difference in PD symptom control between the groups.

Rotigotine

Rotigotine is the latest DA to be approved for use in the USA. This medication comes in a daily patch form. It delivers constant dopaminergic release through the skin. The side-effect profile is similar to the former that of pramipexole and ropinirole, and includes hallucinations, dizziness and impulse control disorder. In patients with dysphagia, rotigotine is a good choice.

Other DAs
Pardoprunox

Pardoprunox is a partial dopamine D2 receptor agonist with full 5-HT$_{1A}$ agonist activity and has demonstrated an anti-PD effect with antidepressant and anxiolytic properties in animal models. It was tested in a double-blinded study in early PD patients [19]. The patients were randomized to either medication or placebo. The medication was taken orally three times daily. The authors used the UPDRS motor scores as the primary endpoint. Secondary endpoints included UPDRS-activities of daily living (ADL) scores and combined UPDRS motor and ADL scores and Clinical Global Impression (CGI) scores. They found that medication resulted in a significant improvement in the UPDRS motor scores when compared with placebo. Secondary endpoints were also reached. Side effects were significantly more frequent in the treatment group than in the placebo group. The most common adverse effects were nausea, dizziness, somnolence and headache. Another study showed similar results [20].

Safinamide

Safinamide is an α-aminoamide with both a dopaminergic and nondopaminergic mechanism of action including monoamine oxidase B (MAO-B) and dopamine reuptake inhibition. This medication has been tested as an add-on therapy in early PD patients [21, 22]. However, there was no significant difference in the efficacy of this medication when compared with placebo.

Isradipine

This calcium-channel blocker has been tested for possible neuroprotection in early PD preclinical models [23]. The results showed toleration of this drug as 94% of patients taking controlled-release isradipine 5 mg, 87% for 10 mg, 68% for 15 mg and 52% for 20 mg. The medication did not have any significant effect on blood pressure or PD motor disability. The most common reasons for dose reductions were lower-extremity edema and dizziness. No significant differences were found between the patients with or without dopaminergic treatment or hypertension.

Rasagiline

Rasagiline is an irreversible MAO-B inhibitor that has been used for symptomatic relief in PD patients. The tolerability and safety of this medication have been proven in early PD [24]. In one study, early PD patients were randomized between taking 1 mg of rasagiline or 1.5 mg of pramipexole daily. The primary outcome was the number of patients experiencing a "clinically significant" adverse event. The mean disease duration was 3.4 months and a mean patient age was 62.6 years. Of the patients taking pramipexole, 44.6% reported a significant adverse event compared with 32.1% of the patients taking rasagiline. Noninferiority of rasagiline was the conclusion reached from these results. There was no significant difference in clinical effectiveness between the groups. Rasagiline had a significant favorable difference in gastrointestinal and sleep adverse events in comparison with pramipexole. In addition, it was given a similar clinician- and patient-rated clinical effectiveness as a monotherapy for the treatment of early PD.

Delayed-start models have been used to test the potential of rasagiline for neuroprotection. A randomized, double-blind, placebo-controlled, delayed-start study to assess rasagiline as a disease-modifying therapy in PD was carried out [25]. This study was divided into two phases. Phase one was a 36-week, double-blind, placebo-controlled phase, and phase two was a 36-week, double-blind, active-treatment phase in which all subjects received the medication. The groups were divided as follows: patients taking 1 mg daily of rasagiline during both phases, patients taking 2 mg of rasagiline daily in both phases, patients taking placebo during the first phase and 1 mg of rasagiline daily during the second phase, and patients taking placebo in the first phase and 2 mg of rasagiline daily in the second phase. Rasagiline 1 mg daily met all the endpoints in the primary analysis. However, rasagiline 2 mg did not meet any of the endpoints [26]. The long-term outcome of early versus delayed rasagiline treatment in early PD has been reported [27]. This study followed PD patients for 6.5 years and found an adjusted mean difference in change from baseline in total UPDRS score of 2.5 units or 16% in favor of the early-start versus delayed-start rasagiline group with statistical significance. The authors suggested that this may be explained by enduring neuroprotection in the early-start group in early PD.

Exercise

Exercise for people with early or midstage PD was studied in a 16-month randomized controlled trial [28]. This study consisted of getting patients with PD at Hoehn and Yahr scale stages 1–3 and randomizing them in a flexibility/balance/function exercise (FBF) program (individualized spinal and extremity flexibility exercise followed by group balance/functional training) versus a supervised aerobic exercise (AE) program (using a treadmill, bike or elliptical trainer). The FBF group was supervised by a physical therapist while the AE program was supervised by an exercise trainer. The supervision was provided 3 days per week for 4 months and then once a month for the rest of the trial. The control group used the National Parkinson Foundation *Fitness Counts* program with one supervised clinic-based group session per month. Blinded assessments were undertaken at months 4, 10 and 16. Overall, 86.8, 82.6 and 79.3% of all the patients completed the 4, 10 and 16 months trials, respectively. At 4 months, the FBF group showed a significant improvement the functional scores when compared with the control group and AE group. Balance was not significantly different in any of the groups at any point. Walking economy (oxygen uptake) was improved in the AE group compared with the FBF group at 4, 10 and 16 months. The FBF group had better scores in the UPDRS-ADL subscale at 4 and 16 months. These findings suggested that AE exercise alone was not sufficient to maintain functionality in the early PD group, although the improvement in oxygen uptake was maintained. This is an important finding as this may change the exercise program in early PD.

Conclusion

The examples outlined in this chapter show the immense challenge and the impressive attempts to obtain more tools – both diagnostic and therapeutic – to be able not only to identify but also to differentiate early PD from late PD and APS. However, none of these trials has been successful in identifying early PD in asymptomatic patients. Only one of the studies mentioned above has indicated the possibility of adding another tool to differentiate early PD from MSA [3]. More research is needed to further resolve these two issues.

References

1. Dalaker TO, Larsen JP, Bergsland N, *et al.* Brain atrophy and white matter hyperintesisites in early Parkisnon's disease. *Mov Disord* 2009; **24**: 2233–41.

2. Jakobson S, Linder J, Forsgren L, et al. Pre- and post-synaptic dopamine SPECT in early phase of idiopathic parkinsonism: a population-based study. *Eur J Nucl Med Mol Imaging* 2010; **37**: 2154–64.

3. Laere KV, Clerinx K, D'Hondt E, de Groot T, Vandenberghe W. Combine striatal binding and cerebral influx analysis of dynamic 11C-raclopride PET improves early differentiation between multiple-system atrophy and Parkinson disease. *J Nucl Med* 2010; **51**: 588–95.

4. Evatt ML, DeLong MR, Kumari M, et al. High prevalence of hypovitaminosis D status in patient with early Parkinson disease. *Arch Neurol* 2011; **68**: 314–19.

5. Shiraishi M, Kobayashi T, Watanabe H, Kamo T, Hasegawa Y. Serum somatostatin in early stage Parkinson's disease. *Acta Neurol Scand* 2010; **121**: 225–9.

6. Charles PD, Dolhun RM, Gill CE, et al. Deep brain stimulation in early Parkinson's disease: Enrollment experience from a pilot trial. *Parkinsonism Relat Disord* 2012; **18**: 268–73.

7. Gill CE, Allen LA, Konrad PE, et al. Deep brain stimulation of early-stage Parkinson's disease: an illustrative case. *Neuromodulation* 2011; **14**: 515–22.

8. Phillips L, Litcofsky KA, Pelster M, et al. Subthalamic nucleus deep brain stimulation impacts language in early Parkinson's disease. *PLoS One* 2012; **7**: e42829.

9. Kahn E, D'Haese PF, Dawant B, et al. Deep brain stimulation in early stage Parkinson's disease: operative experience from a prospective randomized clinical trial. *J Neurol Neurosurg Psychiatry* 2012; **83**: 164–70.

10. Shill HA, Obradov S, Katsnelson Y, Pizinger R. A randomized, double-blind trial of transcranial electrostimulation in early Parkinson's disease. *Mov Disord* 2011; **26**: 1477–80.

11. Hauser RA, Schapira AHV, Rasciol O, et al. Randomized double-blind, multicenter evaluation of pramipexole extended release once daily in early Parkinson's disease. *Mov Disord* 2010; **25**: 2542–9.

12. Schapira AHV, Barone P, Hauser RA, et al. Patient reported convenience of once-daily versus three-times-daily dosing during long-term studies of pramipexole in early and advance Parkinson's disease. *Eur J Neurol* 2013; **20**: 50–6.

13. Poewe W, Rascol O, Barone P, et al. Extended-release pramipexole in early Parkinson disease. *Neurology* 2011; 759–65.

14. Rascol O, Barone P, Hauser RA, et al. Efficacy, safety and tolerability of overnight switching from immediate-to once daily extended-release pramipexole in early Parkinson's disease. *Mov Disord* 2010; **25**: 2326–32.

15. Parkinson Study Group CALM Investigators. Long-term effect of initiating pramipexole vs levodopa in early Parkinson's disease. *Arch Neurol* 2009; **66**: 563–70.

16. Parkinson Study Group PramiBID Investigators. Twice-daily, low-dose parmipexole in early Parkinson's disease: a randomized, placebo-controlled trial. *Mov Disord* 2011; **26**: 37–44.

17. Hauser RA, Reichmann H, Lew M, et al. Long-term, open-label study of once-daily ropinirole prolonged release in early Parkinson's disease. *International J Neurosci* 2011; **121**: 246–53.

18. Watts RL, Lyons KE, Pahwa R, et al. Onset of dyskinesia with adjunct ropinirole prolonged-release or additional levodopa in early Parkinson's disease. *Mov Disord* 2010; **25**: 858–66.

19. Bronzova J, Sampiao C, Hauser RA, et al. Double-blind study of pardoprunox, a new partial dopamine agonist, in early Parkinson's disease. *Mov Disord* 2010; **25**: 738–46.

20. Sampiao C, Bronzova J, Hauser RA, et al. Pardoprunox in early Parkinson's disease: results from 2 large randomized double-blind trials. *Mov Disord* 2011; **26**: 1464–76.

21. Shapira AHV, Stocchi F, Borgohain R, et al. Long-term efficacy and safety of safinamide as add-on therapy in early Parkinson's disease. *Eur J Neurol* 2013; **20**: 271–80.

22. Stocchi F, Borgohain R, Onofrj M, et al. A randomized, double-blind, placebo-controlled trial of safinamide as add-on therapy in early Parkinson's disease patients. *Mov Disord* 2012; **27**: 106–12.

23. Simuni T, Borushko E, Avram MJ, et al. Tolerability of isradipine in early Parkinson's disease: a pilot dose escalation study. *Mov Disord* 2010; **25**: 2863–6.

24. Viallet F, Pitel S, Lancrenon S, Blin O. Evaluation of the safety and tolerability of rasagiline in the treatment of the early stages of Parkinson's disease. *Curr Med Res Opin* 2013; **29**: 23–31.

25. Olanow W, Hauser RA, Jankovick J, et al. A randomized, double-blind, placebo-controlled, delayed start study to assess rasagiline as a disease modifying therapy in Parkinson's disease (the ADAGIO study): rationale, design and baseline characteristics. *Mov Disord* 2008; **23**: 2194–201.

26. Olanow W, Rascol O, Hauser RA, et al. A double blind, delayed-start trial of rasagaline in Parkinson's disease. *N Engl J Med* 2009; **361**: 1268–78.

27. Hauser RA, Lew MF, Hurtig HI, et al. Long-term outcome of early versus delayed rasagiline treatment in early Parkinson's disease. *Mov Disord* 2009; **24**: 564–73.

28. Schenkman M, Hall D, Barón AE, et al. Exercise for people in early- or mid-stage Parkinson disease: a 16-month randomized controlled trial. *Phys Ther* 2012; **92**: 1395–410.

Chapter 27

Controversy: globus pallidus internus versus subthalamic nucleus deep-brain stimulation in the management of Parkinson's disease

Sarah K. Bourne, Sean J. Nagel and Darlene A. Lobel

Introduction

Deep-brain stimulation (DBS) of the subthalamic nucleus (STN) and globus pallidus internus (GPi) is effective for patients with medically intractable Parkinson's disease (PD). The improvement in motor function and quality of life are superior to medical treatment alone [1]. Over 100,000 patients have had DBS, yet the best target in those with PD remains unknown. Many high-volume centers, often for historical reasons, prefer one implant site to the other. This bias continues to hamper research efforts aimed at answering this question and influences interpretation of the results. In this chapter, we discuss the relevant patient factors that should be used in target selection and explore the differences between STN- and GPi-DBS. We favor this tailored approach in our patients until future studies are able to settle the debate. The first step begins with an evaluation of the patient's motor and nonmotor symptoms and their stated goals. This information is compared with outcome studies and a preliminary target is chosen. Other data relevant to the patient, including imaging findings, unique risks and expected postoperative challenges, are then incorporated into a final decision.

Background

Although the groundwork for DBS was set in the previous decade by Benabid and others, the first reports that described the beneficial effects for PD were published in 1993 for STN and in 1994 for GPi [2, 3]. Nearly a decade later in 2003, DBS of the STN and GPi was granted regulatory approval by the US Food and Drug Administration for the treatment of PD; however, although the enthusiasm for DBS as a treatment for PD has only grown, the mechanism through which it works to control symptoms remains obscure. Why electrical stimulation of two anatomically and physiologically distinct targets relieves the cardinal symptoms of PD has only clouded our understanding. The prevailing hypothesis has evolved from a crude excitation/inhibition paradigm to one focused on restoration of circuit specificity through disruption of pathological beta-frequency oscillations that appear to be the hallmark of PD. Although dynamic systems neuroscience has advanced, it seems an integrated theory that is able to reconcile the many disparate findings still remains years away.

Operative anatomy and physiology of the globus pallidus internus and subthalamic nucleus

An appreciation for the unique anatomy and neurophysiology of the GPi and STN is essential for target selection. Microelectrode recording (MER) is a well-described technique that samples neuronal signals along the trajectory to and within the target nucleus. The physiological "noise" is used to resolve the anatomic configuration of the nucleus under study in real time to optimize electrode placement.

Globus pallidus interna

The lateral position of the GPi relative to the STN minimizes the risk that a parasagittal approach will violate the medially located vascular structures. At the same time, this approach is able to capitalize on the posterolateral position of the motor region of the nucleus [4].

The trajectory is planned using an angle of 0–15° in the coronal plane and 30–35° anteriorly in the sagittal plane.

Posteromedial to the GPi is the posterior limb of the internal capsule. Suboptimal electrode placement in this location will induce tetanic contractions. The globus pallidus externus (GPe) lies laterally to the GPi. The internal medullary lamina partitions the internal and external segments. Below the GPi runs the ansa lenticularis anteromedially and the optic tract posteriorly and laterally. The optic tract serves as a landmark to guide electrode depth. Anteriorly, the nucleus basalis lies deep to the GPi.

On entering the GPe, there is an increase in firing activity. The GPe contains neurons that fire tonically at high frequency (50 Hz), interspersed with short pauses. Another population of neurons is identified by low-frequency activity (18 Hz) intermixed with periods of high frequency [5]. The internal medullary lamina is identified by a decrease in firing for 1–2 mm and border cells with regular tonic firing at 5–30 Hz [6]. Parkinson's disease patients have high-frequency firing in the GPi with fewer pauses than recorded from the GPe. The sensorimotor GPi demonstrates driving activity with limb movement. The optic tract, located approximately 1.5 mm below the GPi, will fire when a flashlight is directed at the eyes. The optimal electrode location is far from the internal capsule medially and optic tract inferiorly to prevent side effects at the high voltages sometimes needed to improve motor symptoms [5]. The use of GPi-DBS may have a local inhibitory effect that decreases pathological overactivity or modulates firing patterns [7, 8].

Subthalamic nucleus

Bordering the STN anterolaterally is the internal capsule. Medial and deep to the STN is the red nucleus and third nerve nucleus. Posteriorly run the prelemniscal radiations. The motor units of the STN are arranged within the dorsal, posterolateral sector. The proximity of the internal capsule to the optimal target location complicates electrode insertion. A "routine" MER track will cross the thalamus, recording bursting (15–19 Hz) or tonically active (28 Hz) cells. After passing through the zona incerta, the STN is entered. An MER of the STN is characterized by an increase in background noise. A tract length of 4–5 mm is generally sought before implantation.

Due to the more medial position of the STN compared with the GPi, the trajectory is often angled to avoid the deep vascular structures and lateral ventricle. Enlarged ventricles are especially difficult to avoid. When an extreme lateral trajectory (greater than 30°) is selected, the path of the microelectrode will often miss the thalamus entirely and the STN units recorded may span only 2–3 mm. Imaging may dictate the GPi as a better target in such cases.

Stimulation of the globus pallidus interna and the subthalamic nucleus

Intraoperative stimulation is used to determine voltage requirements for therapeutic effect and voltage-limiting side effects [4]. Reduction of PD symptoms with intraoperative stimulation is less frequent with the GPi. However, intraoperative stimulation of both targets determines the threshold for adverse effects. Stimulation-related side effects emerge when the current spreads to corticobulbar, corticospinal or optic tracts. Stimulation of the deep contacts on the lead may cause visual symptoms during GPi stimulation [4], and STN stimulation of deep contacts may activate the third nerve nucleus or red nucleus, triggering dysconjugate or conjugate gaze paresis.

Stimulation spread to the internal capsule induces contralateral motor contractions. Specific to GPi-DBS, a decreased blood oxygen level-dependent (BOLD) signal is seen in the contralateral motor cortex and subcortical structures such as the striatal and thalamic regions when the electrode location is close to the dorsomedial border of the GPi and the neighboring internal capsule [9]. This may be due to effects on internal capsule fibers and inhibitory corticocortical projection neurons.

The volume of the GPi is approximately three times that of the STN. It has been suggested that stimulation efficacy may be related to the volume of the area stimulated. As the STN is significantly smaller than the GPi, it follows that a larger proportion of the motor region is likely to be stimulated at lower voltages [10]. Stimulation of the smaller STN is also more likely to spread to nearby structures and results in adverse effects [11]. Due to the large size of the GPi, stimulation may not elicit intraoperative side effects during testing [10]. Furthermore, the clinical effect of GPi stimulation is often delayed. Taken together, this limits the predictive value of intraoperative stimulation when the GPi is the target [10]. The microlesional effect that often presages symptom control in the STN even before programming is less evident following MER and lead placement in the GPi. This may also be related to the large nucleus size [12].

Effect of globus pallidus interna and the subthalamic nucleus deep-brain stimulation on motor symptoms

The primary symptomatology in PD patients is marked by tremor predominance in some and disabling rigidity and bradykinesia in others. Both GPi and STN stimulation will improve rigidity, bradykinesia and tremor to varying degrees (Table 27.1) [2, 13, 14]. Yet, a universal approach to target selection based on motor symptoms alone has not been established. For now, the decision should be made collectively and the expected outcome discussed with cautious optimism. Appropriate patient education and management of expectations is associated with improved patient outcomes and quality-of-life scores [15].

Tremor

Tremor-predominant PD may respond better to STN or thalamic DBS than GPi-DBS. After STN-DBS, tremor improvement is estimated to be 90% at 1 year and 75% at 5 years [16, 17]. The use of GPi-DBS results in 80% improvement after 1 year. This disparity in long-term tremor control between the two targets may be related to the size of the GPi. If sufficient current density is unable to spread to the posterior portion of the nucleus, tremor control may be suboptimal [11]. When hand dexterity is studied, it is noted to be dependent on the medication state. Thus, GPi-DBS improves hand dexterity during the on-medications state; conversely, STN-DBS improves hand dexterity in the off-medications state [18].

Table 27.1 Summary of globus pallidus interna (GPi) versus subthalamic nucleus (STN) deep-brain stimulation results based on analysis of relevant factors from patient history and physical and preoperative evaluation

	GPi	STN
Age	Any	<75 years
Cardinal symptoms	Rigidity, bradykinesia predominant	Tremor predominant
Dyskinesias	Occur with low-dose dopaminergic medications	Associated with frequent medication dosing
Cognitive function	Moderate to borderline	Good to moderate; consider staged bilateral procedure
Medications	Low dose	High dose
Other symptoms	Postural instability	Dexterity

Bradykinesia

Bradykinesia, when the predominant symptom, may also respond better to STN-DBS [16]. An improvement of 70–80% is expected after STN-DBS compared with a 30–40% improvement after GPi-DBS [19]. Bradykinesia affects almost any motor function. Parkinson's disease patients may have poor oropharyngeal functions necessary to speak and/or swallow. Jaw velocity during planned movements can be used as a surrogate marker of oropharyngeal function. The use of STN-DBS may result in slowed jaw velocity, while GPi-DBS maintains or improves it [20]. Rigidity improves equally with STN- and GPi-DBS.

Gait and posture

While not cardinal symptoms of PD, postural instability and gait dysfunction affect a significant percentage of patients and respond to STN- and GPi-DBS. In the immediate postoperative period, the improvement is similar, but over time patients with STN-DBS decline. There may be a more durable effect on postural stability with GPi-DBS [21]. Furthermore, control of axial motor symptoms, especially in the off-medication state, is better after GPi-DBS [22]. One study found a significantly greater improvement in the stand–walk–sit test in patients with GPi-DBS compared with those with STN-DBS. Interestingly, this difference in mobility was seen in the off-medication, off-stimulation state [23].

Dyskinesias

Dyskinesias, involuntary movements induced by dopaminergic medications, affect a significant proportion of patients with PD. Dyskinesias may be caused by abnormal patterns of activity within the ventral pallidum. There may be a decrease in dyskinesias following GPi-DBS resulting from interference with such maladaptive patterns of activity or by suppressing GPi output via activation of nearby axons [24]. Deep-brain stimulation of the ventral pallidum may reduce dyskinesias but increase akinesias, whereas dorsal GPi stimulation has been suggested to have the opposite effect [25].

The incidence of levodopa (L-DOPA)-induced dyskinesias varies by age, affecting 50% of young-onset PD patients, compared with 16% of those over the age of 70 [26]. There is no standard levodopa dose that induces dyskinesias; the effect varies from patient to patient. The use of GPi-DBS has a direct antidyskinetic effect [25, 27], and some studies suggest it may be more effective for dyskinesia reduction than STN-DBS [24, 28]. In one study of patients implanted with both STN and GPi electrodes bilaterally, within-subject comparison was possible. The authors reported that, after prolonged medication withdrawal, GPi-DBS significantly reduced apomorphine-induced abnormal involuntary movements, while STN-DBS had no effect [29]. Another study found that GPi-DBS reduced dyskinesias compared with STN-DBS, despite greater medication reduction when the STN was implanted [30]. Other studies have demonstrated a significant reduction in dyskinesias in patients with STN-DBS in both the on- and off-stimulation states. Patients with GPi-DBS require stimulation to be on to experience a reduction of dyskinesias [16].

Long-term symptom control

Some patients with GPi-DBS may show a response reduction with long-term follow-up [25]. This may be related to the variability in clinical outcomes with small differences in lead position [31]. This difference, observed in early studies, has not been replicated and may only be an artifact from early management style [11, 32]. Nevertheless, in a young patient, with a long life expectancy, a potential for a decline in the response rate should be addressed.

Unified Parkinson's Disease Rating Scale (UPDRS) III

The effects of STN- and GPi-DBS are equivalent on general measures of motor function such as the UPDRS-III [23, 33]. However, the degree of motor symptom improvement is target dependent. This effect is evident when comparing on- versus off-stimulation state. A large randomized, controlled, blinded trial evaluating STN- versus GPi-DBS in 299 patients with PD did not find a significant difference in UPDRS-III scores between groups at 24 months when patients were on stimulation but off medication [23]. It did discover a difference in the off-stimulation, off-medication state. Without stimulation or medication, GPi patients had a small improvement in UPDRS-III. This was significantly different from the small decline found in STN patients [23]. Others have reported a similar effect [32]. This may be related to a longer duration of action and washout time for GPi-DBS. A similar effect has been described in the on-stimulation, on-medication state [32]. Additionally, in this state, patients with GPi-DBS demonstrated an improvement in UPDRS-II (activities of daily living) scores, while those with STN-DBS did not [33].

Effect of globus pallidus interna and the subthalamic nucleus deep-brain stimulation on nonmotor symptoms

Deleterious cognitive effects have been reported with STN-DBS in some patients. It is hypothesized that STN-DBS interferes with frontal executive functioning, decreases visual processing speed, and worsens verbal fluency and memory. Conversely, GPi-DBS may be less likely to impair nonmotor function in a clinically meaningful way [34]. Subclinical nonmotor effects are almost certainly occurring with DBS at either target.

Cognition

Cognitive decline occurs in many patients with advanced PD. For this reason, patients submit to a neuropsychological evaluation during the evaluation for surgical treatment. Following STN-DBS, those with minimal or no measurable cognitive changes preoperatively may worsen in the postoperative period. This effect is not as robust after GPi surgery [10]. In a randomized study of patients with GPi- or STN-DBS, slight declines in performance on the Mattis Dementia Scale at 36 months were detected in both groups. However, the decline was significantly greater for STN-DBS [32]. Similarly, at 36 months, performance on the Hopkins Verbal Learning Test was worse after STN-DBS [32]. In a small study that randomized patients to STN- or GPi-DBS, a higher rate of cognitive decline was noted in STN-DBS patients [16]. This effect, it seems, is more pronounced in older patients and in those with moderate baseline cognitive impairment preoperatively. For patients in whom STN-DBS is favored to treat motor symptoms, a staged bilateral procedure may be desirable [35]. Repeat neuropsychological evaluation may be warranted prior to placing the second electrode. At least one study has reported that, following GPi-DBS, confusion scores increased postoperatively. However, not all patients in the study were randomized to a surgical target. Because GPi-DBS is often selected in patients with worse preoperative cognitive function, this finding is most likely related to selection bias [36].

The use of STN-DBS appears to affect verbal fluency negatively. In patients randomized to unilateral STN- or GPi-DBS, STN-DBS decreased letter verbal fluency independent of the stimulation state being on or off.

This suggests that inserting an electrode into STN displaces or damages the neural elements in a clinically relevant manner [37]. Thus, STN-DBS may be associated with improved executive function but worse performance on tasks that test behavioral switching [38]. This higher-order processing is associated with increased activity in the dorsolateral prefrontal cortex (DLPFC): STN-DBS may augment DLPFC activity indirectly via thalamic projections from the substantia nigra reticulata. This increased DLPFC activity differentiates STN from GPi stimulation [39].

Anger

It has been shown that STN-DBS may interfere with the emotional state of PD patients. One study that randomized patients to unilateral STN- or GPi-DBS discovered that patients with STN-DBS had higher scores on the anger subscale of a visual analog mood scale [37]. However, it has also been reported that both STN- and GPi-DBS increase anger scores. This increase was independent of device activity, suggesting an effect related to local effects of the implant or due to events during surgery. Interestingly, in both STN- and GPi-DBS patients, microelectrode passes were directly correlated with anger scores. This further strengthens the argument that there is a surgical effect underlying the emotional change [36].

Mood

Mood is also more likely to be affected by STN-DBS than GPi-DBS [10]. A large randomized, controlled, blinded trial comparing STN- and GPi-DBS found that neither target resulted in a significant change in Beck Depression Inventory (BDI) scores between preoperative evaluation and 24-month follow-up. However, at the 24-month follow-up, BDI scores were slightly improved in the GPi group and worsened in the STN group, with a significant difference between groups [23].

Some negative effects of STN-DBS including depression, anhedonia and abulia may be related to medication withdrawal [40]. Maintaining a constant dose while still reducing dyskinesias may make the GPi a better target for patients dependent on the beneficial effects of their medications [24]. However, in one study, adverse events were less frequent in GPi patients, but those that did develop psychiatric, behavioral or speech adverse events were on higher doses of dopaminergic medication [41]. This suggests that medication dosing postoperatively requires a careful balance.

Quality of life

There may be greater improvement in quality of life with GPi-DBS than with STN-DBS. In one report, quality of life improved by 38% for GPi-DBS versus 15% for STN-DBS at 6 months postoperatively [42]. The GPi patients had a significant improvement in all four subscales of the 39-Item Parkinson's Disease Questionnaire (PDQ-39) (mobility, activities of daily living, stigma and social support), while the STN patients improved only in the stigma subscale.

Effect of globus pallidus interna and the subthalamic nucleus deep-brain stimulation on medication use

Dose reduction or medication elimination is an important goal for many patients with PD that factors into the decision to pursue surgical treatment. The reasons given vary but include side effects, the inconvenience of frequent dosing and cost. The prevailing view is that STN-DBS is associated with a greater medication reduction relative to GPi-DBS, and this in turn is often cited as the rationale to select the STN. Weaver *et al.* [43] reported that both STN- and GPi-DBS patients incurred medication expense savings starting at 6 months after surgery, although the cumulative savings were greater when STN was the target. In a meta-analysis of 45 studies, a net decrease in dopaminergic medication use was shown following STN-DBS but with GPi-DBS [33]. However, provider bias may account for some or all of the differences observed. The use of GPi-DBS may have a direct dyskinetic effect independent of dopaminergic medications. Aggressive medication reduction is then no longer at the forefront during follow-up visits when medication adjustments are made. Therefore, it may be the preferred target in patients whose motor response to dopaminergic medications is favorable but who are limited by dyskinesias [24]. In addition, in some PD patients, the effects of dopaminergic medication on mood and cognition are desirable, and attempts to reduce the dose are met with protest [33].

Not all studies support the widely held belief that STN-DBS is superior compared with GPi-DBS for medication reduction. In one study comparing both targets, patients were dose matched for preoperative dopaminergic medication and no difference was found in postoperative medication reduction between the groups [44]. In this study, postoperative management focused on maximal medication reduction. This lends support to the idea of the physician's role in influencing study outcomes as they relate to medication adjustments after DBS for PD being larger than previously thought. The total daily levodopa-equivalent dose may be of prognostic value for target selection. Patients with a low daily levodopa-equivalent dose (<1000 mg/day) achieved superior motor outcomes with GPi-DBS compared with patients on high-dose dopaminergic medications who responded best to STN-DBS [28]. This finding may be related to the greater medication reduction possible after STN-DBS, which varies between 38 and 56% postoperatively, compared with a 3% reduction in medications after GPi-DBS [16, 45].

Additional factors that influence target selection

Neuroimaging

In select patients, the preoperative imaging findings may drive target selection. The implant trajectory, from entry to target, is in general planned to avoid prominent vascular structures and the ventricles (although the adverse effects of intraventricular trajectories have not been definitively proven). In patients with ventriculomegaly or developmental venous anomalies, the more lateral target and trajectory for GPi electrode placement ($x = \pm 20$–22) may offer an alternative when STN targeting ($x = \pm 11$–12) would necessitate a less-than-ideal transventricular approach, or risk a vascular event caused by traversing a vessel. It has also been demonstrated that trajectories passing closer to the ventricle may result in less accurate electrode placement. Because GPi does not require a trajectory that passes close to the ventricle, its targeting may have a higher degree of accuracy [46].

Optimal visualization of the two nuclei and surrounding anatomy may be best achieved using different MRI sequences for direct targeting purposes. In general, targeting the GPi directly is simpler than the STN. T2 inversion recovery sequences provide good visualization of the GPi. One study found that proton-density-weighted MRI was most accurate in visualizing the GPi, along with critical targeting of landmarks of the optic tract and internal capsule, while susceptibility-weighted imaging was optimal for the STN [47]. Optimal imaging protocol varies based on the scanner type (GE versus Siemens), strength of magnet (1.5 T versus 3 T) and imaging software used to perform planning (Medtronic, BrainLab, FHC).

Positron emission tomography and single-photon-emission computed tomography studies that assess areas of dopamine uptake are evaluated to confirm diagnosis of PD but at this time do not provide sufficient information regarding target selection.

Awake/asleep deep-brain stimulation

Deep-brain stimulation may be performed under general anesthesia using image guidance, with the CereTom®, intraoperative MRI or ClearPoint® system [48]. Advantages of this technique include increased comfort for the patient, who does not have to be awake during the procedure, and greater anatomic accuracy. This technique also benefits patients with poor pulmonary function, whose airway may become compromised during the light sedation commonly used during awake DBS. However, electrode placement performed under general endotracheal anesthesia precludes MER, which may be used to confirm electrophysiological location. Furthermore, this technique yields inconsistent results from macrostimulation to confirm therapeutic efficacy and the absence of adverse effects. Therefore, DBS performed using image guidance alone may be better reserved for GPi electrode placement, as the nucleus is larger than the STN, and electrode placement is more forgiving.

Stereotactic surgery

Frame-based and frameless techniques may be used to guide DBS lead placement in either the GPi or STN. Accuracy of electrode placement is similar between the techniques for either target [49, 50], and some studies suggest that frameless electrode placement may in fact surpass that of frame-based stereotaxy [48]. This is obviously an important question to address because, as the error goes up, so too does the chance that the target is missed; furthermore, a small target is easier to miss.

Programming challenges following globus pallidus interna and the subthalamic nucleus deep-brain stimulation

Because the configuration of the neural components and their relative locations within the motor circuit are different, the strategy to program a DBS lead implanted at one site versus the other will vary. For the same reason, the rate at which the symptoms abate is governed by the target. For example, the therapeutic effect of GPi-DBS may not be observed for several weeks, unlike STN-DBS where the effect is often immediate.

Although patients with PD often have suffered for years if not decades, this additional waiting time may be disheartening. Rigidity tends to improve faster with STN stimulation than with GPi; the effect on tremor and bradykinesia has a more variable time course [51]. Stimulation of the GPi may have an immediate effect on dyskinesias; therefore, it may be preferable to program in the on-medication state [51]. It is not unusual to see an increase in dyskinesias following STN-DBS that prompts physicians to aggressively reduce dopaminergic medications in these patients. This may have contributed to the belief that STN is superior when medication reduction is a major goal of surgery [10].

Target-dependent stimulation-induced side effects may limit the degree of symptom relief. With GPi-DBS, this includes visual complaints related to optic tract stimulation, pseudodystonia from stimulation of the pyramidal tract, nausea and dizziness [25]. The most common side effects after STN stimulation include paresthesias due to prelemniscal stimulation and motor contractions due to stimulation spillover to the internal capsule. In rare cases, STN stimulation may result in hypersexuality, compulsive gambling or other behaviors related to loss of impulse control associated with dysregulation of the limbic circuit [52]. Patients with GPi-DBS may need more frequent implantable pulse generator replacement due to the higher voltage requirements [41]. This should be a consideration in a patient with a high surgical risk who is not a candidate for a rechargeable system.

Operative risks of globus pallidus interna and the subthalamic nucleus deep-brain stimulation

Immediate risks

As would be expected, the inherent operative risks of DBS for two structures approximately 10 mm apart (excluding unwanted stimulation-induced side effects) are similar with perhaps one notable exception – the risk of intraparenchymal hemorrhage. The risk of intraoperative or postoperative hemorrhage may be slightly higher following GPi lead implantation. Binder et al. [53] reported a 7% risk of hemorrhage following lead implantation in the GPi and a 2.2% risk when the STN was the target ($P = 0.001$). However, no significant difference in hemorrhage risk by location was observed in a later study [54]. As postoperative hemorrhage has the potential to lead to long-term disability or death, even a small increase in relative risk should not be discounted and this risk should be disclosed to the patient.

Other immediate risks of surgery are less devastating but still problematic in the short term. Some patients may be more prone to experiencing transient postoperative confusion or delirium following STN-DBS [16]. This may prolong hospitalization and/or compound the risk of being in an unfamiliar environment when disoriented. This risk may be alleviated or lessened when the procedure is staged.

Delayed risks

Patients with STN-DBS may have a higher rate of speech disturbances including dysphonia and dysarthria [22]. Long-term cognitive changes such as memory decline or psychotic symptoms and mood disturbances may also be more common in these patients. It has been postulated that these cognitive changes may be related to the role of STN in cognitive and limbic circuits [22, 41]. These complications may persist for more than 5 years [31]. Stimulation by STN-DBS may be associated with adverse effects on speech and swallowing, as well as with increased hypophonia and hypersalivation. Some of these effects may be related to the reduction of dopaminergic medication postoperatively [40]. In patients with STN- but not GPi-DBS, a high rate of complications in the postoperative period is associated with lower quality-of-life scores in the future [55]. Perhaps related to the beneficial effect of GPi-DBS on gait, there is a higher rate of falls in patients with STN-DBS postoperatively than in those with GPi-DBS [22, 23].

Weight gain has been reported after both STN- and GPi-DBS. Weight gain may be related to the decreased energy expenditure that occurs with improved motor symptom control, changes in eating patterns or other less well-understood factors. One study found that weight gain in GPi-DBS was correlated with a decrease in dyskinesias [56]. Some authors have reported greater weight gain with STN-DBS [57] without a measurable increase in caloric intake [56]. It has been surmised that STN stimulation exerts a central control of energy balance through reciprocal connections with the ventral pallidum [58].

Conclusions

Deep-brain stimulation of the STN and GPi effectively reduces the disabling symptoms of PD in randomized controlled trials. As both sites are proven options, the "paradox of choice" has confounded the decision-making process for surgical teams evaluating patients.

Table 27.2 Summary of studies comparing subthalamic nucleus (STN) and globus pallidus interna (GPi) deep-brain stimulation (DBS) directly

Study	Year	Description	Findings
Deep-Brain Stimulation for Parkinson's Disease Study Group (2001) [7]	2001	91 patients with STN-DBS and 35 patients with GPi-DBS underwent prospective, double-blind, crossover evaluation of UPDRS scores	STN-DBS resulted in 49% and GPi-DBS in 37% improvement in motor scores
Follett et al. (2010) [23]	2010	299 patients randomized to STN-DBS (147) or GPi-DBS (152) underwent blinded assessment at 24 months	Both STN- and GPi-DBS improved motor function with no significant difference between groups. Greater reduction in dopaminergic medication with STN-DBS. STN group had more depression
Okun et al. (2009) [37]	2009	COMPARE trial: 52 patients randomized to unilateral STN-DBS vs GPi-DBS evaluated on cognitive and mood measures at 7 months postoperatively	No difference in primary cognitive and mood outcomes between targets. STN-DBS had greater decline in letter verbal fluency. Greater number of mood and cognitive adverse events with STN-DBS
Anderson et al. (2005) [16]	2005	Blinded assessment of 20 patients randomized to STN-DBS (10) or GPi-DBS (10)	STN had 48% and GPi had 39% improvement in off-medication motor scores. STN trended toward greater reduction in levodopa dose. More cognitive and behavioral complications with STN
Weaver et al. (2005) [32]	2012	Patients randomized to STN-DBS (70) or GPi-DBS (89) assessed in a blinded manner at 36 months	Motor outcomes in the two groups were similar. Dementia scores had a greater decline for STN. Greater decreases in dopaminergic medication for STN
Odekerken et al. (2013) [30]	2013	Randomized, blinded study of STN-DBS (63 patients) vs GPi-DBS (65 patients)	Greater improvement in "off"-phase UPDRS and disability scores with STN-DBS. GPi had greater reduction in dyskinesias

Most early studies touting the success of each target were not randomized and were generally underpowered. This inadvertently introduced significant bias into the discussion, which is still playing out today. Now, however, the influence of surgeon experience, anecdotal evidence and training should carry less weight as the number of peer-reviewed articles has multiplied and subtle differences between the STN and GPi have sharpened. The relative distinctions between the STN and GPi are still under investigation; rigid beliefs that favor one nucleus over the other are crumbling and defectors are found in both camps. We may find that quality-of-life measures, assuming similar risks, matter more than alleviation of select symptoms that guided the decision in the first place. For now, the advantages and disadvantages for each target should be compared with delivering the best possible outcome for each patient (see Table 27.2 for a summary). This should be weighed against what has motivated the patient to pursue motor symptom-specific surgery, medication intolerance and their appreciation of the risks unique to each nucleus. This comes with the inherent understanding by the physician that our knowledge will continue to evolve but does not belie our intentions to optimize outcomes for our patients.

References

1. Weaver FM, Follett K, Stern M, et al. Bilateral deep brain stimulation vs best medical therapy for patients with advanced Parkinson disease: a randomized controlled trial. *JAMA* 2009; **301**: 63–73.
2. Siegfried J, Lippitz B. Bilateral chronic electrostimulation of ventroposterolateral pallidum: a new therapeutic approach for alleviating all parkinsonian symptoms. *Neurosurgery* 1994; **35**: 1126–9; discussion 1129–30.
3. Pollak P, Benabid AL, Gross C, et al. [Effects of the stimulation of the subthalamic nucleus in Parkinson disease]. *Rev Neurol (Paris)* 1993; **149**: 175–6 (in French).
4. Boucai L, Cerquetti D, Merello M. Functional surgery for Parkinson's disease treatment: a structured analysis of a decade of published literature. *Br J Neurosurg* 2004; **18**: 213–22.
5. Gross RE, Krack P, Rodriguez-Oroz MC, Rezai AR, Benabid AL. Electrophysiological mapping for the

implantation of deep brain stimulators for Parkinson's disease and tremor. *Mov Disord* 2006; **21** (Suppl. 14): S259–283.
6. Bour LJ, Contarino MF, Foncke EM, et al. Long-term experience with intraoperative microrecording during DBS neurosurgery in STN and GPi. *Acta Neurochir (Wien)* 2010; **152**: 2069–77.
7. Deep-Brain Stimulation for Parkinson's Disease Study Group. Deep-brain stimulation of the subthalamic nucleus or the pars interna of the globus pallidus in Parkinson's disease. *N Engl J Med* 2001; **345**: 956–63.
8. Cleary DR, Raslan AM, Rubin JE, et al. Deep brain stimulation entrains local neuronal firing in human globus pallidus internus. *J Neurophysiol* 2013; **109**: 978–87.
9. Lai HY, Younce JR, Albaugh DL, Kao YC, Shih YY. Functional MRI reveals frequency-dependent responses during deep brain stimulation at the subthalamic nucleus or internal globus pallidus. *Neuroimage* 2013; **84**: 11–18.
10. Vitek JL. Deep brain stimulation for Parkinson's disease. A critical re-evaluation of STN versus GPi-DBS. *Stereotact Funct Neurosurg* 2002; **78**: 119–31.
11. Okun MS, Foote KD. Subthalamic nucleus vs globus pallidus interna deep brain stimulation, the rematch: will pallidal deep brain stimulation make a triumphant return? *Arch Neurol* 2005; **62**: 533–6.
12. Mann JM, Foote KD, Garvan CW, et al. Brain penetration effects of microelectrodes and DBS leads in STN or GPi. *J Neurol Neurosurg Psychiatry* 2009; **80**: 794–7.
13. Benabid AL, Pollak P, Gross C, et al. Acute and long-term effects of subthalamic nucleus stimulation in Parkinson's disease. *Stereotact Funct Neurosurg* 1994; **62**: 76–84.
14. Ghika J, Villemure JG, Fankhauser H, et al. Efficiency and safety of bilateral contemporaneous pallidal stimulation (deep brain stimulation) in levodopa-responsive patients with Parkinson's disease with severe motor fluctuations: a 2-year follow-up review. *J Neurosurg* 1998; **89**: 713–18.
15. Keitel A, Ferrea S, Sudmeyer M, Schnitzler A, Wojtecki L. Expectation modulates the effect of deep brain stimulation on motor and cognitive function in tremor-dominant Parkinson's disease. *PLoS One* 2013; **8**: e81878.
16. Anderson VC, Burchiel KJ, Hogarth P, Favre J, Hammerstad JP. Pallidal vs subthalamic nucleus deep brain stimulation in Parkinson disease. *Arch Neurol* 2005; **62**: 554–60.
17. Krack P, Batir A, Van Blercom N, et al. Five-year follow-up of bilateral stimulation of the subthalamic nucleus in advanced Parkinson's disease. *N Engl J Med* 2003; **349**: 1925–34.
18. Nakamura K, Christine CW, Starr PA, Marks WJ Jr. Effects of unilateral subthalamic and pallidal deep brain stimulation on fine motor functions in Parkinson's disease. *Mov Disord* 2007; **22**: 619–26.
19. Krack P, Pollak P, Limousin P, et al. Subthalamic nucleus or internal pallidal stimulation in young onset Parkinson's disease. *Brain* 1998; **121**: 451–7.
20. Robertson LT, St George RJ, Carlson-Kuhta P, et al. Site of deep brain stimulation and jaw velocity in Parkinson disease. *J Neurosurg* 2011; **115**: 985–94.
21. St George RJ, Nutt JG, Burchiel KJ, Horak FB. A meta-regression of the long-term effects of deep brain stimulation on balance and gait in PD. *Neurology* 2010; **75**: 1292–9.
22. Rodriguez-Oroz MC, Obeso JA, Lang AE, et al. Bilateral deep brain stimulation in Parkinson's disease: a multicentre study with 4 years follow-up. *Brain* 2005; **128**: 2240–9.
23. Follett KA, Weaver FM, Stern M, et al. Pallidal versus subthalamic deep-brain stimulation for Parkinson's disease. *N Engl J Med* 2010; **362**: 2077–91.
24. Follett KA. Comparison of pallidal and subthalamic deep brain stimulation for the treatment of levodopa-induced dyskinesias. *Neurosurg Focus* 2004; **17**: E3.
25. Volkmann J. Deep brain stimulation for the treatment of Parkinson's disease. *J Clin Neurophysiol* 2004; **21**: 6–17.
26. Kumar N, Van Gerpen JA, Bower JH, Ahlskog JE. Levodopa-dyskinesia incidence by age of Parkinson's disease onset. *Mov Disord* 2005; **20**: 342–4.
27. Krause M, Fogel W, Heck A, et al. Deep brain stimulation for the treatment of Parkinson's disease: subthalamic nucleus versus globus pallidus internus. *J Neurol Neurosurg Psychiatry* 2001; **70**: 464–70.
28. Minguez-Castellanos A, Escamilla-Sevilla F, Katati MJ, et al. Different patterns of medication change after subthalamic or pallidal stimulation for Parkinson's disease: target related effect or selection bias? *J Neurol Neurosurg Psychiatry* 2005; **76**: 34–9.
29. Peppe A, Pierantozzi M, Bassi A, et al. Stimulation of the subthalamic nucleus compared with the globus pallidus internus in patients with Parkinson disease. *J Neurosurg* 2004; **101**: 195–200.
30. Odekerken VJ, van Laar T, Staal MJ, et al. Subthalamic nucleus versus globus pallidus bilateral deep brain stimulation for advanced Parkinson's disease (NSTAPS study): a randomised controlled trial. *Lancet Neurol* 2013; **12**: 37–44.
31. Moro E, Lozano AM, Pollak P, et al. Long-term results of a multicenter study on subthalamic and pallidal stimulation in Parkinson's disease. *Mov Disord* 2010; **25**: 578–86.
32. Weaver FM, Follett KA, Stern M, et al. Randomized trial of deep brain stimulation for Parkinson disease: thirty-six-month outcomes. *Neurology* 2012; **79**: 55–65.

33. Weaver F, Follett K, Hur K, Ippolito D, Stern M. Deep brain stimulation in Parkinson disease: a metaanalysis of patient outcomes. *J Neurosurg* 2005; **103**: 956–67.
34. Borgohain R, Kandadai RM, Jabeen A, Kannikannan MA. Nonmotor outcomes in Parkinson's disease: is deep brain stimulation better than dopamine replacement therapy? *Ther Adv Neurol Disord* 2012; **5**: 23–41.
35. Yaguez L, Costello A, Moriarty J, et al. Cognitive predictors of cognitive change following bilateral subthalamic nucleus deep brain stimulation in Parkinson's disease. *J Clin Neurosci* 2014; **21**: 445–50.
36. Burdick AP, Foote KD, Wu S, et al. Do patient's get angrier following STN, GPi, and thalamic deep brain stimulation. *Neuroimage* 2011; **54** (Suppl. 1): S227–32.
37. Okun MS, Fernandez HH, Wu SS, et al. Cognition and mood in Parkinson's disease in subthalamic nucleus versus globus pallidus interna deep brain stimulation: the COMPARE trial. *Ann Neurol* 2009; **65**: 586–95.
38. Jahanshahi M, Ardouin CM, Brown RG, et al. The impact of deep brain stimulation on executive function in Parkinson's disease. *Brain* 2000; **123**: 1142–54.
39. Limousin P, Greene J, Pollak P, et al. Changes in cerebral activity pattern due to subthalamic nucleus or internal pallidum stimulation in Parkinson's disease. *Ann Neurol* 1997; **42**: 283–91.
40. Volkmann J, Allert N, Voges J, et al. Safety and efficacy of pallidal or subthalamic nucleus stimulation in advanced PD. *Neurology* 2001; **56**: 548–51.
41. Hariz MI, Rehncrona S, Quinn NP, et al. Multicenter study on deep brain stimulation in Parkinson's disease: an independent assessment of reported adverse events at 4 years. *Mov Disord* 2008; **23**: 416–21.
42. Zahodne LB, Okun MS, Foote KD, et al. Greater improvement in quality of life following unilateral deep brain stimulation surgery in the globus pallidus as compared to the subthalamic nucleus. *J Neurol* 2009; **256**: 1321–9.
43. Weaver FM, Stroupe KT, Cao L, et al. Parkinson's disease medication use and costs following deep brain stimulation. *Mov Disord* 2012; **27**: 1398–403.
44. Evidente VG, Premkumar AP, Adler CH, et al. Medication dose reductions after pallidal versus subthalamic stimulation in patients with Parkinson's disease. *Acta Neurol Scand* 2011; **124**: 211–14.
45. Schupbach WM, Chastan N, Welter ML, et al. Stimulation of the subthalamic nucleus in Parkinson's disease: a 5 year follow-up. *J Neurol Neurosurg Psychiatry* 2005; **76**: 1640–4.
46. Burchiel KJ, McCartney S, Lee A, Raslan AM. Accuracy of deep brain stimulation electrode placement using intraoperative computed tomography without microelectrode recording. *J Neurosurg* 2013; **119**: 301–6.
47. O'Gorman RL, Shmueli K, Ashkan K, et al. Optimal MRI methods for direct stereotactic targeting of the subthalamic nucleus and globus pallidus. *Eur Radiol* 2011; **21**: 130–6.
48. Khan FR, Henderson JM. Deep brain stimulation surgical techniques. *Handb Clin Neurol* 2013; **116**: 27–37.
49. Holloway KL, Gaede SE, Starr PA, et al. Frameless stereotaxy using bone fiducial markers for deep brain stimulation. *J Neurosurg* 2005; **103**: 404–13.
50. Bjartmarz H, Rehncrona S. Comparison of accuracy and precision between frame-based and frameless stereotactic navigation for deep brain stimulation electrode implantation. *Stereotact Funct Neurosurg* 2007; **85**: 235–42.
51. Volkmann J, Moro E, Pahwa R. Basic algorithms for the programming of deep brain stimulation in Parkinson's disease. *Mov Disord* 2006; **21** (Suppl. 14): S284–9.
52. Broen M, Duits A, Visser-Vandewalle V, Temel Y, Winogrodzka A. Impulse control and related disorders in Parkinson's disease patients treated with bilateral subthalamic nucleus stimulation: a review. *Parkinsonism Relat Disord* 2011; **17**: 413–17.
53. Binder DK, Rau GM, Starr PA. Risk factors for hemorrhage during microelectrode-guided deep brain stimulator implantation for movement disorders. *Neurosurgery* 2005; **56**: 722–32; discussion 722–32.
54. Ben-Haim S, Asaad WF, Gale JT, Eskandar EN. Risk factors for hemorrhage during microelectrode-guided deep brain stimulation and the introduction of an improved microelectrode design. *Neurosurgery* 2009; **64**: 754–62; discussion 762–3.
55. Volkmann J, Albanese A, Kulisevsky J, et al. Long-term effects of pallidal or subthalamic deep brain stimulation on quality of life in Parkinson's disease. *Mov Disord* 2009; **24**: 1154–61.
56. Sauleau P, Leray E, Rouaud T, et al. Comparison of weight gain and energy intake after subthalamic versus pallidal stimulation in Parkinson's disease. *Mov Disord* 2009; **24**: 2149–55.
57. Mills KA, Scherzer R, Starr PA, Ostrem JL. Weight change after globus pallidus internus or subthalamic nucleus deep brain stimulation in Parkinson's disease and dystonia. *Stereotact Funct Neurosurg* 2012; **90**: 386–93.
58. Rieu I, Derost P, Ulla M, et al. Body weight gain and deep brain stimulation. *J Neurol Sci* 2011; **310**: 267–70.

Chapter 28

Controversy: ablative surgery vs deep-brain stimulation in the management of Parkinson's disease

Gian D. Pal and Leo Verhagen Metman

Introduction

The concept of surgically modulating the central nervous system as treatment for Parkinson's disease (PD) has been in existence since the early 1900s [1]. At that time, lesions were made via craniotomies, initially involving the pyramidal and later the extrapyramidal systems. Lesion therapy as we know it today for PD has its origins in the late 1940s, when Spiegel and Wycis [2] introduced the stereotactic head frame, allowing surgeons to target subcortical structures without using an open, nonstereotactic approach. These pioneers performed and reported on 100 stereotactic pallidoansotomies for PD [3] using the same target that Russell Meyers had used during open surgery [4] and showed improvements in tremor and rigidity. In addition, in the early 1950s, Cooper made a serendipitous discovery (when he was "obliged to sacrifice" the anterior choroidal artery) that pallidotomy could improve the motor symptoms of PD [5, 6]. Pallidotomy continued to be performed through the 1950s [5–8] but then fell out of favor with the introduction of thalamotomy [9]. The ventrolateral thalamic target became favored based on neuroanatomical data [9] as well as, again, on serendipity, when Cooper found that a planned pallidal lesion was actually in the ventrolateral thalamus on autopsy. His report of impressive efficacy of the thalamic lesion on parkinsonian tremor helped drive most contemporary surgeons to choose the thalamus over the pallidum as the surgical target of choice [10].

In 1960, Svennilson et al. [11] kept the practice of pallidotomy alive by demonstrating that posteroventral pallidotomy was an effective therapy for all cardinal features of PD, and that posteriorly placed pallidal lesions produced superior results to those placed more anteriorly [11]. At the time, this work was largely ignored, and thalamotomy continued to be the procedure of choice [10]. With the advent of levodopa (L-DOPA), surgical therapy was largely abandoned until it was eventually recognized that the benefits of medical therapy came at a cost over time, in the form of levodopa-induced dyskinesias and motor fluctuations [12, 13]. In 1992, when Laitinen et al. [14] reintroduced Leksell's posteroventral pallidotomy for PD and reported marked benefits in *all* cardinal motor signs of the disease (not just tremor), pallidotomy became the surgery of choice for patients with PD and motor complications.

The modern era of deep-brain stimulation (DBS) was heralded by the seminal publication in 1987 by Benabid et al. [15], entitled "Combined (thalamotomy and stimulation) stereotactic surgery of the VIM thalamic nucleus for bilateral Parkinson's disease." Shortly thereafter, studies regarding functional anatomy of the basal ganglia [16] and primate models of movement disorders [17] fueled new interest in surgery, and the stage was set for exploration of the subthalamic nucleus (STN) and globus pallidus interna (GPi) as targets for DBS in humans. In 1993, the Grenoble group reported a case of unilateral STN-DBS for akinetic–rigid PD and found that akinesia was alleviated and no hemiballismus was elicited [18]. In their 1998 publication, the same investigators reported outcomes in 20 PD patients with 1 year of bilateral STN-DBS and documented a 60% improvement in motor Unified Parkinson's Disease Rating Scale (UPDRS) "off" scores and a 50% reduction in levodopa requirement [19]. Emboldened by the similar efficacy of thalamotomy and thalamic DBS for tremor [15], Siegfried and

Parkinson's Disease: Current and Future Therapeutics and Clinical Trials, ed. Gálvez-Jiménez et al. Published by Cambridge University Press. © Cambridge University Press 2016.

Lippitz [20] set out to determine whether the efficacy of pallidotomy could be matched by pallidal DBS. In 1994, they reported substantial benefits of GPi-DBS in three PD patients [20].

By the turn of the century, the world now had two viable surgical techniques for the treatment of PD. The availability of lesioning procedures and DBS sparked an inevitable debate – are both procedures comparable from an efficacy and safety standpoint? In this chapter, we intend to shed light on this debate by reviewing the literature. Clearly, there is a paucity of head-to-head controlled trials; in addition, there are many different targets that can be, and have been, lesioned or stimulated, making comparisons all the more complicated. Where possible, we have used level I studies that include randomized controlled studies, if not of head-to-head comparison design, then at least of surgery versus best medical therapy design. In the absence of such controlled studies, we have included larger case–control studies (level II evidence) and case series (level III evidence). We have organized this review per target and will discuss the benefits as well as adverse events associated with each of the two procedures (lesioning and stimulation) in each target. The studies presented here are not meant to be exhaustive but rather are chosen to highlight the key points for each procedure.

The potential controversy

In theory, lesioning and DBS should have similar outcomes. After all, they are quite similar from a procedural standpoint in many ways. A stereotactic head frame or a frameless system along with MRI and/or CT can be used for target planning in both procedures. The target coordinates can be obtained directly using the acquired images or measured indirectly with standard stereotactic measurements. In both procedures, burr holes are created and the target localization can be performed with or without microelectrode recording guidance. Macrostimulation can be used in either procedure to help verify the target and assess benefit [21, 22]. From a conceptual point of view, with both structural (lesioning) and functional (stimulation) methods, aberrant neuronal firing patterns within the pathological circuitry are inactivated.

Of course key differences exist as well. With lesioning, no hardware is left behind, and a second procedure to place the pulse generator and extension leads under anesthesia is not needed, as occurs in DBS. The lesioning surgery therefore is shorter and less expensive. Once the incision has healed, lesioning procedures do not carry long-term risks of infection; they are not associated with fracture, displacement or skin erosion, nor do they require battery changes or time-intensive programming sessions that are typical for DBS. If lesioning were a procedure in the culinary world of rotisserie, it would be advertised as "set it and forget it." However, these exact "advantages" of lesioning at the same time represent significant shortcomings. First, lesioning is by definition a procedure in which tissue is *permanently* destroyed. If the lesion is in the perfect location, then there is no problem. If, on the other hand, a lesion is made too close to an undesirable region such as the internal capsule or optic tract, unwanted side effects may be permanent. In contrast, a DBS lead in the same undesirable location can be reprogrammed, inactivated or repositioned through additional surgery. Secondly, the volume of a lesion is fixed. If the lesion is too generous, side effects will occur and if the lesion is too conservative, the benefit will wane over time, as it will do with progression of the disease. With DBS, on the other hand, the stimulated tissue volume as well as the field of stimulation can be tailored, to some degree, to maximize benefit, minimize side effects and optimize symptom control as the disease progresses. If the slogan for lesioning is "set it and forget it," then the catchphrase for DBS would be "personalized medicine," or better, personalized surgery.

With the above in mind, we will now examine studies on the efficacy and safety of lesioning versus DBS by focusing on the most common targets – the thalamus, pallidum and STN. As we explore the literature on these two treatments, we anticipate that a common theme will emerge where efficacy may be comparable and side effect profiles will drive the decision to favor one therapy over the other.

Lesioning versus deep-brain stimulation: a comparison of efficacy and safety

Thalamus

Thalamotomy versus thalamic DBS

In the aforementioned seminal study that launched the modern era of DBS, Benabid *et al.* [15] performed unilateral thalamotomy in 18 patients, nine with PD and nine with "bilateral tremor of extrapyramidal origin." The tremor response was classified as excellent (tremor resolution) in 16 patients, while the results were "moderate in 1 and bad in 1." In six patients, chronic thalamic DBS was performed, but only three patients were "greatly improved." In one PD patient, combined thalamotomy and contralateral thalamic DBS was performed. The latter was of particular interest as it had been recognized that bilateral thalamotomy was associated with considerable side effects. In this patient, the thalamotomy had an "excellent but transient effect on tremor," while DBS "strongly improved" the contralateral tremor. Of the 18 patients who received thalamotomy, seven had transitory complications, while four had permanent complications that were not specified. In the chronic thalamic DBS group, no complications occurred. This case series showed the promise of thalamotomy and thalamic DBS as a viable treatment for PD tremor but also highlighted potential concerns for each of these surgical therapies.

There has been a single level I study in which thalamotomy was directly compared with thalamic DBS. Schuurman et al. [23] conducted a randomized trial assessing the efficacy of unilateral thalamotomy versus unilateral or bilateral thalamic DBS for the treatment of tremor in 70 patients, mainly in PD, but essential tremor and multiple sclerosis patients with tremor were also included. The primary outcome measure was change from baseline in the Frenchay Activities Index, a scale that measures functional status, with higher scores indicating better function. Of the total group, 17 patients underwent unilateral thalamic stimulation and 21 patients underwent unilateral thalamotomy. At 6 months postoperatively, the stimulation group was significantly better than the lesion group with regard to functional status. This was also true at the 5-year follow-up. In the same study, another group of eight patients received unilateral thalamotomy and then received contralateral thalamic stimulation. When these patients were compared with the 17 patients who received bilateral thalamic stimulation, there was no significant difference in functional outcome at 6 months or 5 years. The authors performed a subgroup analysis by diagnosis and reported a significant difference in functional outcome between the PD patients who received stimulation versus thalamotomy in favor of stimulation. However, it is not clear whether the patients in the stimulation group had bilateral procedures, whereas the thalamotomy group had unilateral or bilateral procedures. This study supports the claim that unilateral thalamic DBS has a better functional outcome than unilateral thalamotomy at 5 years, although tremor scores were comparable.

This study also examined bilateral thalamic targeting. The authors state that "bilateral thalamotomy is not performed due to high complication rates in the past," so bilateral thalamic DBS was not compared with bilateral thalamotomy. Instead, bilateral thalamic DBS was compared with the combination of unilateral thalamotomy with thalamic DBS and there was not a clear difference in functional outcome.

With regard to complications, the authors reported that at 5 years, 8/22 (36%) thalamotomy patients had complications from surgery whereas 2/25 (8%) DBS patients had adverse events. The complications that were more pronounced in the thalamotomy group included cognitive deterioration, dysarthria, and gait and balance disturbance. However, there was one death in the DBS group (perioperative cerebral hemorrhage) and six equipment-related complications, all requiring surgery, including a repeat stereotactic procedure in one case.

We can draw several conclusions about the thalamus as a target for PD based on the information above. Tremor improvement or remission can occur, although the other cardinal features of PD, such as bradykinesia, rigidity and gait will likely not improve. If tremor is particularly prominent on one side compared with the other warranting only unilateral treatment, then thalamic DBS seems to have superior long-term functional outcome compared with thalamotomy, although tremor reduction is comparable.

On the other hand, PD patients with bilateral tremor may opt for a bilateral surgical intervention with the thalamus as the target for tremor control. Although bilateral thalamotomy has been performed in the past, it was during a time where imaging and surgical techniques were less sophisticated. This resulted in less accurate targeting and consequently a greater incidence of side effects. Some data regarding the side effects of bilateral thalamotomy seem to be extrapolated from its use in dystonic patients, where a 10–40% risk of serious complications such as bulbar weakness, dysarthria, cognitive impairment and ataxia has been reported [24]. In 1961, Krayenbuhl et al. [25] performed bilateral thalamotomy in 23 PD patients, with abolition of tremor and rigidity in 15 cases. However, different side effects were seen including worsening of speech in seven cases, worsened gait in four subjects and death in one patient. In 1999, Moriyama et al. [26] reported on nine patients who underwent bilateral thalamotomy for PD, all of whom had a "satisfactory" tremor response. However, four of these patients became "completely bedridden or dependent" within 3 years. Jankovic et al. [27] reported that bilateral thalamotomy may improve severe bilateral tremor but at the expense of moderately severe hypophonia. A similar finding was reported by Wester and Hauglie-Hanssen [28]. According to a report from the American Academy of Neurology [29], bilateral thalamotomy is an option if "the patient is willing to accept the possibility of dysarthria, but because of the significant risk, bilateral thalamotomy would have to be considered doubtful – a type D recommendation based on minimal evidence." Today, bilateral thalamotomy is no longer recommended. Thus, if bilateral tremor is problematic and the thalamus is the target of choice, there are two potential options – bilateral thalamic DBS or a combination of thalamic DBS with thalamotomy. However, given that thalamotomy comes with potential risks that are more likely to be irreversible, bilateral thalamic DBS seems to remain superior to thalamotomy.

Pallidum

Unilateral pallidotomy versus unilateral pallidal DBS
Unilateral pallidotomy

Although thalamic targeting certainly helped with PD tremor, the pallidum became a very attractive target once it was realized that many of the levodopa-responsive symptoms, including bradykinesia, rigidity, tremor and gait changes, had the potential to improve if the pallidum was lesioned or stimulated. Unilateral pallidotomy has not been compared directly with unilateral pallidal DBS is in a head-to-head randomized study. However, Blomstedt et al. [30] analyzed the effect of unilateral pallidotomy and contralateral pallidal stimulation on symptoms within the same PD patients. Five consecutive patients received pallidotomy contralateral to the more symptomatic side of the body. At a mean of 14 months later, the same patients received pallidal DBS on the side contralateral to the site of the pallidotomy. Evaluations were performed at a mean duration of 37 months (range 22–60) after the pallidotomy and 22 months (range 12–33) after pallidal DBS. The scores of appendicular item numbers 20–26 of the UPDRS-III (motor severity) were compared between the side that received pallidotomy and the side that received pallidal DBS. The side contralateral to pallidotomy improved by 32.5%, whereas the side contralateral to the pallidal DBS improved by 25%. Dyskinesias and dystonia items 32–35 of the UPDRS-IV (motor complications) were rated separately for each side. The side contralateral to the pallidotomy improved by 91%, whereas the side contralateral to the pallidal DBS improved by 59%. With regard to safety, no pre- or postoperative complications occurred in connection with the initial pallidotomies. Concerning pallidal DBS procedures, two patients exhibited moderate dysarthria and one patient showed a severe worsening of dysphonia following DBS. The dysarthria was partly reversible with alteration of stimulation, but the dysphonia was irreversible regardless of stimulation changes. The DBS system was affected negatively by external factors in two cases. In one case, the neurostimulator was damaged during electrical welding and resulted in replacement. In the second case, the patient's hearing device interacted with the DBS system creating a headache when this was used. This required cable revision without any improvement.

It should be noted that in this study patients always received pallidotomy contralateral to the more symptomatic side, which could explain the greater improvement. In other words, the first operated, most affected, side may have the greatest improvement regardless of the procedure chosen. The authors concluded that "the effect of pallidotomy to be at least as good and as safe as that of pallidal DBS." To further address the veracity of this statement in the absence of head-to-head studies, we can separately examine trials of unilateral pallidotomy and those of unilateral pallidal DBS.

Two level I studies exist that compared unilateral pallidotomy with best medical care. In 1999, de Bie et al. [31] conducted a prospective, randomized, single-blinded, multicenter trial in which 37 patients were randomized to unilateral pallidotomy within 1 month of enrollment or to best medical care (with pallidotomy 6 months later). The primary outcome was the change in the motor UPDRS "off" score between baseline and 6 months. The pallidotomy patients median motor UPDRS "off" score improved by 31% (from 47 to 32.5), whereas the control group with best medical care slightly worsened by 8% (from 52.5 to 56.5). There was a statistically significant difference between the two groups ($P<0.001$). There were also statistically significant improvements in scores for the pallidotomy group on the Barthel index (a scale measuring activities of daily living [ADLs])($P=0.004$), the ADL section of the UPDRS (UPDRS-II; $P=0.002$), and the Schwab and England Scale ($P<0.001$). During the "on"-phase assessment, median score in the dyskinesia rating scale improved compared with the control group by 50%

($P=0.02$). Patients' symptom diaries in the pallidotomy group revealed that they had more "on" time without dyskinesias compared with the control group by an average of 2.8 h/day ($P=0.02$). Similarly, Vitek et al. [32] conducted a randomized trial with blinded ratings of 36 patients comparing the effects of unilateral pallidotomy ($n=18$) versus medical therapy ($n=18$) over a 6-month period. The primary outcome was change in the total UPDRS score, and it was found that pallidotomy induced a 32% improvement compared with a 5% decline in the control group ($P<0.0001$). Dyskinesias and motor fluctuations significantly improved only in the surgery group, although the study was not powered specifically to detect changes in these secondary indices. In general, the "off" UPDRS motor score has been reported to improve by 31–32% postoperatively [31, 32].

The efficacy of unilateral pallidotomy for improving motor symptoms has also been supported by a number of level III studies [33–42]. In addition to improvement in the symptoms of parkinsonism, pallidotomy has consistently been shown to improve dyskinesias, particularly contralateral to the side of the lesion [33–37, 40, 43]. Thus, unilateral pallidotomy seems to improve parkinsonism, dyskinesias and motor fluctuations, and several additional studies have reported on its safety.

A level II study by Perrine et al. [44] examined the impact on cognitive function. The group assessed change in a neuropsychological battery of tests over a 1-year period as the primary outcome. These tests included the Mini Mental Status Examination (MMSE), Controlled Oral Word Association Test, Trail Making Test (part A and B), Symbol Digit Modalities Test, Stroop test, Wisconsin Card Sorting Test, and the Beck Depression Inventory (BDI). There was no statistically significant difference between the two groups for any neuropsychological test at baseline or on retesting. A level III study by Trepanier et al. [41], on the other hand, reported an improvement in sustained attention but a decline in working memory and frontal executive functioning, along with behavioral changes of a "frontal" nature in about 25% of subjects.

Visual-field defects may be another side effect of pallidotomy, as described in a level III study by Biousse et al. [45]. Using microelectrode guidance, the group reported that 7.5% of patients (3/40) had visual defects, discovered with Goldmann visual-field testing, including contralateral homonymous superior quadrantanopias, likely related to pallidotomy. The authors noted that lesion locations in patients with visual-field defects significantly differed from those in patients with no visual-field defects in that they were more ventral, adjacent to or extending into the optic tract. They reported the mean distance from the ventral edge of the primary lesion to the optic tract was -1.67 ± 0.4 mm in patients with visual-field defects and $+1.3 \pm 0.5$ mm in those without ($P = 0.00015$ by Student's t-test). Thus, the authors changed their technique during the study and increased their lesioning threshold from 0.5 to ≥ 1.0 mA in order to place the lesion at a more distant target from the optic tract. By doing this, they were able to reduce the incidence of visual-field defects from 11% (2/18) to 4.5% (1/22).

In another level III study, Hariz and De Salles [46] analyzed complications of posteroventral pallidotomy in 138 consecutive patients who underwent 152 pallidotomies (12 patients had bilateral pallidotomies). Transient adverse reactions, typically lasting less than 3 months, appeared in 18% of the patients ($n = 25$) including subcortical hematoma (2), meningitis (1), facial paresis (3), leg paresis (2), dysarthria (5), limb dyspraxia (2), seizure (2), sialorrhea (4), fatigue (3) and confusion (5). Long-term complications that lasted more than 6 months were noted in 10% of the patients. Other complications described to have occurred alone or in various combinations in 14 patients included fatigue and sleepiness (2), worsening of memory (4), depression (1), aphonia (1), dysarthria (3), scotoma (1), slight facial and leg paresis (2) and delayed stroke (2).

Unilateral pallidal DBS

Many of the concerns described above that are associated with unilateral pallidotomy are not typically seen with unilateral pallidal DBS. Ideally, we would like to compare unilateral pallidotomy with unilateral pallidal DBS in a randomized fashion, but no such trial exists. In addition, there are no trials directly comparing unilateral pallidal DBS with best medical therapy. However, the efficacy of unilateral pallidal DBS has been well demonstrated through a randomized controlled trial by Zahodne et al. [47] in which pallidal DBS was compared with STN-DBS. In this trial, quality-of-life measures were compared in PD patients who received unilateral pallidal DBS ($n = 22$) and unilateral STN-DBS ($n = 20$). The primary outcome was change in the different domains of the quality of life before and 6 months after surgery in patients randomized to receive either therapy. The 39-Item Parkinson's Disease Questionnaire (PDQ-39) summary index (PDQ-SI) score was used to assess quality of life, with higher scores indicating poorer quality of life. Patients with GPi-DBS had a significant 38.1% average reduction in their PDQ-SI scores postoperatively. Analysis of subscales revealed that GPi-DBS patients improved significantly with regard to mobility, ADLs, stigma and social support. On average, the GPi-DBS group exhibited a 28% improvement in the motor UPDRS "off" score compared with baseline. Scores on the Beck Depression Inventory 2nd edition (BDI-II) improved significantly after GPi-DBS. No significant safety concerns were reported in this trial. In a level III study by Rodrigues et al. [48], the change in quality of life following GPi-DBS was measured in 11 patients, in which four patients received unilateral DBS. Outcome measures included the PDQ-39 questionnaire and motor assessments. The PDQ-39 scores were reduced by 30% in the unilateral patients. There was a reduction in the motor UPDRS "off" scores by 19%.

Safety concerns that exist with unilateral pallidal DBS include concerns that occur with stereotactic surgery in general, risk of hemorrhage, infection and neurological deficits caused by local tissue damage [49]. Furthermore, it has been shown that patients undergoing unilateral DBS (GPi or STN) may have cognitive declines on psychomotor processing speed in PD patients compared with age-matched PD controls [50]. Other side effects reported include worsening of concentration and memory, but the sample sizes of those receiving unilateral procedures are too small to make general conclusions [48]. Although changes in cognition may be seen, these are typically isolated to subscales and are not declines in global cognition. Okun et al. [51] reported on 23 subjects who received unilateral GPi-DBS and found that there was no change of mood or cognitive outcomes from pre- to post-DBS in the optimal setting at a 7-month follow-up. Thus, overall, unilateral pallidal DBS is a well-tolerated procedure.

Bilateral pallidotomy versus bilateral pallidal DBS
Bilateral pallidotomy

While unilateral procedures for asymmetric disease can be of benefit, PD is a progressive bilateral disease, requiring bilateral treatment. Bilateral pallidotomy and bilateral pallidal DBS have been performed to address this issue. There are no level I or level II studies comparing bilateral pallidotomy with best medical therapy or pallidal DBS. A number of level III studies have shown that bilateral pallidotomy may improve the cardinal features of PD and reduce motor fluctuations. Scott et al. [52] reported that bilateral posteroventral pallidotomy produced an improvement in the mean total UPDRS score of 53% (from 88 ± 22 to 41 ± 21). In five patients receiving staged bilateral pallidotomy, Intemann et al. [53] reported that the UPDRS total scores improved by 29% ($P = 0.04$) and motor UPDRS "off" scores improved by 36% in the "off" state ($P = 0.01$). The authors comment that the overall improvements in these scores were strongly influenced by specific improvements in tremor, bradykinesia and medication-induced dyskinesias. Counihan et al. [54] reported on the results of 14 patients undergoing staged bilateral pallidotomy and found that dyskinesias were greatly improved and there were significant reductions in "off" time (67%) and ADL "off" scores (24%), and a nonsignificant reduction in "off" motor score (39%). Additional level III studies also report similar findings [55–62].

However, bilateral pallidotomy is generally not considered to be an acceptable treatment for PD, due to its risk-to-benefit profile. According to the task force of the Movement Disorders Society, "serious concerns have been voiced on the risk of speech, balance, gait, and cognitive problems consequent to bilateral surgery" when discussing pallidotomy [63]. Merello et al. [64] conducted a level I prospective study of PD patients who were randomized either to simultaneous bilateral pallidotomy or simultaneous unilateral pallidotomy with contralateral GPi stimulation. However, the first three patients who received bilateral pallidotomy experienced severe side effects, resulting in termination of the trial. These adverse effects included depression and apathy. There was also a dramatic worsening of speech, drooling, swallowing, freezing, ambulation and falls. The reported side effects of bilateral pallidotomy that have been described in class III studies are summarized in Table 28.1. Studies after 1995 and those with a minimum of five patients are included in the table. A systematic review of the morbidity and mortality following pallidotomy reported the incidence of permanent adverse effects being as high as 60% in bilateral pallidotomy cases [67]. Due to these reported complications of bilateral lesioning procedures and the advent of DBS, bilateral pallidotomy has largely been abandoned.

Although the above studies and findings are certainly compelling, is it possible that bilateral pallidotomy received a worse reputation than it deserves? There certainly are factors that may have negatively influenced the outcome of bilateral pallidotomy. In the early years of pallidotomy, preoperative imaging

Table 28.1 Complications reported in Parkinson's disease patients undergoing bilateral pallidotomy[a]

Study	Procedure	Complications
Iacono et al. (1995) [56]	Staged bilateral pallidotomy (n = 19); contemporaneous bilateral pallidotomy (n = 49)	4.5 months (n = 68): bleeding (2); infection (1)
Scott et al. (1998) [52]	Contemporaneous bilateral pallidotomy	3–4 months (n = 8): worsened speech (3); increased drooling (2); falling (1); impaired verbal recall (2); impaired attention (2); impaired verbal fluency (4); worsened nonverbal IQ (1); worsened speech articulation rate (1); impaired recognition memory (1)
Favre et al. (2000) [58]	Staged bilateral pallidotomy (n = 5); contemporaneous bilateral pallidotomy (n = 17)	Median 7 months (n = 22): dysarthria >50%; worsened balance >35%; dysphagia (8); vision impairment (7); worsened depression (5); cognitive decline (6)
Siegel and Verhagen (2000) [59]	Contemporaneous bilateral pallidotomy	1 month (n = 11): visual-field deficit (1)
Counihan et al. (2001) [54]	Staged bilateral pallidotomy	6 months–1 year (n = 14): worsened gait (2); worsened speech, drooling, dysphagia (1); hypophonia (5); quadrantanopia (1)
Intemann et al. (2001) [53]	Staged bilateral pallidotomy (n = 11); contemporaneous bilateral pallidotomy (n = 1)	3 months (n = 8): worsened speech (4); increased drooling (4); worsened memory (1)
Parkin et al. (2002) [65]	Staged bilateral pallidotomy (n = 6); contemporaneous bilateral pallidotomy (n = 47)	3 months: worsened speech (4); increased drooling (7); increased freezing (6); worsened handwriting (6); eye opening apraxia (3)
de Bie et al. (2002) [66]	Staged bilateral pallidotomy	3 months (n = 10): worsened speech (8); visual-field defect (1); delayed infarct with hemiplegia (1); emotional flattening (3); personality change (1); facial paresis (1); increased drooling (1)
Hua et al. (2003) [61]	Staged bilateral pallidotomy (n = 106); contemporaneous bilateral pallidotomy (n = 3)	3 months (n = 109): fatigue (29); worsened speech (13); increased drooling (21); dysphagia (11); hypersomnia (5)
York et al. (2007) [62]	Staged bilateral pallidotomy	3 months (n = 15): worsened speech (9); swallowing difficulty (3); increased drooling (4); cognitive decline (5); gait/balance problems (6); visual hallucinations (1); flashing light (1); numbness/tingling in feet (1) 2 years (n = 9): worsened speech (7); swallowing difficulty (3); increased drooling (2); cognitive decline (6); gait/balance problems (6)

[a] Studies included report results of at least five Parkinson's disease patients.

was not sophisticated (CT rather than MRI, or, at best, low-resolution MRI). The low-resolution imaging combined with the permanent nature of lesioning contributed to the perceived need for extensive "mapping" of the GPi in many centers. Thus, multiple microelectrode tracks were made, sometimes exceeding six tracks per side [21]. In addition, most surgical reports do not mention details regarding the angles of the chosen trajectories from the burr hole to the target, and it thus remains unknown which cortical areas or subcortical nuclei such as the caudate were pierced by these multiple electrode tracts. Conceivably, many of the adverse events reported were at least in part attributable to excessive penetration of structures other than the pallidum along the trajectories through the frontal lobes.

Bilateral pallidal DBS

On the other hand, the rise in popularity of DBS has also led to the accumulation of a large body of evidence regarding its efficacy and safety that continues to grow and be refined. Regarding bilateral pallidal DBS, several studies have established its use for improving parkinsonism, reducing motor fluctuations and dyskinesias. The Deep-Brain Stimulation for Parkinson's Disease Study Group [68] performed a prospective, double-blinded crossover study in patients with advanced PD in whom electrodes were implanted in the GPi ($n = 38$) and the STN ($n = 96$). Blinded evaluation of 35 patients implanted with bilateral pallidal stimulation at 3 months was associated with a mean improved of 32% and a median improvement of 37% in the motor UPDRS "off" score ($P < 0.001$). Unblinded evaluations of 36 patients at 6 months showed that bilateral GPi-DBS improved motor UPDRS "off" scores by 33.3%; in the "on" state, UPDRS motor scores were improved by 26.8%. Home diary assessments showed that between baseline and the 6-month time point, the percentage of time with poor mobility was reduced from 37 to 24% ($P = 0.01$). In addition, the percentage of time with good mobility and without dyskinesias during the waking day increased from 28 to 64% ($P < 0.001$).

The benefits of pallidal stimulation were also shown by Anderson *et al.* [69] in a randomized, blinded parallel-group study of patients receiving either bilateral pallidal (GPi) ($n = 10$) or bilateral subthalamic ($n = 10$) stimulation. In the GPi stimulation group, evaluation after 12 months showed that off-medication, on-stimulation scores improved by 39%, ADLs improved by 18% and dyskinesias improved by 89%. In another level I study, Follett *et al.* [70] randomized patients to pallidal stimulation ($n = 152$) or subthalamic stimulation ($n = 147$) and compared 24-month outcomes. The primary outcome measure was change in the motor UPDRS "off" scores through a blinded assessment. In the pallidal group, there was a 28.2% improvement in the motor UPDRS in the off-medication, on-stimulation state. There was only a slight improvement, 5.3%, in the motor UPDRS score in the on-medication, on-stimulation state. The efficacy of pallidal stimulation was further demonstrated in a randomized controlled trial by Odekerken *et al.* [71]. In this study, the investigators assessed the level of functional improvement provided by either bilateral GPi or STN stimulation using the Academic Medical Center Linear Disability Scale (ALDS) as the primary outcome. This scale quantifies functional status in performing basic and complex ADLs on a scale of 0–100, with lower scores indicating more disability. This score is interesting because it is weighted by time spent in the "off" phase and "on" phase, capturing disability throughout the day. In the GPi group ($n = 44$), the ALDS score improved by about 4% at 12 months. In the 62 patients who completed the secondary outcome measures, the off-medication, on-stimulation UPDRS motor score improved by 26% and UPDRS-ADL score improved by 21.7% between baseline and 12 months. In the on-medication, on-stimulation state, dyskinesias improved by about 56% as measured by the clinical dyskinesia rating scale.

Thus, a clear benefit for bilateral GPi stimulation has been established with several high-quality studies, as described above. However, as with any surgical therapy, the possibility of complications exists. A variety of adverse effects have been reported with bilateral pallidal DBS, but generally the rates of these events are significantly less compared with bilateral pallidotomy. Serious adverse events such as intracranial hemorrhage have been reported at a rate of between 1% [70] and 9% [68]. Altered mental status/confusion can be seen in as many as 20% of cases, but is often transient and resolves without sequelae [71]. Speech problems may occur in up to 29% of cases [71]. Other rare side effects include, but are not limited to, stroke [69], seizure [68, 71], falls [70, 71], stimulation-induced side effects such as dyskinesia [68, 70, 71], psychiatric symptoms [70], implantation site infections [70, 71] and death [70]. In summary, bilateral pallidal DBS is preferred to pallidotomy for several reasons. Speech changes, falls, and lack of sustained effect are more likely with pallidotomy compared with DBS based on the information available. This is likely because DBS may be more forgiving than pallidotomy. If a lesion is made in a suboptimal place, pallidotomy cannot be reversed, whereas DBS can be adjusted. It is important to note that studies of pallidotomy were conducted during a time where imaging and surgical techniques were not optimized, nor were detailed reports of the results documented or available. Thus, bilateral pallidotomy may have been doomed to fail since its inception. However, all things being equal, the point still remains that DBS is reversible while lesioning is not, making DBS the preferred therapy.

Subthalamic nucleus

Unilateral subthalamotomy versus unilateral subthalamic DBS
Unilateral subthalamotomy

As discussed above, the STN became a target of interest in the world of stereotactic surgery for PD in the early 1990s. Stimulation of the STN gained popularity exponentially, but lesioning this nucleus was initially met with trepidation, as researchers were concerned about inducing hemiballismus as a complication. Consequently, efficacy studies of subthalamotomy did not materialize until the 2000s, when unilateral subthalamotomy was performed and compared directly with other accepted therapies such as pallidotomy. Coban *et al.* [72] conducted a small prospective, randomized, double-blinded study in which they compared four PD patients who underwent unilateral subthalamotomy with six PD patients who underwent unilateral pallidotomy. At 6 months, the motor

UPDRS-III "off" scores improved by 25% in the STN-lesion group compared with 17% in the pallidotomy group, but this difference was not statistically significant. Postoperatively in the "on" state, there was a 42% improvement in dyskinesia disability (as measured by item 33 of the UPDRS-IV) in the pallidotomy group compared with a 50% improvement in the subthalamotomy group. Subthalamotomy was considered comparable to pallidotomy with regard to efficacy. Abnormal involuntary movements were seen in two of the four subthalamotomy cases. In one patient, abnormal involuntary choreic movements were seen during surgery and resolved during the intraoperative course. The second patient developed left hemiballistic movements 3 days after subthalamotomy, which were responsive to pharmacological therapy with valproate.

In a large level III study by Alvarez et al. [73], 89 patients with PD were treated with unilateral subthalamotomy, of which 68 subjects were available for evaluation after 12 months, 36 subjects were evaluated at 24 months and 25 subjects were evaluated at 36 months. Postoperatively, there was a significant reduction in the UPDRS-III "off" scores at 12 (50%), 24 (30%) and 36 (18%) months. The daily levodopa dose was reduced by 45% ($P < 0.001$), 36% ($P < 0.001$) and 28% ($P < 0.05$) at 1, 2 and 3 years, respectively, compared with baseline. In the 33 patients assessed neuropsychologically, there were no significant changes in test scores from baseline values when they were evaluated 24 months after surgery using the MMSE, visuospatial tests and a frontal assessment battery. Adverse events were encountered in 20 of the 89 patients who underwent surgery. These included persistent dyskinesias induced by surgery (14), transient or mild dysarthria (4), infection of the scalp incision (3), seizure (2) and asymptomatic bleeding along the electrode trajectory (3). The dyskinesias were observed within the first 24 h in 52 patients (58.4%) before any antiparkinsonian medication was reintroduced. In 38 of these patients, the dyskinesias resolved spontaneously over the subsequent 4–12 weeks. In the remaining 14 (15%) patients, the dyskinesias persisted. In eight of these patients, dyskinesia was severe and persisted, despite stopping all dopaminergic treatments and after starting tetrabenazine and sulpiride (three patients). The authors concluded that, while unilateral subthalamotomy was associated with significant and sustained motor benefit contralateral to the lesion, the concern for severe, persistent chorea/ballism was present in certain patients.

Unilateral subthalamic DBS

Unilateral STN-DBS has been shown to be quite effective in treating PD, with less concern for complications compared with subthalamotomy. The efficacy of unilateral STN-DBS was well demonstrated through the level I study by Zahodne et al. [47] discussed above, in which quality-of-life measures were compared in unilateral STN-DBS and unilateral GPi-DBS. The primary outcome was change in the different domains of the PDQ-39 6 months after surgery in patients randomized to receive either unilateral STN-DBS ($n = 20$) or GPi-DBS ($n = 22$). Regardless of the target, all subjects had an improved overall quality of life ($P = 0.016$) compared with baseline. Change in UPDRS-III "off" score was a secondary measure. The motor UPDRS "off" score was significantly reduced between baseline and STN surgery (from 43.8 to 32.2, $P < 0.001$). Additional level III studies further support this evidence. Slowinski et al. [74] reported the effects of unilateral STN-DBS in 24 advanced PD patients over a mean follow-up period of 9 months. They found statistically significant improvements in the UPDRS-II score (18%), total UPDRS-III score (31%), the contralateral items of the motor UPDRS "off" score (63%) and Parkinson's Disease Quality of Life (PDQL) questionnaire score (15%) in the on-stimulation state compared with baseline. Patients in the on-stimulation state had a significant improvement in performance in the Purdue Pegboard Test in comparison with the off-stimulation state (38%, $P < 0.05$). In addition, patients were able to reduce the daily levodopa-equivalent dose by 21% ($P = 0.018$). Linazasoro et al. [75] reported on a series of eight PD patients who received unilateral STN-DBS. During a mean follow-up of 12 months, patients experienced 72% improvement in their contralateral motor UPDRS "off" score with stimulation, with a 68% reduction in contralateral dyskinesias. Given the small sample size, these figures should be interpreted with caution, but, nonetheless, the patients significantly benefitted from the therapy. Germano et al. [49] reported on 12 patients who received unilateral STN-DBS and were followed for 12 months. Following DBS, there was a mean improvement in the motor UPDRS "off" score of 26% compared with baseline. When analyzing only the contralateral scores, the side receiving stimulation improved by approximately 50% and ipsilateral scores improved by about 17%. On-medication periods without dyskinesias during the waking day significantly improved and on-medication periods with dyskinesias were reduced.

From a safety standpoint, unilateral DBS is a well-tolerated procedure [49]. A variety of different side effects of unilateral STN-DBS have been reported. Zahonde et al. [47] reported that, on average, STN patients produced 5.7 fewer words on verbal fluency testing compared with the preoperative assessment ($P = 0.01$). In a study by Slowinski et al. [74], side effects related to stimulation (confusion, double vision and swallowing problems) were observed in 25% (6/24) of patients and were easily resolved by stimulation adjustments without permanent sequelae. These patients were followed over a 9-month period and no hardware-related complications occurred. Scalp incision healing problems were observed in one patient and required plastic surgery, while another patient had minor intraventricular bleeding without neurological complications. Nineteen of 24 patients (79%) were discharged less than 24 h following surgery. Neuropsychological testing revealed no significant postoperative changes in auditory–verbal attention, generative naming for semantic categories, visuospatial perception, speeded visuomotor number sequencing, learning, memory or mood ratings. Germano [49] reported that all unilateral STN procedures were well tolerated in 24 patients, and there was no surgical or perioperative occurrence of morbidity or death. There was no intracerebral hemorrhage, infarction or infection, and no patient suffered neurological disability postoperatively over a 24-month period. In addition, no adverse cognitive effects were observed on clinical examination. Patients did not have any stimulation-related side effects, and no electrode had to be withdrawn or repositioned. Although the comparison is imperfect, the data available suggest that unilateral subthalamotomy is comparable to unilateral STN-DBS with regard to efficacy. However, due to the ability to deliver benefit through modulation and potentially fewer permanent side effects, STN-DBS is preferred to unilateral subthalamotomy.

Bilateral subthalamotomy versus bilateral subthalamic DBS

Bilateral subthalamotomy

We can also examine the available evidence for bilateral subthalamotomy and bilateral STN-DBS. In fact, these two procedures have been directly compared. In a level I study conducted by Merello et al. [76], subjects were prospectively randomized to bilateral subthalamotomy ($n = 5$) versus bilateral STN stimulation ($n = 5$) versus the combination of unilateral subthalamotomy with contralateral STN-DBS ($n = 5$) in PD patients. Total UPDRS and motor UPDRS "off" scores improved in all groups without between-group differences when subjects were followed for 12 months. More specifically, the total UPDRS improved by 54% in the bilateral STN-lesion group compared with 60% in the bilateral STN-DBS group. The "off" motor UPDRS scores improved by 52% in the bilateral STN-lesion group compared with 61% in the bilateral STN-DBS group. Despite the comparable improvement with these three therapies, the concern for hemichorea–hemiballism was realized only in the lesioning cases. According to the study, 13% of subthalamotomies were associated with a hemichorea–hemiballismus syndrome. In one case, these symptoms lasted over 3 months and required pallidotomy for resolution. This concern for adverse events has been further supported by a level III study conducted by Alvarez et al. [77] in which the authors reported the effects of bilateral subthalamotomy in 18 patients with idiopathic PD. Contemporaneous subthalamotomy was performed in 11 patients, while seven subjects had a staged procedure. Patients were evaluated using the motor UPDRS "off" score at baseline with subsequent evaluations at 1 and 6 months and every year thereafter for a minimum of 3 years after bilateral subthalamotomy. Bilateral subthalamotomy induced a significant reduction in the "off" motor UPDRS scores (49.5%) at the final assessment. A blinded rating of videotape motor examinations in the off- and on-medication states preoperatively and at 2 years postoperatively also revealed a significant improvement. The mean daily levodopa dose was reduced by 47% at the time of the last evaluation compared with baseline, and levodopa-induced dyskinesias were reduced by 50% Adverse effects included persistent surgery-induced chorea for at least 3 months ($n = 3$), and severe and persistent dysarthria ($n = 3$). There was no permanent cognitive impairment reported in any patient.

Bilateral subthalamic DBS

Several studies have established the efficacy and safety of bilateral STN-DBS. Two class I studies have directly compared STN-DBS with best medical treatment. Deuschl et al. [78] reported on a large, randomized, controlled, multicenter (unblinded) trial of bilateral STN stimulation versus best medical therapy (BMT) in 156 patients. The subjects were randomly assigned in pairs to receive either STN-DBS in combination with BMT or BMT alone. The primary outcome measures were the changes in motor UPDRS "off" score and changes in the health-related quality-of-life score as measured by the PDQ-39. For the motor UPDRS "off" score, 55 of the 78 pairs of patients (71%) had a greater improvement in the stimulator on/off-medication UPDRS-III score compared with the paired non-DBS subject evaluated in the off-medication state ($P < 0.001$). In addition, 50 of the 78 pairs of patients (64%) treated with DBS had a greater improvement in the PDQ-SI score than the patients assigned to BMT ($P = 0.02$). The dyskinesia score improved by 54% in the DBS group (by a mean of 3.4 ± 4.5 points; 95% confidence interval, 2.3–4.5 points), but remained unchanged in the BMT group ($P < 0.001$). Diary records of "on" time without troublesome dyskinesias were significantly improved from a mean of 3.2 to 7.6 h/day and "on" time with troublesome dyskinesias was also improved from 2.0 to 1.0 h/day. Total "off" time was reduced from 6.2 to 2.0 h/day in the DBS group but remained unchanged in the BMT group.

Schupbach et al. [79] randomized 20 patients in pairs to either immediate bilateral STN-DBS ($n = 10$) or optimized medical treatment ($n = 10$). Patients were assessed at multiple time intervals up to 18 months. Quality of life, measured by the PDQ-39, was significantly improved by 24% in the surgical group but did not change in nonsurgical patients, resulting in a significant end-of-study difference in the two groups ($P < 0.05$). After 18 months, off-medication parkinsonian motor signs were reduced by 69% in the surgical group but increased by 29% in the medically treated group ($P < 0.05$). Motor complications of levodopa, as assessed by the UPDRS-IV, improved by 83% in operated-on patients but worsened by 15% in the medically treated group ($P < 0.05$). Williams et al. [80] performed a multicenter, open-label trial in which subjects were randomized to surgery and BMT ($n = 183$) or to BMT alone ($n = 183$). Of the patients assigned to surgery, 98% underwent STN-DBS (only four underwent pallidal DBS), and underwent a bilateral procedure in all but two cases. Subjects were assessed at 1 year for changes in the PDQ-39 compared with baseline. There was a statistically significant improvement in the PDQ-SI score when comparing surgery with medical therapy, 13% versus <1%, respectively. The motor UPDRS "off" score improved by 36% in the surgery group compared with <1% in the medical therapy group. There was an improvement in dyskinesia and a reduction in "off" time that was significant in the surgical group compared with the medical group, as measured by the UPDRS-IV. The earlier study discussed above conducted by Follett et al. [70] randomized PD subjects to either bilateral STN-DBS ($n = 147$) or bilateral pallidal DBS ($n = 152$) and demonstrated the efficacy of both surgical treatments. The primary outcome was the change in the UPDRS-III "off" score at 24 months. This score did not differ by target, and patients on average experienced a 25% improvement at 24 months in the bilateral STN group. There was improvement in secondary outcomes as well, including patients' motor diaries, the stand–walk–sit test, and six of the eight subscales of the PDQ-39. Motor function with troublesome dyskinesias was reduced from 4.0 ± 3.3 h/day to 1.4 ± 2.4 h/day when comparing baseline and 24-month patient diaries. The efficacy of STN-DBS has been further supported by the study of Odekerken et al. [71], which was also discussed above. In this study, using the ALDS as the primary outcome, the investigators showed an improvement of 11% at 12 months in the STN group ($n = 46$). In the 63 patients who completed the secondary outcome measures, the off-medication, on-stimulation motor UPDRS score improved by about 46%, and UPDRS ADLs improved by about 42% between baseline and 12 months. In the on-medication, on-stimulation state, dyskinesias improved by about 23%, as measured by the clinical dyskinesia rating scale.

Bilateral STN-DBS shows clear efficacy based on the above studies, without the major concern of hemichorea–hemiballism as seen with subthalamic lesioning. Krack et al. [81] reported that disabling dyskinesias due to stimulation were seen in seven patients but were permanent in only two. In many cases, use of dorsal contacts can provide an antidyskinetic effect that is not possible with subthalamotomy. Other adverse events have been reported with bilateral STN-DBS, although some events are not specific to the target. Weaver et al. [82] reported a significantly higher incidence of at least one serious adverse event in patients undergoing bilateral DBS (40%) compared with the medically treated group (11%). These were typically surgical-site infections. The DBS group also had significantly more falls. Patients demonstrated small decrements in working memory, processing speed, phonemic fluency and delayed recall. Similarly, others have reported that, although global cognitive functioning may be preserved, frontal cognitive functions and verbal fluency may be impaired with bilateral STN-DBS [83]. Williams et al. [80] reported similar findings, showing that patients undergoing bilateral STN-DBS had a decline in verbal fluency and vocabulary compared with a medical therapy control group. A number of nonmotor adverse events have been reported with bilateral STN-DBS. These include emotional lability [84], apathy [85], impulsive–compulsive behaviors [86], suicide [87] and social maladjustment [79]. The argument can be made that many of these side effects of bilateral STN-DBS may also be seen with bilateral subthalamotomy. However, tissue destruction through lesioning comes with the prospect of making an adverse event permanent, whereas side effects from a modulating therapy such as DBS offers at least the chance to mitigate or modify such occurrences. Because of this, bilateral STN-DBS remains the preferred therapy when compared with bilateral subthalamotomy.

Stimulation versus lesioning: is there really a controversy?

In summary, although lesioning and stimulation have the potential for similar efficacy, there are significant safety concerns for lesioning that limit its utility, as discussed above. Lesioning is a permanent therapy and cannot be modulated. If the correct target is not chosen or the lesion is made too close to nearby structures such as the internal capsule, patients can have permanent side effects. In addition, if patients have recurrence of symptoms due to progression of PD, repeat surgery is needed. Although many centers follow a protocol for lesioning, there is no agreed standard with regard to how large a lesion should be in order to control symptoms. For instance, Bakay and colleagues [88] made thalamic lesions to control tremor that were approximately $3-4 \times 3-4$ mm in size, whereas Van Buren et al. [89] placed lesions that were $6 \times 6 \times 9$ mm in the thalamus. This variability leads to differential outcomes and sometimes necessitates the need for repeat surgery if the lesion size is not adequate. On the other hand, if too generous a lesion is made, neighboring structures will be negatively impacted.

Deep-brain stimulation overcomes many of these limitations of lesioning. Bilateral implantation has been shown to be efficacious, and there are fewer safety concerns with bilateral DBS compared with lesioning [90]. Device-related complications, such as lead migration, infection and breakage, are reported in 1% [70] to 12% [68] of cases, and battery replacements are needed throughout the lifespan of the patient. However, many of these problems can be resolved without permanent sequelae, whereas side effects that are associated with lesioning may be permanent. Furthermore, DBS is an adjustable therapy, so recurrence of symptoms can be potentially addressed without repeat surgery by adjusting stimulation parameters, and side effects of stimulation can easily be modulated. Given these factors, DBS is a superior therapy to lesioning.

Yet there may be a role for lesioning in certain cases. Deep-brain stimulation is a costly procedure and may not be offered as the surgical treatment of choice throughout the world. In addition, immunocompromised patients who are at risk for hardware infection may not be the best candidates for DBS. Elderly patients with poor skin turgor, which can lead to slowed wound healing and potential infection, may also be offered lesion therapy instead of DBS. Deep-brain stimulation is a time-intensive therapy, requiring rigorous evaluation preoperatively and close follow-up in the initial postoperative months, with lifelong monitoring of symptoms, battery life and hardware. Patients with poor follow-up or those with distance limitations from a DBS center may consider lesion therapy instead of DBS. Deep-brain stimulation involves implanted hardware, which has the potential for mechanical breakage or failure, limits access to MRI scanning and requires regular battery replacement through surgery [91].

Although DBS is the preferred therapy over lesioning at this time and there is no true controversy regarding the two therapies, the debate may be rekindled with the advent of newer methods for lesioning, especially when noninvasive procedures become an option. Elias et al. [92] used high-intensity focused ultrasound under MRI guidance to perform a noninvasive thalamotomy in 15 essential tremor patients. The results of the study were positive, but large randomized trials are needed to assess the safety and efficacy of such a procedure. The technique offers advantages over existing noninvasive lesioning procedures (gamma knife) in that the effect is immediate, allowing assessment of benefits and side effects throughout the gradual sonication process, while tissue temperature is monitored "online" through magnetic resonance thermography. In addition, newer imaging techniques including magnetic resonance tractography allow us to visualize targets (including subnuclei in the thalamus) at much higher resolution, enabling more accurate lesioning than in the days of ventriculography and X-rays. Yet despite the possibility of improved techniques for lesioning, the same irreversibility associated with the traditional, invasive methods of lesioning may ultimately limit its widespread utility in movement disorders. As the field of DBS moves forward with novel lead designs, closed-loop DBS systems and current steering, it is safe to predict that DBS will remain the preferred surgical therapy for a long time to come.

References

1. Horsley V. The Linacre Lecture on the function of the so-called motor area of the brain: delivered to the master and fellows of St. John's College, Cambridge, May 6th, 1909. *Br Med J* 1909; **2**: 121–32.
2. Spiegel EA, Wycis HT, Marks M, Lee AJ. Stereotaxic apparatus for operations on the human brain. *Science* 1947; **106**: 349–50.
3. Spiegel EA, Wycis HT, Baird HW 3rd. Long-range effects of electropallidoansotomy in extrapyramidal and convulsive disorders. *Neurology* 1958; **8**: 734–40.
4. Meyers R. Surgical experiments in the therapy of certain 'extrapyramidal' diseases: a current evaluation. *Acta Psychiatr Neurol Suppl* 1951; **67**: 1–42.
5. Cooper IS. Ligation of the anterior choroidal artery for involuntary movements; parkinsonism. *Psychiatr Q* 1953; **27**: 317–19.
6. Cooper IS. Surgical alleviation of parkinsonism; effects of occlusion of the anterior choroidal artery. *J Am Geriatr Soc.* 1954; **2**: 691–718.
7. Guiot G, Brion S. Treatment of abnormal movement by pallidal coagulation. *Rev Neurol (Paris)* 1953; **89**: 578–80.
8. Narabayashi H, Okuma T. Procaine oil blocking of the globus pallidus for treatment of rigidity and tremor of parkinsonism: preliminary report. *Proc Jpn Acad*; 1953; **2** Procaine oil blocking 9: 134.
9. Hassler R. The influence of stimulations and coagulations in the human thalamus on the tremor at rest and its physiopathologic mechanism. *Proc Second Int Cong Neuropathol* 1955; **2**: 637–42.
10. Laitinen LV. Brain targets in surgery for Parkinson's disease. Results of a survey of neurosurgeons. *J Neurosurg* 1985; **62**: 349–51.
11. Svennilson E, Torvik A, Lowe R, Leksell L. Treatment of parkinsonism by stereotatic thermolesions in the pallidal region. A clinical evaluation of 81 cases. *Acta Psychiatr Scand* 1960; **35**: 358–77.
12. Yahr MD. Clinical aspects of abnormal movements induced by L-dopa. In: Barbeau A, McDowell FH, eds. *L-Dopa and Parkinsonism*. Davis Company; 1970; 101–8.
13. Barbeau A. The clinical physiology of side effects in long-term L-DOPA therapy. *Adv Neurol* 1974; **5**: 347–65.
14. Laitinen LV, Bergenheim AT, Hariz MI. Leksell's posteroventral pallidotomy in the treatment of Parkinson's disease. *J Neurosurg* 1992; **76**: 53–61.
15. Benabid AL, Pollak P, Louveau A, Henry S, de Rougemont J. Combined (thalamotomy and stimulation) stereotactic surgery of the VIM thalamic nucleus for bilateral Parkinson disease. *Appl Neurophysiol* 1987; **50**: 344–6.
16. Albin RL, Young AB, Penney JB. The functional anatomy of basal ganglia disorders. *Trends Neurosci* 1989; **12**: 366–75.
17. Bergman H, Wichmann T, DeLong MR. Reversal of experimental parkinsonism by lesions of the subthalamic nucleus. *Science* 1990; **249**: 1436–8.
18. Pollak P, Benabid AL, Gross C, et al. Effects of the stimulation of the subthalamic nucleus in Parkinson disease. *Rev Neurol (Paris)* 1993; **149**: 175–6.
19. Limousin P, Krack P, Pollak P, et al. Electrical stimulation of the subthalamic nucleus in advanced Parkinson's disease. *N Engl J Med* 1998; **339**: 1105–11.
20. Siegfried J, Lippitz B. Bilateral chronic electrostimulation of ventroposterolateral pallidum: a new therapeutic approach for alleviating all parkinsonian symptoms. *Neurosurgery* 1994; **35**: 1126–9; discussion 1129–30.
21. Vitek JL, Bakay RA, Hashimoto T, et al. Microelectrode-guided pallidotomy: technical approach and its application in medically intractable Parkinson's disease. *J Neurosurg* 1998; **88**: 1027–43.
22. Kaplitt MG, Hutchison WD, Lozano AM. Target localization in movement disorders surgery. In: Tarsy D, Vitek JL, Lozano AM, eds. *Surgical Treatment of Parkinson's Disease*. Humana Press; 2003; 87–98.
23. Schuurman PR, Bosch DA, Merkus MP, Speelman JD. Long-term follow-up of thalamic stimulation versus thalamotomy for tremor suppression. *Mov Disord* 2008; **23**: 1146–53.
24. Loher TJ, Pohle T, Krauss JK. Functional stereotactic surgery for treatment of cervical dystonia: review of the experience from the lesional era. *Stereotact Funct Neurosurg* 2004; **82**: 1–13.
25. Krayenbuhl H, Wyss OA, Yasargil MG. Bilateral thalamotomy and pallidotomy as treatment for bilateral parkinsonism. *J Neurosurg* 1961; **18**: 429–44.
26. Moriyama E, Beck H, Miyamoto T. Long-term results of ventrolateral thalamotomy for patients with Parkinson's disease. *Neurol Med Chir (Tokyo)* 1999; **39**: 350–6; discussion 356–7.
27. Jankovic J, Cardoso F, Grossman RG, Hamilton WJ. Outcome after stereotactic thalamotomy for parkinsonian, essential, and other types of tremor. *Neurosurgery* 1995; **37**: 680–6; discussion 686–7.
28. Wester K, Hauglie-Hanssen E. Stereotaxic thalamotomy – experiences from the levodopa era. *J Neurol Neurosurg Psychiatry* 1990; **53**: 427–30.
29. Hallett M, Litvan I. Evaluation of surgery for Parkinson's disease: a report of the Therapeutics

and Technology Assessment Subcommittee of the American Academy of Neurology. The Task Force on Surgery for Parkinson's Disease. *Neurology* 1999; **53**: 1910–21.
30. Blomstedt P, Hariz GM, Hariz MI. Pallidotomy versus pallidal stimulation. *Parkinsonism Relat Disord* 2006; **12**: 296–301.
31. de Bie RM, de Haan RJ, Nijssen PC, et al. Unilateral pallidotomy in Parkinson's disease: a randomised, single-blind, multicentre trial. *Lancet* 1999; **354**: 1665–9.
32. Vitek JL, Bakay RA, Freeman A, et al. Randomized trial of pallidotomy versus medical therapy for Parkinson's disease. *Ann Neurol* 2003; **53**: 558–69.
33. Kondziolka D, Bonaroti E, Baser S, et al. Outcomes after stereotactically guided pallidotomy for advanced Parkinson's disease. *J Neurosurg* 1999; **90**: 197–202.
34. Giller CA, Dewey RB, Ginsburg MI, Mendelsohn DB, Berk AM. Stereotactic pallidotomy and thalamotomy using individual variations of anatomic landmarks for localization. *Neurosurgery* 1998; **42**: 56–62; discussion 62–5.
35. Shannon KM, Penn RD, Kroin JS, et al. Stereotactic pallidotomy for the treatment of Parkinson's disease. Efficacy and adverse effects at 6 months in 26 patients. *Neurology* 1998; **50**: 434–8.
36. Kishore A, Turnbull IM, Snow BJ, et al. Efficacy, stability and predictors of outcome of pallidotomy for Parkinson's disease. six-month follow-up with additional 1-year observations. *Brain* 1997; **120**: 729–37.
37. Krauss JK, Desaloms JM, Lai EC, et al. Microelectrode-guided posteroventral pallidotomy for treatment of Parkinson's disease: postoperative magnetic resonance imaging analysis. *J Neurosurg* 1997; **87**: 358–67.
38. Lang AE, Lozano AM, Montgomery E, et al. Posteroventral medial pallidotomy in advanced Parkinson's disease. *N Engl J Med* 1997; **337**: 1036–42.
39. Kazumata K, Antonini A, Dhawan V, et al. Preoperative indicators of clinical outcome following stereotaxic pallidotomy. *Neurology* 1997; **49**: 1083–90.
40. Uitti RJ, Wharen RE Jr, Turk MF, et al. Unilateral pallidotomy for Parkinson's disease: comparison of outcome in younger versus elderly patients. *Neurology* 1997; **49**: 1072–7.
41. Trepanier LL, Saint-Cyr JA, Lozano AM, Lang AE. Neuropsychological consequences of posteroventral pallidotomy for the treatment of Parkinson's disease. *Neurology* 1998; **51**: 207–15.
42. Blomstedt P, Hariz MI. Are complications less common in deep brain stimulation than in ablative procedures for movement disorders? *Stereotact Funct Neurosurg* 2006; **84**: 72–81.
43. Alkhani A, Lozano AM. Pallidotomy for Parkinson disease: a review of contemporary literature. *J Neurosurg* 2001; **94**: 43–9.
44. Perrine K, Dogali M, Fazzini E, et al. Cognitive functioning after pallidotomy for refractory Parkinson's disease. *J Neurol Neurosurg Psychiatry* 1998; **65**: 150–4.
45. Biousse V, Newman NJ, Carroll C, et al. Visual fields in patients with posterior GPi pallidotomy. *Neurology* 1998; **50**: 258–65.
46. Hariz MI, De Salles AA. The side-effects and complications of posteroventral pallidotomy. *Acta Neurochir Suppl* 1997; **68**: 42–8.
47. Zahodne LB, Okun MS, Foote KD, et al. Greater improvement in quality of life following unilateral deep brain stimulation surgery in the globus pallidus as compared to the subthalamic nucleus. *J Neurol* 2009; **256**: 1321–9.
48. Rodrigues JP, Walters SE, Watson P, Stell R, Mastaglia FL. Globus pallidus stimulation improves both motor and nonmotor aspects of quality of life in advanced Parkinson's disease. *Mov Disord* 2007; **22**: 1866–70.
49. Germano IM, Gracies JM, Weisz DJ, et al. Unilateral stimulation of the subthalamic nucleus in Parkinson disease: a double-blind 12-month evaluation study. *J Neurosurg* 2004; **101**: 36–42.
50. Mikos A, Zahodne L, Okun MS, Foote K, Bowers D. Cognitive declines after unilateral deep brain stimulation surgery in Parkinson's disease: a controlled study using reliable change, part II. *Clin Neuropsychol* 2010; **24**: 235–45.
51. Okun MS, Fernandez HH, Wu SS, et al. Cognition and mood in Parkinson's disease in subthalamic nucleus versus globus pallidus interna deep brain stimulation: the COMPARE trial. *Ann Neurol* 2009; **65**: 586–95.
52. Scott R, Gregory R, Hines N, et al. Neuropsychological, neurological and functional outcome following pallidotomy for Parkinson's disease. A consecutive series of eight simultaneous bilateral and twelve unilateral procedures. *Brain* 1998; **121**: 659–75.
53. Intemann PM, Masterman D, Subramanian I, et al. Staged bilateral pallidotomy for treatment of Parkinson disease. *J Neurosurg* 2001; **94**: 437–44.
54. Counihan TJ, Shinobu LA, Eskandar EN, Cosgrove GR, Penney JB Jr. Outcomes following staged bilateral pallidotomy in advanced Parkinson's disease. *Neurology* 2001; **56**: 799–802.
55. Iacono RP, Lonser RR, Yamada S. Contemporaneous bilateral postero-ventral pallidotomy for early onset "juvenile type" Parkinson's disease. Case report. *Acta Neurochir (Wien)* 1994; **131**: 247–52.
56. Iacono RP, Shima F, Lonser RR, et al. The results, indications, and physiology of posteroventral pallidotomy for patients with Parkinson's disease. *Neurosurgery* 1995; **36**: 1118–25; discussion 1125–7.
57. Vitek JL, Bakay RA, DeLong MR. Microelectrode-guided pallidotomy for medically intractable Parkinson's disease. *Adv Neurol* 1997; **74**: 183–98.

58. Favre J, Burchiel KJ, Taha JM, Hammerstad J. Outcome of unilateral and bilateral pallidotomy for Parkinson's disease: patient assessment. *Neurosurgery* 2000; **46**: 344–53; discussion 353–5.
59. Siegel KL, Metman LV. Effects of bilateral posteroventral pallidotomy on gait of subjects with Parkinson disease. *Arch Neurol* 2000; **57**: 198–204.
60. de Bie RM, Schuurman PR, Esselink RA, Bosch DA, Speelman JD. Bilateral pallidotomy in Parkinson's disease: a retrospective study. *Mov Disord* 2002; **17**: 533–8.
61. Hua Z, Guodong G, Qinchuan L, et al. Analysis of complications of radiofrequency pallidotomy. *Neurosurgery* 2003; **52**: 89–99; discussion 99–101.
62. York MK, Lai EC, Jankovic J, et al. Short and long-term motor and cognitive outcome of staged bilateral pallidotomy: a retrospective analysis. *Acta Neurochir (Wien)* 2007; **149**: 857–66; discussion 866.
63. Movement Disorder Society Task Force. Management of Parkinson's disease: an evidence-based review. *Mov Disord* 2002; **17** (Suppl. 4): S1–166.
64. Merello M, Starkstein S, Nouzeilles MI, Kuzis G, Leiguarda R. Bilateral pallidotomy for treatment of Parkinson's disease induced corticobulbar syndrome and psychic akinesia avoidable by globus pallidus lesion combined with contralateral stimulation. *J Neurol Neurosurg Psychiatry* 2001; **71**: 611–14.
65. Parkin SG, Gregory RP, Scott R, et al. Unilateral and bilateral pallidotomy for idiopathic Parkinson's disease: a case series of 115 patients. *Mov Disord* 2002; **17**: 682–92.
66. de Bie RM, Schuurman PR, Esselink RA, Bosch DA, Speelman JD. Bilateral pallidotomy in Parkinson's disease: a retrospective study. *Mov Disord* 2002; **17**: 533–8.
67. de Bie RM, de Haan RJ, Schuurman PR, et al. Morbidity and mortality following pallidotomy in Parkinson's disease: a systematic review. *Neurology* 2002; **58**: 1008–12.
68. Deep-Brain Stimulation for Parkinson's Disease Study Group. Deep-brain stimulation of the subthalamic nucleus or the pars interna of the globus pallidus in Parkinson's disease. *N Engl J Med* 2001; **345**: 956–63.
69. Anderson VC, Burchiel KJ, Hogarth P, Favre J, Hammerstad JP. Pallidal vs subthalamic nucleus deep brain stimulation in Parkinson disease. *Arch Neurol* 2005; **62**: 554–60.
70. Follett KA, Weaver FM, Stern M, et al. Pallidal versus subthalamic deep-brain stimulation for Parkinson's disease. *N Engl J Med* 2010; **362**: 2077–91.
71. Odekerken VJ, van Laar T, Staal MJ, et al. Subthalamic nucleus versus globus pallidus bilateral deep brain stimulation for advanced Parkinson's disease (NSTAPS study): a randomised controlled trial. *Lancet Neurol* 2013; **12**: 37–44.
72. Coban A, Hanagasi HA, Karamursel S, Barlas O. Comparison of unilateral pallidotomy and subthalamotomy findings in advanced idiopathic Parkinson's disease. *Br J Neurosurg* 2009; **23**: 23–9.
73. Alvarez L, Macias R, Pavon N, et al. Therapeutic efficacy of unilateral subthalamotomy in Parkinson's disease: results in 89 patients followed for up to 36 months. *J Neurol Neurosurg Psychiatry* 2009; **80**: 979–85.
74. Slowinski JL, Putzke JD, Uitti RJ, et al. Unilateral deep brain stimulation of the subthalamic nucleus for Parkinson disease. *J Neurosurg* 2007; **106**: 626–32.
75. Linazasoro G, Van Blercom N, Lasa A. Unilateral subthalamic deep brain stimulation in advanced Parkinson's disease. *Mov Disord* 2003; **18**: 713–16.
76. Merello M, Tenca E, Perez Lloret S, et al. Prospective randomized 1-year follow-up comparison of bilateral subthalamotomy versus bilateral subthalamic stimulation and the combination of both in Parkinson's disease patients: a pilot study. *Br J Neurosurg* 2008; **22**: 415–22.
77. Alvarez L, Macias R, Lopez G, et al. Bilateral subthalamotomy in Parkinson's disease: initial and long-term response. *Brain* 2005; **128**: 570–83.
78. Deuschl G, Schade-Brittinger C, Krack P, et al. A randomized trial of deep-brain stimulation for Parkinson's disease. *N Engl J Med* 2006; **355**: 896–908.
79. Schupbach WM, Maltete D, Houeto JL, et al. Neurosurgery at an earlier stage of Parkinson disease: a randomized, controlled trial. *Neurology* 2007; **68**: 267–71.
80. Williams A, Gill S, Varma T, et al. Deep brain stimulation plus best medical therapy versus best medical therapy alone for advanced Parkinson's disease (PD SURG trial): a randomised, open-label trial. *Lancet Neurol* 2010; **9**: 581–91.
81. Krack P, Batir A, Van Blercom N, et al. Five-year follow-up of bilateral stimulation of the subthalamic nucleus in advanced Parkinson's disease. *N Engl J Med* 2003; **349**: 1925–34.
82. Weaver FM, Follett K, Stern M, et al. Bilateral deep brain stimulation vs best medical therapy for patients with advanced Parkinson disease: a randomized controlled trial. *JAMA* 2009; **301**: 63–73.
83. Witt K, Daniels C, Reiff J, et al. Neuropsychological and psychiatric changes after deep brain stimulation for Parkinson's disease: a randomised, multicentre study. *Lancet Neurol* 2008; **7**: 605–14.
84. Esselink RA, de Bie RM, de Haan RJ, et al. Long-term superiority of subthalamic nucleus stimulation over pallidotomy in Parkinson disease. *Neurology* 2009; **73**: 151–3.
85. Drapier D, Drapier S, Sauleau P, et al. Does subthalamic nucleus stimulation induce apathy in Parkinson's disease? *J Neurol* 2006; **253**: 1083–91.

86. Lim SY, O'sullivan SS, Kotschet K, *et al.* Dopamine dysregulation syndrome, impulse control disorders and punding after deep brain stimulation surgery for Parkinson's disease. *J Clin Neurosci* 2009; **16**: 1148–52.
87. Voon V, Krack P, Lang AE, *et al.* A multicentre study on suicide outcomes following subthalamic stimulation for Parkinson's disease. *Brain* 2008; **131**: 2720–8.
88. Bakay RA, DeLong MR, Vitek JL. Posteroventral pallidotomy for Parkinson's disease. *J Neurosurg* 1992; **77**: 487–8.
89. Van Buren JM, Li CL, Shapiro DY, Henderson WG, Sadowsky DA. A qualitative and quantitative evaluation of parkinsonians three to six years following thalamotomy. *Confin Neurol* 1973; **35**: 202–35.
90. Fox SH, Katzenschlager R, Lim SY, *et al.* The Movement Disorder Society Evidence-based Medicine Review Update: treatments for the motor symptoms of Parkinson's disease. *Mov Disord* 2011; **26** (Suppl. 3): S2–41.
91. Hooper AK, Okun MS, Foote KD, *et al.* Clinical cases where lesion therapy was chosen over deep brain stimulation. *Stereotact Funct Neurosurg* 2008; **86**: 147–52.
92. Elias WJ, Huss D, Voss T, *et al.* A pilot study of focused ultrasound thalamotomy for essential tremor. *N Engl J Med* 2013; **369**: 640–8.

Chapter 29

Controversy: midstage vs advanced-stage deep-brain stimulation in the management of Parkinson's disease

Mallory L. Hacker and David Charles

Introduction

Parkinson's disease (PD) is a chronic neurodegenerative condition characterized by loss of dopaminergic neurons in multiple areas of the brain including the substantia nigra. Substitutive dopaminergic therapy effectively manages the cardinal motor symptoms of PD (i.e. tremor, rigidity and bradykinesia) early in the disease. However, most patients develop progressive levodopa (L-DOPA)-associated motor complications within 5–10 years of medical intervention [1]. These levodopa-associated motor fluctuations and dyskinesias worsen as PD progresses and significantly compromise patient quality of life. Because of the limited window of effective medical treatment and the current lack of therapies that alter disease progression, new PD treatment strategies must be considered.

Deep-brain stimulation (DBS) is an approved adjunctive therapy for advanced PD when medication no longer adequately controls symptoms. It offers superior benefit to medication alone through improvement of motor skills, quality of life and activities of daily living (ADLs), and reduction of levodopa-associated motor complications [2–6]. The success of DBS in advanced PD motivates the question of whether stimulation at earlier stages would extend or even enhance its benefits. Deep-brain stimulation offered sooner in PD has the potential to reduce complications of medical therapy and provide superior improvement to current interventions. However, DBS has not been widely studied in a less advanced PD population, and additional issues must be considered, including patient selection, DBS risks, economic impact and the potential for disease modification by slowing the progression of disability.

Here, we discuss these topics from the perspective of both critics and advocates of earlier applications of DBS therapy for PD.

Deep-brain stimulation is only appropriate for advanced Parkinson's disease

Clinical efficacy

Deep-brain stimulation is an appropriate treatment for advanced PD patients suffering from levodopa-associated motor complications. Deep-brain stimulation combined with standard medical therapy is superior to medication alone to reduce the adverse effects of medication and improve patient quality of life [2, 7, 8]. The benefits of high-frequency electrical stimulation include significantly reduced levodopa-associated dyskinesias and motor fluctuations [9, 10], improved quality of life [2, 11] and reduced need for PD medication [7, 12, 13]. Thus, DBS is now the standard of care for appropriately selected advanced PD patients.

The success of DBS in advanced PD encourages discussions of whether therapeutic benefits could be extended or even enhanced if offered sooner in PD. A recently completed multinational study was the first appropriately powered, randomized, controlled clinical trial to investigate DBS effects in PD subjects with midstage PD [14]. Quality of life in the neurostimulation group improved by 26% 2 years after surgery, with no improvement in the medication group. Between-group scores for motor disability, ADLs, levodopa-associated motor complications, and time with good mobility and no dyskinesias all significantly favored the neurostimulation group. Medication was reduced by 39% in the DBS group but was increased by 21% in the medication-alone group. Overall, neurostimulation plus medical therapy was superior to medication alone in midstage PD patients after 2 years of treatment.

While this large midstage PD trial was well executed, notable limitations to this study should be considered. First, PD research historically suffers from a robust placebo effect, partially due to patients' expected benefit inducing dopamine release [15]. Except for the motor subset of the Unified Parkinson's Disease Rating Scale (UPDRS) assessment, outcome measures for this study were not blinded, and it is possible that the superiority of the DBS group was influenced by the placebo effect. Secondly, subjects were randomized either to undergo DBS surgery or to continue standard medical treatment. This study design inherently established divergent treatment procedures between the two groups. Since the neurostimulation group experienced additional procedures associated with DBS, performance bias may have been introduced into the study and influenced its outcomes [16]. Thirdly, PD is a slowly progressing condition that causes increased disability for several decades after onset. This midstage PD study only reported outcomes after 2 years of treatment, and the results of long-term stimulation in midstage PD remain unknown. Finally, this study was conducted in a younger PD population (average age <53 years; Table 29.1) whose outcomes may not reflect the average midstage PD patient (average onset of PD is 60–65 years [18]). Therefore, these results should be interpreted carefully and verified by independent investigators before definitive conclusions are made about the efficacy of DBS in the general midstage PD population.

Surgical candidacy

Successful DBS therapy relies on careful patient selection [19]. The widespread use of DBS in advanced PD has led to well-defined selection criteria for patients who are predicted to respond favorably to neurostimulation. The best outcomes for DBS are with advanced PD patients who (i) respond well to levodopa; (ii) lack levodopa-resistant axial symptoms; (iii) are not significantly cognitively impaired; (iv) are without active psychiatric conditions; and (v) are younger in age [19]. The current US Food and Drug Administration (FDA)-approved indication for DBS is advanced PD when symptoms are not adequately controlled by medications. Midstage PD patients are often sufficiently treated with medications, a feature that distinguishes them from those currently offered DBS. Ideally, the midstage DBS selection criteria would expand candidacy to include individuals before experiencing comorbidities that might preclude them from receiving the therapy. More research is required to fully understand the optimal DBS selection criteria for patients effectively managed by PD medication.

The potential for misdiagnosis is increased in the initial stage or with younger-onset PD. Parkinson's disease is challenging to diagnose because there is currently no biomarker available. Medical history, neurological examinations and response to dopaminergic medication are clinical measures cumulatively assessed by physicians in order to reach the diagnosis. This is often challenging, because not only is PD a heterogeneous condition but initial PD symptoms are mild and share features of other parkinsonian disorders. Despite symptom overlap, these atypical parkinsonism syndromes typically do not respond to DBS [20]. Therefore, offering stimulation before the disease is advanced might increase the rate of implanting patients who later prove to have a neurodegenerative condition other than PD [21]. A clear advantage to delaying DBS until PD symptoms are not adequately controlled with medications is reducing the chance of exposing patients who will not respond to stimulation to the risks, costs and expectations of DBS.

Deep-brain stimulation risks

Deep-brain stimulation is safe, and device surgery has very low complication rates. However, DBS remains an invasive procedure that involves intracranial implantation of stimulating electrodes and associated hardware. The potential benefits of DBS must be carefully weighed against the risks of surgery, the device and stimulation-associated side effects. These risks are often justified by the potential benefits of DBS for advanced PD patients who suffer from diminished quality of life without other viable treatment options. Noninvasive treatments are available for earlier-stage PD patients, and DBS in this population would expose patients to the risks before exhausting safer therapeutic options. Additionally, implanting sooner in PD would inherently mean that patients would live longer with any lasting adverse device effects compared with if they were offered DBS later in life. Without evidence supporting safe and effective longitudinal outcomes for DBS in earlier PD stages, there are ethical concerns with exposing patients to the risks of surgery while medication remains beneficial.

Table 29.1 Baseline characteristics of patients treated with subthalamic nucleus deep-brain stimulation in randomized controlled trials

Characteristic	Okun et al. (2012) [5]	Williams et al. (2010) [3]	Follett et al. (2010) [4]	Weaver et al. (2009) [7]	Deuschl et al. (2006) [2]	Schuepbach et al. (2013) [14]	Charles et al. (2014) [17]
PD stage	Advanced	Advanced	Advanced	Advanced	Advanced	Middle	Early
n	101	183	147	121	78	124	15
Age (years)	60.6 ± 8.3	59	61.9 ± 8.7	62.4 ± 8.8	60.5 ± 7.4	52.9 ± 6.6	60 ± 6.8
Male (%)	62	68	79	81	64	76	93
Duration of medication treatment (years)	NA	NA	11.1 ± 5.0	10.8 ± 5.4	13.0 ± 5.8	4.8 ± 3.3	2.2 ± 1.4
LEDD (mg/day)	1311 ± 615	NA	1289 ± 585	1281 ± 521	1176 ± 517	918.8 ± 412.5	417.2 ± 306.6
UPDRS-III on medication	18.3 ± 9.5[a]	18.9 ± 11.4[b]	22.4 ± 11.9[a]	22.6 ± 12.6[a]	18.9 ± 9.3[a]	12.5 ± 1.5[a]	11.1 ± 6.9[ac]
UPDRS-III off medication	40.8 ± 10.8	47.6 ± 14.0	NA	43.0 ± 13.5	48.0 ± 12.3	33.2 ± 1.8	25.3 ± 9.0[c]
UPDRS-IV	8.8 ± 3.5	9.0 ± 3.4	9.0 ± 2.9	9.2 ± 0.3	NA	5.6 ± 0.3	2.1 ± 2.1

NA, no data available; LEDD, levodopa-equivalent daily dose.

[a]After medication challenge.

[b]Authors did not indicate use of medication challenge.

[c]Screening visit.

In addition to surgical risks such as stroke (0–2%), intracranial hemorrhage (0–10%), infection (0–15%) and death (0–4.4%) [19], there are also concerns with the DBS hardware. Device-related problems include infection, electrode migration, lead fracture or erosion, and battery failure [22]. Correcting for DBS hardware deficiencies requires more surgery, which correlates with increased risk and additional costs. Even optimally functioning stimulator batteries only last an average of 4–7 years, after which they must be surgically replaced [23]. Since PD patients implanted sooner with DBS would have a longer *in vivo* device time, this population could experience an increased frequency of hardware malfunction or device-related repairs.

Advocates contend that earlier DBS intervention may extend the benefits of stimulation (i.e. motor function, quality of life and ADLs) over a longer period of time. This argument is counterbalanced by the chance of prolonged exposure to adverse effects known to accompany DBS. Although stimulation does not cause neuropsychological decline [24], subthalamic nucleus (STN)-DBS surgery is consistently associated with reduced verbal fluency performance [25]. Deep-brain stimulation is also linked to neuropsychiatric issues and weight gain [26, 27]. A controversial neuropsychiatric concern tied to DBS surgery is an increased risk of suicide [28], although multiple factors independent of the surgery and stimulation could account for this perceived rise in suicidality. Physicians, patients and caregivers considering earlier intervention must fully understand the potential lifelong consequences of DBS.

Economic impact

The increased costs of DBS are attributed to the device, surgery, hospitalization and follow-up visits. These expenses are partially offset by the reduced need for medication after surgery, but studies evaluating the cost-effectiveness of DBS were conducted over relatively short time periods (i.e. less than 5 years after surgery) [12, 13, 29]. Implanting patients sooner in the course of PD would extend their time with the device, which may ultimately increase the number of device-related procedures (i.e. battery replacements) [23]. Additionally, DBS patients require visits with neurologists who are familiar with adjusting stimulation settings and medication regimens to provide optimal clinical benefit. This specialized care often involves travel to distinct centers, which can be more burdensome than visits to local neurologists. This travel may impact both patient and caregiver productivity by requiring more time off work. Additionally, long-term adverse effects of DBS could also force early retirement of the patient and/or the caregiver and negatively impact the economic value of neurostimulation. Therefore, it is not yet known whether or not DBS is cost-effective over longer periods of time.

Disease modification

Many therapies treat PD symptoms, but no intervention has been shown to slow, halt or reverse neurodegeneration, disease progression or increasing disability. Efforts to identify neuroprotective strategies are hindered by the lack of an objective biomarker to track disease progression. Dopaminergic imaging studies quantifying nigral neurons are difficult to interpret because of compensatory mechanisms likely arising both naturally in PD and from the therapeutic interventions used to treat PD symptoms (i.e. dopaminergic medications) [30]. Therefore, neuroprotection can only be inferred by clinical rating scales or patient questionnaires. These measures are highly subjective and are ultimately influenced by multiple variables. Until a validated biomarker for PD is identified, it will be challenging to conduct clinical trials to definitively address neuroprotection.

The FDA approved DBS as an adjunctive therapy for advanced PD in 1997. Despite the wealth of clinical research on DBS in PD, there is no conclusive evidence that stimulation modifies PD progression. Several randomized, controlled trials of DBS in advanced PD show progressive worsening of symptoms over time [9, 31, 32]. Furthermore, despite active and clinically beneficial stimulation, DBS-treated PD patients develop axial, levodopa-resistant symptoms as the disease progresses [33]. This clear advancement of PD in late-stage patients suggests that DBS only treats PD symptoms and does not impact the natural course of the disease.

One study addressed disease progression in PD using fluorodopa positron emission tomography (^{18}F-DOPA PET) to quantify dopaminergic function [34]. Despite clinically efficacious DBS treatment (i.e. reduced PD medication and improved UPDRS scores), advanced PD patients showed a continuing decline in dopaminergic function over 16 months. This study was limited by its small sample size and the absence of a comparative medical therapy control group, but these results suggest that stimulation cannot protect dopaminergic neurons in advanced PD.

Despite lacking overt clinical evidence supporting stimulation-related modification of PD progression, advocates of DBS earlier in the course of PD are motivated by preclinical findings suggesting that active stimulation is neuroprotective [35–39]. Several studies show stimulation applied after dopaminergic lesioning protects nigral neurons [38, 39]. While animal models of PD have been useful tools to understand certain aspects of the disease (such as identifying treatments for dopamine deficiency), they do not fully recapitulate the age-dependent, progressive nature of PD [40]. So far, neuroprotective therapies that show promise in laboratory models have failed to translate into successful interventions in clinical trials. The DBS-induced neuroprotection observed in animal studies could be an artifact that fails to reflect accurately how stimulation influences the basal ganglia in PD.

Deep-brain stimulation should be offered as the standard of care in midstage Parkinson's disease

Clinical efficacy

Randomized controlled trials have demonstrated that DBS effectively relieves medication-induced motor complications in advanced PD patients [2, 7]. Long-term analyses confirm that these benefits are retained for up to 10 years after surgery [33, 41, 42]. Recently, a longitudinal study showed that DBS-mediated improvements in motor function and quality of life translated to enhanced survival and a reduced need for residential nursing care compared with standard medical therapy [43]. Results from this 10-year trial support the idea that the established symptomatic benefits of DBS also have lasting effects for patients via enhanced survival and functional independence. The long-term success of DBS therapy for advanced PD patients raises the intriguing question of whether there could be additional value from stimulation if offered earlier in the disease.

This hypothesis was tested recently in a population of midstage PD patients who still responded to PD medications but who also experienced motor complications [14]. This 2-year, randomized, multinational, parallel-group clinical trial compared STN-DBS plus medical therapy with medication alone in midstage PD patients experiencing levodopa-associated motor complications for 3 years or less (Hoehn and Yahr scale score <3 on medication; Table 29.1). Quality of life was significantly improved in the neurostimulation group over a 2-year period compared with the medication group. Subjects treated with DBS also improved considerably in motor disability, ADLs, levodopa-induced motor complications, and time with good mobility without dyskinesias. Although this was an open-label study, the validity of their findings was supported by blind assessments of the motor subset of the UPDRS. Furthermore, medications were appropriately managed according to current guidelines, as determined by an independent expert panel. This study was the first randomized controlled DBS trial in PD subjects who were still effectively managed by dopaminergic medication. Additional investigations in midstage PD are strongly encouraged to verify the results of this landmark study.

Surgical candidacy

Although DBS is an effective PD treatment, it is currently restricted to use in late-stage patients (disease duration 10–15 years, Table 29.1) [19]. Deep-brain stimulation is only considered in PD patients whose symptoms are no longer adequately controlled with medication (i.e. individuals with severe levodopa-associated side effects) and in those without significant cognitive and psychiatric symptoms. Unrelated to DBS, neuropsychiatric symptoms arise as part of PD and are relentlessly progressive when they occur [44]. Advancing age is also associated with the development of comorbidities, such as cardiac disease, dementia, diabetes and hypertension. Withholding DBS treatment until the late disease stage often excludes PD patients who would otherwise benefit from the therapy.

Because stimulation improves levodopa-dependent PD features, DBS success correlates strongly with patients who are highly responsive to levodopa without significant axial symptoms [45]. By the time patients reach the advanced stages of PD, symptoms develop that are resistant to medication and subsequently also refractory to stimulation [9, 46]. Therefore, DBS intervention sooner in PD, when dopaminergic symptoms predominate, should be considered to maximize the therapeutic benefit of stimulation.

In order to be considered for DBS surgery, advanced PD patients must have exhausted all other medical treatment options. Withholding DBS until this advanced stage can leave patients desperately searching for a viable treatment, and expectations of patients and families often exceed what is therapeutically possible. A difficult issue arises with late-stage DBS that stems from patient and family disappointment after surgery [22]. Unrealistic expectations combined with the stimulation-resistant symptoms that develop in late PD could contribute to the diminished psychosocial outcomes for some DBS patients [47]. Because patients with midstage PD are more responsive to levodopa therapy and experience fewer medication-resistant symptoms, this population is innately poised to achieve a better response to stimulation. Since medication still effectively treats symptoms, midstage PD patients are also less likely to adopt a last-resort mentality reported in some DBS patients with advanced PD [48]. Thus, midstage patients might have more realistic expectations of DBS outcomes compared with advanced PD patients.

Deep-brain stimulation risks

Overall perioperative adverse event rates are 18–23%, but the majority of these events are transient and resolve without sequelae [2–4]. Furthermore, DBS is an adjustable therapy – stimulation settings can be fine-tuned to maximize the clinical benefit and also minimize the occurrence and magnitude of stimulation-associated side effects. Unlike other surgical treatments, DBS is reversible, such that the device can be turned off or even removed if necessary. The surgical procedure for DBS has improved since the technique was introduced in the 1980s. Since DBS has emerged as an effective therapy for late-stage PD, the device technology and experience of surgical teams has also continually progressed. These advances account for reduced complication rates, especially with regard to intracerebral hemorrhage (<2%) and incidence of lead fracture or migration [19]. There are few reports of perioperative adverse event rates for DBS in earlier PD stages, but similar implanting procedures and target brain regions suggest that surgical complications would be comparable to later stages. A midstage PD study reported surgical complication rates similar to those accepted for advanced-stage PD [14]. This midstage PD data suggests there is no increased surgical risk associated with implanting the device sooner in PD.

Although DBS improves motor symptoms and complications of PD, cognitive domains are also impacted by surgery and/or neurostimulation. These post-surgery cognitive changes often resolve over the long term, but one cognitive dysfunction that is commonly reported is reduced verbal fluency scores after

STN-DBS. This cognitive decline is believed to be due to effects of microlesions from the surgical procedure and is not a result of neurostimulation [8]. Reduced verbal fluency after DBS surgery is often relatively mild, and in some cases, patients and families are unable to detect the declines that are reported by neuropsychological tests [49]. Preexisting cognitive impairment is a predictor of poorer cognitive performance after surgery [24, 50]. The contradictory reports on cognitive assessments after DBS are further confounded by underlying PD progression, which likely accounts for the reported cognitive decline [46]. For most patients, the dramatic benefits in quality of life and motor symptoms far exceed the risks of mildly reduced verbal fluency.

An increased risk of postoperative suicide in STN-DBS patients has been suggested [28], but recent analysis of data from a prospective, randomized, controlled study found no increase in suicidal behavior after STN-DBS surgery [51]. Instead, the authors pointed to the increasing evidence supporting the hypothesis that risk factors such as rapid and significant decreases in dopaminergic medication as well as substantial medical and psychiatric comorbidities may contribute to suicidal behaviors in the PD population. If this model is true, midstage PD patients would be expected to have reduced risk for suicidal ideation because they require less medication (Table 29.1) and have less comorbidity than in advanced PD. Alternatively, others suggest that PD patients who choose to undergo surgery have a higher risk for suicidal behavior than patients who opt against surgery [14]. This hypothesis is supported by studies in mid- and advanced-stage PD that report similar suicidal risk between treatment groups, which was higher than the risk in the general PD population [4, 14]. Investigators in the midstage PD study developed a suicidal risk monitoring procedure to offer surveillance and immediate intervention in order to address suicidal ideation [14]. Based on the currently available reports, there is no evidence confirming that STN-DBS increases suicidal risk. Thus, this speculative risk does not justify withholding DBS from patients sooner in PD

Economic impact

Parkinson's disease causes a significant economic burden on the individual patient due to its progressive nature over many years. Direct costs of PD (i.e. medication and patient care) significantly increase over time as PD progressively advances. Although DBS is initially an expensive procedure, it may prove to be a cost-effective alternative to standard medical therapy. The use of STN-DBS considerably reduces the requirement for PD medication [12, 13], which results in savings after 2 years that are projected to extend long term [12, 52]. It is reasonable to hypothesize that implanting sooner may extend and improve this economic benefit, due to more years with reduced medication costs.

There are also indirect measures of the economic impact of PD therapies to consider. The average onset age of PD is 60–65 years [17], which affects a population transitioning into retirement. Parkinson's disease patients experience decreasing productivity and uniformly become disabled from gainful employment. Improving quality of life and reducing symptoms may extend workable years and delay the retirement that PD often forces prematurely. Deep-brain stimulation improves patient quality of life and ADLs for late-stage PD patients [29], and these measures are also improved by stimulation in midstage PD [14]. The enhanced quality of life provided by DBS could also potentially provide patients with more-active and enjoyable retirement years if implanted sooner, rather than waiting until more-severe disability develops. A longitudinal study recently showed that DBS significantly reduced the need for residential nursing care and enhanced the survival of advanced PD patients [43]. Additionally, patient access to programming is becoming more obtainable, as increasing numbers of community-based general neurologists are adopting DBS therapy. Caregiver burden is also not increased as a result of DBS therapy [53]. Extending patient and caregiver vocational productivity (i.e. during midstage PD) and reducing the cost of nursing care (i.e. during advanced PD) may offer significant economic benefit for PD patients considering DBS.

Disease modification

The sustained clinical benefit of DBS for up to 10 years after surgery [33, 41–43] raises the question of whether stimulation alters the progressive disability caused by PD. Several animal PD models suggest that active STN stimulation protects nigral dopaminergic neurons [38, 54]. However, neuroprotection in PD remains controversial, due to the lack of a biomarker to objectively measure disease progression.

The most encouraging evidence supporting the hypothesis that DBS slows the rate of nigral dopaminergic neurodegeneration comes from preclinical models of PD. The neurotoxins 1-methyl-4-phenyl-1,2,3,6-tetrahydropyridine (MPTP) and 6-hydroxydopamine

(6-OHDA) selectively kill striatal dopaminergic neurons and cause parkinsonian-like symptoms in animal models [55, 56]. Several independent preclinical studies have reported that active STN stimulation increases the total dopaminergic neuron number in the striatum compared with nonstimulated controls [35–39]. Three key findings from these animal studies suggest that STN-DBS may protect or reduce the loss of dopaminergic neurons:

1. *Dopaminergic neuroprotection requires active STN stimulation.* Use of STN-DBS in 6-OHDA-treated rats improved motor function and increased dopaminergic neuron survival [35, 36]. Initial studies in PD animal models showed that DBS is neuroprotective, but these reports did not control for potential tissue damage-related effects associated with device implantation. This concern was addressed by comparing animals with active DBS with those that were not receiving stimulation but also had the device surgically implanted [37, 39]. Active STN stimulation significantly increased the ratios of dopaminergic neurons compared with controls (i.e. nonstimulated and nonimplanted animals) [37]. The requirement for active DBS for neuroprotection in animal models parallels the active stimulation-dependent improvement of motor symptoms in advanced PD patients [57].

2. *Stimulation applied after the onset of dopaminergic cell death inhibits further cell loss.* Early DBS animal studies were performed with neurotoxin and stimulation applied concurrently [35, 36]. This experimental strategy was unable to rule out the possibility that neuron survival resulted from impaired toxin uptake or metabolism somehow related to stimulation. Recent studies more accurately parallel when stimulation is therapeutically provided for PD patients (i.e. after the onset of dopaminergic neurodegeneration). By first determining the time course and severity of nigral dopaminergic neuron death after subacute 6-OHDA administration, Spieles-Engemann et al. [39] showed that 2 weeks of continuous DBS applied after 50% of the dopaminergic neurons were lost prevented further neuron death. Similar results were reported in an MPTP primate model of PD [38, 54]. These findings demonstrate that STN stimulation after the onset of dopaminergic cell loss can reduce further neuron death. This work addresses criticisms of prior studies and more closely models when DBS intervention is applied clinically.

3. *Severity of dopaminergic cell loss strongly influences efficacy of stimulation on neuroprotection.* An interesting phenomenon noted in preclinical studies is the inverse relationship between the severity of dopaminergic lesioning and the success of stimulation-mediated neuroprotection. After severe dopaminergic lesioning (85% cell loss), stimulation was unable to prevent further loss of the remaining dopaminergic neurons [58]. However, DBS applied following subacute lesioning (50% cell death) significantly improved dopaminergic cell survival in both nonhuman primates and rats [38, 39]. These findings suggest that with more severe dopaminergic injury, there are fewer surviving neurons and thus fewer cells to be impacted by stimulation. This correlation supports the hypothesis that DBS intervention sooner in PD has greater potential to protect or reduce dopaminergic neuron degeneration than when applied to advanced-stage patients.

Despite promising results from animal studies, there is limited clinical evidence supporting the hypothesis that DBS alters PD progression. Two independent studies reported no significant decline in motor symptoms after 4 years of stimulation [59, 60]. Since PD is relentlessly progressive in every case and motor function always gradually declines, this lack of symptom progression over several years may suggest that DBS is delaying progression. However, disease modification was not stated as a study endpoint, and these trials also lacked medication-only controls to allow progression rates to be compared. Conversely, an ^{18}F-DOPA PET study of DBS in advanced PD noted a decline in dopaminergic function over 16 months [34]. While this result implies that DBS lacks the ability to halt PD progression, the study was conducted in advanced PD subjects and also lacked a medication-only control group. There was insufficient evidence to determine whether any intermediate disease modification occurred (i.e. not completely halting progression but instead slowing the disease). The authors acknowledged that their study focused only on advanced PD patients and remarked that earlier intervention might delay the onset of drug-induced motor complications [34]. Since DBS is offered only in late-stage PD, it is possible that stimulation is applied too late to impact disease progression. Many reports indicate that 30–50% of striatal dopaminergic neurons have already degenerated at the time of initial PD diagnosis (i.e. when motor symptoms emerge prompting a visit to the physician) [61].

After the onset of motor symptoms, dopaminergic neurons rapidly degenerate within the first 5 years of diagnosis [62]. By late-stage PD, 90% of these neurons have degenerated, leaving few neurons to be protected by any potential disease-modifying therapy. The question of whether DBS can delay advancing disability in PD has not been investigated appropriately, with current research limited to conflicting and inconclusive reports. There is a clear need for adequately powered, randomized, controlled clinical trials designed to address this question.

Future direction: deep-brain stimulation for very-early-stage Parkinson's disease?

Although patients with midstage PD experience dyskinesias and other motor fluctuations, these motor complications are often not yet disabling. Advanced PD, however, is associated with a host of disabling features including dyskinesias, motor fluctuations, neuropsychological decline and medication-resistant symptoms. Most importantly, the outcomes of applying DBS in the very early stages (i.e. before the onset of motor complications) are unknown. The next frontier for DBS research is addressing whether stimulation offered early enough in PD could delay the onset of advancing disability, dyskinesias and other motor fluctuations, and the overall decline in quality of life. Many of the arguments for offering DBS in midstage PD translate into rationale supporting clinical research to test stimulation in early-stage PD:

1. *Prolonged benefits of neurostimulation.* Deep-brain stimulation is an established treatment for advanced PD, and initial research on midstage PD also suggests that DBS is superior to medications alone for appropriately selected patients. If stimulation is also shown to be safe and effective for early-stage PD, the benefits of DBS could be offered to a healthier cohort who stand to experience many more years of favorable stimulation-related outcomes.
2. *More DBS-responsive symptoms.* It is well known that DBS improves symptoms that respond to levodopa (i.e. dopaminergic-dependent processes), and early-stage patients possess significantly more dopaminergic neurons than even midstage patients [62]. Very-early-stage PD patients are a population that is poised to receive the greatest benefit from DBS, because they have the most stimulation-responsive neurons remaining.
3. *Greatest potential for neuroprotection.* Preclinical experiments strongly indicate that STN-DBS has the potential to prevent dopaminergic degeneration, and this neuroprotection is greatest when stimulation is applied following acute lesioning (i.e. there are more remaining neurons to be impacted by DBS) [38, 39]. Therefore, in order to maximize the potential neuroprotection of any therapy, intervention must be applied as soon as possible after PD is definitively diagnosed.

We recently completed a pilot study of DBS in the very earliest stage of PD tested to date to gather preliminary safety and tolerability data and to inform the design of a large-scale phase 3 trial [17, 63–68]. This is the first prospective, randomized, single-blinded clinical trial of DBS in subjects with early-stage PD responding well to medical therapy and prior to the onset of dyskinesias or other motor fluctuations (Table 29.1). Motor ability, quality of life and neuropsychological function were assessed every 6 months in subjects treated with standard medical therapy or DBS plus medications for 2 years. Eligible subjects were 50–75 years of age, idiopathic PD Hoehn and Yahr stage 2 off medication, and had been treated successfully with dopaminergic therapy for more than 6 months but less than 4 years. Subjects with dyskinesias, motor fluctuations or previous brain injury or operations were excluded. Comprehensive psychiatric and neuropsychological assessments were performed to ensure that subjects were not psychiatrically ill or cognitively impaired at the time of enrollment. Thirty-seven subjects were enrolled and 30 were randomized (seven failed at screening). This study's very low dropout rate (one patient, 3.3%) was likely a result of the multiphase informed consent process that was used to ensure that subjects fully understood the risks and their role in the study [64].

Since this was the first controlled study of DBS in very-early-stage PD, it was unclear prior to this study whether the mild symptoms of early PD would permit proper lead placement. Intraoperative techniques that assist with the identification of the optimal target for the DBS lead include microelectrode neurophysiological recordings of the STN and surrounding structures and neurological examination of stimulation-mediated symptom relief. This early PD pilot study demonstrated that the STN can be accurately targeted and implanted in PD patients with only mild symptoms [66]. More importantly, early PD subjects received clinical benefits from DBS over the ensuing 2-year study [17, 68].

This pilot study was conducted to gather preliminary safety and tolerability data necessary to inform the design of a large-scale, pivotal study concerning safety and efficacy of DBS in very-early-stage PD. This objective led the FDA to limit the number of subjects enrolled to 30, and thus the pilot study was not powered to make definitive determinations about PD progression between treatment groups. As expected, there were few significant differences between treatment groups. At 24 months, DBS subjects did not experience worsening of motor function (UPDRS-III off treatment, primary endpoint) compared with the optimal drug therapy group [17]. Average scores of the UPDRS-IV (motor complications) and 39-Item Parkinson's Disease Questionnaire (PDQ-39; measuring quality of life) were better in the stimulation group, but this did not reach statistical significance. Perioperative adverse event rates were comparable to those described for advanced PD [66]. This study met its primary endpoint, finding that subjects receiving stimulation did not experience unexpected PD worsening when compared with the medication control group.

Subjects also underwent neuropsychological analyses, and these results indicated DBS is generally safe with regard to cognitive function in subjects with early-stage PD [67]. The DBS group scores were reduced on specific measures (i.e. attention, executive functioning and verbal fluency) at 12 months compared with the medication-only group, but these between-group differences were mostly resolved by 24 months. Impaired phonemic word fluency is the most commonly reported STN-DBS-related cognitive effect in patients with advanced PD [25, 50], but this adverse effect is mild and is greatly outweighed by the benefits of DBS in motor response and quality of life. In the early PD pilot study, declines in verbal fluency in early PD subjects were minimal (most prominent at 12 months). These analyses indicated that early-stage PD patients did not experience abnormal psychological decline at higher rates than previously published for midstage or advanced patients.

A patient-centered composite endpoint was developed that analyzes clinically important worsening on two meaningful outcomes for PD patients – motor symptoms and complications of medical therapy [68]. Evaluation of this endpoint using data from the pilot trial of DBS in early-stage PD suggests that subjects treated with optimal drug therapy were two to five times more likely to experience clinically important worsening than those treated with DBS plus optimal drug therapy [68]. This analysis supports utilization of this patient-centered outcome in future trials of DBS in early-stage PD.

This early PD pilot study provides the foundation for investigations of the efficacy of DBS in early-stage PD. Future prospective trials should be appropriately powered and should also make the best attempt to achieve a double-blind, placebo-controlled design. This could be achieved by implanting both treatment groups with therapeutically functional DBS systems, which would provide two notable experimental controls: (i) this design would attempt to blind subjects to treatment assignment; and (ii) groups would be distinguished only by inactive or active stimulation, which would allow assessment of whether active STN stimulation or device implantation impacts the study outcomes. Alternatively, a double-blind, placebo-controlled design could also be achieved with a sham DBS implant control group compared with an active DBS implant group. This design would also attempt to blind subjects to treatment assignment, while also removing the potential confound of a microlesioning effect in the control group, thus allowing a more pure comparison of DBS with medical therapy. While it is not appropriate to offer DBS in early-stage PD as the standard of care, there is now sufficient evidence to support a large-scale clinical trial to address whether DBS is superior to medication for this population.

Despite decades of clinical success, the mechanism of DBS-mediated benefits remains elusive. As more is understood about how stimulation of distinct neurons in the basal ganglia improves PD symptoms, scientists can begin to draw from existing knowledge of molecular pathways and circuits to potentially identify genetic factors to predict those who will benefit from DBS. Parkinson's disease is a complex, heterogeneous condition, and it is likely that subsets of patients will respond to medical and surgical treatments differently based on their genetics. Polymorphisms in genes controlling mitochondrial function, dopaminergic signaling, neuronal plasticity or cell survival could potentially be used to predict favorable treatment outcomes for PD patients considering DBS surgery. Characterization of the molecular mechanisms responsible for DBS success will provide a huge leap forward for PD research and should uncover new avenues for therapeutic intervention.

Conclusions

Deep-brain stimulation for PD is currently approved to treat advanced-stage patients who are not adequately controlled by medication. Research over the last decade demonstrates that DBS is superior to medication alone for treating appropriately selected PD patients, and it is likely that the randomized, controlled trial of DBS in midstage PD [14] will transform the application of DBS toward patients who still respond to medication and are newly experiencing dyskinesias or other motor fluctuations. Critics of DBS at earlier PD stages have concerns with exposing patients to the risks of DBS when safer therapies remain effective [69–72]. Advocates point to the demonstrated success of DBS in later stages, as well insight from animal studies and the potential for disease modification. Clearly, more research is needed to address these controversial areas surrounding offering DBS sooner in the course of PD.

Despite the proven success of DBS for treatment of mid- and late-stage PD, there is currently insufficient evidence to support offering DBS to early-stage PD patients as the standard of care. A small-scale study comparing DBS with optimal drug therapy in early-stage PD subjects is complete, but this trial was not powered to address whether DBS is an effective treatment in early-stage PD [17]. It remains to be seen whether stimulation at very early PD stages will also be superior to medication, and whether it will delay the onset of dyskinesias and other motor fluctuations, delay the development of disability, extend work productivity and/or provide a better quality of life. The FDA has approved a large-scale, randomized, double-blinded, multicenter, phase 3, pivotal clinical trial testing DBS in early-stage PD designed to answer these questions.

References

1. Obeso JA, Rodriguez-Oroz MC, Chana P, et al. The evolution and origin of motor complications in Parkinson's disease. *Neurology* 2000; **55** (Suppl. 4): S13–20; discussion S21–3.
2. Deuschl G, Schade-Brittinger C, Krack P. A randomized trial of deep-brain stimulation for Parkinson's disease. *N Engl J Med* 2006; **355**: 896–908.
3. Williams A, Gill S, Varma T, et al. Deep brain stimulation plus best medical therapy versus best medical therapy alone for advanced Parkinson's disease (PD SURG trial): a randomised, open-label trial. *Lancet Neurol* 2010; **9**: 581–91.
4. Follett KA, Weaver FM, Stern M, et al. Pallidal versus subthalamic deep-brain stimulation for Parkinson's disease. *N Engl J Med* 2010; **362**: 2077–91.
5. Okun MS, Gallo BV, Mandybur G, et al. Subthalamic deep brain stimulation with a constant-current device in Parkinson's disease: an open-label randomised controlled trial. *Lancet Neurol* 2012; **11**: 140–9.
6. Odekerken VJ, van Laar T, Staal MJ, et al. Subthalamic nucleus versus globus pallidus bilateral deep brain stimulation for advanced Parkinson's disease (NSTAPS study): a randomised controlled trial. *Lancet Neurol* 2013; **12**: 37–44.
7. Weaver F, Follett K, Stern M, et al. Bilateral deep brain stimulation vs best medical therapy for patients with advanced Parkinson disease: a randomized controlled trial. *JAMA* 2009; **301**: 63–73.
8. Okun M, Fernandez H, Wu S, et al. Cognition and mood in Parkinson's disease in subthalamic nucleus versus globus pallidus interna deep brain stimulation: the COMPARE trial. *Ann Neurol* 2009; **65**: 586–95.
9. Krack P, Batir A, van Blercom N, et al. Five-year follow-up of bilateral stimulation of the subthalamic nucleus in advanced Parkinson's disease. *N Engl J Med* 2003; **349**: 1925–34.
10. Simonin C, Tir M, Devos D, et al. Reduced levodopa-induced complications after 5 years of subthalamic stimulation in Parkinson's disease: a second honeymoon. *J Neurol* 2009; **256**: 1736–41.
11. Schüpbach WM, Maltête D, Houeto JL, et al. Neurosurgery at an earlier stage of Parkinson disease: a randomized, controlled trial. *Neurology* 2007; **68**: 267–71.
12. Charles PD, Padaliya BB, Newman WJ, et al. Deep brain stimulation of the subthalamic nucleus reduces antiparkinsonian medication costs. *Parkinsonism Relat Disord* 2004; **10**: 475–9.
13. Weaver FM, Stroupe KT, Cao L, et al. Parkinson's disease medication use and costs following deep brain stimulation. *Mov Disord* 2012; **27**: 1398–403.
14. Schuepbach WM, Rau J, Knudsen K, et al. Neurostimulation for Parkinson's disease with early motor complications. *N Engl J Med* 2013; **368**: 610–22.
15. Dumitriu A, Popescu BO. Placebo effects in neurological diseases. *J Med Life* 2010; **3**: 114–21.
16. Paradis C. Bias in surgical research. *Ann Surg* 2008; **248**: 180–8.
17. Charles PD, Konrad PE, Davis TL, et al. Subthalamic nucleus deep brain stimulation in early stage Parkinson's disease. *Parkinsonism Relat Disord* 2014; **20**: 731–7.
18. Twelves D, Perkins KSM, Counsell C. Systematic review of incidence studies of Parkinson's disease. *Mov Disord* 2003; **18**: 19–31.
19. Bronstein JM, Tagliati M, Alterman RL, et al. Deep brain stimulation for Parkinson disease: an expert consensus and review of key issues. *Arch Neurol* 2011; **68**: 165.

20. Shih LC, Tarsy D. Deep brain stimulation for the treatment of atypical parkinsonism. *Mov Disord* 2007; **22**: 2149–55.
21. Lang AE, Houeto J, Krack P, *et al*. Deep brain stimulation: preoperative issues. *Mov Disord* 2006; **21** (Suppl. 14): S171–96.
22. Okun MS, Rodriguez RL, Mikos A, *et al*. Deep brain stimulation and the role of the neuropsychologist. *Clin Neuropsychol* 2007; **21**: 162–89.
23. Anheim M, Fraix V, Chabardès S, *et al*. Lifetime of Itrel II pulse generators for subthalamic nucleus stimulation in Parkinson's disease. *Mov Disord* 2007; **22**: 2436–9.
24. Funkiewiez A. Long term effects of bilateral subthalamic nucleus stimulation on cognitive function, mood, and behaviour in Parkinson's disease. *J Neurol Neurosurg Psychiatry* 2004; **75**: 834–9.
25. Parsons TD, Rogers SA, Braaten AJ, Woods SP, Tröster AI. Cognitive sequelae of subthalamic nucleus deep brain stimulation in Parkinson's disease: a meta-analysis. *Lancet Neurol* 2006; **5**: 578–88.
26. Rieu I, Derost P, Ulla M, *et al*. Body weight gain and deep brain stimulation. *J Neurolog Sci* 2011; **310**: 267–70.
27. Voon V, Kubu C, Krack P, Houeto J, Tröster AI. Deep brain stimulation: neuropsychological and neuropsychiatric issues. *Mov Disord* 2006; **21** (Suppl. 14): S305–27.
28. Voon V, Krack P, Lang AE, *et al*. A multicentre study on suicide outcomes following subthalamic stimulation for Parkinson's disease. *Brain* 2008; **131**: 2720–8.
29. Kleiner-Fisman G, Herzog J, Fisman D, *et al*. Subthalamic nucleus deep brain stimulation: summary and meta-analysis of outcomes. *Mov Disord* 2006; **21** (Suppl. 14): S290–304.
30. Appel-Cresswell S, La Fuente-Fernandez de R, Galley S, McKeown MJ. Imaging of compensatory mechanisms in Parkinson's disease. *Curr Opin Neurol* 2010; **23**: 407–12.
31. Rodriguez-Oroz MC. Bilateral deep brain stimulation in Parkinson's disease: a multicentre study with 4 years follow-up. *Brain* 2005; **128**: 2240–9.
32. Wider C, Pollo C, Bloch J, Burkhard PR, Vingerhoets FJG. Long-term outcome of 50 consecutive Parkinson's disease patients treated with subthalamic deep brain stimulation. *Parkinsonism Relat Disord* 2008; **14**: 114–19.
33. Zibetti M, Merola A, Rizzi L, et al. Beyond nine years of continuous subthalamic nucleus deep brain stimulation in Parkinson's disease. *Mov Disord* 2011; **26**: 2327–34.
34. Hilker R, Portman A, Voges J, Staal M. Disease progression continues in patients with advanced Parkinson's disease and effective subthalamic nucleus stimulation. *J Neurol* 2005; **76**: 1217–21.
35. Maesawa S, Kaneoke Y, Kajita Y, *et al*. Long-term stimulation of the subthalamic nucleus in hemiparkinsonian rats: neuroprotection of dopaminergic neurons. *J Neurosurg* 2004; **100**: 679–87.
36. Temel Y, Visser-Vandewalle V, Kaplan S, *et al*. Protection of nigral cell death by bilateral subthalamic nucleus stimulation. *Brain Res* 2006; **1120**: 100–5.
37. Harnack D, Meissner W, Jira J, *et al*. Placebo-controlled chronic high-frequency stimulation of the subthalamic nucleus preserves dopaminergic nigral neurons in a rat model of progressive Parkinsonism. *Exp Neurol* 2008; **210**: 257–60.
38. Wallace BA, Ashkan K, Heise CE, *et al*. Survival of midbrain dopaminergic cells after lesion or deep brain stimulation of the subthalamic nucleus in MPTP-treated monkeys. *Brain* 2007; **130**: 2129–45.
39. Spieles-Engemann AL, Behbehani MM, Collier TJ, *et al*. Stimulation of the rat subthalamic nucleus is neuroprotective following significant nigral dopamine neuron loss. *Neurobiol Dis* 2010; **39**: 105–15.
40. Olanow CW, Kieburtz K, Schapira AH. Why have we failed to achieve neuroprotection in Parkinson's disease? *Ann Neurol* 2008; **64**(Supp. 2): S101–10.
41. Moro E, Lozano A, Pollak P, *et al*. Long-term results of a multicenter study on subthalamic and pallidal stimulation in Parkinson's disease. *Mov Disord* 2010; **25**: 578–86.
42. Castrioto A, Lozano A, Poon Y, *et al*. Ten-year outcome of subthalamic stimulation in Parkinson disease: a blinded evaluation. *Arch Neurol* 2011; **68**: 1550–6.
43. Ngoga D, Mitchell R, Kausar J, *et al*. Deep brain stimulation improves survival in severe Parkinson's disease. *J Neurol Neurosurg Psychiatry* 2013; **85**: 17–22.
44. Aarsland D, Marsh L, Schrag A. Neuropsychiatric symptoms in Parkinson's disease. *Mov Disord* 2009; **24**: 2175–86.
45. Welter ML, Houeto JL, Tezenas du Montcel S, *et al*. Clinical predictive factors of subthalamic stimulation in Parkinson's disease. *Brain* 2002; **125**: 575–83.
46. Rodriguez-Oroz MC, Moro E, Krack P. Long-term outcomes of surgical therapies for Parkinson's disease. *Mov Disord* 2012; **27**: 1718–28.
47. Schermer M. Ethical issues in deep brain stimulation. *Front Integr Neurosci* 2011; **5**: 17.
48. Bell E, Bell E, Maxwell B, *et al*. Deep brain stimulation and ethics: perspectives from a multisite qualitative study of Canadian neurosurgical centers. *World Neurosurg* 2011; **76**: 537–47.
49. Ardouin C, Pillon B, Peiffer E, *et al*. Bilateral subthalamic or pallidal stimulation for Parkinson's disease

affects neither memory nor executive functions: a consecutive series of 62 patients. *Ann Neurol* 1999; **46**: 217–23.

50. Massano J, Garrett C. Deep brain stimulation and cognitive decline in Parkinson's disease: a clinical review. *Front Neurol* 2012; **3**: 66.

51. Weintraub D, Duda JE, Carlson K, *et al*. Suicide ideation and behaviours after STN and GPi DBS surgery for Parkinson's disease: results from a randomised, controlled trial. *J Neurol Neurosurg Psychiatry* 2013; **84**: 1113–18.

52. Meissner W, Schreiter D, Volkmann J, *et al*. Deep brain stimulation in late stage Parkinson's disease: a retrospective cost analysis in Germany. *J Neurol* 2005; **252**: 218–23.

53. Oyama G, Okun MS, Schmidt P, *et al*. Deep brain stimulation may improve quality of life in people with Parkinson's disease without affecting caregiver burden. *Neuromodulation* 2013; **17**: 126–32.

54. Temel Y, Kessels A, Tan S, *et al*. Behavioural changes after bilateral subthalamic stimulation in advanced Parkinson disease: a systematic review. *Parkinsonism Relat Disord* 2006; **12**: 265–72.

55. Kopin IJ. MPTP: an industrial chemical and contaminant of illicit narcotics stimulates a new era in research on Parkinson's disease. *Environ Health Perspect* 1987; **75**: 45–51.

56. Schwarting RK, Huston JP. The unilateral 6-hydroxy-dopamine lesion model in behavioral brain research. Analysis of functional deficits, recovery and treatments. *Prog Neurobiol* 1996; **50**: 275–331.

57. Deep-Brain Stimulation for Parkinson's Disease Study Group. Deep-brain stimulation of the subthalamic nucleus or the pars interna of the globus pallidus in Parkinson's disease. *N Engl J Med* 2001; **345**: 956–63.

58. Luquin M, Saldise L, Guillén J, *et al*. Does increased excitatory drive from the subthalamic nucleus contribute to dopaminergic neuronal death in Parkinson's disease? *Exp Neurol* 2006; **201**: 407–15.

59. Visser-Vandewalle V, van der Linden C, Temel Y, *et al*. Long-term effects of bilateral subthalamic nucleus stimulation in advanced Parkinson disease: a four year follow-up study. *Parkinsonism Relat Disord* 2005; **11**: 157–65.

60. Rodriguez-Oroz M, Obeso J, Lang A, *et al*. Bilateral deep brain stimulation in Parkinson's disease: a multicentre study with 4 years follow-up. *Brain* 2005; **128**: 2240–9.

61. Cheng H, Ulane CM, Burke RE. Clinical progression in Parkinson disease and the neurobiology of axons. *Ann Neurol* 2010; **67**: 715–25.

62. Kordower JH, Olanow CW, Dodiya HB, *et al*. Disease duration and the integrity of the nigrostriatal system in Parkinson's disease. *Brain* 2013; **136**: 2419–31.

63. Gill CE, Allen LA, Konrad PE, *et al*. Deep brain stimulation for early-stage Parkinson's disease: an illustrative case. *Neuromodulation* 2011; **14**: 515–22.

64. Charles PD, Dolhun RM, Gill CE, *et al*. Deep brain stimulation in early Parkinson's disease: enrollment experience from a pilot trial. *Parkinsonism Relat Disord* 2012; **18**: 268–73.

65. Charles D, Tolleson C, Davis T, Gill C. *et al*. Pilot study assessing the feasibility of applying bilateral subthalamic nucleus deep brain stimulation in very early stage Parkinson's disease: study design and rationale. *J Parkinson's Dis* 2012; **2**: 215–23.

66. Kahn E, D'Haese P-, Dawant B, *et al*. Deep brain stimulation in early stage Parkinson's disease: operative experience from a prospective randomised clinical trial. *J Neurol Neurosurg Psychiatry* 2012; **83**: 164–70.

67. Tramontana MG, Molinari AL, Konrad PE, *et al*. Neuropsychological effects of deep brain stimulation in early stage Parkinson's disease. *J Parkinsons Dis* 2015; **5**: 151–63.

68. Hacker ML, Tonascia J, Turchan M, *et al*. Deep brain stimulation may reduce the relative risk of clinically important worsening in early stage Parkinson's disease. *Parkinsonism Relat Disord* 2015; **21**: 1177–83.

69. Finder SG, Bliton MJ, Gill CE, Davis TL, Konrad PE, Charles PD. Potential subjects' responses to an ethics questionnaire in a phase I study of deep brain stimulation in early Parkinson's disease. *J Clin Ethics* 2012; **23**: 207–16.

70. Finder SG, Bliton MJ. Fortitude and Community: Response to Yee and Ford. *J. Clin Ethics* 2012; **23**: 221–3.

71. Charles D, Konrad PE, Davis TL, Neimat JS, Hacker ML, Finder SG. Deep brain stimulation in early stage Parkinson's disease. *Parkinsonism Relat Disord* 2015; **21**: 347–8.

72. Hacker M, Charles D, Finder S. Deep brain stimulation in early stage Parkinson's disease may reduce the relative risk of symptom worsening. *Parkinsonism Related Disord* 2016; **22**: 112–13.

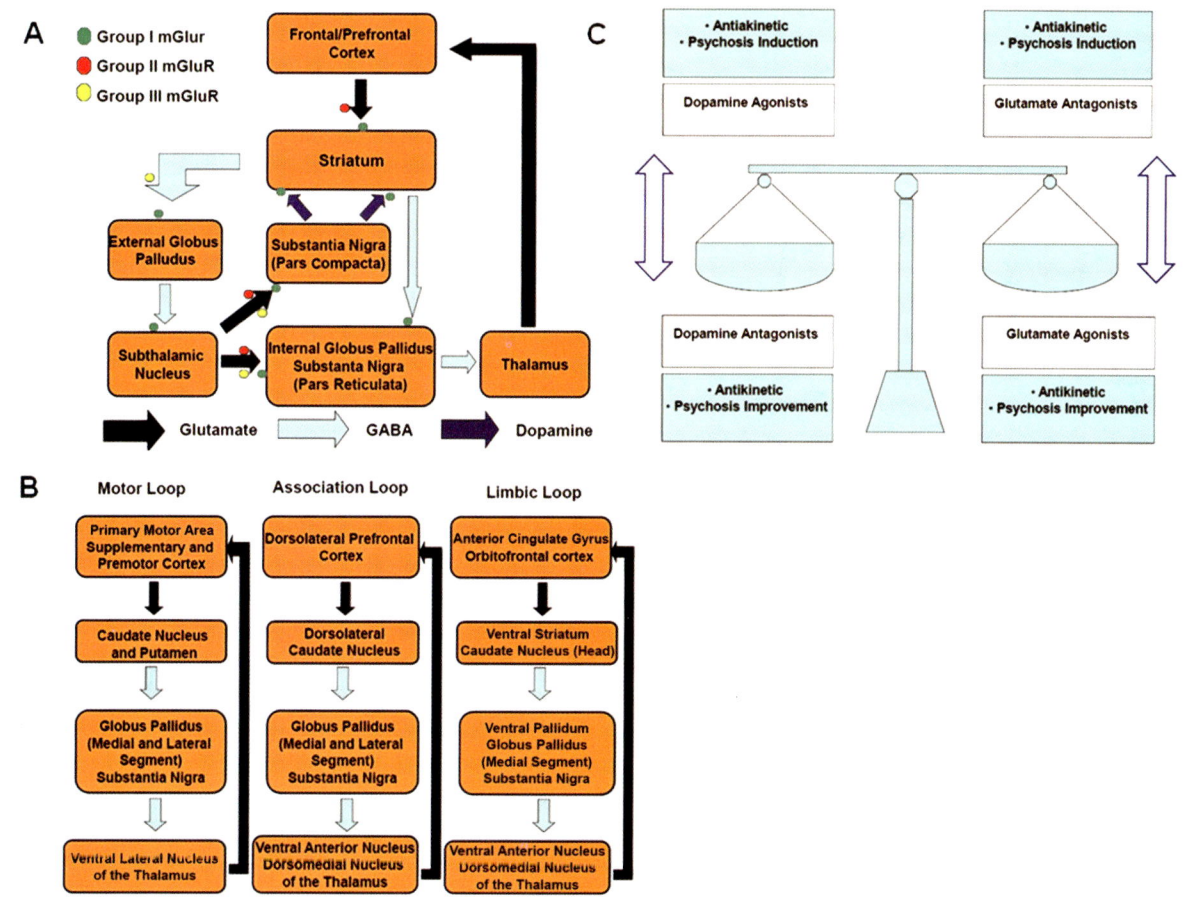

Figure 3.1 (A) Expression of different glutamate receptor subtypes, demonstrating the complexity expected in any attempt to modulate glutamatergic neurotransmission. (B) Illustration of the corticostriatal circuits, demonstrating the role of glutamatergic neurotransmission in motor, limbic and associative loops. (C) An early schematization of the dopaminergic/glutamatergic imbalance in Parkinson's disease and psychosis, as a tribute to the first pharmacologist who developed amantadine and memantine.

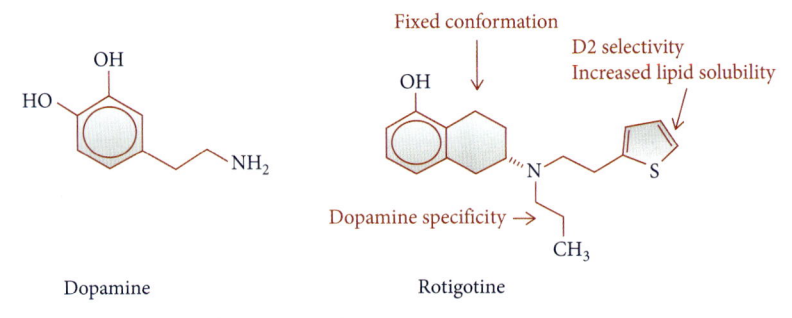

Figure 6.1 Structure of dopamine and rotigotine.

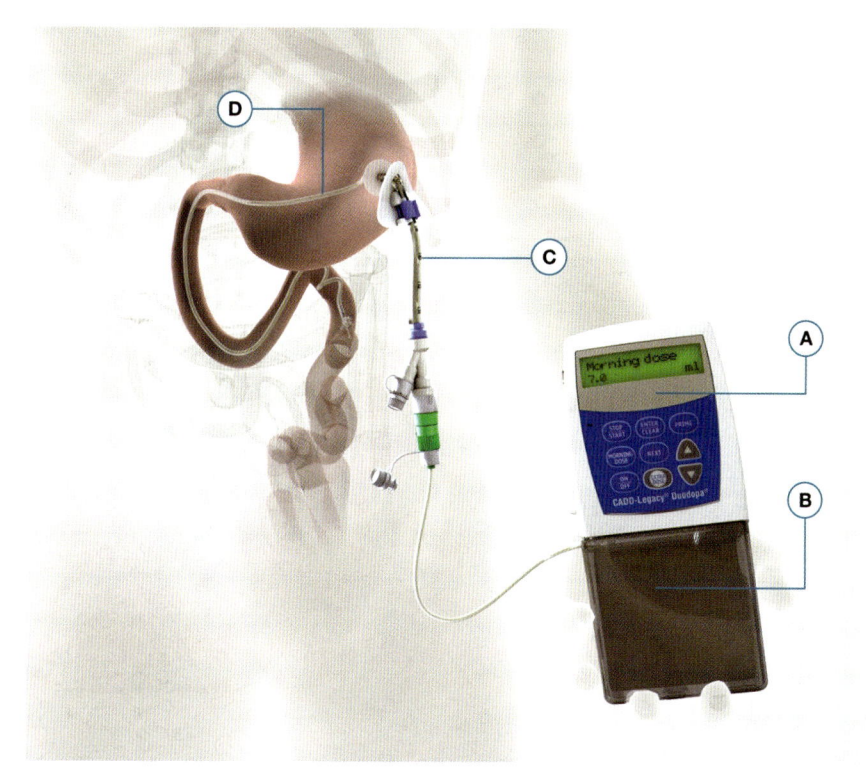

Figure 7.2 The levodopa/carbidopa gel (LCIG) infusion system. (A) Pump. (B) LCIG cassette. (C) Percutaneous endoscopic gastrostomy. (D) Intestinal tube.
(Permission for publication from AbbVie Inc.)

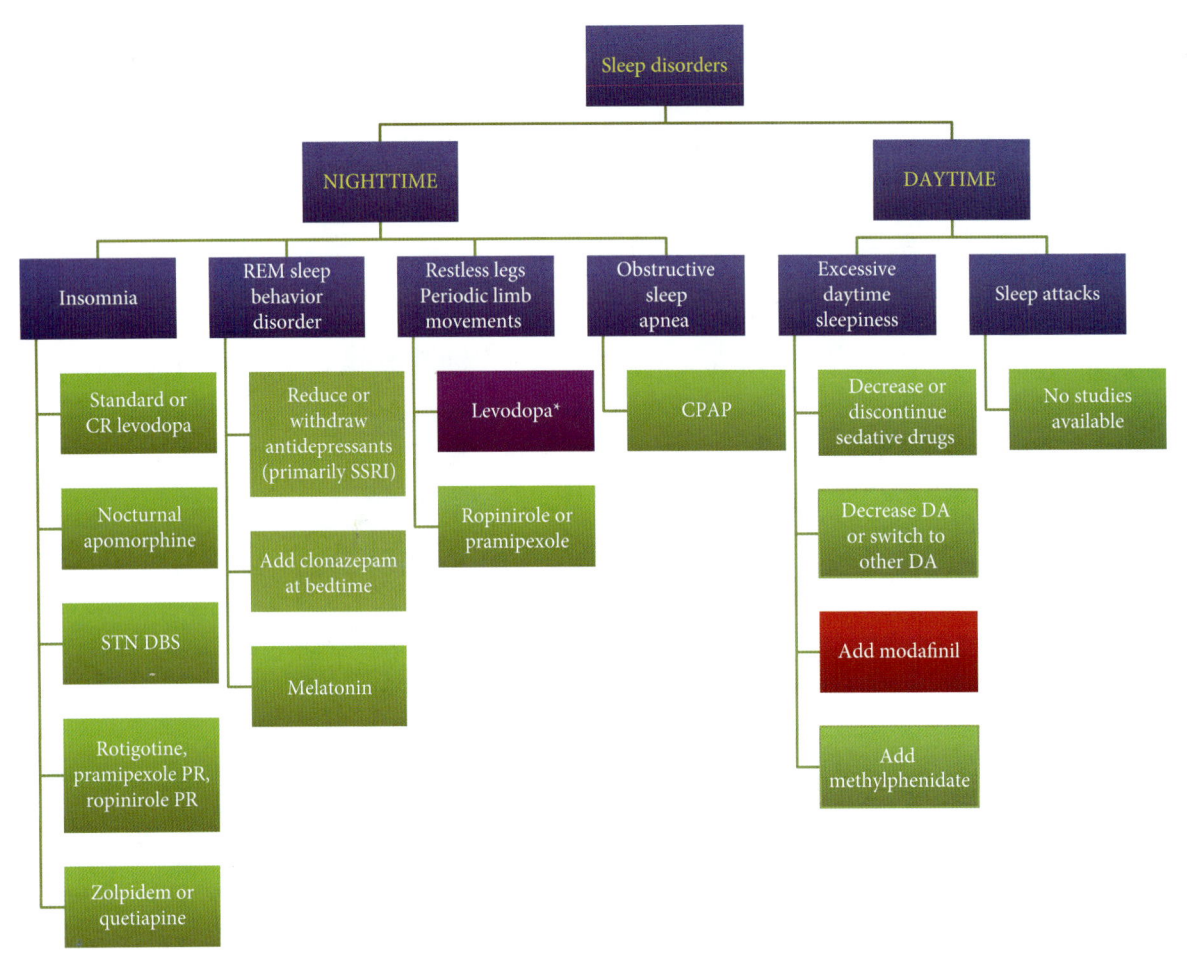

Figure 15.1 Summary flowchart for the treatment of sleep disorders in Parkinson's disease resulting from evidence-based data. Levels of recommendation are based on the American Academy of Neurology practice parameters [53]: level A recommendations are in red, level B recommendations are in violet; level U recommendations are in green. CPAP, continuous positive airway pressure; DA, dopamine agonist; DBS, deep-brain stimulation; PR, prolonged release; SSRI, selective serotonin reuptake inhibitor; STN, subthalamic nucleus. *This option refers only to periodic limb movement disorder.

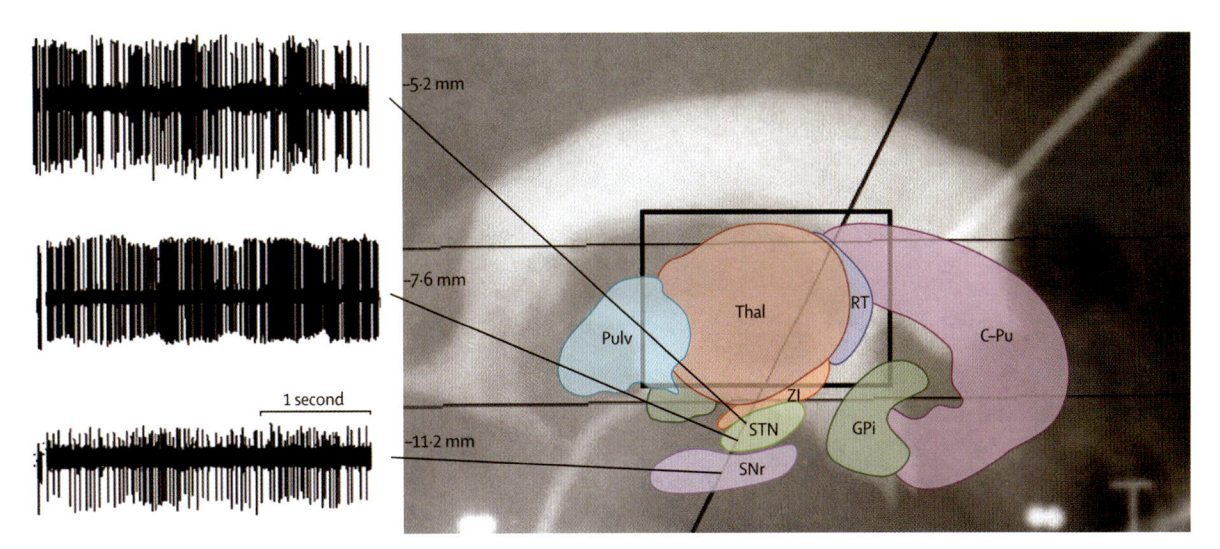

Figure 19.2 Stereotactic localization of the subthalamic nucleus using firing patterns from microelectrode recordings. The microelectrode trajectory (black oblique line) encounters the thalamus and then the zona incerta, followed by a rich, irregular burst of neural activity in the kinesthetic neurons of the subthalamic nucleus (STN; 5.2 and 7.6 mm below the commissural line in this patient), and high-amplitude, regular and unresponsive neural activity in the substantia nigra pars reticulata (SNr; 11.2 mm below the commissural line). C-Pu, caudate and putamen (striatum); GPi, internal globus pallidus; Pulv, pulvinar; RT, reticularis thalami; Thal, thalamus; ZI, zona incerta.
Reproduced with permission from Benabid AL *et al*. Deep brain stimulation of the subthalamic nucleus for the treatment of Parkinson's disease. *The Lancet Neurology*. 2009;8[1]: 67–81 [32].

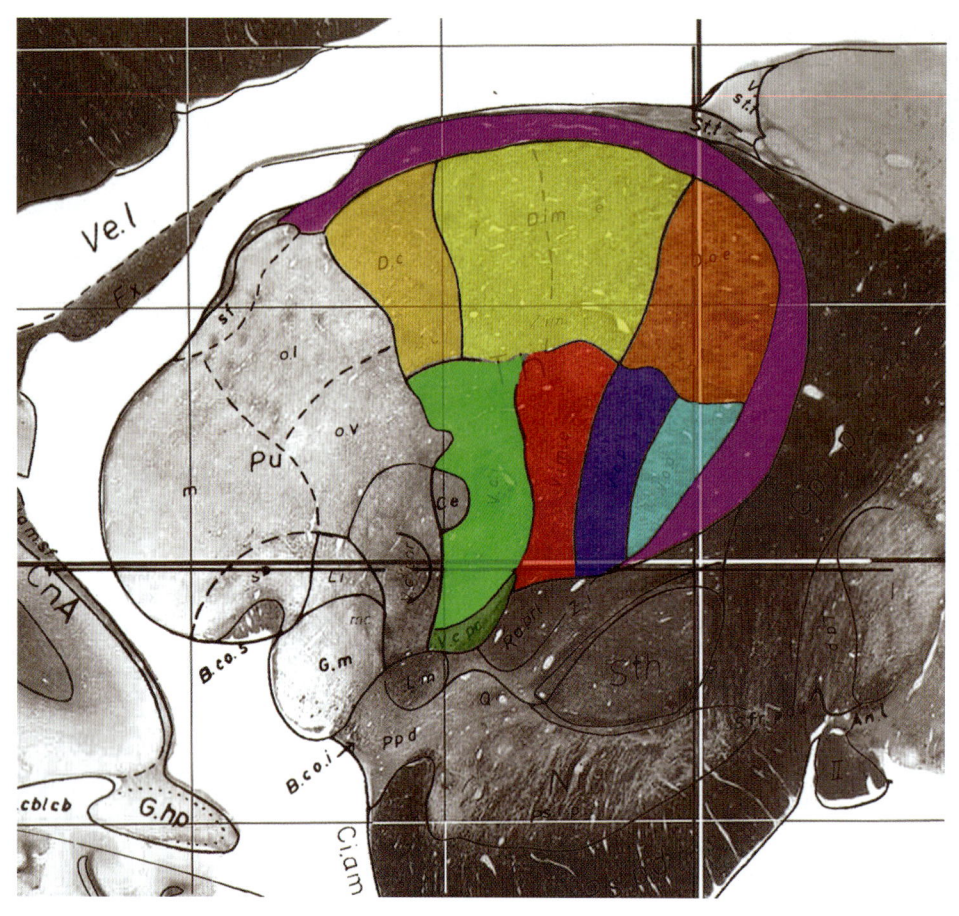

Figure 20.1 A sagittal slice through the thalamus taken 14.5 mm from the midline. The ventral intermediate nucleus, shown in red, is the target for tremor therapy in deep-brain stimulation (DBS). The initial target for the DBS lead is 14.5 mm from the midline and is then fine-tuned using intraoperative neurophysiological mapping techniques. From [17].

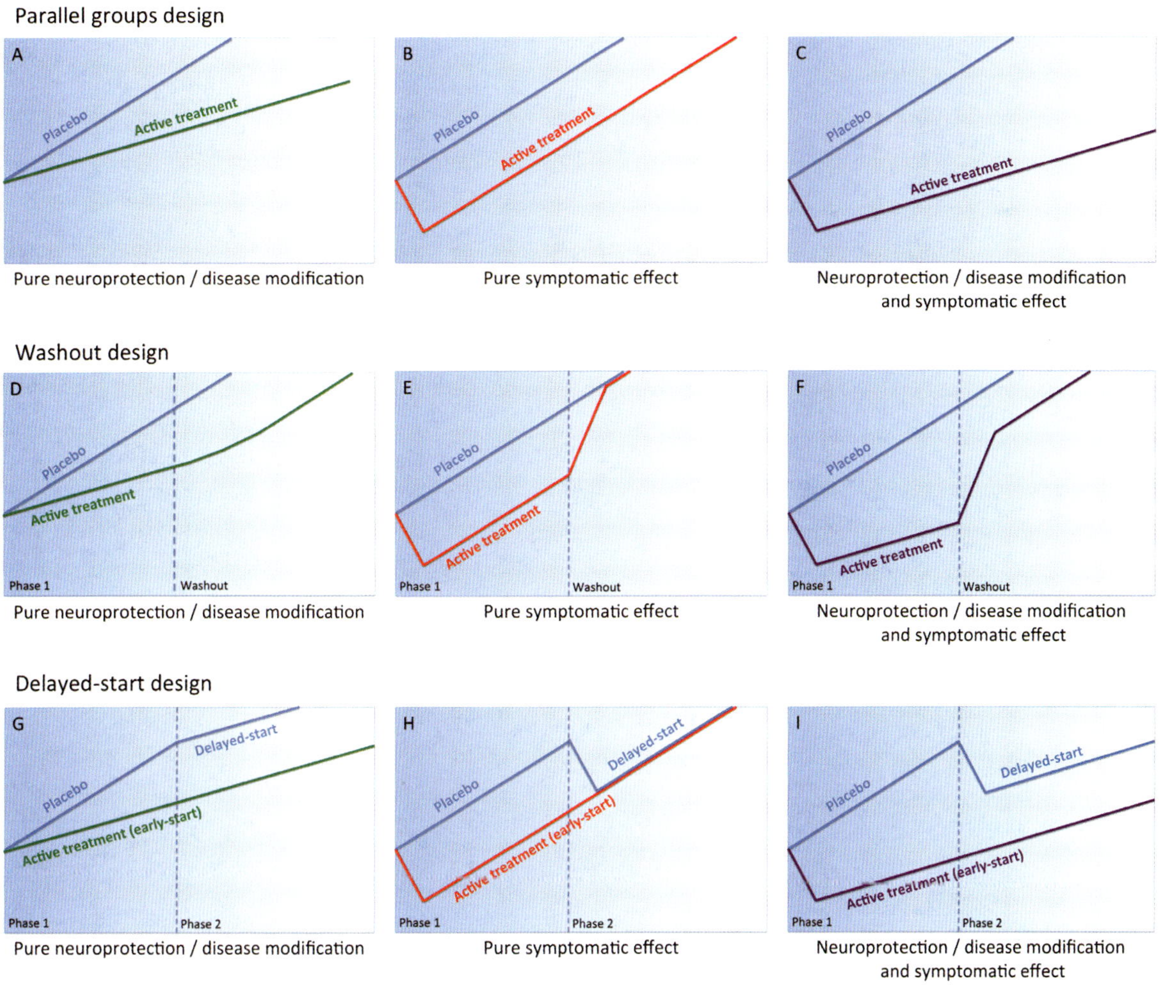

Figure 25.1 Schematic representation of the theoretical effect of neuroprotective, symptomatic, or mixed neuroprotective and symptomatic treatments compared with placebo in different study designs. The x-axis represents time and the y-axis represents the measure of progression, for instance Unified Parkinson's Disease Rating Scale (UPDRS) score. The parallel-group design (A–C), washout design (D–F) and delayed-start design (G–I) are illustrated. The placebo group is depicted as a blue line. The green lines (A, D, G) represent a pure neuroprotective agent, the red lines (B, E, H) represent a pure symptomatic agent, and the purple lines (C, F, I) represent a mixed symptomatic and neuroprotective agent (see text for details). Of note, the curves are artificially simplified; in particular, a beneficial clinical effect of the placebo (i.e. a placebo effect) is not reflected.

Chapter 30

Lessons and challenges of trials for cognitive and behavioral complications of Parkinson's disease

Daniel Weintraub and Lama M. Chahine

Introduction

There has been increasing recognition that Parkinson's disease (PD) is much more than a motor disorder; it is also often associated with neuropsychiatric symptoms (NPSs) that lead to as much, if not more, morbidity as the motor manifestations, and which also have a significant negative impact on quality of life. These include cognitive decline, affective disorders, psychosis, impulse control disorders (ICDs), anxiety symptoms and apathy. While early clinical trials in PD focused on the management of motor symptoms, recent years have seen several trials for the NPSs of PD. Major advances in the evidence available for treatment of depression in PD have been made, but much remains to be learned. For other NPSs, only a few pharmacological agents have been proven beneficial for symptomatic control. The limited armamentarium available to treat most of the NPSs is the result of a variety of factors, including but not limited to challenges in attaining adequately powered studies, defining trial eligibility and utilizing appropriate outcome measures. This chapter summarizes key issues pertaining to the design and implementation of clinical trials aimed at identifying effective treatments for NPSs in PD.

Summary of available evidence to date

A comprehensive review of all the options available to treat NPS is beyond the scope of this chapter and is discussed elsewhere in this book (see Chapters 11–13). What follows is a brief summary focusing either on agents for which there is robust evidence of benefit or agents that hold promise.

Mild cognitive impairment and dementia

Dementia is a common problem in PD, occurring in up to 80% of patients [1]. In PD, cognitive decline is a significant contributor to functional impairment and is associated with reduced quality of life and increased caregiver burden. The pathophysiology of PD dementia (PDD) is complex and likely multifactorial. While PDD is considered one of the nondopaminergic, long-term complications of PD [2], some studies have shown that striatal dopamine function correlates with executive function and may be most important in the initial stages of cognitive decline [1]. However, it is the degeneration of cholinergic neurons, present early in PD [1], that has been the biological basis for the majority of clinical trials for dementia to date.

Of the acetylcholinesterase inhibitors studied in PD, only rivastigmine is of demonstrated benefit, thus leading to its approval by the US Food and Drug Administration (FDA) for the treatment of PDD. The main trial to study rivastigmine in PDD [3] was a multicenter, randomized (2:1) parallel-group, double-blinded, placebo-controlled trial of 24 weeks' duration, with 362 individuals with PDD in the treatment arm, and 172 in the placebo arm. Parkinson's disease dementia was diagnosed based on the *Diagnostic and Statistical Manual of Mental Disorders, 4th Edn, Text Revision* (DSM-IV-TR; now DSM-V) criteria for PDD [4]. Primary endpoints were the Alzheimer's Disease Assessment Scale–Cognitive (ADAS-Cog) subscale and the Alzheimer's Disease Co-operative Study-Clinical, Global Impression of Change (ADCS-CGIC) scale. A mean (±standard deviation) improvement of 2.1 (± 8.2) on the ADAS-Cog subscale occurred in the treatment group, whereas the placebo group showed a worsening of 0.7 (± 7.5) points. Rivastigmine also

Parkinson's Disease: Current and Future Therapeutics and Clinical Trials, ed. Gálvez-Jiménez et al. Published by Cambridge University Press. © Cambridge University Press 2016.

provided significant benefits over placebo with respect to all secondary efficacy variables. Premature study discontinuation occurred in 131 patients, mostly due to adverse events (27.3% in treatment group and 17.1% in placebo group). Adverse events leading to withdrawal from the study were nausea and vomiting. Of note, while significant differences in motor function were not observed between the treatment and placebo arm, tremor was severe enough to cause withdrawal from the study in 1.7% of patients in the rivastigmine group (and none of the patients in the placebo group). A post-hoc analysis demonstrated that those in the rivastigmine group had significantly better outcomes in basic and high-level-function activities of daily living (ADLs) compared with the placebo group at 24 weeks [5]. Based on the study by Emre et al. [3], in the Movement Disorders Society (MDS) Evidence-Based Medicine Review of treatments for the nonmotor symptoms of PD [6], rivastigmine was considered efficacious for the treatment of PDD. Other findings from this study, namely improved neuropsychiatric symptoms as measured by the 10-Item Neuropsychiatric Inventory (NPI) and lower rates of hallucination in the rivastigmine arm [3], have prompted consideration of rivastigmine for use in the treatment of psychotic symptoms in PD.

Regarding other acetylcholinesterase inhibitors, evidence for donepezil is inconclusive; while several randomized trials for donepezil in PD have been conducted [7–9], the majority had small sample sizes (fewer than 20 per arm). In the largest trial of donepezil to date for treatment of cognition in PDD (diagnosed based on DSM-IV criteria) [10], participants were randomized 1:1:1 to double-blinded treatment with donepezil 5 mg, donepezil 10 mg or placebo. There were two co-primary efficacy end points: (i) change from baseline to week 24 in total score for the ADAS-Cog; and (ii) overall change score at week 24 for the Clinician's Interview Based Impression of Change with caregiver/study partner input (CIBIC). Secondary endpoints included measures of specific cognitive domains and the NPI. Overall, 550 patients from 108 sites across 13 countries were randomized. The mean change from baseline to week 24 in the ADAS-Cog was not significant for donepezil in the intent-to-treat population by the predefined statistical model. Post-hoc ADAS-Cog analysis, removing the treatment-by-country interaction term from the model, revealed a significant, dose-dependent benefit with donepezil (difference from placebo −2.08, $P = 0.002$ for 5 mg; −3.31, $P < 0.001$, for 10 mg). Significantly better CIBIC scores compared with placebo occurred in the 10 mg group (3.7 vs 3.9, $P = 0.113$, for 5 mg; 3.6 vs 3.9, $P = 0.040$, for 10 mg). Significant benefits in secondary endpoints of cognition were present, but there was no significant benefit in ADLs. In terms of adverse events, there was a higher incidence of cholinergic-related events in the donepezil-treated groups (e.g. nausea, vomiting and diarrhea) and higher discontinuation rates related to adverse events. There were higher rates of worsening parkinsonism in the donepezil-treated patients, but the difference was not significant, without apparent dose dependency and no impact on the Unified Parkinson's Disease Rating Scale (UPDRS) motor scale score.

The rationale for examining the utility of N-methyl-D-aspartate (NMDA) receptor antagonists such as memantine in PDD stems from in vitro and animal data suggesting that this class of agents may be neuroprotective, perhaps by interfering with glutamate-mediated excitotoxity [11], as well as the relative success of this agent in the treatment of Alzheimer's disease [12]. However, evidence for memantine was felt to be insufficient in the MDS Evidence-Based Medicine Review [6], particularly in light of the conflicting evidence found in the randomized control trials (RCTs) investigating it [13, 14]. A possible benefit of memantine on psychiatric symptoms (as assessed by the NPI) has been suggested in subgroup analyses of patients with dementia with Lewy bodies [14] and warrants further consideration.

In terms of other pharmacological classes that may be of utility in PDD, in a controlled study [15], the selective norepinephrine reuptake inhibitor atomoxetine, while not efficacious for the treatment of clinically significant depressive symptoms, was associated with improvements in global cognitive performance and daytime sleepiness. The biological plausibility of this is based on several lines of evidence. There is a putative role of norepinephrine in cognition [16], particularly in relation to prefrontal cortex functioning, including attention and executive abilities. The latter likely accounts in large part for the efficacy of atomexetine for attention-deficit disorder (an FDA-approved indication). Early involvement of the brainstem noradrenergic nucleus (the locus coeruleus) in PD is well established [17]. Thus, this agent may be of utility for treating cognitive dysfunction, particularly of the frontal/executive type [17], in PD, and examination of this question in a RCT may be warranted.

Approximately 25–30% of nondemented PD patients have mild cognitive impairment (PD-MCI), and accumulating evidence suggests that a substantial subset of PD-MCI patients go on to develop PDD [18]. At the time of writing, no large randomized trials for treatment of PD-MCI have been published, although an exploratory, 12-week placebo-controlled RCT showed benefits of the monoamine oxidase B (MAO-B) inhibitor rasagiline on attention and executive functions [19]. There is an ongoing trial examining the impact of rasagiline on PD-MCI [20]. Results of an open-label trial of atomoxetine in 12 nondemented PD patients with executive dysfunction [21] suggest that consideration for study of this drug for the treatment of nonamnestic MCI in PD is warranted as well.

Regarding nonpharmacological therapies, preliminary data suggest that cognitive training or rehabilitation can improve executive abilities [22] and speed of processing [23] in nondemented patients, but it remains unknown whether there are any acute or long-term cognitive benefits to treating PD-MCI patients with these modalities.

Depression

Depression is common in PD patients and has significant consequences including functional disability, higher rates of caregiver stress, decreased quality of life and poorer outcomes [24]. Several RCTs for depression in PD have been published. Selective serotonin reuptake inhibitors (SSRIs) and bupropion are commonly used clinically. While bupropion is used to treat depression in PD and has the advantage of minimal adverse sexual side effects and good tolerability from a motor standpoint, evidence for its efficacy is lacking. On the other hand, several RCTs for SSRIs in PD depression have been conducted, although the size of the trials and other limitations did not provide sufficient evidence for conclusions to be drawn in the last MDS Evidence-Based Medicine Review [6], and an early meta-analysis suggested that the benefit of SSRI treatment is less in PD than in non-PD depression [25]. However, since that time, the RCT Study of Antidepressants in Parkinson's Disease (SAD-PD) has provided class I evidence for use of one SSRI, paroxetine, and the serotonin and norepinephrine reuptake inhibitor venlafaxine (extended release), in the treatment of depression in PD [26]. This was a 12-week, multicenter study in which 115 PD patients were randomized; of note, the sample size was only half of the projected enrollment. The final analyses included 42, 34 and 39 patients in the paroxetine, extended-release venlafaxine and placebo groups. The mean (± standard deviation) paroxetine dosage at week 12 was 24 ± 11 mg/day, and that of extended-release venlafaxine was 121 ± 75 mg/day. Depression was diagnosed based on DSM-IV criteria, and subsyndromal depression wasbased on the 17-item Hamilton Depression Rating Scale (HDRS-17) score, which was also the primary outcome measure. Secondary outcomes included the Montgomery–Åsberg Depression Rating Scale (MADRS), Beck Depression Inventory (BDI-II), Geriatric Depression Scale (GDS) and NIMH Clinical Global Impression (CGI) scores. Significant improvements in HRDS-17 scores were noted in the paroxetine and venlafaxine group (–13.0 and –11.0 points difference between baseline and 12 weeks, respectively) compared with the placebo group (–6.0 points). Significant beneficial effects of paroxetine and venlafaxine were also noted for the secondary depression outcomes examined. While over 85% of patients in each group reported adverse events, there were no significant differences in overall frequency of adverse events between groups. Insomnia was less common in the paroxetine group compared with the venlafaxine group. Venlafaxine was associated with an 8.5 mmHg increase in seated systolic blood pressure, and paroxetine with a 1.3 kg increase in weight. Importantly, significant differences in UPDRS motor scores were not different between the treatment arms and placebo.

While tricyclic antidepressants (TCAs) are often avoided in older adults because of concerns about side effects (particularly related to anticholinergic activity), several RCTs have investigated the utility of TCAs in PD depression, and both nortriptyline and desipramine were considered likely efficacious in the MDS Evidence-Based Medicine Review [6]. Menza et al. [27] compared nortriptyline with paroxetine in a double-blinded, randomized, placebo-controlled trial. Eighteen PD patients with depression or dysthymia as diagnosed by DSM-IV criteria received paroxetine, 17 received nortriptyline and 17 received placebo. The primary endpoint was the HDRS-17 score. Overall, 65% of patients completed the study, with no between-group differences in discontinuation rates. Nortriptyline was superior to placebo regarding change in HDRS-17 score, while paroxetine was not. Both medications were well tolerated, with no differences in study discontinuation rates and cognitive outcomes. However, paroxetine, but not nortriptyline, was associated with a higher average number of side effects than placebo, including fatigue and orthostatic hypotension.

In another RCT comparing citalopram and desipramine in 48 PD patients [28], the study completion rate was 94%. The primary endpoint was MADRS scores, and both treatment arms showed significant improvement in overall MADRS scores compared with placebo. Adverse events were twice as common in the desipramine group.

Among other considerations, the occurrence of "off"-time depressive and other NPSs as manifestations of the PD "off" period prompted investigation of dopamine agonists for the treatment of depression in PD, and efficacy has been demonstrated. In a 12-week, randomized, placebo-controlled study of pramipexole [29], the 139 patients randomized to the pramipexole group who were included in the final analysis had significant improvements in BDI (the primary endpoint) and UPDRS scores compared with the 148 in the placebo group. Importantly, secondary analyses (i.e. path analysis) showed that approximately 80% of the treatment effect was due to the effect of pramipexole on depressive symptoms rather than on motor symptoms. Adverse events were not significantly more common in the treatment group. Pramipexole was also compared with sertraline in a 14-week, randomized trial using the HDRS-17 as the primary endpoint, with similar results [30]. While there are some data to suggest that ropinirole improves depression in PD [31], no RCTs with depression as a primary endpoint have been conducted for this agent, and there are insufficient data to ascertain whether the antidepressant effect of dopamine agonists in PD is a class effect or is specific to pramipexole.

Nonselective monoamine oxidase inhibitors (MAOIs) were previously widely used for treatment of depression in the general population, but their used decreased dramatically as safer drugs were developed. Subsequently, rasagiline, a selective MAOI that specifically targets the B-isoform, was developed and is widely used in PD as an adjunct to levodopa (L-DOPA) therapy [32]. Preliminary data suggest that rasagiline may have antidepressant effects that are independent of its motor benefit [33]. The ADAGIO (Attenuation of Disease Progression with Azilect Given Once-daily) study [34] was a double-blind, placebo-controlled, delayed-start trial of rasagiline in de novo PD. In an analysis of patients taking an antidepressant any time during the 36-week phase 1, in which patients were randomized to rasagiline (1 or 2 mg/day) or placebo, NPSs were assessed by the MDS-UPDRS-experiences of daily living (EDLs), original UPDRS and Parkinson's Fatigue Scale (PFS). Sixteen percent (191/1174) of patients were treated with antidepressants, approximately 75% with an SSRI, during phase 1. The EDL depression and cognition item scores improved significantly in the rasagiline group compared with the placebo group ($P = 0.045$ and $P = 0.002$, respectively). The PFS ($P < 0.001$) and daytime sleepiness ($P = 0.006$) scores also improved significantly in the rasagiline group compared with placebo. The effect on depression remained significant after controlling for improvement in motor symptoms ($P = 0.009$). There were no serious adverse events in the combined rasagiline and antidepressant group suggestive of serotonin syndrome. Thus, rasagiline augmentation of antidepressant treatment was associated with improvement in mood, cognition, fatigue and daytime sleepiness in de novo PD. These findings suggest a role for the dopamine system in clinically significant NPSs in early PD (D. Weintraub, unpublished data).

Nonpharmacological treatments for depression, including cognitive behavioral therapy (CBT), may be as efficacious and preferred by patients [35]. Given the relative burden of frequent in-person visits, studies on telephone- and web-based administration of CBT are also being pursued. Another nonpharmacological interventions for depression for which sufficient data are lacking but which is a promising avenue of active investigation is transcranial magnetic stimulation [6]. Regarding the effects of deep-brain stimulation (DBS) on depression in PD, in a randomized trial examining the effects of subthalamic nucleus (STN)- versus globus pallidus interna (GPi)-DBS, the primary outcome was motor improvement, but the BDI was examined as a secondary outcome. The BDI scores [36] improved by 0.6 points and increased by 1.3 points in the GPi and STN arms ($P = 0.02$). This has led some to wonder whether the NPS outcomes might be better with GPi versus STN lead placement for DBS surgery.

Psychosis

Psychosis is uncommon in early and untreated PD but may occur in up to as many as 60% of patients over the disease course [37]. It is particularly associated with older age and dementia [37]. As with other NPSs, psychosis in PD causes significant caregiver burden and increases the probability of nursing home admission [38, 39]. The most common manifestations are visual hallucinations, but other symptoms include illusions, hallucinations in other sensory modalities and delusions. The pathophysiology of psychosis in

PD is complex and multifactorial, but a contribution from both the underlying neurodegenerative disease process as well as exogenous dopaminergic medication exposure is probable. To this end, the majority of treatment trials for PD psychosis have targeted the dopaminergic system alone or in combination with the serotonergic system, although agents targeted selectively at the serotonergic system are being investigated as well, as detailed below.

The strongest evidence for treatment of psychosis in PD exists for clozapine, which has activity at both dopaminergic and serotonergic receptors. The PSYCLOPS (PSychosis and CLOzapine in PD Study) [40] was a 4-week, placebo-controlled, double-blinded RCT that examined clozapine in 60 PD patients. Primary outcome measures were the CGI for psychosis and the UPDRS for parkinsonism; the Brief Psychiatric Rating Scale (BPRS) and Scale for the Assessment of Positive Symptoms (SAPS) were also examined. In total, 54 participants completed the trial. At a mean dose of 24.7 mg/day for those in the clozapine group resulted in significantly more improvement in CGI, BPRS and SAPS scores. There was no significant worsening of motor symptoms in either group and, in fact, a significant beneficial effect on tremor was noted in the clozapine group. In one patient, clozapine was discontinued due to leucopenia. A 4 beats/min increase in heart rate and a 0.7 kg increase in weight were noted in the clozapine group, but otherwise side effects and adverse events were no different between the groups. Based on the results of the PSYCLOPS and two reports based on 4-week, open-label extensions of it, the MDS Evidence-Based Medicine Review [6] determined that clozapine is efficacious for the treatment of psychosis in PD. On the other hand, the evidence for quetiapine was considered insufficient based on the presence of conflicting data and several methodological concerns of the studies published, including small sample sizes and low-quality ratings [6]. Despite this, quetiapine is the most widely used antipsychotic in PD, prescribed in over two-thirds of cases [41], whereas clozapine accounts for less than 2% of prescriptions, likely due to the burden of blood monitoring that is required [41]. Of note, regarding other atypical antipsychotics, based on available evidence, olanzapine was deemed unlikely to be efficacious [6] and is thus recommended against. An open-label study [42] of aripiprazole in 14 PD patients with psychosis has raised concerns that the motor side effects of this drug may make it unsuitable for use in PD as well.

Given the significant safety concerns regarding the use of atypical antipsychotics in PD patients, including worsening of parkinsonism and increased mortality [43], alternative treatments are clearly needed. A promising agent in this regard is the selective serotonin 5-HT2A inverse agonist pimavanserin [44]. In a 6-week, placebo-controlled RCT of pimavanserin, the primary outcome was change in the total Parkinson's Disease-adapted Scale for Assessment of Positive Symptoms (SAPS-PD) score from baseline to day 43. Importantly, the assessment was conducted by a centralized blinded rater. In an attempt to minimize confounding by the placebo response, after screening and before baseline, participants entered a 2-week lead-in period during which nonpharmacological brief psychosocial therapy adapted for PD was administered. Overall, 199 patients were randomized and 185 were included in the final analysis. The 95 randomized to the treatment arm had significant improvements in SAPS-PD scores compared with the 90 in the placebo arm (difference of −3.06). Significant improvements in CGI and caregiver burden were also seen. Of note, an improvement in nighttime sleep (a secondary outcome assessed by the Scale for Outcomes of Parkinson's disease [SCOPA]-sleep scale), without worsening in daytime sleepiness, was found. No significant differences in motor function were observed between the treatment groups. Serious adverse events occurred in 11% of the pimavanserin arm and in 4% of the placebo arm.

As mentioned above, consideration of rivastigmine for use in the treatment of psychotic symptoms in PD has been prompted by lower rates of hallucinations among patients randomized to a rivastigmine treatment arm in a trial of that agent for treatment of PDD [3].

Others

Impulse control disorders, including compulsive gambling, buying, sexual behavior and eating, occur in 13.6% of patients with PD [45], and are the result of medications (and not the underlying disease itself) [46]. Thus, while a reduction in the dosage or cessation of the inciting medication, usually a dopamine agonist, is the cornerstone of therapy for ICDs, given the symptomatic benefits seen from dopaminergic medications, pharmacologic treatments of ICDs have been pursued. A 17-week, double-blind, placebo-controlled, crossover RCT of amantadine was considered by the MDS Evidence-Based Medicine Review [6] to provide insufficient evidence based on the small sample size (*n* = 17, with five patients dropping out) and other methodological issues. The other pharmacological agent being investigated in an RCT for treatment of ICDs in PD is naltrexone. In this study, PD patients (*n* = 50) with an ICD were enrolled in an 8-week, randomized (1:1), double-blinded, placebo-controlled study of naltrexone 50–100 mg/day (flexible dosing). The primary outcome measure was remission based on the Clinical Global Impression of Change (CGIC) score, and the secondary outcome was change in symptom severity using the Questionnaire for Impulsive–Compulsive Disorders in Parkinson's Disease – Rating Scale (QUIP-RS) ICD score. Forty-five patients (90%) completed the study. There was no significant between-group difference in remission status (odds ratio = 1.6, 95% confidence interval [CI] = 0.5–5.2, Wald χ^2 [d.f.] = 0.5 [1], P = 0.5), but naltrexone treatment led to a significantly greater decrease in QUIP-RS ICD score over time compared with placebo (regression coefficient for interaction term in linear mixed-effects model = –0.9, F [d.f.] = 4.3 [1.49], P = 0.04). Cohen's effect size (d = 0.61) indicated a medium to large treatment effect on the QUIP-RS ICD score (D. Weintraub, unpublished data). An RCT of CBT for impulse control behaviors in PD [47] shows the promise of this modality, and larger trials are needed.

Anxiety is common in PD, occurring in approximately 40% of patients. While there are no RCTs for treatment of anxiety in PD, anxiety was a secondary outcome in four RCTs examining treatments for depression in PD (two of the antidepressants discussed above [27, 28], one of atomoxetine [15] and one of CBT [35]). A pooled analysis of these trials [48] showed that the pooled effect size for antidepressants on anxiety in PD was large (d = 1.13) but nonsignificant (95% CI = –0.67 to 2.94). Subgroup analyses were conducted, and a large and significant effect size of TCAs (d = 1.40, 95% CI = 0.09–2.70) but not SSRIs (d = 0.85, 95% CI = –0.40 to 2.09) was found. Overall, TCAs, atomoxetine and CBT all demonstrated a significant and large secondary effect on anxiety outcomes [48].

Apathy is also a common NPS, with approximately 40% of patients affected. In a 6-month, double-blinded, placebo-controlled RCT [49], the effect of rivastigmine on apathy in 30 nondemented, nondepressed patients with PD was assessed. The primary end point was change in the Lille Apathy Rating Scale (LARS), and measures of functional impact and quality of life were secondary endpoints. There was a significant reduction in apathy in the treatment group; 37% of the patients in the rivastigmine group and 83% of the patients in the placebo group were classified as apathetic at 6 months. Significant improvements in functional ability (but not quality of life) were also noted. This was independent of effects of rivastigmine on cognition. Regarding other classes of drugs that are of promise in the treatment of apathy in PD, the selective D2/D3 agonist piribedil has also been preliminarily investigated in a small, placebo-controlled, randomized study [50] of PD patients with apathy following withdrawal of dopamine agonist medications post-DBS and shows promise.

Lessons and challenges from clinical trials for neuropsychiatric manifestations in Parkinson's disease

A summary of the key challenges and possible solutions in clinical trials for NPSs in PD is shown in Table 30.1.

Patient population

Increasingly, studies are using clinical characteristics, biomarkers or genetic profiles to subtype patients who may have a differential response to a specific treatment, potentially leading to an increased likelihood of demonstrating an active-treatment effect. This attempt to homogenize the study population in some way, and minimize the variability in response, has been applied in studies of psychiatric conditions such as alcohol dependence. In terms of study design, patients can be enrolled simply on the basis of having a particular characteristic, or the study population can be stratified on that characteristic. A potential example of this for NPSs in PD relates to the finding from secondary analyses that patients in the PDD rivastigmine placebo-controlled study [3] who experience psychosis at baseline had a more robust response to rivastigmine treatment compared with patients without psychosis. Thus, future cognitive studies in PDD patients might consider focusing the study population on those patients with psychosis in addition to having PDD, or stratifying the study population on the basis of having psychosis.

Placebo response

While placebo-controlled trials are considered the "gold standard" of trial design, large placebo effects, as has been seen in trials for several NPSs including depression [25] and psychosis [51], may make it more difficult to detect a significant benefit for the drug being investigated. This is an issue that affects psychiatric

Table 30.1 Key challenges and possible solutions in clinical trials for neuropsychiatric symptoms (NPSs) in Parkinson's disease (PD)

Challenges	Potential solutions
Placebo effect masking a clinically significant benefit	Better understanding of placebo response for different NPSs in PD
Achieving sample size necessary for adequately powered study	Consideration of run-in period during which placebo effect is induced "up front" (further study of this is required as well)
Optimizing trial duration (balance between cost and accounting for natural history of NPSs in question)	Centralized ratings
Maximizing participant retention throughout the study	Multicenter collaboration to increase sample sizes and power of clinical trials
Site heterogeneity in research infrastructure, resources and expertise for specific NPSs	Development of regional subspecialty centers for patient care and clinical research
Overlap of NPSs in PD	Using biomarkers to enrich samples and decrease heterogeneity in study populations
Confounding by motor manifestations and "on"/"off" fluctuations	Incorporation of biomarkers (such as biofluid or imaging biomarkers) as outcome measures to give biological plausibility to clinical outcomes
Generic diagnostic criteria and rating scales may not account for disease-specific considerations	Development and validation of PD-specific diagnostic criteria for use as inclusion criteria
	Development and validation of PD-specific rating scales for use as outcome measures
	Assessment of NPSs in PD "on" and "off" states for studies focused on nonmotor fluctuations

treatment studies in the general population too, and increasingly so [52]. To address this issue, in the trial of pimavanserin for the treatment of psychosis in PD [44], the investigators included a novel 2-week run-in phase of daily psychosocial interaction to reduce the placebo effect encountered during the active-treatment phase. However, details of this intervention were not described, and placebo run-ins have not been shown to clearly diminish the placebo response during the controlled phase of psychiatric studies in the general population. Further study of such approaches to ascertain whether they successfully mitigate the placebo response is essential. This is of particular importance in light of data suggesting that, at least in studies for symptomatic treatment of PD motor symptoms or for neuroprotection, a strong placebo response is present throughout the study (and not just early on) [53].

Sample size considerations

While several clinical trials have been conducted for the treatment of NPSs in PD, the majority, particularly early on, have been marred by small sample sizes and short durations of follow-up. This is in part due to the challenge of recruiting and retaining patients with a neurodegenerative disease, often with cognitive impairment, in an intervention study for psychiatric symptoms. Efforts to increase sample size have in some instances led to potentially deleterious heterogeneity in the sample being studied. An example of this is the inclusion of patients with both dementia with Lewy bodies and PDD in clinical trials of memantine for dementia [54]. While these two disorders share similar pathological findings and may be considered on a spectrum, at least pathologically, key clinical differences exist between them, and including patients with both diseases in the same study certainly introduces heterogeneity that, at a minimum, needs to be accounted for during analyses.

Increased collaboration among sites in the USA and internationally has significantly improved the sample sizes possible for clinical trials in PD. In addition, efforts are underway to increase PD patient participation through initiatives such as the Fox Trial Finder [55]. Identifying sites with the subspecialized expertise (among both clinician investigators and other research staff) required to diagnose and treat NPSs must be balanced against the need for participation of multiple sites. The study by Dubois *et al.* [10] investigating donepezil for treatment of PDD is an important lesson in considerations for site selection in international multicenter studies, as well as in planning analyses such that lower-recruiting sites are weighted differently (statistically). Another example of the detrimental heterogeneity that may be introduced by inclusion of sites from different countries is the success of pimavanserin when study sites were limited to one country [44], as opposed to inclusion of international sites in prior trials of this agent that had failed. Other factors likely account for the success of the pimavanserin trial as well, such as centralized ratings for key outcome measures. Central ratings may minimize the need for site-specific subspecialty expertise. On the other hand, for patient care purposes, identifying regional subspecialty centers to which patients can be referred should subspecialty care be needed but not be offered at sites in their immediate vicinity may be of benefit (such a model is used for the provision of movement disorders services at the six regional Parkinson's Disease Research, Education and Clinical Centers [PADRECCS] in the US Department of Veterans Affairs health care system).

As our understanding of the pathophysiology of NPSs evolves, treatments become more targeted and biomarkers are developed, sample size requirements may decrease accordingly. For example, if biomarkers emerge that increase our ability to predict which PD-MCI patients are at high risk of conversion to PDD, identification of such patients would be expected to yield enriched samples that increase the ability to detect clinically meaningful benefits from the therapeutic intervention in question.

Trial duration

The duration of trials for NPSs must take into consideration the natural history of these symptoms in PD. For example, the annual rate of conversion from MCI to PDD needs to be determined and then accounted for in determining the necessary duration of a trial aimed at demonstrating the benefit of an intervention to reduce this risk. Other considerations include the rapidity with which the intervention in question exerts its effects. For example, trial durations must account for antidepressants, such as SSRIs, that may require 8–12 weeks to have full effects. As mentioned above, biomarkers, by enriching the population being studied, may also shorten the trial duration required to detect a meaningful effect.

Diagnostic criteria

Traditionally, the diagnostic criteria used for NPS studies have used DSM-IV-TR (now DSM-5) criteria [4]. This presents a problem for various reasons. Most of these criteria stipulate absence of an underlying medical or neurological condition that accounts for a primary neuropsychiatric disorder. In addition, these criteria do not factor in the overlap of the various NPSs that can occur in PD, such as anxiety and depression [56]. Confounding or compounding by motor symptoms are also considerations. Parkinson's disease-specific diagnostic criteria are thus essential.

The proposition of new or revised diagnostic criteria for PDD [1, 57], PD-MCI [58], depression [24], apathy [59, 60], psychosis [38] and various ICDs [61] and related disorders (such as dopamine dysregulation syndrome [62]) is a positive step in this direction. However, validation of these diagnostic criteria and their ongoing revision as necessary [63] is also needed, as is development of such criteria for other NPSs. Future diagnostic criteria may include biomarkers as supportive or perhaps even core criteria, as has been proposed for Alzheimer's disease. Biomarkers may also contribute to identification of patients with subtypes of NPs that will benefit from specific targeted therapies to be studied in clinical trials. Thus, future entry criteria into clinical trials for NPSs may include (formalized and validated) diagnostic criteria as well as biomarker findings.

Outcome measures

In PD, outcome measures of importance may include those that take into consideration symptom severity, their functional impact, quality of life and caregiver burden.

Questionnaire- or examination-based rating scales have been the mainstays of primary outcomes in NPS clinical trials. Rating scales may include those administered to the patient, physician or caregiver, and some are self-completed, which is contingent on insight into the problem. Depending on the NPS and the intervention in question, one of these or perhaps a combination or even composite of all three may be of benefit as a primary outcome. For example, in the rivastigmine trial for treatment of PDD [3], there were two primary endpoints, a rating scale to assess severity of symptoms (the ADAS-Cog, as required by the FDA), and another (ADCS-CGIC), a clinical global impression, as a more overarching measure geared toward function as well. Of note, co-primary outcomes have implications for sample size. It is possible that composite measures may be most sensitive to *clinically meaningful* benefits or adverse effects. Composite endpoints have the added advantage of possibly increasing the event rate and thus the statistical power of the study. However, composite endpoints can be misleading. In order for a composite endpoint to be meaningful, its constituents must all be of relatively equal importance, and the magnitude of effect must not differ markedly across components.

In general, rating scales of NPSs need to account for: (i) the overlap of NPSs (for example, the overlap of apathy and depression); (ii) the impact of motor symptoms; and (iii) the impact of bradyphrenia (particularly in relation to timed cognitive tasks). Ideally, assessments that account for "on–off" phenomena (such as administration of rating scales in both the "on" and "off" state) should occur. In trials assessing specific NPSs, secondary measures of other NPSs that are often comorbid may be of benefit in identifying additional uses of the agent under study, and for hypothesis generation. An example of this was the benefit noted of pimavanserin on nighttime sleep [44].

In RCTs, the subjective nature of these scales is mitigated to some extent by blinding. Central rating of NPSs, such as occurred in one of the trials of pimavanserin for psychosis in PD [44], may help minimize administration and response bias, among other types of bias (which tend to increase the standard deviations of ratings and decrease power). The future is likely to hold more objective measures, such as structural and functional imaging and biofluid biomarkers, for use in clinical trials of NPSs.

Many of the commonly used patient-administered scales were not developed specifically for PD but have been validated against clinician rating or some other disease measure. A critical review of rating scales for several of the NPSs in PD has been carried out [64–67]. Since the time the last of these were conducted, several PD-specific scales have been developed including for psychosis [68] and ICDs [61]. A PD-specific anxiety rating scale is also under development [69]. Where recommended scales are available, they should be used, and for the NPSs for which optimal rating scales are deficient, development of scales is needed.

The standard RCT is an efficacy study, but the primary outcome measures using this study design do not account for the higher rates of adverse events observed in the active-treatment group, an issue of particular significance in studies of older patients or those with neurodegenerative diseases. The higher discontinuation rates observed in the active-treatment arms of RCTs [3] suggest that consideration of time to treatment discontinuation as a primary outcome may be warranted, as was utilized in a trial of antipsychotics for the treatment of psychosis or agitation in AD (the CATIE-AD [Clinical Antipsychotic Trials of Intervention Effectiveness – Alzheimer's Disease] trial [68, 70]). In this study, even though antipsychotics were superior to placebo in treating symptoms of psychosis or agitation, this effect was negated by the earlier time to discontinuation in the active-treatment group due to adverse events.

Conclusions

Neuropsychiatric manifestations in PD are common and contribute significantly to morbidity and caregiver burden. In addition, with the expected increase in the prevalence of PD in the future will come increased numbers of patients with several of the NPSs that increase with age, including depression, psychosis and cognitive impairment. For all these reasons, identification of efficacious treatments for NPSs is essential. Several challenges exist in the designing of trials to study treatments for NPSs. Future goals in this regard may include: (i) better understanding of the placebo response in trials of NPSs and efforts to minimize this; (ii) planning adequately powered studies and utilizing multicenter studies where feasible to achieve sufficient sample sizes; (iii) implementing trial durations that take into consideration the natural history of the disease, particularly in trials aimed at disease modification; (iv) continuing to define diagnostic criteria for each of the NPSs and validating these criteria; and (v) developing valid and clinically meaningful measures of psychiatric symptoms, including biomarkers to diagnose and measure severity and response, which may allow for smaller sample sizes and be of greater clinical significance.

References

1. Emre M, Aarsland D, Brown R, et al. Clinical diagnostic criteria for dementia associated with Parkinson's disease. *Mov Disord* 2007; **22**: 1689–707; quiz 1837.

2. Kehagia AA, Barker RA, Robbins TW. Cognitive impairment in Parkinson's disease: the dual syndrome hypothesis. *Neurodegener Dis* 2013; **11**: 79–92.

3. Emre M, Aarsland D, Albanese A, et al. Rivastigmine for dementia associated with Parkinson's disease. *N Engl J Med* 2004; **351**: 2509–18.

4. American Psychiatric Association. *Diagnostic and Statistical Manual of Mental Disorders*, 5th edn. Arlington, VA: American Psychiatric Publishing, 2013.

5. Olin JT, Aarsland D, Meng X. Rivastigmine in the treatment of dementia associated with Parkinson's disease: effects on activities of daily living. *Dement Geriatr Cogn Disord* 2010; **29**: 510–15.

6. Seppi K, Weintraub D, Coelho M, et al. The Movement Disorder Society Evidence-Based Medicine Review Update: treatments for the non-motor symptoms of Parkinson's disease. *Mov Disord* 2011; **26** (Suppl. 3): S42–80.

7. Leroi I, Brandt J, Reich SG, et al. Randomized placebo-controlled trial of donepezil in cognitive impairment in Parkinson's disease. *Int J Geriatr Psychiatry* 2004; **19**: 1–8.

8. Ravina B, Putt M, Siderowf A, et al. Donepezil for dementia in Parkinson's disease: a randomised, double

blind, placebo controlled, crossover study. *J Neurol Neurosurg Psychiatry* 2005; **76**: 934–9.

9. Aarsland D, Laake K, Larsen JP, Janvin C. Donepezil for cognitive impairment in Parkinson's disease: a randomised controlled study. *J Neurol Neurosurg Psychiatry* 2002; **72**: 708–12.

10. Dubois B, Tolosa E, Katzenschlager R, et al. Donepezil in Parkinson's disease dementia: a randomized, double-blind efficacy and safety study. *Mov Disord* 2012; **27**: 1230–8.

11. Lipton SA, Rosenberg PA. Excitatory amino acids as a final common pathway for neurologic disorders. *N Engl J Med* 1994; **330**: 613–22.

12. McShane R, Areosa Sastre A, Minakaran N. Memantine for dementia. *Cochrane Database Syst Rev* 2006; (2): CD003154.

13. Leroi I, Overshott R, Byrne EJ, Daniel E, Burns A. Randomized controlled trial of memantine in dementia associated with Parkinson's disease. *Mov Disord* 2009; **24**: 1217–21.

14. Emre M, Tsolaki M, Bonuccelli U, et al. Memantine for patients with Parkinson's disease dementia or dementia with Lewy bodies: a randomised, double-blind, placebo-controlled trial. *Lancet Neurol* 2010; **9**: 969–77.

15. Weintraub D, Mavandadi S, Mamikonyan E, et al. Atomoxetine for depression and other neuropsychiatric symptoms in Parkinson disease. *Neurology* 2010; **75**: 448–55.

16. Trillo L, Das D, Hsieh W, et al. Ascending monoaminergic systems alterations in Alzheimer's disease. translating basic science into clinical care. *Neurosci Biobehav Rev* 2013; **37**: 1363–79.

17. Del Tredici K, Braak H. Dysfunction of the locus coeruleus-norepinephrine system and related circuitry in Parkinson's disease-related dementia. *J Neurol Neurosurg Psychiatry* 2013; **84**: 774–83.

18. Pedersen KF, Larsen JP, Tysnes OB, Alves G. Prognosis of mild cognitive impairment in early Parkinson disease: the Norwegian ParkWest study. *JAMA Neurol* 2013; **70**: 580–6.

19. Hanagasi HA, Gurvit H, Unsalan P, et al. The effects of rasagiline on cognitive deficits in Parkinson's disease patients without dementia: a randomized, double-blind, placebo-controlled, multicenter study. *Mov Disord* 2011; **26**: 1851–8.

20. US National Institutes of Health. Parallel-group study to assess the effect of rasagiline on cognition in patients with Parkinson's disease. Available at: http://clinicaltrials.gov/show/NCT01723228.

21. Marsh L, Biglan K, Gerstenhaber M, Williams JR. Atomoxetine for the treatment of executive dysfunction in Parkinson's disease: a pilot open-label study. *Mov Disord* 2009; **24**: 277–82.

22. Sammer G, Reuter I, Hullmann K, Kaps M, Vaitl D. Training of executive functions in Parkinson's disease. *J Neurol Sci* 2006; **248**: 115–19.

23. Edwards JD, Hauser RA, O'Connor ML, et al. Randomized trial of cognitive speed of processing training in Parkinson disease. *Neurology* 2013; **81**: 1284–90.

24. Marsh L, McDonald WM, Cummings J, Ravina B, NINDS/NIMH Work Group on Depression and Parkinson's Disease. Provisional diagnostic criteria for depression in Parkinson's disease: report of an NINDS/NIMH Work Group. *Mov Disord* 2006; **21**: 148–58.

25. Weintraub D, Morales KH, Moberg PJ, et al. Antidepressant studies in Parkinson's disease: a review and meta-analysis. *Mov Disord* 2005; **20**: 1161–9.

26. Richard IH, McDermott MP, Kurlan R, et al. A randomized, double-blind, placebo-controlled trial of antidepressants in Parkinson disease. *Neurology* 2012; **78**: 1229–36.

27. Menza M, Dobkin RD, Marin H, et al. A controlled trial of antidepressants in patients with Parkinson disease and depression. *Neurology* 2009; **72**: 886–92.

28. Devos D, Dujardin K, Poirot I, et al. Comparison of desipramine and citalopram treatments for depression in Parkinson's disease: a double-blind, randomized, placebo-controlled study. *Mov Disord* 2008; **23**: 850–7.

29. Barone P, Poewe W, Albrecht S, et al. Pramipexole for the treatment of depressive symptoms in patients with Parkinson's disease: a randomised, double-blind, placebo-controlled trial. *Lancet Neurol* 2010; **9**: 573–80.

30. Barone P, Scarzella L, Marconi R, et al. Pramipexole versus sertraline in the treatment of depression in Parkinson's disease: a national multicenter parallel-group randomized study. *J Neurol* 2006; **253**: 601–7.

31. Pahwa R, Stacy MA, Factor SA, et al. Ropinirole 24-hour prolonged release: randomized, controlled study in advanced Parkinson disease. *Neurology* 2007; **68**: 1108–15.

32. Rascol O, Brooks DJ, Melamed E, et al. Rasagiline as an adjunct to levodopa in patients with Parkinson's disease and motor fluctuations (LARGO, Lasting effect in Adjunct therapy with Rasagiline Given Once daily, study): a randomised, double-blind, parallel-group trial. *Lancet* 2005; **365**: 947–54.

33. Korchounov A, Winter Y, Rossy W. Combined beneficial effect of rasagiline on motor function and depression in de novo PD. *Clin Neuropharmacol* 2012; **35**: 121–4.

34. Olanow CW, Rascol O, Hauser R, et al. A double-blind, delayed-start trial of rasagiline in Parkinson's disease. *N Engl J Med* 2009; **361**: 1268–78.

35. Dobkin RD, Menza M, Allen LA, et al. Cognitive-behavioral therapy for depression in Parkinson's

36. Follett KA, Weaver FM, Stern M, *et al.* Pallidal versus subthalamic deep-brain stimulation for Parkinson's disease. *N Engl J Med* 2010; **362**: 2077–91.
37. Forsaa EB, Larsen JP, Wentzel-Larsen T, *et al.* A 12-year population-based study of psychosis in Parkinson disease. *Arch Neurol* 2010; **67**: 996–1001.
38. Ravina B, Marder K, Fernandez HH, *et al.* Diagnostic criteria for psychosis in Parkinson's disease: report of an NINDS, NIMH work group. *Mov Disord* 2007; **22**: 1061–8.
39. Fenelon G, Alves G. Epidemiology of psychosis in Parkinson's disease. *J Neurol Sci* 2010; **289**: 12–17.
40. Parkinson Study Group. Low-dose clozapine for the treatment of drug-induced psychosis in Parkinson's disease. *N Engl J Med* 1999; **340**: 757–63.
41. Weintraub D, Chen P, Ignacio RV, Mamikonyan E, Kales HC. Patterns and trends in antipsychotic prescribing for Parkinson disease psychosis. *Arch Neurol* 2011; **68**: 899–904.
42. Friedman JH, Berman RM, Goetz CG, *et al.* Open-label flexible-dose pilot study to evaluate the safety and tolerability of aripiprazole in patients with psychosis associated with Parkinson's disease. *Mov Disord* 2006; **21**: 2078–81.
43. Marras C, Gruneir A, Wang X, *et al.* Antipsychotics and mortality in parkinsonism. *Am J Geriatr Psychiatry* 2012; **20**: 149–58.
44. Cummings J, Isaacson S, Mills R, *et al.* Pimavanserin for patients with Parkinson's disease psychosis: a randomised, placebo-controlled phase 3 trial. *Lancet* 2013; **383**: 533–40.
45. Weintraub D, Koester J, Potenza MN, *et al.* Impulse control disorders in Parkinson disease: a cross-sectional study of 3090 patients. *Arch Neurol* 2010; **67**: 589–95.
46. Weintraub D, Papay K, Siderowf A, Parkinson's Progression Markers Initiative. Screening for impulse control symptoms in patients with de novo Parkinson disease: a case–control study. *Neurology* 2013; **80**: 176–80.
47. Okai D, Askey-Jones S, Samuel M, *et al.* Trial of CBT for impulse control behaviors affecting Parkinson patients and their caregivers. *Neurology* 2013; **80**: 792–9.
48. Troeung L, Egan SJ, Gasson N. A meta-analysis of randomised placebo-controlled treatment trials for depression and anxiety in Parkinson's disease. *PLoS One* 2013; **8**: e79510.
49. Devos D, Moreau C, Maltete D, *et al.* Rivastigmine in apathetic but dementia and depression-free patients with Parkinson's disease: a double-blind, placebo-controlled, randomised clinical trial. *J Neurol Neurosurg Psychiatry* 2013; **85**: 668–74.
50. Thobois S, Lhommee E, Klinger H, *et al.* Parkinsonian apathy responds to dopaminergic stimulation of D2/D3 receptors with piribedil. *Brain* 2013; **136**: 1568–77.
51. Friedman JH, Ravina B, Mills R. A multicenter, placebo controlled, double blind trial to examine the safety and efficacy of pimavanserin in the treatment of psychosis in Parkinson's disease. *Neurology* 2010; **74**: A299.
52. Walsh BT, Seidman SN, Sysko R, Gould M. Placebo response in studies of major depression: variable, substantial, and growing. *JAMA* 2002; **287**: 1840–7.
53. Goetz CG, Wuu J, McDermott MP, *et al.* Placebo response in Parkinson's disease: comparisons among 11 trials covering medical and surgical interventions. *Mov Disord* 2008; **23**: 690–9.
54. Aarsland D, Ballard C, Walker Z, *et al.* Memantine in patients with Parkinson's disease dementia or dementia with Lewy bodies: a double-blind, placebo-controlled, multicentre trial. *Lancet Neurol* 2009; **8**: 613–18.
55. Michael J. Fox Foundation. Fox Trial Finder. Available at: https://foxtrialfinder.michaeljfox.org/.
56. Starkstein SE, Dragovic M, Dujardin K, *et al.* Anxiety has specific syndromal profiles in Parkinson disease: a data-driven approach. *Am J Geriatr Psychiatry* 2013; **22**: 1410–17.
57. Dubois B, Burn D, Goetz C, *et al.* Diagnostic procedures for Parkinson's disease dementia: recommendations from the Movement Disorder Society task force. *Mov Disord* 2007; **22**: 2314–24.
58. Litvan I, Aarsland D, Adler CH, *et al.* MDS Task Force on mild cognitive impairment in Parkinson's disease: critical review of PD-MCI. *Mov Disord* 2011; **26**: 1814–24.
59. Robert P, Onyike CU, Leentjens AF, *et al.* Proposed diagnostic criteria for apathy in Alzheimer's disease and other neuropsychiatric disorders. *Eur Psychiatry* 2009; **24**: 98–104.
60. Drijgers RL, Dujardin K, Reijnders JS, Defebvre L, Leentjens AF. Validation of diagnostic criteria for apathy in Parkinson's disease. *Parkinsonism Relat Disord* 2010; **16**: 656–60.
61. Weintraub D, Mamikonyan E, Papay K, *et al.* Questionnaire for impulsive-compulsive disorders in Parkinson's disease – rating scale. *Mov Disord* 2012; **27**: 242–7.
62. Giovannoni G, O'sullivan JD, Turner K, Manson AJ, Lees AJ. Hedonistic homeostatic dysregulation in patients with Parkinson's disease on dopamine replacement therapies. *J Neurol Neurosurg Psychiatry* 2000; **68**: 423–8.
63. Barton B, Grabli D, Bernard B, *et al.* Clinical validation of Movement Disorder Society-recommended diagnostic criteria for Parkinson's disease with dementia. *Mov Disord* 2012; **27**: 248–53.

64. Schrag A, Barone P, Brown RG, *et al*. Depression rating scales in Parkinson's disease: critique and recommendations. *Mov Disord* 2007; **22**: 1077–92.
65. Fernandez HH, Aarsland D, Fenelon G, *et al*. Scales to assess psychosis in Parkinson's disease: Critique and recommendations. *Mov Disord* 2008; **23**: 484–500.
66. Leentjens AF, Dujardin K, Marsh L, *et al*. Apathy and anhedonia rating scales in Parkinson's disease: critique and recommendations. *Mov Disord* 2008; **23**: 2004–14.
67. Leentjens AF, Dujardin K, Marsh L, *et al*. Anxiety rating scales in Parkinson's disease: critique and recommendations. *Mov Disord* 2008; **23**: 2015–25.
68. Voss T, Bahr D, Cummings J, *et al*. Performance of a shortened Scale for Assessment of Positive Symptoms for Parkinson's disease psychosis. *Parkinsonism Relat Disord* 2013; **19**: 295–9.
69. Martinez-Martin P, Rojo-Abuin JM, Dujardin K, *et al*. Designing a new scale to measure anxiety symptoms in Parkinson's disease: item selection based on canonical correlation analysis. *Eur J Neurol* 2013; **20**: 1198–203.
70. Schneider LS, Tariot PN, Dagerman KS, *et al*. Effectiveness of atypical antipsychotic drugs in patients with Alzheimer's disease. *N Engl J Med* 2006; **355**: 1525–38.

Chapter 31

Lessons and challenges of trials for other nonmotor complications of Parkinson's disease

Federico E. Micheli and Carlos Zúñiga-Ramírez

Introduction

Nonmotor symptoms have a high impact on both function and quality of life in patients who suffer from Parkinson's disease (PD). Recent research points to a systemic disease rather than a disorder limited to the central nervous system as previously thought. Understanding the pathophysiology of these symptoms is one of the largest challenges of this disease as we need to learn how to diagnose and treat them adequately. Unfortunately, therapeutic interventions are not as effective as expected (Figure 31.1). Frequently, positive findings from interventions in animal models produce negative results when transferred to humans. This might occur when animal models are not evaluated correctly or when the phenomenological behavior is different in humans. This chapter reviews some of the most important studies reporting how to treat the most common nonmotor symptoms.

Sialorrhea

Drooling is present in 80% of patients with PD and is secondary to disturbances in swallowing the saliva that accumulates in the mouth rather than to increased production.

Marks et al. [1] performed a 4-month, randomized trial in PD patients. Those who had had PD for more than 15 years and presented hypersalivation were divided into three groups for speech/language therapy, therapy with botulinum toxin type A injections in the salivary glands and a control group. In the group treated with speech/language therapy, the basic mechanisms of salivation, functionality and swallowing exercises were explained from a table filled out by the subject about salivation. Separately, this group was given a device that made a sound at a determined time reminding them to swallow. A total of 28 patients were included; however, a significant number withdrew due to a fear of needles in the botulinum toxin group. According to the final results, both the speech/language therapy and the botulinum toxin injections were effective in reducing sialorrhea, the latter being measured by a salivation scale. The strengths of this study are the findings that re-education and a heightened awareness of the mechanics of swallowing are effective in the management of hypersalivation, even though the poor methodological and statistical design of the study, the number of losses of subjects in one of the branches of the study and the small number of recruited participants warrant further studies to corroborate these findings.

Botulinum toxin may reduce saliva production by inhibiting the release of acetylcholine at the parasympathetic autonomic level and at the postganglionic sympathetic level. Mancini et al. [2] performed a 3-month, randomized, double-blinded, placebo-controlled study in 20 subjects (14 with PD and six with multiple-system atrophy [MSA]), which consisted of ultrasound-guided applications of 450 U of botulinum toxin A (Dysport®) or placebo in the parotid and submandibular glands. They were assessed using salivation scales (Drooling Severity Scale, Drooling Frequency Scale and Drooling Score). The patients in both groups had a history of PD of more than 7 years. Improvements in the reduction of sialorrhea lasted 1 month, and there was no significant benefit after 3 months of application. The trial demonstrated the safety and effectiveness of this therapy in the management of drooling. However, the heterogeneity of the

---

Parkinson's Disease: Current and Future Therapeutics and Clinical Trials, ed. Gálvez-Jiménez et al. Published by Cambridge University Press. © Cambridge University Press 2016.

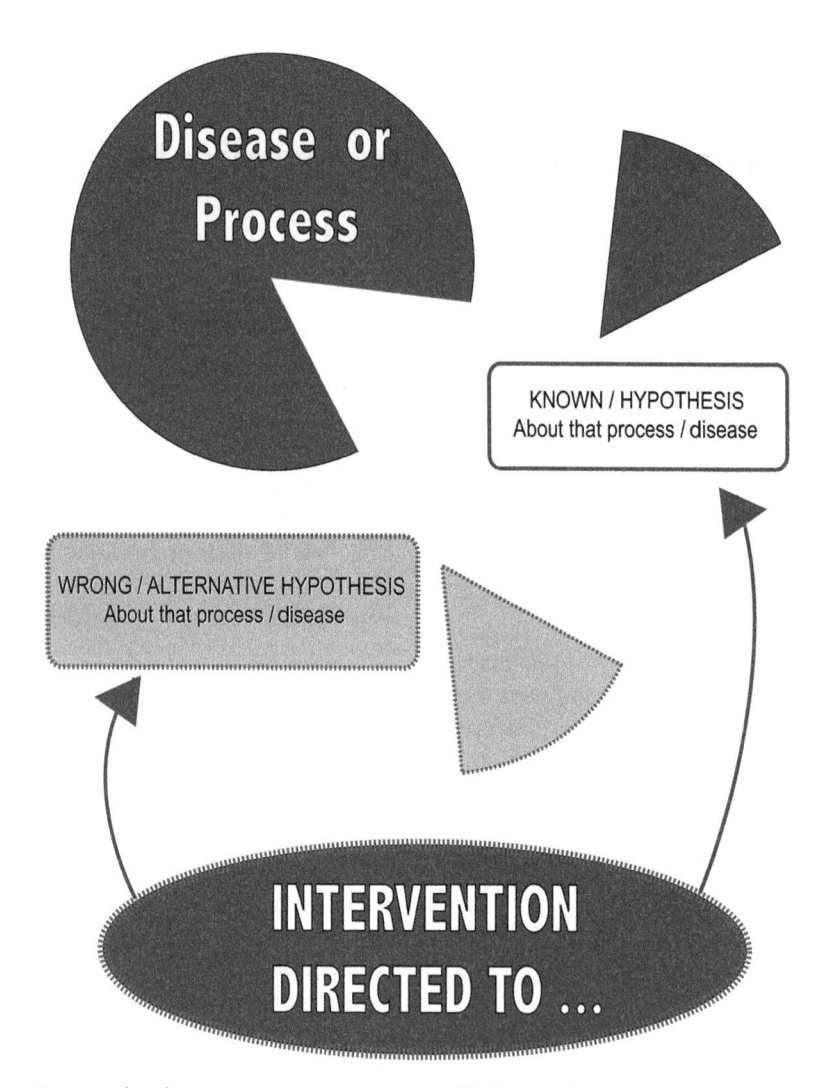

Figure 31.1 Therapeutic approach to the common nonmotor symptoms of Parkinson's disease.

tested groups as well as the small size of the sample could have caused biased results.

Lagalla *et al.* [3] performed a randomized, double-blinded, placebo-controlled study using 50 U of botulinum toxin type A (Botox®) in 32 PD subjects with an average age of 70 and more than 12 years with the disease. Visual analog scales were used to evaluate the severity of hypersalivation. They referenced the frequency of salivation as well as the secondary, frequent familial and social stresses, and the items in the Unified Parkinson's Disease Rating Scale (UPDRS)-II that evaluate sialorrhea and dysphagia. One month after the injections, a significant difference was observed for all scores except for the item for dysphagia on the UPDRS-II. Eighty-eight percent of the subjects tested with botulinum toxin and 31% of those with placebo were satisfied with the results. An objective evaluation of the quantity of saliva, measured by the weight of five oral cotton rolls placed in the mouth for 5 min without swallowing, demonstrated a significant reduction in cases treated with the toxin compared with those treated with placebo. Although the authors confirmed the benefits of the toxin for hypersalivation associated with PD, the length of the study and a more objective analysis of the target should be improved. In addition, the mental or emotional state of the subjects, which directly affects the responses measured from the visual analog scales, was not reported. Lastly, a higher proportion of the subjects with PD at Hoehn and Yahr stage IV were in the group treated with placebo (25 vs 12%, placebo vs botulinum toxin; respectively), which might unbalance the findings, making the toxin seem more effective in the more disabled subjects than it actually is.

Botulinum toxin type B has also been studied in subjects with PD and sialorrhea, as it is believed to have better selectivity and higher potential at the autonomic level. In 2004, Ondo et al. [4] performed a randomized, double-blinded, placebo-controlled study on 16 patients with PD injecting 2500 U of botulinum toxin type B or placebo in the parotid and submandibular glands. Participants were evaluated using salivation scales (Drooling Severity Scale, Drooling Frequency Scale and Drooling Score), visual analog scales and a global impression of change. The subjects had suffered from PD for more than 12 years. At 1 month after the injection, the majority of the subjects treated with botulinum toxin B showed significant improvements on all applied scales. In addition, they were studied using scintigraphy with ^{99m}TC-pertechnetate to evaluate saliva production in the salivary glands. They found a greater than 30% reduction in saliva production in four out of six patients treated with the toxin when compared with two out of seven subjects treated with placebo. The weaknesses of the study were the low number of subjects included and the short evaluation time (1 month), as well as significant differences in age, disease duration and UPDRS-II and –III scores. Botulinum toxin type B was similarly effective to what has been reported for type A for the treatment of hypersalivation.

In 2009, Lagalla et al. [5] published another randomized placebo-controlled study in subjects with PD and moderate to severe sialorrhea. They were treated either with 4000 U of botulinum toxin type B (Neurobloc®) or placebo in the parotid glands. Subjects were evaluated at baseline and 1 month after intervention. They were then questioned monthly by telephone to see if the effects were sustained. The participants were evaluated according to the Frequency and Drooling Severity Scale, by similar scales for familial and social stress, a Global Impression Scale and the UPDRS-II items for dysphagia and sialorrhea. Thirty-six subjects with a PD history of more than 12 years were randomly assigned to either the botulinum toxin or placebo (18 per arm). Subjects treated with botulinum toxin type B showed significant favorable changes in practically all of the scales employed 1 month after treatment. Almost 78% of the participants treated with the toxin expressed a moderate to dramatic improvement with sialorrhea, lasting for 19 weeks. This study employed good methodology and demonstrated the effectiveness of botulinum toxin type B for the management of sialorrhea in patients with PD. The type of evaluations utilized were practically the same as those in the study published by the same team in 2006 with botulinum toxin type A, with visual analog scales and two items from the UPDRS-II. It is possible that the data could have been better analyzed by using Fisher's exact test instead of a χ^2 test and the beneficial results of the toxin evaluated more objectively by using monthly oral cotton roll test measurements weighing the saliva content.

In 2012, Chinnapongse et al. [6] conducted a randomized, double-blinded, placebo-controlled study in 17 centers in the USA on 54 participating subjects who suffered from PD and problematic sialorrhea. The population was divided into four groups: placebo (15 subjects), and botulinum toxin type B (Myobloc®) of 1500 U (14 subjects), 2500 U (12 subjects) and 3500 U (13 subjects). Toxin was applied to the parotid and submandibular glands (250 U per gland, fixed dose for the latter). The principal objective of the study was to evaluate the safety of the drug, although the main scale for evaluating the effect was the Drooling Frequency and Severity Scale (DFSS). After 8 weeks, there was a significant decrease in saliva in all the subjects treated with botulinum toxin type B when compared with placebo and measured by the DFSS. The effect of the toxin lasted for about 100 days. This study showed the effectiveness of botulinum type B for problematic sialorrhea in patients with PD as well as demonstrating the safety and the duration of the effect lasting over 3 months. The challenge for future studies will be to assess whether the effect is sustained throughout the years with continued use.

There have been other interventions evaluated in the management of sialorrhea associated with PD. In 2007, Thomsen et al. [7] evaluated the safety, tolerability and effectiveness of an ipratropium bromide spray through sublingual administration in subjects with PD. Ipratropium bromide is a muscarinic antagonist that does not cross the blood–brain barrier and, when administered locally, has no systemic side effects. This was a randomized, double-blinded, crossover, placebo-controlled study with intervals of drug/placebo application of no less than 4 h during 2 weeks, followed by 1 week of washout and switch to the other intervention. The primary objective was to assess the reduction of saliva production as measured by three to five cotton dental rolls placed in the mouth for 5 min and weighed. Fifteen subjects were evaluated without finding any significant differences between ipratropium bromide and placebo in either the severity or frequency of sialorrhea. It is possible that the small size of the group and the statistical management of categorical variables as if they were continuous could have affected the final results.

Another anticholinergic that has been tested for the treatment of hypersalivation is glycopyrrolate, a drug that does not cross the blood–brain barrier. Arbouw et al. [8] tested this drug through oral administration (1 mg three times daily) in subjects with PD and problematic sialorrhea in a randomized, double-blinded, placebo-controlled, crossover study that lasted for 4 weeks. Twenty-three subjects were randomly chosen and the effect of the drug was measured on a sialorrhea scale of 9 points. Responders demonstrated a 30% reduction on the sialorrhea scale. Almost 40% of the subjects treated with glycopyrrolate responded to the intervention compared with less than 5% of those treated with placebo. The subjects treated with glycopyrrolate showed an average improvement in the sialorrhea score of 0.8 points. Both results were statistically significant. The rate of adverse effects between one intervention and another did not demonstrate any differences. A larger sample size, validation of the employed scale and an exploratory dosage study are some of the future needs for this kind of therapy.

Recently, Lloret et al. [9] used intraoral tropicamide films in subjects with PD. This was a randomized, double-blinded, placebo-controlled study and was divided into four groups: tropicamide at concentrations of 0.3, 1 or 3 mg, and placebo. A visual analog scale was used together with oral cotton rolls placed in the mouth for 5 min and then weighed, to measure the severity of the sialorrhea. The visual analog scale baseline was the primary measurement of effectiveness at 20 min after treatment. The first phase of the study consisted of 12 subjects receiving treatment on different days separated by a 7-day washout. The second phase objectively measured the content of saliva in the mouth at baseline and at 75 min after treatment. Only six subjects completed the analysis at the second phase of the study. The trial demonstrated significant benefits only when utilizing 1 mg of tropicamide and at 120 min after its application. There was no significant difference observed in neither the tropicamide dosage nor placebo or in the volume of saliva obtained in the other different groups. A small sample size plus large time assessments of a short half-life drug could interfere with the outcomes of this study.

Dysphagia

This complication leads to the principal cause of death in patients with PD: aspiration pneumonia. The hyolaryngeal muscular complex with poor contractions of the submentonian muscles is believed to produce this complication.

In 2010, Troche et al. [10] conducted a randomized, double-blinded, placebo-controlled study with 60 subjects with PD and mild to moderate dysphagia. They employed an expiratory muscle strength training (EMST) device designed to generate equal resistance to expiratory pressure or, for the placebo group, a device that did not produce the resistance. The primary objective of the study was to verify improvements on the Penetration–Aspiration Scale. This was a 4-week study where the participants had to do five sets of five repetitions five times a week. Subjects were examined in a blinded manner by language/speech therapists using videofluoroscopy. There was a significant improvement in the Penetration–Aspiration Scale score for the EMST subjects when compared with those in the placebo group (a 0.57 reduction of points in the scale vs a 0.61 point increase for treated vs not treated, respectively). This scale is categorical, consists of 8 points, where 1 implies no aspiration and 8 demonstrates aspiration and risk in swallowing. The subjects treated with the EMST device had an average baseline of 2.64, which was reduced to 2.07, and those treated with placebo had an average baseline of 2.59, which increased to 3.3. Eleven subjects treated with the EMST device showed score improvements on the Penetration–Aspiration Scale in contrast to the five treated with placebo. It would be interesting to observe whether the results showed positive changes in the subjects who had a greater severity of dysphagia, and whether the score obtained from the scale showed a large divergence from the results. It is possible that the mild grade of severity in the tested subjects did not affect their Penetration–Aspiration Scale score considerably, which caused the minimal numerical results.

Manor et al. [11] published a randomized, double-blinded study that compared video-assisted swallowing therapy (VAST) against conventional rehabilitation swallowing therapy in 42 subjects (21 in each group) with PD and dysphagia. Patients were evaluated by fiber-optic endoscopy and by a speech specialist. Endoscopy qualifies five variables: bolus flow time, bolus location when the swallowing reflex is triggered, residue location, and the penetration and aspiration of food and liquid. The following other swallowing evaluation scales were also employed: swallowing disturbance questionnaire, swallowing quality of life, swallowing quality of care and pleasure of eating. Each group started with five rehabilitation sessions and finished with a sixth, 4 weeks after the fifth intervention. For those treated with VAST, their videoendoscopy was shown to them, informing them about swallowing mechanisms, the problems they had and how to correct them. The most frequent abnormality found was food residue left in the pharynx. This complication diminished in both groups but achieved significant improvement only for the VAST group when compared with the conventional rehabilitation group. There were no statistical differences in the other items that were analyzed by fiber-optic endoscopy. The VAST group also showed more favorable results on the other scales that were employed.

Surface electrical stimulation therapy for treating dysphagia has also been evaluated in two recent open-label studies. The first was by Baijens et al. [12], which consisted of a pilot study with ten subjects with PD and mild to severe dysphagia as well as ten healthy control subjects of the same age and gender. Surface electrical stimulation was applied in three different positions with VitalStim®, using a frequency of 80 Hz and a pulse width of 700 μs. Stimulation was applied on the suprahyoid, infrahyoid or a combination of the two muscles. After 90–120 min from having taken dopaminergic therapy, videofluoroscopic images were captured while the participants were being electrically stimulated. There were no significant differences between the subjects with PD and the control group during the fluoroscopic evaluation. It is possible that the small size of the group, the lack of blindness and an important placebo effect created an inadequate context to reach the formulated hypothesis.

In the second study, Heijnen et al. [13] included three groups of patients with PD and dysphagia. The subjects participated in physical therapy, motor electrical stimulation and electrical stimulation of the suprahyoid muscles. The electrical impulses were performed with VitalStim®, using a frequency of 80 Hz and a pulse width of 700 μs. The evaluations were made according to the Dysphagia Severity Scale, Quality of Life in Swallowing Disorders (SWAL-QOL) and MD Anderson Dysphagia Inventory. The study demonstrated overall benefits for swallowing in the three groups, but there were no significant differences among them. The loss of participants near to 20%, an unblinded study, a nonparametric distribution of the data and the lack of sensitivity to change from the scales employed could all have contributed to a loss in the differentiation for the results obtained from the groups.

Constipation

This disorder is present in 80–90% of the population with PD, and may be secondary to several problems including a decrease in gastric and intestinal motility secondary to dopaminergic and anticholinergic drugs, as well as from the disease, a decline in fluid intake, a reduction in body movements as a result of the disease, anorectal dysfunction and pelvic floor dysinergia, among others.

Sullivan et al. [14] conducted a double-blinded, randomized, placebo-controlled pilot study using tegaserod for the treatment of constipation in PD. Fifteen subjects (eight with tegaserod 6 mg and seven with placebo, three times daily) were evaluated using the Subject's Global Assessment of Relief for 4 weeks after the initial intervention. Subsequently, a tendency toward a significant statistical improvement for constipation was noted in the tegaserod group (Subject's Global Assessment of Relief score of 9.1 before treatment and 8.3 after with tegaserod vs a score of 6.2 before treatment and 8.7 after with placebo). The small group size and a gender imbalance among the participants warrant a study on a larger scale to test the effectiveness of this drug.

Zangaglia et al. [15] published a randomized, double-blinded, placebo-controlled study on the use of macrogol in patients with PD and constipation. Subjects took either 7.3 g of macrogol diluted in water or placebo for 8 weeks. The patients filled out a diary with the following information: stool frequency, straining and stool consistency. Fifty-seven subjects were included in the study (29 on macrogol and 28 with placebo), of which 14 did not finish (nine macrogol and five placebo). Stool frequency increased in a significant way in both groups; however, stool frequency was better for the macrogol group (5.6 vs 3.4 at 4 weeks and 6.6 vs 3.7 at 8 weeks for macrogol versus placebo, respectively) when compared over the same time period. Straining improved in both groups at week 4; however, at 8 weeks the study showed no differences between the groups, although there was a tendency toward improvement for the group managed with macrogol. Furthermore, stool consistency improved in a significant way during the two stages of the study for those treated with macrogol when compared with placebo. The use of higher doses and the frequency of the use of laxatives throughout the duration of the study were smaller for the group that was treated with macrogol, although these differences were not statistically significant. A withdrawal rate of greater than 20% and a possible lack of dietary control as well as an arbitrary management of laxatives could mislead the results obtained from this study.

Ondo et al. [16] conducted a randomized, double-blinded, placebo-controlled study of lubiprostone for constipation in PD. The study lasted for 6 weeks. Thirty patients were randomized for the trial of lubiprostone 48 μg daily and 31 for placebo, of which five from the first group and four from the second withdrew. The patients in the lubiprostone group wrote in diaries that showed significant improvements in global impression, stool frequency, visual analog scale score and constipation questionnaires. Although almost 50% of the population displayed stool softening, it did not become a serious problem or cause them to end the treatment.

Weight

Weight change is a documented fact with PD. Some causes that may contribute to the weight loss are: mitochondrial respiratory chain dysfunction, hypothalamic dysfunction, the presence of Lewy bodies on nonmotor circuits, an increase in energy expenditure, early satiety from gastric hypomotility, bulbar dysfunction, olfactory disorders, depression and the loss of the mechanisms related to dopaminergic reward function due to depletion, among others.

To date, there are no direct interventions for the management of weight loss in PD, although there is a subanalysis of the COMPARE (Cognition and Mood in Parkinson Disease in Subthalamic Nucleus Versus Globus Pallidus Interna Deep Brain Stimulation) study [17] that detailed weight changes in patients with PD. From these, 23 patients were treated with globus pallidus interna deep-brain stimulation (GPi-DBS) (10 bilateral, 13 unilateral) and 21 with subthalamic nucleus (STN)-DBS (15 bilateral, six unilateral). Thirty-one evaluated subjects (70%) gained weight 6 months after DBS, 10 subjects (23%) lost weight and three (7%) showed no weight change. When analyzed according to the target, of those who received GPi stimulation, 16 (70%) gained weight (10.65 ± 6.98 lb), six (24%) lost weight (7.77 ± 4.55 lb) and in one participant (4%) there was no change.

For those treated with DBS-STN, 15 subjects (71%) gained weight (7.2 ± 5.55 lb), four subjects (19%) lost weight (4.5 ± 2.38 lb) and two participants (10%) did not show changes. There were no significant changes between the groups; however, it is worth noting that the percentage of subjects who received uni- or bilateral treatments within those groups showed a trend for significant differences ($P = 0.06$). As data was analyzed retrospectively, misclassification bias can occur. The relatively small sample and the lack of DBS unilateral or bilateral stratification for subjects could also have caused biases in this study.

Urinary symptoms

Urinary dysfunction is the most frequent complaint in patients with PD, affecting up to 70% of patients in the early stages of the disease and 90% for those in the advanced stages. They include mainly urinary urgency, nocturia, increased urinary frequency, incontinence, detrusor hyper- or hyporeflex found in urodynamic findings, decreased bladder capacity and anomalies of the external urinary sphincter. There have been some studies done to evaluate the management of these disorders.

Kabay et al. [18] conducted an open study of electrical stimulation on the posterior tibial nerve to improve bladder capacity in 32 subjects with PD who had had almost 7 years with the disease. Cystometric analysis was performed before and after stimulation. The mean volume of the first involuntary detrusor contraction was 145.2 ± 41.1 ml. There was an important change after the stimulation, increasing the average by 244.7 ± 51.7 ml. A greater than 50% volume increase of the first involuntary detrusor contraction was observed in 20 of the 32 participants. Similarly, the maximum cystometric capacity average was 204.8 ± 40.5 ml before stimulation and 301.2 ± 51.5 ml with stimulation. An improvement of greater than 50% for maximum cystometric capacity was observed in 15 of the 32 participants. In addition, stimulation was effective for the relief of detrusor pseudodyssynergia in five of the seven participants. Posterior tibial nerve stimulation proves to be a useful therapy for some urinary complications in patients with PD; however, a double-blinded study with a "sham procedure," and a larger sample size of the test group are required.

Kulaksizoglu et al. [19] reported an open study using botulinum toxin type A (Dysport®) on 16 patients with PD and an overactive bladder. They were interviewed using the SEAPI (stress incontinence, emptying, anatomy, protection and inhibition) Incontinence Quality of Life Assessment Questionnaire, as well as other urodynamic studies. The caregivers were asked to describe the burden of urinary symptoms in quality of life, as evaluated with a visual analog scale. Five hundred units of the toxin was diluted in 30 ml of saline solution and applied with a flexible fiberscope on 30 points at a depth of 4 mm, respecting the bladder dome. An initial visit was made and then at 3, 6, 9 and 12 months post-application. There was an important improvement on the SEAPI scale as well as in the maximum bladder capacity, lasting for up to 12 months (SEAPI baseline: 32; 3 months: 11, 6 months: 10, 9 months: 16, 1 year: 26; and maximum bladder capacity baseline: 217.8 ml; 3 months: 355.1 ml; 6 months: 399 ml; 9 months: 401.4 ml; 1 year: 295.2 ml). Six subjects presented continuous urinary incontinence, which improved within the first 3–6 months as measured by the number of daily diaper changes. The visual analog scale from the caregiver improved for the first 9 months but reached the same score a year after the application. A double-blinded, placebo-controlled study with a larger number of participants and stratified by other variables including age, gender, the presence of prostate disorders, mental status, diabetes and dopaminergic and/or anticholinergics daily dosage would be helpful for this purpose.

Vaughan et al. [20] conducted an open study that consisted of exercise-based behavioral therapy in PD patients with urinary incontinence. The study included five visits, at 2-week intervals, over 8 weeks. During the visits, it was explained to the patients how to contract and relax the pelvic floor muscles, manage liquid intake and constipation and exercise pelvic floor muscles, and they were given strategies for urge suppression. The primary objective was to observe a weekly change in incontinence. Out of the 24 subjects selected, only 17 completed the study. Of this group, 12 (71%) achieved a greater than 50% reduction in urinary incontinence frequency and seven (41%) were continent by the end of the study. This demonstrates some interesting results because the subjects improved their problems without the help of pharmaceuticals. However, there are various reasons why we should be cautious of the results: there was no control group, the evaluations were not blinded, withdrawal from the study was greater than 20% and there was no formal statistical evaluation due to the number of participants.

Erectile dysfunction

Erectile dysfunction affects about 60% of male patients with PD, almost twice as much as the general population. Dopamine depletion at the mesolimbic level is suspected to be involved with libido and erection.

Hussain et al. [21] published a randomized, double-blinded, placebo-controlled, crossover study of sildenafil on erectile dysfunction in 12 patients with PD and 12 with MSA lasting for 24 weeks. Participants were evaluated using the International Index for Erectile Dysfunction Questionnaire, a quality-of-life questionnaire and a questionnaire for the patient's bedpartner. The average given dose was 50 mg 1 h prior to have sexual intercourse, using it no more than three times a week. Ten subjects with PD and six with MSA completed the study. Nine out of ten subjects with PD reported a good response. There were no changes in the quality-of-life scale, although there was improvement of sexual life. This improvement was confirmed by the survey given to the couple. Similar results were found for participants with MSA. The three groups presented significant hypotension as a side effect. It is possible that the small size of the group, the treatment of ordinal variables as if they were continuous and the lack of statistics for other variables including age and grade of erectile dysfunction could bias the results.

An RCT of sildenafil for PD-related ED by Safarinejad et al. [22] was positive, but this paper was later retracted by the publisher for reasons that are not clear.

Orthostatic hypotension

Orthostatic hypotension is one of the most frequent autonomic complications in PD. More than 90% of PD patients present this complication, although only 10% are symptomatic.

Abate et al. [23] conducted a randomized, double-blinded, placebo-controlled study using indomethacin intravenous infusions (50 mg over 30 min of infusion) and oral ingestion (50 mg three times daily) for the treatment of orthostatism in 12 participants with PD. After intravenous application, indomethacin caused an increase in supine systolic and diastolic blood pressure, a small fall in pressure when standing and an enhanced blood pressure response to the cold pressor test. When the drug was taken orally, a reduction in the fall of the mean arterial pressure, when standing, was detected. Although the study was not described in great detail, it was one of the first to demonstrate the usefulness of prostraglandin inhibitors for improving blood pressure.

Schoffer *et al.* [24] conducted a randomized, double-blinded, crossover study comparing domperidone and fludrocortisone for the management of orthostatic hypotension in 17 PD cases. Participants, besides being instructed in nonpharmacological measures for orthostatism, were treated with fludrocortisone 0.1 mg daily and two placebo tablets for 3 weeks, followed by a week of washout, and then with domperidone 10 mg three times daily for a further 3 weeks. They were evaluated according to the Composite Autonomic Symptom Scale (COMPASS-OD), Clinical Global Impression of Change (CGI), blood pressure measurements and the tilt test. Both medications demonstrated benefits for the management of orthostatic hypotension. Domperidone demonstrated a greater effect. The changes evaluated on the COMPASS-OD and CGI scales were statistically significant in both groups of the study. The study found that nonpharmacological treatment for the management of orthostatic hypotension did not produce significant results. The small sample size, the different ways of measuring orthostasis (taking blood pressure at the bedside vs the tilt test) and the loss of four participants during the first intervention are some of the limitations of this study.

Pain

Pain is present in more than 50% of patients with PD. The etiology is not clear; however, it is believed that monoaminergic depletion can reduce central pain inhibitory mechanisms. Few studies have focused on the treatment of pain, which is a major cause of disability and worsening of quality of life.

Djaldetti *et al.* [25] conducted an open study on 23 patients. Duloxetine 60 mg was administered at night and assessment was made using the Beck Depression Inventory (BDI), 39-Item Parkinson's Disease Questionnaire (PDQ-39), Brief Pain Inventory, Visual Analog Scale for Pain and Short Form McGill Pain Questionnaire, as well as quantitative sensory testing with a Peltier-based contact temperature stimulation device. Three subjects abandoned the study due to secondary side effects from the drug, 13 subjects reported improvement and the seven remaining patients reported no benefits from the medication. Significant changes were found on the Brief Pain Inventory, Visual Analog Scale for Pain and Short Form McGill Pain Questionnaire. There were no significant differences observed in temperature perception before or after the intervention. The study used a small group of patients, and it was not placebo controlled or blinded; however, it showed that some drugs with monoaminergic modulation properties seem to be useful in the management of this type of symptomatology.

Dellapina *et al.* [26] tested the usefulness of STN-DBS in pain management among subjects with PD. The study was divided in two parts: in the first, eight subjects with PD and neuropathic pain were evaluated by a visual analog scale and the Neuropathic Pain Symptoms Inventory (NPSI) before and after surgery. In the second part, 16 patients with PD were evaluated in a short, randomized, crossover trial before and after STN stimulation. Heat pain thresholds were measured with a Peltier-based contact temperature stimulation device. In addition, different cortical areas activated by pain were compared in subjects with and without neuropathic pain. This was done using $H_2^{15}O$ positron emission tomography. Patients with PD and neuropathic pain showed significant improvement on the visual analog scale score after stimulation (7.5 vs 5.4) as well as a trend for significant improvement on the NPSI. For subjects with neuropathic pain, the activation of cerebral stimulation profoundly elevated the pain threshold (STN-DBS off: 40.3 ± 4.2 °C vs on: 41.6 ± 4.3 °C). In addition, subjects with neuropathic pain showed activation of the prefrontal, somatosensory and premotor cortex during the off-stimulation periods through imaging studies. The right prefrontal cortex was activated among these subjects when the stimulator was activated. For pain-free subjects, activation while the stimulation device was turned off was observed in the left thalamus, right inferotemporal cortex and left anterior cingulum. When the DBS was turned on, activation was seen around the right cerebellar hemisphere as well as the somatosensitive cortex. It is interesting to observe the effect that DBS has on pain treatment for patients with PD and how this may be manifested in different areas of the cerebral cortex for individuals who have neuropathic pain and those who do not. A larger number of subjects will be required to study these effects in the future.

Marques *et al.* [27] conducted a randomized, double-blinded, crossover study assessing pain and tolerance thresholds using levodopa (L-DOPA) and STN-DBS in 19 patients with PD. They were evaluated in three different conditions with 1 week of difference between each: medication off/stimulation off, medication off/stimulation on and medication on/stimulation off. Participants were evaluated without having taken oral medication for 10 h and with the stimulator off, and then with levodopa (1.5 times the habitual dose) or placebo. At this time, the stimulator was either left on or turned off. A thermotest, which is capable of raising the temperature by 1 °C/s on the area where the device is applied, was used for evaluation starting with a baseline temperature of 30 °C. Tolerance thresholds were measured by a digital pressure algometer. Both levodopa and STN-DBS achieved a significant increase in pain and tolerance thresholds to mechanical stimuli. When the stimuli were thermal, neither of the two therapies was able to change the thresholds in a significant way. While it was possible to achieve benefits with both therapies for the mechanical pain and tolerance thresholds, there was a trend for a nonstatistical change for either alone. The authors questioned how they obtained positive results concerning some pain modalities and at the same time negative results for others. Rather than a scientific explanation regarding pain segmental ways, these results could be explained simply by chance or a type I error due to the small sample size.

Daytime sleepiness

Excessive daytime sleepiness is present in more than 50% of the population with PD. There are several probable causes including depression, cognitive changes, medications, central monoaminergic depletion, hypothalamus dysfunction, insomnia, sleep fragmentation and other sleep disorders such as rapid eye movement (REM) sleep behavior disorder, restless legs syndrome, periodic limb movements during sleep and sleep apnea, among others.

Högl et al. [28] conducted a randomized, double-blinded, crossover, placebo-controlled study in patients with PD and excessive daytime sleepiness (10 or more points on the Epworth Sleepiness Scale [ESS]). This 6-week study was divided into 2 weeks with modafinil (100 mg the first week and 200 mg the second) or placebo, followed by 2 weeks of washout and a further 2 weeks with modafinil or placebo according to the randomization. There were 12 subjects included who were evaluated using the ESS, Maintenance of Wakefulness Test, Sleep logs and BDI. Modafinil significantly improved ESS when compared with placebo (a change of score of 3.42 vs 0.83, respectively). The remainder of the methods employed demonstrated no significant statistical differences. While the study was built on an adequate methodological design, the small sample group could be the reason for the poor results in this trial.

Adler et al. [29] studied the effects of modafinil on excessive daytime sleepiness in patients with PD who scored 10 or more on the ESS in a randomized, double-blinded, placebo-controlled, crossover trial. Subjects received either 200 mg of modafinil or placebo for 3 weeks, followed by 1 week of washout and then the alternate treatment for 3 more weeks. The primary objective was to change the ESS score and make a comparison of both interventions. The Excessive Daytime Sleep Rating Scale, Modified Fatigue Assessment Inventory, Excessive Daytime Fatigue Rating Scale and Clinical Global Impression of Change (CGIC), among others, were also used. Twenty subjects completed the study. Those on modafinil showed significant changes on the ESS when compared with placebo. The difference in the ESS score was 4.4 points, signaling a carryover effect between the testing periods for the groups. There were no significant changes in the scores of the other scales. Although the difference between groups was positive, there was a trend for nonstatistical significance ($P = 0.039$), participants were only assessed in a subjective way and the number of subjects studied was small.

Ondo et al. [30] conducted a randomized, placebo-controlled clinical study in parallel groups in order to evaluate the efficiency of modafinil in patients with PD and who scored more than 10 on the ESS. The primary objective was to evaluate the changes in the ESS score between subjects treated with modafinil (200–400 mg daily, depending on tolerance) or placebo. The Fatigue Severity Scale, Hamilton Depression Scale, global impressions and Medical Outcome Survey Short Form 36 (SF-36) were also used. In addition, a multiple sleep latency test was given. Two groups of 20 participants were evaluated: three did not complete the study (two in the placebo group and one in the modafinil group). The modafinil dose was increased from 200 to 400 mg over 2 weeks and reevaluated 4 weeks later. No significant differences were found in any of the scales used, nor was there a favorable change in the multiple sleep latency test for the participants who used modafinil. Possible reference bias, a small sample group, a strong placebo effect and a subjective assessment using the ESS may have influenced the final results.

Postuma et al. [31] published a randomized, placebo-controlled clinical study of parallel groups in order to evaluate the usefulness of caffeine for the management of excessive daytime sleepiness (ESS score of 10 or more points) in patients with PD. This was a 6-week study: during the first 3 weeks, 100 mg caffeine doses were administered twice daily and the dose was then increased to 200 mg twice daily. Motor severity, Fatigue Severity Scale, Pittsburgh Sleep Quality Index, BDI, SF-36, PDQ-39 and CGIC scales were also used. Sixty-one participants were randomized (31 on placebo, 30 on caffeine), but four of them violated the protocol (two from each group). At 6 weeks, there was a nonsignificant reduction of 1.71 points in the ESS score among subjects using caffeine. There was a significant improvement on the CGIC scale of 0.64 points in the group treated with caffeine when compared with placebo. A significant improvement in the UPDRS motor scale and the global scale was seen in those on caffeine treatment. There were no significant differences in the rest of the scales used. Further studies evaluating the effects of caffeine according to age, progression of the disease and daily dosage of dopaminergics, among other variables, should be able to differentiate the real effect of this drug on the disease.

Sleep disorders

More than 90% of patients with PD have some sleep disturbances, which are varied and may be present many years before having any motor manifestations of the disease.

Medeiros *et al.* [32] conducted a randomized, double-blinded, placebo-controlled study in parallel groups with melatonin 3 mg for patients with PD and insomnia. Eighteen subjects completed the study and were analyzed with the Pittsburgh Sleep Quality Index (PSQI) and the ESS, as well as with polysomnography. The patients received treatment for 28 consecutive days. Subsequently, they were evaluated and an improvement in the PSQI was found for those treated with melatonin when compared with those on placebo (PSQI: 8.3 initial and 4.5 final on melatonin vs 9.9 initial and 9.9 final on placebo), although there was a trend toward no statistical significance ($P = 0.03$). The small group size in this study creates difficulties for the interpretation of the data.

Dowling *et al.* [33] published a multisite, randomized, double-blinded, placebo-controlled crossover trial using melatonin in doses of 5 and 50 mg in patients with PD and sleeping disturbances. Forty subjects completed the study. They were evaluated by polysomnography and actigraphy, as well as the PSQI, General Sleep Disturbance Scale, Standford Sleepiness Scale and ESS, and with diaries. The patients were treated in any one of the three arms of the study for 2 weeks, followed by a week of washout and were then crossed with another group. The subjects had an average age of 61 years and on average had had the disease for 7.5 years. Those treated with 50 mg of melatonin daily found a significant difference in sleep time when compared with the other groups; however, this extra effect was only 10 min more. On the other hand, the subjects treated with 5 mg of melatonin daily showed significant differences in the General Sleep Disturbance Scale when compared with either the 50 mg of melatonin or placebo group. The study showed no other significant differences, finding moderate results for the quality of sleep and a possible random error because of the effects found with the 5 mg group and not with the 50 mg melatonin group.

Menza *et al.* [34] published a 6-week, multisite, randomized, double-blinded, placebo-controlled trial of eszopiclone (3 mg in subjects younger than 65 years and 2 mg in subjects 65 years or older) in patients with PD and insomnia. The subjects filled out diaries for total sleep time. Other secondary endpoints of the study were evaluated with the Wake After Sleep Onset test, number of awakenings, Sleep Impairment Index, PDQ-8, CGIS-severity, CGIS-improvement, Fatigue Severity Scale, Multidimensional Caregiver Burden Inventory and Center for Epidemiologic Studies Depression Scale, as well as the Likert scale for sleep quality and daytime alertness. Thirty subjects who had PD for an average of 4.5 years and with an average age of 56 and an average of less than 2 on the Hoehn and Yahr scale were included in the study. Thirty-seven percent of the cases dropped out because of lack of improvement. There was a significant difference in the number of awakenings, sleep quality and CGIS-improvement for those treated with eszopiclone when compared with placebo. There were negative results for the rest of the variables analyzed. With a greater than 20% drop out, positive results with a tendency toward no statistical significance and the short-term period with PD for the patients analyzed cast doubts about the efficacy of the drug in this particular situation.

Larsson *et al.* [35] conducted a multicenter, randomized, double-blinded, placebo-controlled study of memantine (20 mg/day) in patients with PD dementia (PDD) or dementia with Lewy bodies (DLB) and REM sleep behavior disorder (RBD). The study lasted for 24 weeks. Patients were evaluated with the Stavanger Sleep Questionnaire and ESS. Fifty-seven subjects were recruited but only 47 finished the study. Memantine appeared to demonstrate an improvement for cases with RBD. Despite this, the ESS showed no changes. The RBD was not confirmed with polysomnography, which could have caused a misclassification bias. This and other methodological limitations, such as a small group size and being a subanalysis of another study where the primary outcome was not to evaluate sleep disorders in this population, question the usefulness of this drug for this disorder.

Di Giacopo *et al.* [36] conducted a double-blinded, randomized, crossover, placebo-controlled pilot study of transdermal rivastigmine (4.6 mg daily) in patients with PD and RBD in whom clonazepam and melatonin treatments had failed. The study consisted of a 3-week intervention followed by 1 week of washout and a further 3 weeks of an alternative treatment. Twelve subjects were included but only ten completed the study. The disorders were confirmed in all subjects by polysomnography. The patients had an average age of 68 years and had had PD for about 9 years. Six subjects had a significant reduction in the frequency of weekly episodes of RBD, which were monitored in a diary by a bedside partner. There were no changes in the disorder in four of the subjects. The small size of the group as well as the losses suffered throughout the study encourage the development of a better trial for this population in order to verify the results.

Conclusions

Diverse interventions are being studied for the management of nonmotor complications in PD. To date, it can be concluded that:

- Botulinum toxins type A and B are effective in the management of sialorrhea in patients with PD, and the lack of collateral systemic effects makes this type of treatment desirable.
- Rehabilitation in the management of swallowing mechanisms may improve dysphagia, although there is a lack of studies with solid methodology that strengthen these results.
- Macrogol and lubiprostone may be an effective intervention for the management of constipation in PD, although more studies are required to confirm this.
- There are no studies at this time directed toward the management of weight disorders in PD.
- Randomized, double-blinded, placebo-controlled trials (RCTs) are needed for urinary symptoms of PD.
- Sildenafil seems to be an effective drug for the management of erectile dysfunction in PD.
- Domperidone and fludrocortisone may be useful in the management of orthostatic hypotension associated with the disease; however, there is a lack of definitive studies with clear objectives.
- Deep-brain stimulation of the STN may be effective for the treatment of pain associated with the disease, although more studies are required in order to evaluate these effects.
- There are no studies to date for the solid management of excessive daytime sleepiness.
- More studies with a higher level of methodology are required to evaluate pharmacological interventions for insomnia and other sleep disorders in PD.

References

1. Marks L, Turner K, O'Sullivan J, Deighton B, Lees A. Drooling in Parkinson's disease: a novel speech and language therapy intervention. *Int J Lang Commun Disord* 2001; **36** (Suppl.): 282–7.
2. Mancini F, Zangaglia R, Cristina S, *et al.* Double-blind, placebo-controlled study to evaluate the efficacy and safety of botulinum toxin type A in the treatment of drooling in parkinsonism. *Mov Disord* 2003; **18**: 685–8.
3. Lagalla G, Millevolte M, Capecci M, Provinciali L, Ceravolo MG. Botulinum toxin type A for drooling in Parkinson's disease: a double-blind, randomized, placebo-controlled study. *Mov Disord* 2006; **21**: 704–7.
4. Ondo WG, Hunter C, Moore W. A double-blind placebo-controlled trial of botulinum toxin B for sialorrhea in Parkinson's disease. *Neurology* 2004; **62**: 37–40.
5. Lagalla G, Millevolte M, Capecci M, Provinciali L, Ceravolo MG. Long-lasting benefits of botulinum toxin type B in Parkinson's disease-related drooling. *J Neurol* 2009; **256**: 563–7.
6. Chinnapongse R, Gullo K, Nemeth P, Zhang Y, Griggs L. Safety and efficacy of botulinum toxin type B for treatment of sialorrhea in Parkinson's disease: a prospective double-blind trial. *Mov Disord* 2012; **27**: 219–26.
7. Thomsen TR, Galpern WR, Asante A, Arenovich T, Fox SH. Ipratropium bromide spray as treatment for sialorrhea in Parkinson's disease. *Mov Disord* 2007; **22**: 2268–73.
8. Arbouw ME, Movig KL, Koopmann M, *et al.* Glycopyrrolate for sialorrhea in Parkinson disease: a randomized, double-blind, crossover trial. *Neurology* 2010; **74**: 1203–7.
9. Lloret SP, Nano G, Carrosella A, Gamzu E, Merello M. A double-blind, placebo-controlled, randomized, crossover pilot study of the safety and efficacy of multiple doses of intra-oral tropicamide films for the

short-term relief of sialorrhea symptoms in Parkinson's disease patients. *J Neurolog Sci* 2011; **310**: 248–50.

10. Troche MS, Okun MS, Rosenbek JC, et al. Aspiration and swallowing in Parkinson disease and rehabilitation with EMST A randomized trial. *Neurology* 2010; **75**: 1912–19.

11. Manor Y, Mootanah R, Freud D, Giladi N, Cohen JT. Video-assisted swallowing therapy for patients with Parkinson's disease. *Parkinsonism Relat Disord* 2013; **19**: 207–11.

12. Baijens LW, Speyer R, Passos VL, et al. The effect of surface electrical stimulation on swallowing in dysphagic Parkinson patients. *Dysphagia* 2012; **27**: 528–37.

13. Heijnen BJ, Speyer R, Baijens LW, Bogaardt HC. Neuromuscular electrical stimulation versus traditional therapy in patients with Parkinson's disease and oropharyngeal dysphagia: effects on quality of life. *Dysphagia* 2012; **27**: 336–45.

14. Sullivan KL, Staffetti JF, Hauser RA, Dunne PB, Zesiewicz TA. Tegaserod (Zelnorm) for the treatment of constipation in Parkinson's disease. *Mov Disord* 2006; **21**: 115–16.

15. Zangaglia R, Martignoni E, Glorioso M, et al. Macrogol for the treatment of constipation in Parkinson's disease. A randomized placebo-controlled study. *Mov Disord* 2007; **22**: 1239–44.

16. Ondo WG, Kenney C, Sullivan K, et al. Placebo-controlled trial of lubiprostone for constipation associated with Parkinson disease. *Neurology* 2012; **78**: 1650–4.

17. Locke MC, Wu SS, Foote KD, et al. Weight changes in subthalamic nucleus vs globus pallidus internus deep brain stimulation: results from the COMPARE Parkinson disease deep brain stimulation cohort. *Neurosurgery* 2011; **68**: 1233–7.

18. Kabay SC, Kabay S, Yucel M, Ozden H. Acute urodynamic effects of percutaneous posterior tibial nerve stimulation on neurogenic detrusor overactivity in patients with Parkinson's disease. *Neurourol Urodyn* 2009; **28**: 62–7.

19. Kulaksizoglu H, Parman Y. Use of botulinim toxin-A for the treatment of overactive bladder symptoms in patients with Parkinson's disease. *Parkinsonism Relat Disord* 2010; **16**: 531–4.

20. Vaughan CP, Juncos JL, Burgio KL, et al. Behavioral therapy to treat urinary incontinence in Parkinson disease. *Neurology* 2011; **76**: 1631–4.

21. Hussain IF, Brady CM, Swinn MJ, Mathias CJ, Fowler CJ. Treatment of erectile dysfunction with sildenafil citrate (Viagra) in parkinsonism due to Parkinson's disease or multiple system atrophy with observations on orthostatic hypotension. *J Neurol Neurosurg Psychiatry* 2001; **71**: 371–4.

22. Safarinejad MR, Taghva A, Shekarchi B, Safarinejad S. Safety and efficacy of sildenafil citrate in the treatment of Parkinson-emergent erectile dysfunction: a double-blind, placebo-controlled, randomized study. *Int J Impot Res* 2010; **22**: 325–35. Retraction: *Int J Impot Res* 2011; **23**: 94.

23. Abate G, Polimeni RM, Cuccurullo F, Puddu P, Lenzi S. Effects of indomethacin on postural hypotension in Parkinsonism. *Br Med J* 1979; **2**: 1466.

24. Schoffer KL, Henderson RD, O'Maley K, O'sullivan JD. Nonpharmacological treatment, fludrocortisone, and domperidone for orthostatic hypotension in Parkinson's disease. *Mov Disord* 2007; **22**: 1543–9.

25. Djaldetti R, Yust-Katz S, Kolianov V, Melamed E, Dabby R. The effect of duloxetine on primary pain symptoms in Parkinson disease. *Clin Neuropharmacol* 2007; **30**: 201–5.

26. Dellapina E, Ory-Magne F, Regragui W, et al. Effect of subthalamic deep brain stimulation on pain in Parkinson's disease. *Pain* 2012; **153**: 2267–73.

27. Marques A, Chassin O, Morand D, et al. Central pain modulation after subthalamic nucleus stimulation: a crossover randomized trial. *Neurology* 2013; **81**: 633–40.

28. Högl B, Saletu M, Brandauer E, et al. Modafinil for the treatment of daytime sleepiness in Parkinson's disease: a double-blind, randomized, crossover, placebo-controlled polygraphic trial. *Sleep* 2002; **25**: 905–9.

29. Adler CH, Caviness JN, Hentz JG, Lind M, Tiede J. Randomized trial of modafinil for treating subjective daytime sleepiness in patients with Parkinson's disease. *Mov Disord* 2003; **18**: 287–93.

30. Ondo WG, Fayle R, Atassi F, Jankovic J. Modafinil for daytime somnolence in Parkinson's disease: double blind, placebo controlled parallel trial. *J Neurol Neurosurg Psychiatry* 2005; **76**: 1636–9.

31. Postuma RB, Lang AE, Munhoz RP, et al. Caffeine for treatment of Parkinson disease A randomized controlled trial. *Neurology* 2012; **79**: 651–8.

32. Medeiros CA, Carvalhedo de Bruin PF, Lopes LA, et al. Effect of exogenous melatonin on sleep and motor dysfunction in Parkinson's disease. *J Neurol* 2007; **254**: 459–64.

33. Dowling GA, Mastick J, Colling E, et al. Melatonin for sleep disturbances in Parkinson's disease. *Sleep Med* 2005; **6**: 459–66.

34. Menza M, Dobkin RD, Marin H, et al. Treatment of insomnia in Parkinson's disease: a controlled trial of eszopiclone and placebo. *Mov Disord* 2010; **25**: 1708–14.

35. Larsson V, Aarsland D, Ballard C, Minthon L, Londos E. The effect of memantine on sleep behaviour in dementia with Lewy bodies and Parkinson's disease dementia. *Int J Geriatr Psychiatry* 2010; **25**: 1030–8.

36. Di Giacopo R, Fasano A, Quaranta D, et al. Rivastigmine as alternative treatment for refractory REM behavior disorder in Parkinson's disease. *Mov Disord* 2012; **27**: 559–61.

Chapter 32

Lessons and challenges of trials involving ancillary therapies for the management of Parkinson's disease

Chris J. Hass, Elizabeth L. Stegemöller, Madeleine E. Hackney and Joe R. Nocera

Introduction

Progressive impairment, particularly related to gait, postural control and cognitive decline, are not effectively treated by the current pharmacological and surgical management of Parkinson's disease (PD). This has led many patients and treating physicians to explore concomitant therapeutic modalities such as aerobic exercise, resistance training, physical therapy, massage, dance and music therapy, tai chi and others to aid in reducing symptomatology and improving patient quality of life. Over the last 15 years, the research community has also experienced an explosion of efforts into studying the efficacy of these treatments on motor and nonmotor symptoms, as well as their ability to enhance patient well-being. For example, in the decade preceding 2004, there were roughly 10–15 papers published per year related to exercise in PD. From 2004 to 2013, this number skyrocketed to an average of 50 papers per year. With this progression of efforts, the quality and ingenuity of treatments have expanded from small pilot studies of walking and weight training to large multi-center trials investigating robotic-assisted cycling and exercises paired with brain-stimulation techniques. In general, many of the abovementioned accessory treatments have proven moderately effective. However, issues with study designs, small sample sizes and heterogeneous outcome measures coupled with the trials and tribulations of prescribing these treatments to the heterogeneous PD community have largely prevented a major contribution of these therapies to advances in the treatment of PD. Although the evidence from the animal literature is quite compelling with respect to neuroprotective and neuroplastic benefits of exercise, as well as the ability of different exercises to result in differential effects on the nervous system, these effects in humans have been more difficult to demonstrate. In this chapter, we will outline the effectiveness of the more popular movement and behavioral therapies on the treatment of motor and nonmotor features of PD.

Aerobic exercise

Aerobic exercise improves a wide range of functional outcomes in individuals with PD. Indeed, individuals with PD benefit from aerobic exercise as much as healthy older adults [1, 2]. In fact, aerobic exercise interventions may represent one of the best ways to prevent disability and secondary complications associated with PD [3]. For example, multiple studies examining 16-week aerobic exercise training regimens have reported improvements in oxygen consumption (VO_2) consistent with a healthier and more efficient cardiovascular system, improved scores on the Unified Parkinson's Disease Rating Scale (UPDRS), and improved performance on physical function performance tests and movement initiation [4]. Specifically, Bergen et al. [5] demonstrated a 26% improvement in peak VO_2 among PD patients follow aerobic training. Additionally, improved walking economy has been noted in individuals with PD who participated aerobic activity [6]. When compared with other forms of exercise, aerobic interventions have demonstrated a greater improvement on select facets of physical function. For example, when compared with a medical Chinese exercise (qigong), Burini et al. [7] demonstrated that aerobic training exerted a significant impact on moderately disabled PD patients in functional parameters

Parkinson's Disease: Current and Future Therapeutics and Clinical Trials, ed. Gálvez-Jiménez et al. Published by Cambridge University Press. © Cambridge University Press 2016.

including, the 6-min walk test, Borg scale and cardiorespiratory outcomes (peak VO_2).

Studies from animal models suggest that aerobic exercise may not only have effects on physical function – it may also interfere with the disease process itself. For example, treadmill or wheel running initiated soon after a unilateral 6-hydroxydopamine (6-OHDA) lesion reduced neurochemical loss, lessened forelimb motor deficits and reduced dopamine loss when compared with sedentary lesioned rats [8]. Forced-exercise paradigms, in which the animal has to maintain a running velocity that is greater than their preferred running speed, have also been studied. Results from forced-exercise paradigms in animals demonstrate short- and long-term improvements in forelimb akinesia, stride length and step length, as well as sparing of striatal dopamine compared with sedentary lesioned animals [8, 9]. Similarly, Poulton and Muir [10] reported that forced treadmill running ameliorated dopamine loss in 6-OHDA rats.

Forced aerobic exercise in the human PD condition has demonstrated equally intriguing results. Ridgel *et al.* [11] randomly assigned ten mild to moderate PD patients to either 8-weeks of forced exercise or voluntary exercise. Patients in the forced-exercise group pedaled on a stationary tandem bicycle with the assistance of a trainer at a rate 30% greater than their preferred voluntary rate. Patients randomized to the voluntary group pedaled at their preferred rate. The results demonstrated that the forced-exercise group improved their UPDRS motor score by 35%. Interestingly, improvements in coordination of grasping forces during the performance of a functional bimanual dexterity task improved significantly in the forced-exercise group, suggesting improved central motor function.

Another promising aerobic intervention for PD patients is treadmill/gait training. Patients with PD who have undergone gait training on a treadmill have shown improvements in UPDRS motor scores, increases in gait speed and cadence during walking, and reductions in the number of falls [12, 13]. Research examining progressive speed-dependent treadmill training showed an improvement in gait speed and stride length of walking in early PD when compared with conventional gait therapy [14].

Unfortunately, despite being classified as a movement disorder, cognitive deficits are present in a large percentage of PD patients and greatly impact on function and quality of life. Cognitive deficits in PD affect complex working memory (WM), the ability to store and manipulate information held in memory, and the ability to store information despite distraction [15]. In addition, a wide range of executive function abilities including planning, inhibitory processes and set-shifting, are impaired in PD [16–18]. Interestingly, recent work from the healthy older-adult literature [19, 20] suggests that aerobic exercise and/or cardiovascular fitness may reverse age-related cognitive decline and facilitate a healthy cortex. For example, Colcombe *et al.* [21] demonstrated that older adults with greater levels of cardiovascular fitness have significantly less atrophy of the gray matter in the frontal cortex, which typically shows the greatest age-related decline [22]. Furthermore, greater aerobic fitness is associated with sparing of age-related deterioration of the anterior and posterior white-matter tracts. Several other randomized controlled trials report that aerobic exercise has its greatest effects on improving the frontal cognitive processes, which are greatly impacted in PD.

While the above studies illustrate that aerobic exercise combats cognitive decline in healthy aging, the potential impact of aerobic exercise on cognitive changes in PD have not been studied thoroughly. Preliminary data are indeed encouraging, as results from a case study by Nocera *et al.* [23] demonstrated that a patient with PD improved on cognitive outcomes including executive and language processes following an aerobic exercise intervention. This work suggests improvements in brain health in PD similar to that of older adults who participate in aerobic exercise. However, larger randomized trials are warranted to evaluate the efficacy of aerobic exercise for ameliorating declines in cognitive performance in people with PD.

The work described above suggests that aerobic exercise can be an effective way to prevent disability in PD patients, as it targets critical functional areas impacted by the disease process. However, it appears critical that the type of aerobic exercise be tailored to the specific needs of the patient. Furthermore, care must be taken to have a complete understanding of the fall risk and cardiac symptomatology of the patient such that safe guards can be implemented and the risk lessened. Future studies need to address issues that currently plague the data in this arena including sample size, optimal state and timing of medication, as well as how more alternative, perhaps forced-exercise, models, can be implemented and have an impact on those further along in the disease process.

Resistance training

While improvements in cognitive and physical function are observed following traditional aerobic exercise (treadmill walking, cycling), recent reviews suggest that the most supportive evidence for therapeutic benefits are based on interventions incorporating strength training [24, 25]. Decrements in muscular strength have negative consequences on the performance of activities of daily living (ADLs) such as getting out of a chair or putting away groceries on a shelf above chest height. These decrements and others lead to reduced physical activity, deconditioning, increased frailty and dependence on the services of others. The quantity and quality of muscle mass and strength impacts numerous aspects of daily performance in older adults and people with PD such as walking speed, stair negotiation, avoiding obstacles, chair rise, and recovering from slips and trips. Recent comprehensive reviews suggest that the progression of these losses may be attenuated or at least slowed through regular resistance training exercise [24, 25]. We suggest that resistance training is a safe, effective and noninvasive way of reducing the symptoms of the disease that gives patients an active role in the management of their disease, yet we know little about the mechanisms by which such benefits are achieved.

Several of the neural consequences and symptoms of PD reinforce the rationale for providing resistance training to patients [26]. First, loss of muscle strength is frequently observed, particularly in the muscles surrounding the hip, knee and ankle in both the unmedicated and medicated state. Furthermore, loss of muscle strength contributes to bradykinesia and reduced balance capabilities during dynamic locomotor tasks. In addition to loss of strength, PD researchers observe a reduction in the ability to produce force rapidly, which is particularly important when trying to take a recovery step after a stumble or reaching out the arm to grab a handrail to prevent a fall. Torque production has also been shown to vary with movement velocity, with particular deficits between the more- and less-affected side becoming pronounced at fast movement speeds. Aberrant muscle activation patterns are frequently observed during single joint and functional movement tasks. These abnormal activation patterns are likely related to impairments in variability, intensity and frequency of the corticospinal activation of the muscle. It is unclear, however, if these changes that are seen in muscular performance are solely related to changes at the periphery (muscle mass), impaired corticospinal activation, consequences of overall diminished activity or a combination of all of the above [26]. The peripheral and central neural adaptations that occur with resistance training may improve these decrements. Indeed, evidence suggests that resistance training can enhance cortical plasticity, improve descending activation from the motor cortex, enhance activation of basal ganglia nuclei, alter functional properties of spinal cord circuitry and cross-transfer training effects from the trained to untrained limb [26]. Despite recommendations for the inclusion of strength training into PD treatment more than 20 years ago [27], very few well-controlled investigations exist on this topic.

The extant literature suggests that resistance training can improve muscle mass, muscle strength and muscular endurance as well as neuromuscular function for patients with PD. Importantly, concomitant with these enhancements were observed reductions in parkinsonian motor disability. For example, Corcos et al. [28] observed a 7-point reduction in UPDRS motor scores following 24 months of twice-weekly resistance training. Also of note was that physical training was done at the participants' own gym and not in a strict laboratory setting. Due to disease-related cost and travel limitations, gym- and laboratory-based exercise interventions may not be accessible for all individuals. Importantly, we have shown that home-based exercise intervention focusing on lower-extremity strength can also improve muscle performance that carries over to enhanced balance, as measured by computerized dynamic posturography [29]. As with any exercise modality, it is important to the patient to see that becoming bigger, stronger and faster carries over to enhance functional performance.

Work from our laboratories and others have shown that resistance training in PD can lead to improvements in gait, gait initiation, chair rise, stair stepping and postural control [30, 31]. Gait speed, step length and head posture all improve following training, as well as functional gait outcomes such as walking endurance during the 6-min walk and improved timed performance on timed up-and-go and stair ascent and descent. Resistance training also improves anticipatory postural adjustments during gait initiation leading to larger and faster steps. Similarly, resistance training improves not only the speed of chair rise, but also the biomechanical mechanisms for safe and efficient performance. After resistance training, people with PD also demonstrate an improved ability to maintain balance during quiet and destabilizing balance conditions. Lastly, these improvements in muscular and functional performance lead to improvements in patient-perceived quality of life.

As with many therapeutic interventions, the present state of knowledge is impacted by several limitations that influence our ability to prescribe resistance training to our patients. First, the extant literature is plagued by small sample sizes and a potpourri of outcome measures that, while supporting a broad range effect, also limit our understanding of mechanisms and the ability to target disease-specific manifestations. Furthermore, the true benefits of resistance training are likely masked by evaluation of PD patients in the optimally medicated state. This practice has several ramifications, including masking the effects of training on the disease itself, as well as reducing effect sizes, which influences statistical findings and the conclusions with respect to efficacy. While much of the research has focused on motor benefits in PD, non-motor features of the disease may also be impacted by resistance training. For example, resistance training in older adults facilitates general cognition. In fact, resistance training has a more beneficial effect on cognition that involves executive control, which, as stated previously, is particularly impacted by PD. The influence of resistance training on affective domains relevant to PD such as depression and apathy are also poorly studied. The long-term effects of progressive resistance exercise are yet to be determined, as well as the interactive effects of resistance training when it is included as part of a comprehensive exercise program including aerobic training and stretching. Furthermore, the optimal prescription of resistance training including the number and types of exercises (machines vs free weights, number of repetitions and sets) is understudied. Lastly, future research should evaluate the benefits of resistance training in the context of the different clinical subtypes of individuals with PD. In spite of these limitations, the literature supports the recommendation of resistance training for patients with PD.

Tai chi

In the healthy older-adult literature, tai chi exercise has gained attention as an attractive intervention because of its potential to reduce falls and improve postural control and walking abilities, while also being safe and at a low cost. Tai chi was first evaluated as a complementary therapy for PD motor symptoms with a case study examining the progress of two 66-year-old males with PD who demonstrated balance improvements after a 3-month fitness program, which involved balance, unsupervised activity at a fitness center and twice-weekly tai chi sessions [2]. A later study, with more focus on tai chi specifically, revealed that an intensive 5-day tai chi program in 17 individuals with mild to moderate PD resulted in improvements in mobility and flexibility, as well as satisfaction and enjoyment with the program [32]. Hackney and Earhart [33] studied 13 individuals with PD who completed 20 1 h lessons of tai chi and compared them with an untreated control group. The findings demonstrated that those who participated in tai chi developed improvements in the Berg balance scale, disease severity, mobility, static balance, endurance and backward walking.

To date, the strongest evidence that tai chi may improve motor impairments related to PD has been provided by a randomized controlled trial that assigned 195 participants to one of the following groups: tai chi, resistance training or stretching (24 weeks, 1 h, twice weekly) [34]. Follow-up analysis revealed that the tai chi group performed consistently better than the resistance training and stretching groups in maximum excursion during a postural stability test. The tai chi group also performed significantly better when compared with the stretching group in measures of gait and strength, scores on functional reach and timed up-and-go tests, and motor scores on the UPDRS. Additionally, the tai chi group improved compared with the resistance training group in stride length and functional reach. Lastly, tai chi lowered the incidence of falls compared with stretching but not resistance training, and the effects were maintained 3 months later. A noteworthy flaw in this study, however, is that the resistance training was very low intensity.

Interestingly, not all PD-related motor outcomes have benefitted from tai chi. For example, Amano et al. [35] investigated the effect of tai chi exercise on dynamic postural control during gait initiation and gait performance in people with idiopathic PD. In this multisite investigation, two separate tai chi groups completed 16-weeks of supervised tai chi exercise, while the control groups consisted of either a placebo (i.e. qigong) or nonexercise. The results indicated that tai chi did not significantly improve the UPDRS motor score, selected gait initiation parameters or gait performance. Combined results from both tai chi groups in this study suggested that 16 weeks of class-based tai chi were ineffective in improving gait initiation or gait performance, or reducing parkinsonian disability in people with PD.

Because tai chi is a form of physical activity that demands high cognitive involvement, it may serve as an effective modality for nonmotor symptoms of PD beyond the proven motor outcomes. Interestingly, Lam et al. [36] demonstrated that 1 year of tai chi training significantly improved not only balance function but also visual attention in older adults at risk of progressive cognitive decline. They hypothesized that "apart from being a form of physical activity, Tai Chi demands memory training for the complex motor sequences, as well as coordinated pathway between attention, voluntary motor action, postural control, verbal, and visual imagery which provides increased cognitive stimulation." Additionally, tai chi appears to lower feelings of stress and increase vigor in patient populations. Specific to PD, we demonstrated the tai chi three times weekly for 16 weeks significantly improved scores on the 39-Item Parkinson's Disease Questionnaire (PDQ-39) summary index, as well as the emotional well-being subscore when compared with a control group.

A difficult and important element to implementing any life style intervention is to ensure adherence and track attrition. Previous studies examining the use of tai chi in various populations have reported success with participants adhering to the program [33]. In a study by Nocera et al. [37], 92% attendance was reported. Equally important to consider is that previous studies have been unable to determine ideal dosage and length of tai chi intervention in PD. Future research is needed to address how tai chi implementation can be maximized for optimal effectiveness in the general PD population.

In summation, tai chi appears to appear to reduce balance impairments in patients with mild to moderate PD, with additional benefits of improved functional capacity and reduced falls. Furthermore, tai chi may have implications for the nonmotor symptoms associated with PD. Importantly, it also appears to be well tolerated by individuals with PD, as few adverse events have been reported, and adherence and self-reported satisfaction are high. It is important to note, however, that not all studies have concluded physical improvement with tai chi exercise in people with PD. Future research is needed to identify the ideal dose response and which motor and nonmotor aspects of PD can be maximized with tai chi.

Massage/acupuncture

Patients with PD also resort to other complementary and alternative medicines in hopes of improving quality of life and motor symptoms. Indeed, previous reports suggest that 40% of patients use some form of alternative therapy, with massage therapy and acupuncture being among the most common [38]. Several studies have shown that routine massage therapy services have led to improvement in performance of ADLs, improved sleep quantity and quality, and lower levels of stress hormones [39]. Unfortunately, mechanism-based research in this area is lacking. Conversely, acupuncture stimulation in PD models suggests that acupuncture may have neuroprotective benefits through the release of various neuroprotective agents such as brain-derived neurotrophic factor, glial cell line-derived neurotrophic factor and cyclophilin A [40]. In an 8-week duration human trial, acupuncture led to a reduction in disease severity and reduced depressive symptoms [41]. However, sham-controlled clinical trials that adhere to the CONSORT (Consolidated Standards of Reporting Trials) and STRICTA (Standards for Reporting Interventions in Clinical Trials of Acupuncture) guidelines are strongly needed to confirm the precise effect of acupuncture on PD [42].

Creative arts therapies

The use of creative arts therapies in the treatment of PD has become popular over the last decade. Complementary therapies including music therapy and dance therapy provide treatment for both the motor and nonmotor complications of PD while tailoring to patient-specific needs and interests. While research remains limited in these areas, support is gaining for the incorporation of creative arts therapies in treatment of PD.

Music therapy

Music therapy is the use of music within a therapeutic relationship to address physical, emotional, cognitive and social needs of individuals. When treating people with PD, music therapists often focus on two main areas; improving movement and voice performance.

To improve movement performance, the music therapist may incorporate the use of various instruments. Music therapists are skilled at adapting instruction and use of the instruments to meet specific therapeutic needs. For example, a person with PD may be learning to play the piano or guitar to improve fine motor and bilateral coordination, or a person with PD may be playing jingle bells fixed to their walker to increase the range of motion for hip flexion. In both examples, one of the most beneficial elements to music therapy is the use of external cues. Abundant evidence demonstrates the benefits of rehabilitative exercise that exploits external cueing [43, 44]. External cuing has improved movement initiation [45, 46], while additional research has shown that people with PD have faster reaction times when externally cued compared with self-initiated movement [47]. Synchronizing movement to rhythm may also enhance movement speed [48]. Yet there remains little explanation regarding the neurophysiological basis for these improvements. Currently, it is suggested that the use of external cues accesses a cerebellar–premotor cortical circuitry, bypassing the basal ganglia–supplementary motor area circuitry typically active during self-initiated movements [39]. Thus, music therapy programs that include external cues in combination with consistent rhythmic auditory stimulation are recommended for people with PD.

Auditory cues, another focus of music therapy, have also been shown to facilitate gait. Research has consistently shown that gait training with regular external rhythmic auditory cues improved gait velocity, stride length, step cadence, timing of EMG patterns and mobility in people with PD. Less is known, however, about the effects of music on gait in PD. Often, the results attributed to the facilitation of gait with auditory cues are extended to include music because of the similarity between the stimuli. However, only one study has examined the effects of music on gait training in people with PD, and this similarly revealed improved gait velocity, stride time and cadence. Interestingly, however, the use of auditory cues during more complex walking tasks such as dual-task walking and obstacle crossing demonstrates similar positive effects on gait, but listening to music while completing these challenging walking tasks may be attention demanding and has negative effects on gait [8, 49]. This evidence provides a conundrum, as there are several anecdotal reports of people with PD using music to walk in various environmental conditions, such as the mall or park, that involve dual tasking. Perhaps the focus of the attentional demand should be an area of consideration. In environments where minimizing external distractions is needed for effective ambulation, focusing on walking with music may be beneficial. Persons with PD may be able to focus more on the walking by synchronizing movement with the music. In contrast, in environments where attention is needed to complete additional tasks while walking, focusing on the additional task may be more beneficial. In these cases, music may indeed be distracting and have a negative effect on performance. Continued research on the appropriate environment in which to use music to facilitate gait is needed and will aid in determining appropriate music therapy strategies for gait disturbances in people with PD.

Group singing has also been used in music therapy for speech impairments in PD. Previous research has revealed mixed reports on the effectiveness of group singing in PD. Improvements in maximum inspiratory and expiratory pressure, voice range, speech intelligibility and vocal intensity have been reported after group singing interventions [50]. However, Shih *et al.* [51] revealed that group singing did not demonstrate improvements in objective measures of voice and speech impairment. A possible explanation for these differences in results may be attributed to the type of instruction being provided. When participating in group singing, specific elements such as learning the words, melody and rhythm could be emphasized over the proper singing technique (i.e. breath support and posture). Thus, the effects of group singing may match the training emphasis: improved working memory for learning a song versus improved voice for proper singing technique. Given that people with PD experience both cognitive and voice deficits, a combination of both may prove to be most beneficial. Yet no study has examined the effects of group singing on cognitive abilities in people with PD. There are additional elements that music may influence (social, quality of life) that have yet to be examined in group singing. Overall, the effects of group singing in people with PD have been underexplored, and there remains a need to better understand the potential benefits of group singing on the voice and on additional related measures. However, the fact that group singing may be able to target multiple treatment aspects such as cognition, socialization and voice performance at one time makes exploring how to most effectively incorporate group singing into the music therapy treatment of persons with PD intriguing.

Music therapists may also directly treat additional areas such as relaxation, cognition, emotional well-being and socialization. Music has been found to activate specific neural pathways associated with emotion and may enhance social relationships. In a study of seated exercises performed to musical cues, 14 participants with PD experienced improvements in the PDQ-39 subscales of emotional well-being, stigma, bodily discomfort, mobility and ADLs [52]. Additionally, music therapy involving rhythmic body movements demonstrably improved scores on the Parkinson's Disease Quality of Life questionnaire [53]. While research supporting the use of music therapy in the treatment of nonmotor symptoms is limited, treating the whole person is very valuable and is recommended in the treatment of people with PD. In fact, it is virtually impossible for a music therapist to treat only one independent objective given the innate emotional and social context associated with music that is nearly impossible to remove. Thus, music therapists tailor the therapeutic experience by using patient-specific music to treat the whole person.

Dance therapy

Effective motor rehabilitation should be safe, be participant friendly, promote high adherence and have demonstrated efficacy in improving disease severity, mobility and quality of life. Traditional exercise programs often suffer from high attrition rates because of high patient task demand and lack of social interaction. Ideally, exercise activities should engage and sustain interest, because 60% of all Americans older than 65 do not achieve the recommended daily amounts of physical activity. Activity levels in individuals with PD are further reduced [54].

However, dance, which is a robust activity that involves mental and physical engagement while coordinating movements to music, when used as a therapeutic tool, may garner adherence through an enjoyable activity. Social and partnered dance could foster community involvement and social support while – crucially – necessitating the practice of dynamic balance and adjustment to environment, both of which are key to rehabilitating balance and axial impairments [55]. Group social dance can enhance motivation to be active and pursue healthy, exercise-related behaviors in older individuals [56, 57]. Older adults who participated in dance also demonstrated improved balance and functional mobility [58]. Greater improvements have been noted in balance and complex gait tasks in older adults who participated in an Argentine tango group than in a walking group [59]. While unconventional as an approach to balance and gait problems for older and/or physically challenged individuals, dance may be appropriate and pleasurable as a therapeutic activity because of its benefits to physical, mental and emotional states.

Recently, a series of studies have investigated the effects of adapted Argentine tango dance (adapted tango) for individuals with PD (Hoehn and Yahr stages 2–4]). Participants experienced significant gains in mobility, balance and quality of life, improvements that were maintained 1 month later [60–62]. After participating in 1 year of tango classes offered in the community, participants with PD also demonstrated decreased disease severity [63]. Recently, a study demonstrated that a 12-week adapted tango program, which was disseminated to several novice instructors and offered in the community, improved spatial cognition as well as disease severity in participants with mild to moderate PD. These improvements were maintained 3 months after cessation of the intervention [64].

Other forms of dance besides tango have been investigated for efficacy for those with PD. A study that investigated the feasibility of Irish set dancing, in comparison with standard physiotherapy, found the dancing safe and feasible. Furthermore, participants tended to improve more in gait, balance and freezing of gait after dancing than after the standard care [65]. Dance may have an immediate effect on mobility in those with PD, as improvements have been found with as little as 2 weeks of tango [66] and contact improvisation training [67]. The UPDRS score, i.e. disease severity, has also been improved in the very short term – after single dance sessions – in before/after contemporary dance class assessments [68]. This same study also reported improved health-related quality of life (HRQoL) for the PD participants as well as for their caregivers.

Other studies examining dance for its therapeutic effects on PD also noted improvements in HRQoL that often accompanied improved motor function. Improvements in HRQoL were found in a participant with PD (Hoehn and Yahr stage 5) who was severely mobility impaired, which demonstrated that even those with end-stage disease could benefit from and enjoy a modified dance class [69]. In a mixed-methods study examining the effects of a ballet class that included participants with PD, the participants reported being highly motivated and valued dance as being important [70]. In a study of modern dance with physically active PD participants, in addition to improvements in balance, social interaction was evident, as participants were observed staying after class to socialize with peers. Modern dance in the guise of the very popular Dance for PD® class format, started by the Mark Morris Dance Company, has also been shown to positively influence HRQoL in those with PD. A study found improvements in social support after 10 weeks, and improvements in activity participation were noted after 12 months of tango dance.

Although several studies have demonstrated the effectiveness of dance for improving both mobility and HRQoL, there is a need for a clinical trial to definitively determine the effectiveness of dance. Importantly, it is also necessary to conduct studies to determine the underlying mechanisms of rehabilitative dance for those with PD. Some possibilities will be introduced in the following paragraphs.

Movement strategies involving strong cognitive involvement and planning are associated with mobility improvements [71]. While learning and practicing dance, one focuses on critical movement aspects (e.g. longer steps or quicker movements), an attentional strategy that may help individuals with PD to achieve nearly normal speed and amplitude [72]. For individuals with PD, having complex movements broken down into simpler elements by the teacher, which would be done in any dance pedagogy, may facilitate motor performance [71]. A dancing partner may enhance balance, as even light touch contact can augment postural control. Improvements achieved via dance may also have resulted because dance addresses PD motor impairments through exploiting external auditory cues, which enhance motor therapy.

Participation, defined as involvement in a life situation, is related to mobility-related HRQoL, and the ability to do functional tasks like rising from a chair. Participation in a year-long program of tango led to participants recovering lost activities, beginning new ones and having the ability to engage in more complex activities [73]. Potentially, individuals with PD have benefitted in HRQoL through dance by the removal of barriers to participation (e.g. availability of dance programs, motor challenges of the steps).

Older adults have benefitted from regular aerobic activity in terms of plasticity-related changes in synaptogenesis, angiogenesis and neurogenesis. There is a strong link between activity, mental engagement and neural pathways. Dancing, whether it be tango, contemporary or folk dance, involves complex, unfamiliar tasks like walking backwards, allowing for problem solving and movement improvisation, possibly targeting mobility issues in individuals with PD through increased mental engagement and strategy development. The creativity involved in a dance form might tap into mechanisms of neural plasticity for novices just beginning classes for therapy. The exposure to novel steps and choreographic patterns could be fodder for expanding neural areas and improving neural pathways. The neuroprotection and neurorestoration that may be derived from consistent, task-specific and frequent exercise could be provided by dance, and may extend into improved mobility and, ultimately, the ability to accomplish ADLs.

Participant-friendly, adapted tango had a low attrition rate (14%), demonstrating patient acceptance and feasibility with a diverse patient population [66]. Several mobility programs are effective (e.g. movement strategies, dance, tandem biking, tai chi) for people with PD. A better mechanistic understanding of beneficial exercise effects could improve the design of targeted motor rehabilitation interventions for particular symptoms (e.g. freezing, bradykinesia and various disease stages of PD). This information would be of great clinical significance to individuals with motor impairment of all etiologies, as well as due to PD. Exercise programs for individuals with PD that are self-guided may not be as helpful as programs that involve a therapist or instructor [74]. Gait and balance are increasingly recognized as especially important for determinants of HRQoL as well as mortality. Tango and other dance forms may improve the axial impairment that greatly affects mobility – and therefore participation – and ultimately HRQoL in those with PD.

Art therapy

Research on the effects of art therapy in people with PD has primarily been limited to case reports, although more recent work has produced larger efficacy trials. The process of creating art, whether it is through brush stroke or molding of clay, allows patients to express their emotions, leading to an apparent reduction in stress and enhanced relaxed meditative states. For example, Elkis-Abuhoff *et al.* [75] observed significant decreases in somatic and emotional symptoms following manipulation of a ball of clay in a large group of patients. Viewing drama and participating in interactive drama projects have also been proposed to improve patients' engagement and a positive sense of self and community. This early evidence suggests that art therapy may also be a complementary treatment modality for patients.

Conclusions

In conclusion, the use of creative arts therapies in the treatment of people with PD shows promise, with initial research showing positive effects. However, there is a substantial lack of research examining the associated brain activity with creative arts therapies. For therapies such as music, dance and art therapy to be validated and incorporated into the treatment of PD, future research in this area is greatly needed. Studies of the human response to music, dance and art remain challenging, however. To elicit controlled responses, much of the creative and personal aspects of music, dance and art are limited. Researchers in this area face an interesting and intriguing quest to determine the neurophysiological basis for mediums such as music, dance and art that can influence the physical, emotional and social well-being at the same time.

Summary

Individuals with PD exhibit cardinal features of the disease that manifest as impaired motor ability, non-motor impairment and ultimately a decreased quality of life. While drug therapy and deep-brain stimulation have proven to provide some positive benefits on clinically observed motor function, there are inherent limitations as well as negative side effects. The current research suggests that exercise therapies may be the most effective strategy for improving function in individuals with PD. Various forms of exercise including multiple aerobic paradigms, strength training programs and perhaps less conventional exercises modules like tai chi, dance and music therapy have all be attributed to improved gait performance, cardiovascular health, functional performance and in some cases multitasking. While this review has focused primarily on examining therapies in isolation, the optimal approach would probably incorporate multiple modes of engagement, each aimed at improving quality of life in areas that meet the needs of the patient. And while the combination of therapies is difficult from a research/statistical standpoint, a few studies have suggested that multicomponent interventions do cast a wider net of positive outcomes. In an effort to evolve our understanding of and clinical application to PD, research should continue to explore novel approaches to exercise interventions based on sound neuroplasticity-based mechanisms so that disease symptoms can be ameliorated and performance and quality of life can be optimized.

References

1. Ashburn A, Fazakarley L, Ballinger C, *et al.* A randomised controlled trial of a home based exercise programme to reduce the risk of falling among people with Parkinson's disease. *J Neurol Neurosurg Psychiatry* 2007; **78**: 678–84.
2. Kluding P, McGinnis PQ. Multidimensional exercise for people with Parkinson's disease: a case report. *Physiother Theory Pract* 2006; **22**: 153–62.
3. Kwolek A. [Rehabilitation of patients with Parkinson disease]. *Neurol Neurochir Pol* 2003; **37** (Suppl. 5): 211–20 (in Polish).
4. Schenkman M, Hall D, Kumar R, Kohrt WM. Endurance exercise training to improve economy of movement of people with Parkinson disease: three case reports. *Phys Ther* 2008; **88**: 63–76.
5. Bergen JL, Toole T, Elliott RG 3rd, *et al.* Aerobic exercise intervention improves aerobic capacity and movement initiation in Parkinson's disease patients. *NeuroRehabilitation* 2002; **17**: 161–8.
6. Schenkman M, Hall DA, Baron AE, *et al.* Exercise for people in early- or mid-stage Parkinson disease: a 16-month randomized controlled trial. *Phys Ther* 2012; **92**: 1395–410.
7. Burini D, Farabollini B, Iacucci S, *et al.* A randomised controlled cross-over trial of aerobic training versus Qigong in advanced Parkinson's disease. *Eura Medicophys* 2006; **42**: 231–8.
8. Tillerson JL, Caudle WM, Reveron ME, Miller GW. Exercise induces behavioral recovery and attenuates neurochemical deficits in rodent models of Parkinson's disease. *Neuroscience* 2003; **119**: 899–911.
9. Rochester L, Burn DJ, Woods G, Godwin J, Nieuwboer A. Does auditory rhythmical cueing improve gait in people with Parkinson's disease and cognitive impairment? A feasibility study. *Mov Disord* 2009; **24**: 839–45.
10. Poulton NP, Muir GD. Treadmill training ameliorates dopamine loss but not behavioral deficits in hemi-parkinsonian rats. *Exp Neurol* 2005; **193**: 181–97.
11. Ridgel AL, Vitek JL, Alberts JL. Forced, not voluntary, exercise improves motor function in Parkinson's disease patients. *Neurorehabil Neural Repair* 2009; **23**: 600–8.
12. Miyai I, Fujimoto Y, Yamamoto H, *et al.* Long-term effect of body weight-supported treadmill training in Parkinson's disease: a randomized controlled trial. *Arch Phys Med Rehabil* 2002; **83**: 1370–3.
13. Protas EJ, Mitchell K, Williams A, *et al.* Gait and step training to reduce falls in Parkinson's disease. *NeuroRehabilitation* 2005; **20**: 183–90.
14. Pohl M, Rockstroh G, Ruckriem S, Mrass G, Mehrholz J. Immediate effects of speed-dependent treadmill training on gait parameters in early Parkinson's disease. *Arch Phys Med Rehabil* 2003; **84**: 1760–6.
15. Baddeley A. Working memory: looking back and looking forward. *Nat Rev Neurosci* 2003; **4**: 829–39.

16. Altgassen M, Phillips L, Kopp U, Kliegel M. Role of working memory components in planning performance of individuals with Parkinson's disease. *Neuropsychologia* 2007; **45**: 2393–7.
17. Koerts J, Leenders KL, Brouwer WH. Cognitive dysfunction in non-demented Parkinson's disease patients: controlled and automatic behavior. *Cortex* 2009; **45**: 922–9.
18. Muslimovic D, Post B, Speelman JD, Schmand B. Cognitive profile of patients with newly diagnosed Parkinson disease. *Neurology* 2005; **65**: 1239–45.
19. Kramer AF, Erickson KI. Capitalizing on cortical plasticity: influence of physical activity on cognition and brain function. *Trends Cogn Sci* 2007; **11**: 342–8.
20. Kramer AF, Hahn S, Cohen NJ, et al. Ageing, fitness and neurocognitive function. *Nature* 1999; **400**: 418–19.
21. Colcombe SJ, Erickson KI, Scalf PE, et al. Aerobic exercise training increases brain volume in aging humans. *J Gerontol A Biol Sci Med Sci* 2006; **61**: 1166–70.
22. Raz N, Williamson A, Gunning-Dixon F, Head D, Acker JD. Neuroanatomical and cognitive correlates of adult age differences in acquisition of a perceptual-motor skill. *Microsc Res Tech.* 2000; **51**: 85–93.
23. Nocera JR, Altmann LJ, Sapienza C, Okun MS, Hass CJ. Can exercise improve language and cognition in Parkinson's disease? A case report. *Neurocase* 2010; **16**: 301–6.
24. Latham NK, Bennett DA, Stretton CM, Anderson CS. Systematic review of progressive resistance strength training in older adults. *J Gerontol A Biol Sci Med Sci* 2004; **59**: 48–61.
25. Mian OS, Baltzopoulos V, Minetti AE, Narici MV. The impact of physical training on locomotor function in older people. *Sports Med* 2007; **37**: 683–701.
26. David FJ, Rafferty MR, Robichaud JA, et al. Progressive resistance exercise and Parkinson's disease: a review of potential mechanisms. *Parkinsons Dis* 2012; **2012**: 124527.
27. Glendinning DS, Enoka RM. Motor unit behavior in Parkinson's disease. *Phys Ther* 1994; **74**: 61–70.
28. Corcos DM, Robichaud JA, David FJ, et al. A two-year randomized controlled trial of progressive resistance exercise for Parkinson's disease. *Mov Disord* 2013; **28**: 1230–40.
29. Nocera J, Horvat M, Ray CT. Effects of home-based exercise on postural control and sensory organization in individuals with Parkinson disease. *Parkinsonism Relat Disord* 2009; **15**: 742–5.
30. Hass CJ, Buckley TA, Pitsikoulis C, Barthelemy EJ. Progressive resistance training improves gait initiation in individuals with Parkinson's disease. *Gait Posture* 2012; **35**: 669–73.
31. Hass CJ, Collins MA, Juncos JL. Resistance training with creatine monohydrate improves upper-body strength in patients with Parkinson disease: a randomized trial. *Neurorehabil Neural Repair* 2007; **21**: 107–15.
32. Li F, Harmer P, Fisher KJ, et al. Tai Chi-based exercise for older adults with Parkinson's disease: a pilot-program evaluation. *J Aging Phys Act* 2007; **15**: 139–51.
33. Hackney ME, Earhart GM. Tai Chi improves balance and mobility in people with Parkinson disease. *Gait Posture* 2008; **28**: 456–60.
34. Li F, Harmer P, Liu Y, et al. A randomized controlled trial of patient-reported outcomes with tai chi exercise in Parkinson's disease. *Mov Disord* 2014; **29**: 539–45.
35. Amano S, Nocera JR, Vallabhajosula S, et al. The effect of Tai Chi exercise on gait initiation and gait performance in persons with Parkinson's disease. *Parkinsonism Relat Disord* 2013; **19**: 955–60.
36. Lam LC, Chau RC, Wong BM, et al. A 1-year randomized controlled trial comparing mind body exercise (Tai Chi) with stretching and toning exercise on cognitive function in older Chinese adults at risk of cognitive decline. *J Am Med Dir Assoc* 2012; **13**: 568.e15–20.
37. Nocera JR, Amano S, Vallabhajosula S, Hass CJ. Tai Chi exercise to improve non-motor symptoms of Parkinson's disease. *J Yoga Phys Ther* 2013; **3**. DOI:10.4172/2157-7595.1000137.
38. Rajendran PR, Thompson RE, Reich SG. The use of alternative therapies by patients with Parkinson's disease. *Neurology* 2001; **57**: 790–4.
39. Donoyama N, Ohkoshi N. Effects of traditional Japanese massage therapy on various symptoms in patients with Parkinson's disease: a case-series study. *J Altern Complement Med* 2012; **18**: 294–9.
40. Zeng BY, Salvage S, Jenner P. Current development of acupuncture research in Parkinson's disease. *Int Rev Neurobiol* 2013; **111**: 141–58.
41. Cho SY, Shim SR, Rhee HY, et al. Effectiveness of acupuncture and bee venom acupuncture in idiopathic Parkinson's disease. *Parkinsonism Relat Disord* 2012; **18**: 948–52.
42. Lee HS, Park HL, Lee SJ, et al. Scalp acupuncture for Parkinson's disease: a systematic review of randomized controlled trials. *Chin J Integr Med* 2013; **19**: 297–306.
43. Nieuwboer A, Rochester L, Muncks L, Swinnen SP. Motor learning in Parkinson's disease: limitations and potential for rehabilitation. *Parkinsonism Relat Disord* 2009; **15** (Suppl. 3): S53–8.
44. Kadivar Z, Corcos DM, Foto J, Hondzinski JM. Effect of step training and rhythmic auditory stimulation on functional performance in Parkinson patients. *Neurorehabil Neural Repair* 2011; **25**: 626–35.

45. Dibble LE, Nicholson DE, Shultz B, et al. Sensory cueing effects on maximal speed gait initiation in persons with Parkinson's disease and healthy elders. *Gait Posture* 2004; **19**: 215–25.

46. Jiang Y, Norman KE. Effects of visual and auditory cues on gait initiation in people with Parkinson's disease. *Clin Rehabil* 2006; **20**: 36–45.

47. Ballanger B, Thobois S, Baraduc P, et al. "Paradoxical kinesis" is not a hallmark of Parkinson's disease but a general property of the motor system. *Mov Disord* 2006; **21**: 1490–5.

48. Howe TE, Lovgreen B, Cody FW, Ashton VJ, Oldham JA. Auditory cues can modify the gait of persons with early-stage Parkinson's disease: a method for enhancing parkinsonian walking performance? *Clin Rehabil* 2003; **17**: 363–7.

49. Nanhoe-Mahabier W, Delval A, Snijders AH, et al. The possible price of auditory cueing: influence on obstacle avoidance in Parkinson's disease. *Mov Disord* 2012; **27**: 574–8.

50. Elefant C, Baker FA, Lotan M, Lagesen SK, Skeie GO. The effect of group music therapy on mood, speech, and singing in individuals with Parkinson's disease – a feasibility study. *J Music Ther* 2012; **49**: 278–302.

51. Shih LC, Piel J, Warren A, et al. Singing in groups for Parkinson's disease (SING-PD): a pilot study of group singing therapy for PD-related voice/speech disorders. *Parkinsonism Relat Disord* 2012; **18**: 548–52.

52. Clair A, Lyons KE, Hamburg J. A feasibility study of the effects of music and movement of physical function, quality of life, depression, and anxiety in patients with Parkinson's Disease. *Music Med* 2011; **4**: 49–55.

53. Pacchetti C, Mancini F, Aglieri R, et al. Active music therapy in Parkinson's disease: an integrative method for motor and emotional rehabilitation. *Psychosom Med* 2000; **62**: 386–93.

54. Toth MJ, Fishman PS, Poehlman ET. Free-living daily energy expenditure in patients with Parkinson's disease. *Neurology* 1997; **48**: 88–91.

55. Hirsch MA, Toole T, Maitland CG, Rider RA. The effects of balance training and high-intensity resistance training on persons with idiopathic Parkinson's disease. *Arch Phys Med Rehabil* 2003; **84**: 1109–17.

56. Federici A, Bellagamba S, Rocchi MB. Does dance-based training improve balance in adult and young old subjects? A pilot randomized controlled trial. *Aging Clin Exp Res* 2005; **17**: 385–9.

57. Palo-Bengtsson L, Winblad B, Ekman SL. Social dancing: a way to support intellectual, emotional and motor functions in persons with dementia. *J Psychiatr Ment Health Nurs* 1998; **5**: 545–54.

58. Song R, June KJ, Kim CG, Jeon MY. Comparisons of motivation, health behaviors, and functional status among elders in residential homes in Korea. *Public Health Nurs.* 2004; **21**: 361–71.

59. McKinley P, Jacobson A, Leroux A, et al. Effect of a community-based Argentine tango dance program on functional balance and confidence in older adults. *J Aging Phys Act* 2008; **16**: 435–53.

60. Hackney ME, Earhart GM. Health-related quality of life and alternative forms of exercise in Parkinson disease. *Parkinsonism Relat Disord* 2009; **15**: 644–8.

61. Hackney ME, Earhart GM. Effects of dance on gait and balance in Parkinson's disease: a comparison of partnered and nonpartnered dance movement. *Neurorehabil Neural Repair* 2010; **24**: 384–92.

62. Hackney ME, Kantorovich S, Levin R, Earhart GM. Effects of tango on functional mobility in Parkinson's disease: a preliminary study. *J Neurol Phys Ther* 2007; **31**: 173–9.

63. Duncan RP, Earhart GM. Randomized controlled trial of community-based dancing to modify disease progression in Parkinson disease. *Neurorehabil Neural Repair* 2012; **26**: 132–43.

64. McKee KE, Hackney ME. The effects of adapted tango on spatial cognition and disease severity in Parkinson's disease. *J Mot Behav* 2013; **45**: 519–29.

65. Volpe D, Signorini M, Marchetto A, Lynch T, Morris ME. A comparison of Irish set dancing and exercises for people with Parkinson's disease: a phase II feasibility study. *BMC Geriatr* 2013; **13**: 54.

66. Hackney ME, Earhart GM. Short duration, intensive tango dancing for Parkinson disease: an uncontrolled pilot study. *Complement Ther Med* 2009; **17**: 203–7.

67. Marchant D, Sylvester JL, Earhart GM. Effects of a short duration, high dose contact improvisation dance workshop on Parkinson disease: a pilot study. *Complement Ther Med* 2010; **18**: 184–90.

68. Heiberger L, Maurer C, Amtage F, et al. Impact of a weekly dance class on the functional mobility and on the quality of life of individuals with Parkinson's disease. *Front Aging Neurosci* 2011; **3**: 14.

69. Hackney ME, Earhart GM. Effects of dance on balance and gait in severe Parkinson disease: a case study. *Disabil Rehabil* 2010; **32**: 679–84.

70. Houston S, McGill A. A mixed-methods study into ballet for people living with Parkinson's. *Arts Health* 2013; **5**: 103–19.

71. Morris ME, Iansek R, Kirkwood B. A randomized controlled trial of movement strategies compared with exercise for people with Parkinson's disease. *Mov Disord* 2009; **24**: 64–71.

72. Morris ME, Huxham F, McGinley J, Dodd K, Iansek R. The biomechanics and motor control of

gait in Parkinson disease. *Clin Biomech (Bristol, Avon)* 2001; **16**: 459–70.

73. Foster ER, Golden L, Duncan RP, Earhart GM. Community-based Argentine tango dance program is associated with increased activity participation among individuals with Parkinson's disease. *Arch Phys Med Rehabil* 2013; **94**: 240–9.

74. Dereli EE, Yaliman A. Comparison of the effects of a physiotherapist-supervised exercise programme and a self-supervised exercise programme on quality of life in patients with Parkinson's disease. *Clin Rehabil* 2010; **24**: 352–62.

75. Elkis-Abuhoff DL, Goldblatt RB, Gaydos M, Convery C. A pilot study to determine the psychological effects of manipulation of therapeutic art forms among patients with Parkinson's disease. *Int J Art Ther* 2013;**18**: 113–21.

Index

AAV2-neurturin, 273, 276
acamprosate, 17
acceptability, rating scales, 232
accordion-pill carbidopa-levodopa, 86
acetylcholine deficiency, 141
activities of daily living (ADLs), 122, 199, 351
acupuncture, 353
acute anticholinergic syndrome, 10
ADAGIO study, 26, 30, 269, 272, 274, 275, 328
ADAS-cog scale, 325, 326, 332
ADCS-CGIC scale, 325, 332
adenosine A2a antagonists, 86
    istradefylline, 86–87
    preladenant, 87
    tozadenant, 87–88
ADS-5102, 89
advanced stage PD
    COMT inhibitors, 78, 80
    DBS, 313–16
    levodopa treatment summary, 72–73
adverse effects
    anticholinergics, 9–10
    apomorphine, 57
    bilateral pallidal DBS, 304
    bilateral pallidotomy, 303
    DBS, 314, 317
    donepezil, 326
    dopamine agonists, 41–43
    intranasal apomorphine, 53
    rasagiline, 27
    rivastigmine, 326
    rotigotine transdermal system, 52
    selegiline, 27
    STN DBS, 198, 199–202, 306
    subthalamotomy, 305
    surgery, 308
    thalamotomy vs thalamic DBS, 299
    tolcapone, 79
    VIM DBS, 211, 212
AE program, 285
aerobic exercise, 349–50
AFQ056, 89–90
agoraphobia, 130
AIMS scale, 233
akathisia, 165, 166
akinetic crisis, 16
akinetic rigid syndromes, 2
ALDS scale, 304, 307
alertness, 151, 218
alpha-blockers, 103
alpha-synuclein, 253–54, 268

Alzheimer's disease, 76, 111, 117, 125, 128, 141
    beta-amyloid and tau proteins, 255
AM IMPAKT study, 56
amantadine, 13–20, 101
    ADS-5102, 89
    compulsive behaviour treatment, 17
    dyskinesias treatment, 14
    ICDs, 329
    levodopa and, 69
amitriptyline, 101
amnestic multiple-domain MCI, 122
amnestic single-domain MCI, 111, 122
amphetamine, 135
amyloid, beta, 255, 268
analgesics, 165, 167
anger, 291
animal models, 270–71
    dopaminergic neuroprotection, 318
    exercise, 350
    lack of, 266
    toxin-induced, 271
    transgenic, 271
antibodies measures, 257
anticholinergics, 5–10, 132
    adverse effects and contraindications, 9–10
    current use in PD management, 7–9
    future use, 10
    levodopa synergy, 9
    pharmacokinetics and pharmacodynamics, 6–7
    psychosis effects, 141
    sialorrhea, 101
    urinary dysfunction, 102
antidepressants, 27, 104, 112, 130, 133, 167
    tricyclic, 103, 133, 327
antidyskinetics, 89–90
antiglutamatergics, 13–20
    akinetic crisis and neuroleptic malignant syndrome, 16
    cognitive improvement, 16
    dyskinesia studies, 16
    evidence-based results and meta analyses, 14–16
    four main effects, 18
    ICD and other compulsive disorders, 17–18
    psychosis induction, 17
antihypertensives, 104
antimuscarinics, 5
antipsychotics, 132, 141
anxiety, 128, 129–31, 330
    categories, 130

apathy, 128–29, 330
    DBS and, 147
    definitions, 128
    depression and dementia, 129
    syndrome, 129
    treatment, 129
apomorphine, 53–54, 80, 155
    adverse effects, 57
    ICDs, 57
    intranasal, 53
    long-term therapy effects, 57
    motor effects, 54–56
    non-motor effects, 56–57
    pain relief, 166
    pharmacokinetics, 54
    sexual dysfunction, 104
    subcutaneous, 100
    transdermal patch, 52
aripiprazole, 132, 329
art therapy, 356
aspiration pneumonia, 340
ataxia, limb, 183
atomoxetine, 124, 326
atropine, 5, 101
attention deficit disorder, 326
attention training, 113
atypical parkinsonism, 66, 196, 243, 281
auditory cues, 354
auditory hallucinations, 131
autonomic dysfunction, 93. *See also* constipation; gastroparesis; orthostatic hypotension; sialorrhea
    defecatory, 100
    drug treatment, 95
    sexual, 104–6
    thermoregulatory, 106
    urinary, 102–4
axial symptoms, anticholinergic effects on, 8

back pain, 166
bapineuzemab, 255
Barthel index, 300
Beck Depression Inventory (BDI), 291
behavioral disturbances, 127. *See also* depression; fatigue; impulse control disorders (ICD); psychosis
    anxiety, 128, 129–31, 330
    apathy, 128–29, 330
    deep brain stimulation and, 146–48
    drug treatment, 148
    personality, 128
    treatment-related, 139–40

361

Index

behavioral treatment, urinary dysfunction, 102, 343
benign prostatic hypertrophy, 103
benign tremulous parkinsonism, 213
benserazide, 23, 67, 76
benzodiazepines, 130
benztropine, 7
beta-amyloid, 255, 268
bilateral GPi DBS, 303–4
bilateral pallidotomy, 302
bilateral posteroventral pallidotomy, 302
bilateral subthalamic DBS, 306–8
bilateral subthalamotomy, 306
bilateral thalamotomy, 179, 299, 300
biofeedback, 100
BioFIND study, 251
biomarkers, 268
   CSF and blood, 250–53
   definition, 249
   dopamine-based, 253–58
   future directions, 259–60
   ideal characteristics for PD, 251
   in clinical trials, 250
   metabolomics, 259
   neuroimaging, 250, 267
   neuroprotective trials, 266, 268
   proteomics, 259
   transcriptomics, 258–59
biperiden, 7
bisacodyl, 99
blood biomarkers, 250–53
   dopamine-based, 253–58
Botox, 100, 103, 338
botulinum toxin, 93, 95, 98, 100, 101, 103
botulinum toxin type A, 337–39
   urinary dysfunction, 342
botulinum toxin type B, 339
bradykinesia, 2, 289
brain function, measurement in trials, 246
brain network imaging, 243
bromocriptine, 34, 35
bupropion, 133, 327

cabergoline, 35, 37, 155, 156
caffeine, 157, 345
calcium channel antagonists, 90
CALM-PD study, 38, 244, 250, 267, 272, 275
CAPIT protocol, 195
CAPSIT protocol, 177, 195–96, 197
car accidents, 41, 152, 154
carbidopa, 23, 67, 68, 69, 70, 76
   accordion pill, 86
   intestinal gel, 70–71, 83–84
cardiac pacing, 97
Carlsson, Arvid, 1
carpal tunnel syndrome, 166
catechol-o-methyl transferase (COMT) inhibitors, 67–68, 76–81
catheterization, 103
CATIE-AD trial, 333
caudal Zona incerta (cZi), 218
central fatigue, 134
central pain, 165, 167
centremedian-parafascicular complex (CM-Pf), 221

CEP-1347, 273, 276
cerebellothalamic tract, 219
cerebrospinal fluid (CSF) biomarkers, 250–53
   dopamine-based, 253–58
CGI scale, 344
Charcot, Professor, 5
Charles Bonnet's syndrome, 141
chewing gum, 101
cholinergic system, 5–6
cholinesterase inhibitors, 112, 123–24, 129, 132, 141
CIBIC scale, 326
cisapride, 98, 99
CISI-PD scale, 233
citalopram, 328
classical test theory (CTT), 231
CLEOPATRA-PD study, 40
clinical trials. See also neuroprotective trials
   biomarkers in, 250
   design, 270–71
   early stage PD, 280–85
   functional imaging markers in, 244–46
   NPS, 330–33
clinician-based rating scales, 232–34
clonazepam, 156
closed-loop devices, 224
clozapine, 132, 141, 329
Cochrane review
   anticholinergics, 8
   monoamine oxidase inhibitors, 25
coenzyme Q10, 256, 273, 277
cog wheeling, 3
cognitive behavioral therapy (CBT), 134, 328
cognitive impairment, 293. See also mild cognitive impairment (MCI)
   background, 111–12
   drug treatment, 112, 123–24, 124
   epidemiology, 122
   exercise and, 350
   future directions, 118
   GPi DBS, 191
   GPi vs STN DBS, 290
   neuropsychological profile and bedside assessment, 122–23
   non-drug interventions, 116–18, 125
cognitive improvement, 16, 352
cognitive rehabilitation, 113, 116–17
cognitive stimulation, 114, 117
colchicine, 100
COMPARE study, 342
COMPASS-OD scale, 344
compensatory rehabilitation, 112, 117
composite endpoints, 332
compulsive disorders, 17–18
COMT inhibitors. See catechol-o-methyl transferase (COMT) inhibitors
consistency, rating scales, 232
constant voltage stimulator, 225
constipation, 98–100, 341–42
   drug treatment, 95
continuous drug delivery (CDD), 48
controlled release levodopa, 67
Cotzias, George, 1
cranial electrotherapy stimulation (CES), 168

creatine, 272, 276
creative arts therapies, 353–57
CSP 468 study, 190
CVT-301, 86
cyclic GMP phosphodiesterase type 5 inhibitors, 105
cystometric analysis, 342

DAICE-ET survey, 52
Dai-Kenchu-To (DKT), 100
dance therapy, 355–56
darifenacin, 103
DAT scans, 267, 281
DATATOP study, 24, 27, 90, 251, 254, 255, 271, 272
DAWS (DAg withdrawal syndrome), 43, 144–45
daytime sleep disorders, 41, 152–53, 345–46
deep brain stimulation (DBS), 83, 118, 146–48, 157–58. See also globus pallidus internus (GPi) DBS; subthalamic nucleus (STN) DBS; ventral intermediate nucleus (VIM) DBS
   advanced stage PD, 313–16
   advantages and drawbacks, 298
   alternative targets, 202
   awake/asleep, 292
   centremedian-parafascicular complex, 221
   development, 176
   early stage PD, 282–83, 320–22
   hemorrhage risk, 182
   introduction, 297
   mid stage PD, 316–20
   novel stimulation paradigms and devices, 224–25
   nucleus basalis of Meynert, 221–22
   other targets, 216
   pain relief, 162, 166, 167
   pedunculopontine nucleus, 216–18, 218
   posterior subthalamic area, 218–19
   post-operative surveillance, 147
   substantia nigra, 219–21
   vs. surgery controversy, 308–9
   thalamic, 298–300
defecatory dysfunction, 100
delayed-start design, 265, 269–70, 274
delirium, 141
delusions, 131, 135, 140
dementia, 111, 112, 122, 128, 135, 325–27. See also Alzheimer's disease
   DBS and, 196
   depression and apathy, 129
   with Lewy bodies, 128, 131
   NBM DBS and, 222
   psychosis and, 131
Denny-Brown, Derek, 1
depression, 132–34, 327–28
   anxiety and, 130
   apathy and dementia, 129
   categories, 128
   DBS and, 147, 196
   fatigue and, 127
   GPi vs STN DBS, 291
   pain and, 164, 167

Index

pramipexole effects on, 39
treatment, 133–34
desmopressin, 97, 103
despiramine, 328
detrusor areflexia, 103
dextromethorphan, 16
DFSS scale, 339
Diagnostic and Statistical Manual (DSM) IV TR, 127, 128, 130, 132, 332
Diagnostic and Statistical Manual (DSM) V TR, 142
diet, 97
high-fiber, 98
disease modification, 265
disease-modifying treatments, 90
DJ-1 gene, 254
DM-1992, 86
docusate, 99
domperidone, 54, 57, 93, 95, 96, 97, 344
donepezil, 123, 124, 331
cognitive impairment, 112, 113, 326
DOPA decarboxylases, inhibitors, 63, 66
dopamine
based biomarkers, 253–58
compulsive misuse, 147
dopamine agonist withdrawal syndrome (DAWS), 43, 144–45
dopamine agonists, 34–35
adverse effects, 41–43
continuous drug delivery, 48
early stage PD, 283–85
ICDs and, 142, 143
intranasal, 53
levodopa and, 69
major clinical trials, 275
most common daily usage, 37–41
pharmacodynamics, 36–37
pharmacokinetics, 37
rationale for use in PD, 35–36
sexual dysfunction, 104
subcutaneous, 53–58
transdermal, 48–53, 58
dopamine dysregulation syndrome, 66, 142, 143–44
dopamine receptors, classes, 36
dopamine system
functional imaging, 242–44
integrity, 245
dopaminergic areas of the brain, 153
dopaminergic neuroimaging, 266–67
dopaminergic neuroprotection, 319
doxepin, 156
drooling, 100. *See also* sialorrhea
droxidopa, 94, 95, 96
duloxetine, 167, 344
duodenal delivery methods, 70
dysarthria, 211
dysautonomia scale, 236
dyskinesias. *See also* motor symptoms
amantadine effects on, 14
antidyskinetics, 89–90
antiglutamatergic studies, 16
DBS, 190
development in PD, 13
GPi vs STN DBS, 289
levodopa-induced, 13, 65, 89, 289

pallidotomy effect on, 179
rating scales, 233
STN DBS and, 199
thalamotomy effect on, 178
dysphagia, 340–41
Dysport, 101, 104, 337, 342
dystonia
anticholinergic effects on, 8
pain related to, 165–66

early stage PD
clinical trials, 280–85
DBS, 282–83, 320–22
definition, 280
exercise, 285
medications, 283–85
MRI scanning, 281
nuclear imaging, 281–82
severity and onset of symptoms, 280
somatostatin levels, 282
treatment summary, 72
vitamin D deficiency, 282
EARLYSTIM trial, 196
economic impact, 315, 318
edemas, pedal and peripheral, 42
effect size (ES), 231
EFNS classification, 23, 28, 30
elderly
anticholinergic adverse effects, 9
summary of treatments in early stage PD, 72
electrical stimulation, 342
cranial electrotherapy, 168
gastric, 98
surface therapy, 341
tDCS, 118
electroconvulsive therapy (ECT), 133, 135, 224
ELLDOPA study, 65, 134, 250, 267, 272, 274
emotional incontinence, 135
EMST device, 340
entacapone, 67, 68, 77, 78–79
epidural spinal cord stimulation (eSCS), 222–24
Epworth sleepiness scale, 153, 154, 345
EQ-5D scale, 237
erectile dysfunction, 104–5, 343
drug treatment, 95
erythromycin, 98
erythropoietin, 97
eszopiclone, 155, 346
excessive daytime sleepiness (EDS), 152, 157, 345
excitotoxicity, 123
executive dysfunction, 111, 122
exercise. *See* physical exercise
external cues, 354

fatigue, 134–35
depression and, 127
scales, 236
Fatigue Assessment inventory, 134
FBF program, 285
FD-PET, 266
feasibility, rating scales, 232
fiberoptic endoscopy, 340
fibrosis, 69

FILOMEN study, 78
fipamezole, 89
Fitness Counts program, 285
fludrocortisone, 94, 95, 344
fluorodopa PET (Fdopa PET), 316
fMRI scanning, 243
forced aerobic exercise, 350
freezing of gait, 221
scale (FOGQ), 235
Frenchay Activities Index, 179, 299
FSS scale, 236
functional imaging, 242
dopamine system integrity, 242–44
functional imaging markers, 244
in clinical trials, 244–46
outcome measures development, 246–47
futility studies, 270

gait abnormalities, 3, 221, 289
gait improvement, 351, 354
gait training, 350, 354
galantamine, 123, 124
gambling, pathological, 142
gastric electrical stimulation, 98
gastrointestinal symptoms scale, 236
gastroparesis, 56, 97–98
drug treatment, 95
gel electrophoresis, 2D, 259
generalized anxiety, 130
Global Biomarkers Standardization Consortium (GBSC), 260
globus pallidus externus (GPE), 288
globus pallidus internus (GPi) DBS, 146, 147, 187, 287
anatomy and physiology, 287–88
background, 287
bilateral, 303–4
complications, 190–92
mechanism, 187–88
medication reduction, 292
motor symptoms, 289–90
neuroimaging, 292
non-motor symptoms, 290–91
operation risks, 293
outcomes, 189
patient selection, 188
programming challenges following, 292
stimulation, 288
vs. STN DBS, 190, 192, 294
technique, 188–89
unilateral, 301–2
glucose metabolism, 267
glutamate receptors, 15, 16
glutamatergic neurotransmission, 13, 14
glutathione, 256
glycopyrrolate, 93, 95, 101, 340
group singing, 354

hallucinations, 131, 140, 141
auditory, 131
minor, 140
presence and passage, 131
visual, 131, 141
HDRS-17 scores, 327
health-related quality of life scales, 236–37, 238

363

Index

hedonistic homeostatic dysregulation, 144
hemiballism, 182, 183
hemorrhage, 182, 293
   intracranial, 201
hepatotoxicity, 79
Hoehn and Yahr staging (HY), 4, 232, 280
homovanillic acid (HVA), 253
Hopkins verbal learning test, 290
5HT2A, 141
5HT4 agonists, 99
Human Plasma Proteome Project (HPPP), 260
hypersexuality, 104, 142
hypomania, 142, 147
hypotension. *See also* orthostatic hypotension
   postural, 42, 105

illusions, 140
immunotherapy, 254
impulse control disorders (ICD), 13, 17–18, 329
   apomorphine and, 57
   characterization, 142
   dopamine agonists, 35, 42
   rotigotine role in, 52
   scales, 236
   treatment related, 142–43
incontinence
   urge incontinence, 102
   urinary, 343
indomethacin, 97, 343
inflammation markers, 256–58
infusion levodopa therapy, 70–72
inosine, 90, 256, 257
insomnia, 151, 155–56
interpretability, in rating scales, 231
intranasal dopamine agonists, 53
ionotropic glutamates, 15, 16
ipratropium bromide, 101, 339
IPX066, 69, 84–85
ischemic stroke, 201
isradipine, 90, 284
istradefylline, 86–87
item response theory (IRT), 231
iTRAQ analysis, 259

Lactobacillus casei Shirota, 99
lactulose, 99
L-amino acid decarboxylase (L-AAD), 76, 81
LARGO study, 26, 80
latent trait theories (LTT), 231
lateral pain system, 162
laxatives, 99
lazabemide, 25
L-deprenyl. *See* selegiline
LEAPS study, 275
lesioning, 178. *See also* surgery
   size of lesion, 308
levodopa, 63, 76. *See also* carbidopa
   advanced-stage PD treatment summary, 72–73
   amantadine and, 69
   anticholinergic synergy, 9
   COMT inhibitors and, 67–68
   controlled release, 67
   dopamine agonists and, 69
   early-stage PD treatment summary, 72
   history of PD therapy, 63–64
   infusion therapy, 70–72
   insomnia and, 155
   major trials, 272, 274–75
   monoamine oxidase inhibitors and, 68
   motor complications, 34, 35, 65
   non-motor complications, 65–66
   novel approaches to delivery, 83–86
   novel formulations, 69–70
   pain management, 344
   peripheral neuropathy and, 168, 169
   pharmacokinetics and pharmacodynamics, 64–65, 67, 68
   radiolabeled, 242
   rasagiline adjunct therapy, 25–26
   sleep disorders and, 156
   standard oral therapy, 66–67
levodopa induced dyskinesias (LIDs), 13, 65, 89, 289
levodopa test, 67
Levodopa-Carbidopa Intestinal Gel (LCIG), 70–71, 83–84
Lewy bodies, 253
   dementia with, 128, 131
Lewy, Freidrich, 1
limb ataxia, 183
liquid paraffin, 99
lisuride, 52, 58
local field potential (LFP) recording, 177
long-duration response, 64
lubiprostone, 93, 100, 342

macroelectrode mapping, 177, 188, 189, 198
macrogol, 93, 99, 341
magnetic stimulation, 100
MALDI-TOF MS, 259
malondialdehyde, 256
mania, 142, 147
MAO inhibitors. *See* monoamine oxidase inhibitors
massage therapy, 353
Mattis Dementia Scale, 290
MCI. *See* mild cognitive impairment (MCI)
MDS-UPDRS, 233, 266
   M-EDL, 235
   nM-EDL, 235
medial pain system, 162
M-EDL scale, 235
melatonin, 155, 156, 346
memantine, 16, 17, 123, 346
   clinical trial, 331
   cognitive impairment, 113, 326
memory performance, 111
messenger RNAs (mRNAs), 258
metabolomics, 259
metabotropic glutamates, 15, 16
methylphenidate, 135, 157
metoclopramide, 98
MFI scale, 236
microelectrode mapping, 177, 188, 189, 198
microelectrode recording (MER), 287, 288, 292

microglial activation, 256
mid stage PD, DBS, 316–20
midodrine, 94, 95, 96
mild cognitive impairment (MC)
   types, 122
mild cognitive impairment (MCI), 111, 122, 325–27. *See also* cognitive impairment
   types, 111
minimally important change (MIC), 231, 232
minimally important difference (MID), 232, 233
minocycline, 272, 276
minor hallucinations, 140
mirabegron, 103
mirtazepine, 133
MitoQ study, 273
mitoquinone, 273
modafinil, 135, 157, 345
monoamine oxidase inhibitors, 23. *See also* rasagiline; selegiline
   background, 23
   COMT inhibitors and, 81
   future role, 28
   levodopa and, 68
   major trials, 271–74
   serotonin syndrome, 27–28
MONOCOMB study, 25
Montreal Cognitive Assessment (MoCA), 123
mosapride, 98, 99
motor changing rate (MCR), 52
motor complications and dyskinesia scales, 233
motor cortex stimulation (MCS), 222
motor impairment and disability scales, 233
motor symptoms. *See also* dyskinesias
   apomorphine effects on, 54–56
   drug treatment, 124
   GPi DBS vs. STN DBS, 289–90
   levodopa and, 34, 35, 65
   post-surgery, 183
   prevention of, 35
   rating scales, 233, 235
   ropinorole and, 39
   rotigotine and, 40, 50
   Tai-Chi and, 352
movement disorders
   categories, 2
   first recognition, 1
   improving, 353
Movement Disorders Society (MDS)
   definitions, 23, 29
   guidelines, 30
MPTP model, 271
MRI scanning, 243, 281
   fMRI, 243
multidomain scales, 233, 238
multimodal imaging, 244, 247
multiple domain MCI, 111, 122
multiple-system atrophy (MSA), 282, 343
muscle strength, loss of, 351
musculoskeletal pain, 164, 165
music therapy, 353–55

Index

naltrexone, 330
ND0611, 70
nebicapone, 77, 80
Neria line, 54, 57
NET-PD LS-1 study, 272
NET-PD study, 272, 275
neural stimulation, 115, 118
neurodegeneration, measurement in trials, 245
neuroimaging. *See also* PET scanning
    biomarkers, 250, 267
    dopaminergic, 266–67
    GPi DBS vs STN DBS, 292
    neuroinflammation, 243
neuroleptic malignant syndrome, 16
neuroleptics, 112
neuromodulation, 104
neuromuscular complications, 168–69
neuropathic pain, 164, 165, 166
neuroprotection, 265, 316, 320
    dopaminergic, 319
neuroprotective trials. *See also* clinical trials
    animal models, 270–71
    biomarkers, 266, 268
    clinical measures, 266
    dopaminergic neuroimaging, 266–67
    future directions, 277
    glucose metabolism, 267
    limitations, 265–66
    results from major studies, 271, 272, 273, 271–77
    structural imaging, 268
neuropsychiatric symptoms (NPS), 325. *See also* non-motor symptoms
    clinical trials, 330–33
    scales, 235
neuropsychological tests, 116
neurturin, 273, 276
neutrophin-3, 100
NHP scale, 237
NICE guidelines, 25, 35
nighttime sleep disorders, 151–52
NMDA receptor antagonists, 112
NMDA receptors, 123
nM-EDL, 235
NMS Questionnaire, 235
nociceptive pain, 164
nocturia, 102
NOMESAFE study, 78
non-amnestic multiple-domain MCI, 122
non-amnestic single-domain MCI, 111, 122
non-invasive brain stimulation, 224
non-motor off symptoms, 127, 130
non-motor symptoms, 337. *See also* autonomic dysfunction; behavioral disturbances; cognitive impairment; neuropsychiatric symptoms (NPS); sleep disorders
    apomorphine and, 56–57
    GPi vs STN DBS, 290–91
    levodopa, 65–66
    post-surgery, 183
    rating scales, 238
    ropinirole and, 39
    rotigotine and, 40
    rotigotine RTS and, 51
    scales, 234, 235–36
    therapeutic approach, 338
Non-Motor Symptoms Scale (NMSS), 40, 51, 55, 234
nortriptyline, 327
NPS. *See* neuropsychiatric symptoms (NPS)
NSAIDs, 165
nuclear imaging, 281–82
nucleus basalis of Meynert (NBM), 221–22

obstructive sleep apnoea (OSA), 152, 157
octreotide, 97
off phase, 65, 166, 179, 195
6-OHDA model, 271, 319, 350
olanzapine, 132, 329
on phase, 65
opicapone, 68, 77, 80
optic tract, 188
orthostatic hypotension, 42, 93–94, 343–44
    definition, 93
    drug treatment, 95, 94–97
    drugs causing, 94
    non-pharmacological management, 94
    symptoms, 93
osmotic laxatives, 99
outcome measures. *See also* clinical trials; rating scales
    functional imaging markers, challenges, 245–46
    functional imaging markers, development, 246–47
oxidative stress, markers, 255–56
oxybutynin, 102

pain, 162–68, 169–70, 344–45
    classification and treatment, 164, 165
    epidural spinal cord stimulation, 222
    non-pharmacologic management, 167
    risk factors in PD, 164
pallidal DBS. *See* globus pallidus internus (GPi) DBS
pallidothalamic tract, 219
pallidotomy, 167, 187, 297. *See also* surgery
    bilateral, 302
    introduction, 175
    outcomes, 179–81, 182
    pain and, 162
    posteroventral, 297, 301, 302
    revitalization, 176
    target confirmation, 177
    unilateral, 300–301
panic attacks, 130
parallel group studies, 268
paranoid delusions, 131
pardoprunox, 284
paresthesias, 211
Parkinson, James, 1, 162
Parkinson's Progression Markers Initiative (PPMI), 251
Parkinson's disease. *See also* advanced stage PD; early stage PD
    atypical, 66, 196, 243, 281
    behavioral effects of treatment, 139–40, 148
    benign tremulous, 213
    cholinergic system and, 5–6
    clinical diagnosis, 63
    experimental pharmacological treatment, 83–91
    first recognition, 1
    mid stage PD, 316–20
    pathological changes, 4
    stages, 3
    summary of treatments for advanced stage, 72–73
    summary of treatments for early stage, 72
    symptoms, 2–3
    UK Brain Bank Criteria, 281
paroxetine, 133, 327
passage hallucinations, 131
patient-reported outcomes (PRO), 231, 234–36
PD Sleep Scale, 154
PDQ-39, 84, 199, 237, 301, 307
PDQ-8, 237
PDQL scale, 237
PDSS scale, 236
PDSS-2 scale, 41, 236
PDYS-26 scale, 235
peak VO2, 349
pedal edema, 42
pedunculopontine nucleus (PPN), 6, 216–18, 218
pelvic floor muscle exercises, 102
Penetration-Aspiration scale, 340
percutaneous endoscopic gastrostomy (PEG), 70
pergolide, 35, 37, 104, 155
periodic limb movement disorder (PLMD), 152
periodic limb movements of sleep (PLMS), 156
peripheral edema, 42
peripheral neuropathy, 166, 168–69
personality, 128
PET scanning, 242, 243, 246, 250
    Fdopa PET, 316
    FD-PET, 266
    REAL-PET study, 244, 250, 267, 272, 275
PFS-16 scale, 236
phencyclidine, 14
physical exercise, 114, 117–18, 165, 167, 349
    aerobic, 349–50
    dance, 355–56
    early stage PD, 285
    resistance training, 351–52
    Tai-Chi, 352–53
physiological fatigue, 134
pimavanserin, 132, 142, 329
PIMS scale, 237
pimvanserin, 331
piribedil, 35, 36, 37, 41
    mechanism of action, 41
    motor systems efficacy, 41
    non-motor systems efficacy, 41
    transdermal patch, 52
Pittsburgh Sleep Quality Index, 154
placebo response, 330
pneumonia, aspiration, 340
polyethylene glycol (PEG) 3350, 99
polysomnography, 154, 347

Index

portable pumps, 54
posterior subthalamic area (PSA), 218–19
postural hypotension, 42, 105
posture, 289
PPMI study, 254, 255
pramipexole, 35, 36, 37–39, 133, 156
   adverse effects, 41
   depression, 328
   early stage PD, 283–84
   formulations, 283
   major trials, 272, 275
   mechanism of action, 37
   motor symptoms efficacy, 38–39
   non-motor symptoms efficacy, 39
   pharmacokinetics, 50
PRECEPT study, 90, 273, 276
preladenant, 87
presence hallucinations, 131
PRESTO trial, 25
primary pain, 164, 165
probiotics, 99
procyclidine, 7
prodromal syndrome, 280
PROGENI study, 280
progression biomarkers, 260
proteomics, 259
PROUD study, 272, 275
prucalopride, 98, 99
psychiatric complications, dopamine agonists, 34
psychosis, 131–32, 328–29
   dopamine agonists, 42
   drug treatment causing, 132
   induction, 17
   medications causing, 131
   symptoms, 328
   treatment-related, 140–42
PSYCLOPS study, 329
psyllium, 98
punding, 66, 142
purines, 256
pyridostigmine, 96, 100

QE3 study, 273
Quality of Life (QoL), 55
   DBS and, 318
   GPi vs STN DBS, 291
   health-related scales, 236–37, 238
   PDQ-39, 84, 199
   unilateral pallidal DBS, 301
quetiapine, 132, 142, 329
QUIP-RS scale, 143, 235, 330

radicular pain, 165, 166
radiofrequency thermolesion, 178
radiotherapy, 102
ramelteon, 156
rasagiline, 68
   adverse effects, 27
   clinical trials, 26, 272, 274
   cognitive impairment, 112, 113, 327
   depression, 328
   early stage PD, 285
   EFNS/MDS guidelines, 30
   levodopa adjunct therapy, 25–26
   MDS guidelines, 30
   selegiline comparisons, 27
   sleep disturbances, 156
Rasch measurement theory, 231
rating scales, 231–32, 249
   classification, 231
   clinician-based, 232–34
   development and validation, 231
   global severity and disability, 232
   global severity and multidomain, 238
   main psychometric attributes, 232
   motor complications and dyskinesias, 233
   motor impairment and disability, 233
   motor symptoms and disabilities, 235
   multidomain, 233
   non-motor symptoms, 234, 235–36, 238
   NPS clinical trials, 332
   patient-reported outcomes, 234–36
   quality of life, 236–37, 238
RDRS scale, 234
REAL-PET study, 244, 250, 267, 272, 275
RECOVER study, 40, 51
rectal laxatives, 99
REM sleep disorder, 128, 141, 152, 153, 347
   treatment, 156
repetitive transcranial magnetic stimulation (rTMS), 104, 118, 168
reproducibility, rating scales, 232
rescue therapy, 54, 55
resistance training, 351–52
responsiveness, in rating scales, 231, 233
rest tremor, 3, 208
restless legs syndrome (RLS), 152, 156, 165, 166
restorative rehabilitation, 112, 113, 114
rigidity, 3
rivastigmine, 123, 124, 156
   apathy, 330
   cognitive impairment, 112, 113
   dementia, 325
   psychosis, 329
   sleep disorders, 347
ropinirole, 35, 36, 37, 39–40, 156
   early stage PD, 284
   major trials, 272, 275
   mechanism of action, 39
   motor systems efficacy, 39
   non-motor symptoms efficacy, 39
   pharmacokinetics, 50
rotigotine, 35, 36, 37, 40–41
   early stage PD, 284
   insomnia and, 155
   mechanism of action, 40
   motor systems efficacy, 40
   non-motor symptoms efficacy, 40
   pharmacokinetics, 50
rotigotine transdermal system (RTS), 49, 58
   impulse control disorders and, 52
   long-term effects, 51
   motor symptoms, 50
   non-motor symptoms, 51
   pharmacokinetics, 49–50
   side effects, 52

safinamide, 88–89, 284
SAPS-PD scores, 329
schizophrenia, 131, 142
SCOPA-AUT scale, 236
SCOPA-Cog scale, 234
SCOPA-Motor, 233
SCOPA-PC scale, 234
SCOPA-PS, 237
SCOPA-Sleep scale, 154, 236
SEAPI scale, 343
secondary pain, 164, 165
seizures, 201
selegiline, 24, 68
   adverse effects, 27
   efficacy, 24
   EFNS/MDS guidelines, 30
   insomnia from, 153
   major trials, 271, 272, 274
   MDS guidelines, 30
   neuroprotective potential, 24–25
   orally disintegrating tablet, 27
   rasagiline comparisons, 27
SEND-PD scale, 236
senna, 99
serotonin receptors, 141
serotonin syndrome, 27–28
sertraline, 328
SES scale, 233
sexual dysfunction, 104–6. *See also* erectile dysfunction
   drugs contributing to, 104
SF-36 scale, 237
shopping, compulsive, 142
sialorrhea, 8, 100–102, 337–40
   drug treatment, 95
sildenafil, 105, 343
SINDEPAR study, 272, 274
single-domain MCI, 111, 122
SIP scale, 237
skin nodules, 57
sleep attacks, 153, 157
sleep disorders, 134, 151, 346–47. *See also* REM sleep disorder
   daytime, 41, 152–53, 345–46
   diagnosis, 153
   dopamine agonists, 41
   EDS, 152, 157, 345
   guidelines, 155
   management, 154–58
   nighttime, 151–52
   pathopathology, 153
   PPN DBS and, 218
   scales, 236
smoking, 128
social phobia, 130
solanezumab, 255
solifenacin, 103
somatostatin, 282
SPECT scanning, 242, 243, 250
speech impairments, 354
speech-language therapy, 337
spinal cord, degeneration, 163
SSRIs, 130, 133, 327, 328
Stalevo®, 78, 81
standard error of measurement (SEM), 233
standardized response mean (SRM), 231
STEADY-PD study, 90

Index

stereotactic surgery, 167, 175, 177, 198, 292, 297. *See also* deep brain stimulation (DBS)
stimulant laxatives, 99
stimulants, 135
stimulation related side effects, 201
stool softeners, 99
striatum, 5
STRIDE-PD study, 65, 68, 79
structural imaging, 243, 268
subcutaneous apomorphine, 100
subcutaneous dopamine agonists, 53–58
substantia nigra (SNr), 219–21
subthalamic nucleus (STN) DBS, 146, 147, 157, 287
   advantages, 195
   adverse effects, 198, 199–202
   anatomy and physiology, 288
   background, 287
   bilateral, 306–8
   future uses, 202
   vs. GPi DBS, 190, 192, 294
   indications and patient selection, 195–96
   introduction and history, 195
   mechanism of action, 199
   medication reduction, 291–92
   motor symptoms, 289–90
   neuroimaging, 292
   non-motor symptoms, 290–91
   operation risks, 293
   outcomes and efficacy, 199
   pain management, 344
   PPN DBS and, 218
   procedure, 198–99
   programming challenges following, 292
   stimulation, 288
   timing of, 196
   unilateral, 305–6
subthalamotomy, 181–82, 183, 219. *See also* surgery
   bilateral, 306
   unilateral, 304–5
suicide, 147, 201, 318
supine hypertension, 96, 97
surface electrical stimulation therapy, 341
surgery, 175, 297–98. *See also* deep brain stimulation (DBS); pallidotomy; stereotactic surgery; subthalamotomy; thalamotomy
   advantages and drawbacks, 298
   vs. DBS controversy, 308–9
   epidural spinal cord stimulation, 222–24
   indications, 176
   lesioning technique, 178
   motor cortex stimulation, 222
   non-invasive brain stimulation, 224
   outcomes, 178–82
   patient preparation, 177
   patient selection, 176
   safety and side effects, 182–83
   target confirmation, 177–78
   target planification, 177
surrogate markers, 249, 260
swallowing therapy, 340
sweating, excessive, 106
SWEDDs, 243, 266
synuclein alpha, 253–54, 268

tai-chi, 352–53
tango dancing, 355, 356
tau protein, 255, 268
TCH346 study, 273, 276
tegaserod, 98, 99, 341
TEMPO study, 26, 30, 272, 274
testosterone replacement therapy, 105
thalamic DBS, 298–300
thalamotomy, 206, 297. *See also* surgery
   introduction, 175
   non-invasive, 308
   outcomes, 178–79, 182
   vs. thalamic DBS, 298–300
thermolesion, 176, 178
thermoregulatory dysfunction, 106
tocopherol, 271, 272
tolcapone, 67, 77, 79–80
tolterodine, 102
toxin-induced models, 271
tozadenant, 87–88
transcranial direct current stimulation (tDCS), 118
transcranial ultrasound, 243
transcriptomics, 258–59
transdermal dopamine agonists, 48, 58
   apomorphine, 52
   delivery routes, 49
   lisuride, 52
   piribedil, 52
   rotigotine, 49–52
transgenic models, 271
TRAP pneumonic, 2
treadmill/gait training., 350
tremors
   anticholinergic effects, 8
   benign tremulous parkinsonism, 213
   GPi vs STN DBS, 289
   rest tremor, 208
   thalamotomy vs thalamic DBS, 299
   VIM DBS treatment, 206, 208, 210
tricyclic antidepressants, 103, 133, 327
trihexyphenidyl, 5, 7, 101
tropicamide, 101, 340
trospium, 102

Unified Dyskinesia Rating Scale, 89, 234
unilateral GPi DBS, 301–2
unilateral pallidotomy, 300–301
unilateral subthalamic DBS, 305–6
unilateral subthalamotomy, 304–5
United Kingdom Brain Bank criteria, 281

UPDRS scores, 24, 26, 67, 266, 269
   bilateral pallidal DBS, 303
   bilateral pallidotomy, 302
   bilateral STN DBS, 307
   bilateral subthalamotomy, 306
   GPi DBS, 189, 290
   MDS-UPDRS, 266
   pallidotomy, 300
   resistance training, 351
   STN DBS, 196, 199, 290
   subscales, 233
   unilateral pallidotomy, 300
   unilateral STN DBS, 305
   unilateral subthalamotomy, 305
   VIM DBS, 209
urate, 256
urge incontinence, 102
uric acid precursor, 90
urinary dysfunction, 102–4, 342–43
   drug treatment, 95
urinary incontinence, 343

validity, rating scales, 232
variability between laboratory measures, 260
venlafaxine, 133, 327
ventral intermediate nucleus (VIM) DBS, 206
   adverse effects, 211, 212
   BTP treatment, 213
   neuroanatomy, 206
   neurophysiology, 207
   procedure, 207
   rebound effect, 211
   stimulation parameters, 211
   surgery results, 208–11
verbal fluency, 317
video-assisted swallowing therapy (VAST), 340
visual analog scales (VAS), 340
visual field defects, 301
visual hallucinations, 131, 141
visuospatial deficits, 111
VitalStim®, 341
vitamin B12 deficiency, 168
vitamin D deficiency, 282
VMAT2, 267

washout period, 265, 268, 274
wearing-off, 76, 80
weight gain, 293
weight loss, 342
WINCS, 224
WOQ scale, 235

xanthine, 253
XP 21279, 69, 85–86

younger patients, treatments in early stage, 72

zona incerta (Zi), 218, 219